The Dementias

Blue Books of Practical Neurology
(*Volumes 1–14 published as BIMR Neurology*)

1 **Clinical Neurophysiology**
Eric Stålberg and Robert R. Young

2 **Movement Disorders**
C. David Marsden and Stanley Fahn

3 **Cerebral Vascular Disease**
Michael J. G. Harrison and Mark L. Dyken

4 **Peripheral Nerve Disorders**
Arthur K. Asbury and R. W. Gilliat

5 **The Epilepsies**
Roger J. Porter and Paolo I. Morselli

6 **Multiple Sclerosis**
W. I. McDonald and D. H. Silberberg

7 **Movement Disorders 2**
C. David Marsden and Stanley Fahn

8 **Infections of the Nervous System**
Peter G. E. Kennedy and Richard T. Johnson

9 **The Molecular Biology of Neurological Disease**
Roger N. Rosenberg and A. E. Harding

10 **Pain Syndromes in Neurology**
Howard L. Fields

11 **Principles and Practice of Restorative Neurology**
Robert R. Young and Paul J. Delwaide

12 **Stroke: Populations, Cohorts, and Clinical Trials**
Jack P. Whisnant

13 **Movement Disorders 3**
C. David Marsden and Stanley Fahn

14 **Mitochondrial Disorders in Neurology**
Anthony H. V. Schapira and S. DiMauro

15 **Peripheral Nerve Disorders 2**
Arthur K. Asbury and P. K. Thomas

16 **Contemporary Behavioral Neurology**
Michael R. Trimble and Jeffrey L. Cummings

17 **Headache**
Peter J. Goadsby and Stephen D. Silberstein

18 **The Epilepsies 2**
Roger J. Porter and David Chadwick

19 **The Dementias**
John H. Growdon and Martin N. Rossor

The Dementias

Edited by

John H. Growdon, M.D.
Professor of Neurology, Harvard Medical School, Boston; Neurologist, Massachusetts General Hospital, Boston

and

Martin N. Rossor, M.D., F.R.C.P.
Senior Lecturer in Neurology, Institute of Neurology, London; Consultant Neurologist, The National Hospital for Neurology and Neurosurgery and St. Mary's Hospital, London

Forewords by

Robert Katzman, M.D.
Research Professor of Neurosciences and Co-Director, Alzheimer Disease Research Center, University of California, San Diego, School of Medicine, La Jolla

and

Sir Martin Roth, M.D., Sc.D. (Hon), F.R.C.P., F.R.C.Psych., F.R.S.
Fellow of Trinity College, Cambridge, United Kingdom; Professor Emeritus of Psychiatry, Cambridge University

BUTTERWORTH HEINEMANN

Boston Oxford Johannesburg Melbourne New Delhi Singapore

Every effort has been made to ensure that the drug dosage schedules within this text are accurate and conform to standards accepted at time of publication. However, as treatment recommendations vary in the light of continuing research and clinical experience, the reader is advised to verify drug dosage schedules herein with information found on product information sheets. This is especially true in cases of new or infrequently used drugs.

Recognizing the importance of preserving what has been written, Butterworth–Heinemann prints its books on acid-free paper whenever possible.

Butterworth–Heinemann supports the efforts of American Forests and the Global ReLeaf program in its campaign for the betterment of trees, forests, and our environment.

Library of Congress Cataloging-in-Publication Data

The dementias / [edited by] John H. Growdon, Martin Rossor.
p. cm. -- (Blue books of practical neurology ; 19)
Includes bibliographical references and index.
ISBN 0-7506-9920-5
1. Dementia. 2. Alzheimer's disease--Diagnosis. 3. Alzheimer's disease--Treatment. 4. Neurology--Research. 5. Brain--Degeneration. I. Growdon, John H. (John Herbert) II. Rossor, M. (Martin) III. Series.
[DNLM: 1. Dementia--etiology. 2. Dementia--diagnosis. 3. Dementia--therapy. 4. Alzheimer Disease--diagnosis. 5. Alzheimer Disease--therapy. W1 BU9749 v. 19 1998 / WM 220 D376387 1998]
RC521.D4577 1998
616.8'3--dc21
DNLM/DLC
for Library of Congress 98-15850
CIP

British Library Cataloguing-in-Publication Data
A catalogue record for this book is available from the British Library.

The publisher offers special discounts on bulk orders of this book.
For more information, please contact:
Manager of Special Sales
Butterworth–Heinemann
225 Wildwood Avenue
Woburn, MA 01801-2041
Tel: 781-904-2500
Fax: 781-904-2620

For information on all Butterworth–Heinemann publications available, contact our World Wide Web home page at: http://www.bh.com

10 9 8 7 6 5 4 3 2 1

Printed in the United States of America

Contents

Contributing Authors

Harry Allen, M.B., B.S., M.R.C.Psych.
Consultant in Old Age Psychiatry, Manchester Royal Infirmary, Manchester, United Kingdom

M. Flint Beal, M.D.
Ann Parish Titzell Professor and Chairman, Department of Neurology, Cornell University Medical College, New York; Neurologist-in-Chief, The New York Hospital–Cornell Medical Center

Giuliano Binetti, M.D.
Alzheimer's Disease Research Unit, Centro San Giovanni di Dio Fatebenefratelli, Istituto di Ricovero e Cura a Carattere Scientifico, Brescia, Italy

Alistair Burns, M.D., F.R.C.P., F.R.C.Psych.
Professor of Old Age Psychiatry, University of Manchester, Withington Hospital, Manchester, United Kingdom

Helena Chang Chui, M.D.
Raymond and Betty McCarron Professor of Neurology, University of Southern California, Los Angeles; Chair of Neurological Sciences, Rancho Los Amigos Medical Center, Downey, California

Christopher M. Clark, M.D.
Assistant Professor of Neurology, University of Pennsylvania School of Medicine, Philadelphia; Director, Memory Disorders Clinic, Hospital of the University of Pennsylvania, Philadelphia

John Collinge, M.D., F.R.C.P.
Professor of Molecular Neurogenetics, Imperial College School of Medicine at St. Mary's, London; Honorary Consultant Neurologist, St. Mary's Hospital, London

Marc Cruts, Ph.D.
Postdoctoral Fellow, Laboratory of Neurogenetics, Department of Biochemistry, University of Antwerp, Antwerp, Belgium

Jeffrey L. Cummings, M.D.
Augustus Rose Professor of Neurology and Psychiatry, University of California, Los Angeles, UCLA School of Medicine

Douglas Ewbank, Ph.D.
Associate Director, Population Aging Research Center, University of Pennsylvania, Philadelphia

Teresa Gómez-Isla, M.D.
Research Associate in Neurology, University of Minnesota Medical School—Minneapolis

Steven M. Greenberg, M.D., Ph.D.
Assistant Professor of Neurology, Harvard Medical School and Massachusetts General Hospital, Boston

John H. Growdon, M.D.
Professor of Neurology, Harvard Medical School, Boston; Neurologist, Massachusetts General Hospital, Boston

Bradley T. Hyman, M.D., Ph.D.
Associate Professor of Neurology, Harvard Medical School, Boston; Associate in Neurology, Massachusetts General Hospital, Boston

Michael C. Irizarry, M.D.
Instructor in Neurology, Harvard Medical School, Boston; Assistant in Neurology, Massachusetts General Hospital, Boston

Clifford R. Jack, Jr., M.D.
Professor of Radiology, Mayo Medical School, Rochester, Minnesota; Department of Diagnostic Radiology, Mayo Clinic and Mayo Foundation, Rochester

Angus M. Kennedy, M.D., M.R.C.P.
Consultant Neurologist, West London Neuroscience Center, Charing Cross Hospital and The Chelsea Westminster Hospital, London

Virginia M.-Y. Lee, Ph.D.
Professor of Pathology and Laboratory Medicine and Co-Director, Center for Neurodegenerative Disease Research, University of Pennsylvania School of Medicine, Philadelphia

Graham G. Lennox, F.R.C.P.
Senior Lecturer and Honorary Consultant in Clinical Neurology, University of Nottingham Medical School, Queen's Medical Centre, Nottingham, United Kingdom

Morgan L. Levy, M.D.
Clinical Instructor of Psychiatry, University of California, Los Angeles, UCLA School of Medicine, Neuropsychiatric Institute; Neurosciences Research Fellow, West Los Angeles Veterans Affairs Medical Center

David M. A. Mann, Ph.D., F.R.C.Path.
Reader in Neuropathology, Department of Pathological Sciences, University of Manchester, Manchester, United Kingdom

Bruce L. Miller, M.D.
Professor of Neurology, Harbor-UCLA Medical Center, University of California, Los Angeles, UCLA School of Medicine

David Neary, M.D., F.R.C.P.
Professor of Neurology, University of Manchester, Manchester, United Kingdom; Consultant Neurologist, Manchester Royal Infirmary

George William Rebeck, Ph.D.
Assistant Professor of Neurology, Harvard Medical School and Massachusetts General Hospital, Boston

Karen Ritchie, M.Psych. Ph.D.
Research Director, Epidemiology of Neurodegenerative Pathologies of the Central Nervous System, Institut National de la Sante et la Recherche Medicale, Montpellier, France

Martin N. Rossor, M.D., F.R.C.P.
Senior Lecturer in Neurology, Institute of Neurology, London; Consultant Neurologist, The National Hospital for Neurology and Neurosurgery, London

Harvey J. Sagar, D.M., F.R.C.P.
Professor and Head of Department of Clinical Neurology, The University of Sheffield and Royal Hallamshire Hospital, Sheffield, United Kingdom

Dennis J. Selkoe, M.D.
Professor of Neurology and Neuroscience, Harvard Medical School, Boston; Co-Director, Center for Neurologic Diseases, Brigham and Women's Hospital, Boston

Julie Snowden, Ph.D.
Clinical Scientist (Neuropsychologist), Cerebral Function Unit, Department of Neurology, Manchester Royal Infirmary, Manchester, United Kingdom

John Q. Trojanowski, M.D., Ph.D.
Professor of Pathology and Laboratory Medicine and Co-Director, Center for Neurodegenerative Disease Research, University of Pennsylvania School of Medicine, Philadelphia

Christine Van Broeckhoven, Ph.D.
Professor and Head of Neurogenetics Laboratory, Department of Biochemistry, University of Antwerp, Antwerp, Belgium

Jean-Paul G. Vonsattel, M.D.
Departments of Neurology and Pathology, The C.S. Kubik Laboratory for Neuropathology, James Homer Wright Pathology Laboratories, Massachusetts Alzheimer Disease Research Center, Massachusetts General Hospital, Boston

Peter J. Whitehouse, M.D., Ph.D.
Professor of Neurology, Case Western Reserve University School of Medicine and University Hospitals of Cleveland Alzheimer Center

Foreword

Interest in Alzheimer's disease and related dementing diseases is a very recent phenomenon. In the 1970s, the term *Alzheimer's disease* was virtually unknown to the public, but today one hears about new breakthroughs in Alzheimer's disease research in newspapers or on television news programs almost on a weekly basis. Whereas in 1966 only 10 articles were published on Alzheimer's disease (as noted by a search of MEDLINE), and the number only rose to 52 in 1976, 826 citations were noted in 1986. In 1996, the citations of newly published articles had risen to 2,277, making it increasingly difficult to remain current with the clinical and scientific advances. These advances have been fueled in large part by the ability of investigators to apply molecular biological and genetic methods to this disorder. One major factor increasing interest in dementing illnesses has been the demographic revolution of the twentieth century. The prevalence of the dementia syndrome and the prevalence of Alzheimer's disease increase exponentially between the ages of 65 and 85, such that somewhere between one-fourth and one-half (depending on whose survey one uses) of those aged 85 years or older are demented. During this century the number of elderly persons with Alzheimer's disease has increased at least 20-fold.

Clinicians whose practice includes older adults increasingly have to treat patients with Alzheimer's disease or their caregiver spouse. Moreover, drugs for treating Alzheimer's disease, such as acetylcholinesterase inhibitors, antioxidants including vitamin E, nonsteroidal anti-inflammatory drugs, and estrogen replacement for postmenopausal women, have either been approved by the U.S. Food and Drug Administration or are under intensive investigation in drug trials. Thus, it becomes increasingly important for the clinician to understand the recent scientific advances in regard to Alzheimer's disease. The editors of this volume have brought together an extraordinary group of experts to define the scientific advances primarily in Alzheimer's disease (Part II) and the new treatments being developed (Part III).

This volume reviews the dementias with the needs of the clinician in mind. The clinical section (Part I) focuses not on Alzheimer's disease but on "related disorders," the less common dementing syndromes due to other neurodegenerative disorders. Part II deals with disease mechanisms and reviews the exciting recent scientific advances in the study of Alzheimer's disease.

In the 1960s, when the classic prospective clinical-pathologic study by Blessed, Tomlinson, and Roth demonstrated that "senile" dementia in the elderly was predominately due to Alzheimer's disease, with multiple vascular infarcts as the second most common etiology, the major focus of clinicians concerned with the accurate diagnosis of Alzheimer's disease was its differentiation from vascular dementia. With the control of hypertension and the introduction of potent antiplatelet aggregation agents to reduce the risk of stroke, the incidence of large cerebral infarcts has plummeted. Many dementia centers find that Alzheimer's disease now accounts for more than 80% of cases of dementia. A significant number of cases, however, show evidence of brain atrophy with pathologic features other than those of Alzheimer's disease. These cases are due to other neurodegenerative disorders, some not yet well defined.

For many years, Pick's disease, defined by the presence of neuronal Pick bodies and frontotemporal atrophy, was considered the second most common neurodegenerative disease producing dementia. Brains with Pick bodies are uncommon, however, and account for only 1–2% of autopsied dementia cases. Patients with frontotemporal dementia are more common than those with Pick's disease. In autopsy series, dementias with so-called nonspecific pathology (e.g., brains showing marked diffuse atrophy with subcortical gliosis or atrophy of frontotemporal regions without Pick bodies) represent a larger number of cases. These cases may present clinically as frontotemporal dementia with behavioral disturbances or progressive aphasia, with the symptoms of subcortical dementia, or with motor neuron disease associated with dementia. Familial cases with these clinical and pathologic presentations have been found to be linked to polymorphisms in a specific region on chomosome 17; an intensive search for this gene is now underway in over a dozen laboratories.

The existence of dementia associated with neocortical Lewy bodies, noted by Kosaka in 1979, was not generally recognized until the late 1980s. Neocortical Lewy bodies do not have the halo on hematoxylin and eosin stains associated with the Lewy bodies typically found in the substantia nigra in Parkinson's disease, nor are they stained by silver, thioflavin S, or other special stains used on the Alzheimer's disease brains; hence, their presence in dementia cases had been ignored by skilled pathologists until ubiquitin stains, which dramatically highlight Lewy bodies, began to be applied to the Alzheimer brains. It then became apparent that as many as 10–20% of cases that had been diagnosed pathologically as Alzheimer's disease, having the requisite number of neocortical plaques and subcortical neurofibrillary tangles to meet diagnostic criteria for Alzheimer's disease, had predominantly Lewy bodies rather then neurofibrillary tangles in the-neocortex. In addition, a small number of dementia cases are found without neuritic plaques or neurofibrillary tangles but with widespread Lewy bodies, the so-called diffuse Lewy body disease. We termed our cases with Alzheimer changes and Lewy bodies at autopsy the *Lewy body variant of Alzheimer's disease*, particularly as two genes, the 717 mutation of the amyloid precursor protein gene and the apolipoprotein E-ε4 allele, are risk factors for both phenotypically "pure" Alzheimer's disease and those with the Lewy body variant. Nevertheless, this latter term has not been widely accepted, and at this time, we abide by a consensus agreement to use the term *dementia with Lewy bodies*, which is the subject of Chapter 3. The relationship of this entity to the one-third of Parkinson's patients who develop dementia, many showing Alzheimer features as well as neocortical Lewy bodies at autopsy, is discussed in Chapter 4.

All of these neurodegenerative diseases are progressive and ultimately fatal. One might question whether the discovery of these newly defined dementia syndromes and diseases in the 1980s and 1990s is of clinical importance. The answer is clearly, "Yes!" As new drug therapies are developed, it will become critical to identify the disorder accurately. For example, the level of acetylcholinesterase is lower in the neocortex in subjects who have both plaques and Lewy bodies than in those with plaques and neurofibrillary tangles, and there is some suggestion that the acetylcholinesterase inhibitors are more effective in those subjects as compared to Alzheimer's disease patients without Lewy bodies. It seems likely that auxiliary tests such as apolipoprotein E allele determination, the level of *tau* protein in cerebrospinal fluid, single photon emission computed tomography and positron emission tomography, and perhaps functional magnetic resonance imaging—tests that may be useful for differentiating Alzheimer's disease from other neurodegenerative disorders presenting as dementia—will increase in importance. The clinician needs to follow closely the advances in what was once an esoteric field.

Robert Katzman

Foreword

This foreword summarizes an enquiry into Alzheimer's disease (AD) and related disorders that has been pursued over a period of more than 40 years and that links the traditional clinical and pathologic investigations with the recent advances in molecular biology.

Until the late 1970s, dementia was regarded as a dark and unpromising area for enquiry in neurology, psychiatry, and medicine. That this is no longer the case has become increasingly plain. Significant advances in knowledge along a wide front have made dementia a focus of interest for clinical and scientific investigators in many disciplines. Valuable lessons can be learned from the manner in which the indifference and neglect in the middle of the century were transformed in the case of AD into the clinical interest and productive research manifest at the present time.

For approximately 10 years before his first publication, Alois Alzheimer had been studying the postmortem brains of patients who probably had the disease he was to describe. Soon after his arrival in Munich, he used Bielschowsky's silver impregnation method on postmortem tissue from a case of dementia without vascular changes. It is not surprising that from the arrestingly beautiful pictures of the neurofibrillary tangle he published in his 1907 paper, he concluded that in his precociously demented 51-year-old patient he had discovered a new structure and a new disease. He was partly in error in this inference. As we were to learn, Alzheimer had described the pathology of the commonest form of "senile" as well as presenile dementia. But this does not significantly detract from the importance of his contribution.

Kraepelin's response to Alzheimer's finding was ambivalent. Although he referred to *Alzheimer's disease* in the eighth edition of his textbook (1909–1915), he found it difficult to accept the "tangle" as defining a distinct disorder. He doubted whether Alzheimer pathology represented anything specifically new. In his text, however, he allowed to prevail his intuition that there was a spark of originality in Alzheimer's account and credited him with the discovery of a new disorder. Yet skepticism about Alzheimer's finding was to reverberate down the next few decades until the 1950s. For 2–3 decades after Kraepelin expressed his reservations, eminent pathologists (Grünthal and Gellerstedt among others) argued that as "Alzheimer" changes, including the tangle, were common in brains of mentally intact aged, there must be some other or additional form of pathology that caused this form of dementia.

Historical Background

These neuropathologic concepts probably contributed to the development of unitary clinical concepts of classification and diagnosis of the mental disorders of the aged. The unitary ideas subsumed depressive, manic, and paranoid states with other syndromes, without organic psychiatric features. All were conceived as different manifestations of senile degeneration of the brain. These views survived unchallenged, causing neglect of the dementias until the middle of the twentieth century.

British textbooks of the time reflect the apathy and indifference to the subject. Dementia occupied only four of 980 pages in Russell Brain's 1951 edition of *Diseases of the Nervous System*. Henderson and Gillespie devoted 10 of 600 pages to the dementias. In that text, grafted onto a background of "organic brain degeneration" with "senile dementia" there were "senile delirium," "senile depression," and "senile paranoid states," all issuing from degeneration of the brain. The apparent explanation for such diffuse clinical concepts was provided by qualitative forms of pathologic investigation of the brain, which reported that some plaques and tangles were found in all the syndromes named [1]. The clinical manifestations of AD were seemingly limitless.

Enquiries into Classification and Diagnosis

A clear pattern of association between clinical observations and pathologic findings emerged after the application of stricter criteria in clinical diagnosis and the introduction of quantitative methods of assessment of the postmortem brain. Two cohorts of elderly people admitted to Graylingwell Hospital were examined. With the aid of "operational criteria," they were divided into five groups: affective psychosis, senile dementia (i.e., AD), late paraphrenia, confusional-delirious states, and vascular dementia. Examination of outcome at 2 years showed that more than 60% of patients with the affective disorders had been discharged, less than 20% had died, and less than 10% were inpatients. Eighty percent of those patients diagnosed with senile dementia (AD) were dead. Most paraphrenic patients had survived mainly as inpatients. The confusional-delirious group were evenly divided between those who had died (mainly with chronic refractory physical disease) and those who had been discharged. Survival of the vascular dementia patients (of whom almost four-fifths had died) was slightly greater than that of patients with AD in the early follow-up stage, and there was an excess of males as compared with the preponderance of females in AD. The findings have been published in full [2,3]. Two investigations by other workers using the same criteria reported follow-up findings from the different medical centers that were almost identical to those published in 1955.

Subsequently, a range of neuropsychological tests was developed that was also able to separate senile and vascular groups on the one hand and the depressive and paraphrenic groups on the other, with very little overlap. Among the confusional-delirious group, approximately 50% had survived, and their scores fell mainly within the distribution of scores in patients with "confusional" illness.

Enquiries into the Correlation of Measurements of Psychological Function and Diagnosis with Quantified Measurements of Postmortem Neuropathology

In Newcastle in the 1960s, the next stage of fresh enquiries sought to ascertain whether (1) the classification that had been arrived at would be upheld by quantitative neuropathologic studies in those who came to postmortem and (2) to determine whether measures of dementia in life correlated with measures of pathology postmortem. A large cohort of psychiatric patients and controls was investigated during life. The clinical and psychometric investigations were repeated at intervals to limit the period that elapsed between the final examination and death. A clinical diagnosis was made with the aid of the same criteria used in the previous study, the scores on quantified tests of cognitive function and for dementia were administered, and several parameters of brain pathology were measured postmortem.

In summary, the main findings [4,5] were as follows: (1) The plaque counts of those in the AD and vascular groups were significantly different from those in the functional and delirious cases. (2) When dementia scores were plotted against plaque counts, the correlation coefficient was 0.77 and highly significant. Neuritic plaques predominated in this material. (3) There was a clearly defined threshold effect of an average of 12 plaques per field; this defined a transition point beyond which 85% of cases proved to have been demented during life. (4) Correlations between tangles and dementia scores in a later study proved to be higher than those with senile plaques. (5) The single feature that distinguished patients with dementia from controls was the incidence of widespread tangles throughout the cortex [6]. (6) When the variance with respect to dementia score attributable to counts of plaques and tangles was deducted from the total, virtually no variance remained to be explained by parameters such as ventricular size and brain weight (Roth and Garside, unpublished observations, 1981).

A similar threshold effect is manifest in other forms of degenerative disorder of the central nervous system. In the case of parkinsonism, 80% of dopaminergic neurons have disappeared from the nigrostriatal system by the time the patient presents with symptoms and signs. Threshold effects are also discernible in the dementia-parkinsonism syndrome manifest in professional boxers and in the precocious dementia of patients with Down syndrome [7].

At a later stage in a Cambridge study, a significant outfall was compared with normal controls of large pyramidal cells from the frontal and temporal cortex and proved to be inversely correlated with tangle counts. The correlation of structural changes with indices of the cholinergic deficit in the brains of AD patients also proved significant.

Enquiries into the Molecular Biology of Alzheimer Changes with Special Reference to the Neurofibrillary Tangles

In 1982, I approached Sir Aaron Klug to seek his help and support for development of an enquiry into which clinicopathologic investigations of patients with AD and normal aged persons could be followed and which structural studies of the paired helical filaments of neurofibrillary changes could be undertaken with the methods he had developed. The selective focus on the tangle required some explanation.

The discovery of mutations in proteins encoded by genes on chromosomes 21 (amyloid precursor protein [APP]) and 1 and 14 (presenilins) as well as an association between AD and possession of the apolipoprotein E-ε4 allele have favored the theory that beta-amyloid (Aβ) protein deposition is central in the degenerative process of AD. But assays of Aβ in the brains of those with AD and comparison with the levels in mentally intact controls revealed amyloid to discriminate only weakly between them [8]. Aβ is extracellular and there is no evidence that it is toxic or destructive to neurons in vivo. In contrast, the neurofibrillary tangle is the only component of brain pathology of AD that is intracellular from the time it is formed. Among the changes in the brains of those with AD, tangles have proved to be the structure most highly correlated with the progressive cognitive and personality deterioration that are central features of the disease.

Molecular Structure of the Paired Helical Filament (of the Tangle) and Its Immunochemistry

Ignorance of the nature of the link between the plaque and tangle and that between Aβ and *tau* protein impedes enquiry into the pathogenesis of AD. The results of some recent genetic studies, however, have partly filled the gap in knowledge. Although many mutations in APP and presenilins cosegregate with AD, no mutations have been discovered in the *tau* gene (on chromosome 17q21). Nevertheless, several families with a hereditary form of dementia have been found to show linkage to markers on chromosome 17q21–22 [9,10]. The pathology is characterized by typical neurofibrillary degeneration in the total absence of Aβ deposits. An autosomal dominant gene defined in these studies has therefore been shown capable of causing a form of dementia with abundant and typical *tau* pathology in the absence of Aβ pathology. It seems justifiable to conclude that *tau* pathology is independently capable of causing a dementia analogous to AD.

In one of his papers, Francis Crick recommended that if one wishes to investigate function, one should explore the structural characteristics of the relevant tissues or organisms involved as a first step. Although Michael Kidd in 1963 had published some observations on the neurofibrillary tangle with the aid of electron microscopy, the resolution achieved proved inadequate for revealing their composition.

With the support of Sir Aaron Klug, we mounted a project in which Wischik and Crowther applied the novel techniques that had been developed by Aaron

Klug in the Medical Research Council Laboratory of Molecular Biology for image reconstruction of macromolecular complexes such as virus particles. With the aid of visual diffraction and computer-assisted reconstruction, Wischik and Crowther established that the paired helical filament (PHF) consisted of a double helical stack of subunits with the overall appearance of a ribbon twisted into a left-handed helix, each consisting of two symmetric C-shaped subunits with three domains.

Individual PHFs consisted of distinct components: a fuzzy coat that was easily removed by solvents, and a proteolytically resistant inner core. This inner core exhibited the entire double helical stack that had been defined with image reconstruction techniques and retained the morphologic appearances of PHFs [11]. At this stage, Wischik extracted a 12.5-kd peptide fragment from an enriched PHF core fraction. Protein sequencing of this fragment enabled Goedert and colleagues [12] to identify the peptide as being derived from the microtubule-associated *tau* protein. A monoclonal antibody raised against core PHFs recognized this fragment of *tau* but failed to interact with full-length *tau* molecules. This was explained by the fact that the core of the PHF contains only the tandem repeat region of the full-length *tau* molecule that arises from C-terminal truncation at Glu391. The antibody specifically recognizes this epitope at the site of truncation, but it is not accessible in full-length *tau* protein.

Discrimination among a number of other structures was made possible with the aid of antibodies originally developed by Wischik, Novak, and Milstein [13]. These served to distinguish intracellular tangles recognized by BR-133 (N-terminal epitope) from extracellular tangles recognized by mAb6.423 and 7.51 (truncated *tau* and repeat region *tau*, respectively). These antibodies were also able to discriminate full-length *tau*, which is soluble, from the truncated portion of the molecule found in the core of the PHF, which is highly resistant to solvents.

With the aid of the assays developed by Charles Harrington [14], these antibodies have been shown capable of discriminating between the brains of patients with AD and mentally intact aged persons [15]. In the normal aged, the soluble pool of full-length *tau* is found to constitute 97% of the total amount of this protein in the brain. In contrast, patients with AD have only 13% of the normal soluble *tau* remaining, with 87% replaced by insoluble truncated *tau*. The protein is also redistributed from the axons into the somatodendritic component of neurons.

Bondareff and Mena traced the development of the tangle in the brain through a sequence of changes. In the first stage, amorphous aggregates of truncated *tau* assemble inside the neuron. As the *tau* becomes truncated and therefore insoluble, neuronal dysfunction commences. As the expanding tangle bursts through the neuronal cell membrane, it becomes a "ghost" tangle. Each ghost represents the tombstone of a neuron that has been destroyed. *tau* protein is normally involved in axonal transport. In AD, transport and synaptic connections are disrupted by the substantial redistribution of truncated *tau* and the normal soluble *tau*.

The Normal Soluble Version of *tau* Protein, Its Truncated Insoluble Form, and Its Role in the Destruction of Neurons

The amount of PHF *tau* is highly correlated with the number of tangles, neuritic plaques, and dystrophic neurites, and is inversely correlated with the number of intact pyramidal neurons in the different cortical areas. It is also correlated with the degree of cognitive impairment and personality deterioration, central features of AD as recorded in life. The changes as a whole reflect a major qualitative transformation of the brain of the mentally intact aged person into the brain of the individually mentally deteriorated in senescence due to AD.

Truncated *tau* fragments in vitro readily bind full-length *tau* molecules. When the latter becomes truncated, the bound *tau* captures more *tau* molecules. Repetition of this process leads to an exponential increase in *tau* capture and truncation, culminating in the production of the highly insoluble polymer that constitutes the PHF [16,17].

The "Autocatalytic" Process Involved in the Assembly of Paired Helical Filaments and Attempts at Arresting *tau* Capture as a Possible Approach to Treating Alzheimer's Disease

The autocatalytic process described here is likely to prove a major factor underlying the cerebral and mental degeneration in AD. Even if the rate at which degeneration progresses were pharmacologically decreased by only 10%, the rate of cell elimination would be decreased and the process of mental deterioration markedly retarded.

The assembly of *tau-tau* aggregates in vitro provides a target for therapeutic intervention. Our group in Cambridge has found that certain desmethyl diaminophenothiazines are capable of selectively and specifically inhibiting *tau-tau* aggregation. Evidence has been adduced that certain inhibitors of specific *tau-tau* interaction can pull apart the subunits of PHFs isolated from the brain. It may therefore prove possible to develop pharmacologic agents capable of retarding the accumulation of truncated insoluble *tau* protein fragments into PHF in an effort to mitigate the symptoms of AD. It is too early to assess the chances of success in this venture.

Sir Martin Roth

References

1. Newton RD. J Mental Sci 1948;94:225–249.
2. Roth M. The natural history of mental disorders in old age. J Mental Sci 1955;101:281–301.
3. Roth M. The association of clinical and neurological findings and its bearing on the classification and aetiology of Alzheimer's disease. Br Med Bull 1986;42:42–50.
4. Roth M, Tomlinson BE, Blessed G. Correlation between scores for dementia and counts of 'senile plaques' in cerebral grey matter of elderly subjects. Nature 1966;209:109–110.
5. Blessed G, Tomlinson BE, Roth M. The association between quantitative measures of dementia and of senile change in the cerebral grey matter of elderly subjects. Br J Psychiatry 1968;114:797–811.
6. Tomlinson BE, Blessed G, Roth M. Observations on the brains of demented old people. J Neurol Sci 1970;11:205–242.
7. Roth M, et al. Convergence and Cohesion of Recent Neurobiological Findings in Relation to Alzheimer's Disease and Their Bearing on Its Aetiological Basis. In M Bergener, M Ermini, HB Stahelin (eds), Thresholds in Aging. London: Academic Press, 1985;117–146.
8. Harrington CR, Mukaetova-Ladinska EB, Hills R, et al. Measurement of distinct immunochemical presentations of *tau* protein in Alzheimer disease. Proc Natl Acad Sci U S A 1991;88:5842–5846.

9. Bird TD, Wijsman EM, Nochlin D, et al. Chromosome 17 and hereditary dementia: linkage studies in three non-Alzheimer families and kindreds with late-onset FAD. Neurology 1997;48:949–954.
10. Spillantini MG, Goedert M, Crowther RA, et al. Familial multiple system taupathy with presenile dementia: a disease with abundant neuronal and glial *tau* filaments. Proc Natl Acad Sci U S A 1997; 94:4113–4118.
11. Wischik CM, Crowther RA, Stewart M, Roth M. Subunit structure of paired helical filaments in Alzheimer's disease. J Cell Biol 1985;100:1905–1912.
12. Goedert M, Wischik CM, Crowther RA, et al. Cloning and sequencing of the cDNA encoding a core protein of the paired helical filament of Alzheimer disease: identification as the microtubule-associated protein *tau*. Proc Natl Acad Sci U S A 1988;85:4051–4055.
13. Wischik CM, Novak M, Thogersen HC, et al. Isolation of a fragment of tau derived from the core of the paired helical filament of Alzheimer disease. Proc Natl Acad Sci 1988;85:4506–4510.
14. Harrington CR, Louwagie J, Rossau R, et al. Influence of apolipoprotein E genotype on senile dementia of the Alzheimer and Lewy body types. Am J Pathol 1994;145:1472–1484.
15. Mukaetova-Ladinska EB, Harrington CR, Roth M, Wischik CM. Biochemical and anatomical redistribution of *tau* protein in Alzheimer's disease. Am J Pathol 1993;143:565–578.
16. Wischik CM, Edwards PC, Lai RY, et al. Selective inhibition of Alzheimer disease–like *tau* aggregation by phenothiazines. Proc Natl Acad Sci U S A 1996;93:11213–11218.
17. Wischik CM, Lai RY, Harrington CR. Modelling Prion-Like Processing of Tau Protein in Alzheimer's Disease for Pharmaceutical Development. In J Avila, R Brandt, K Kosik (eds), Brain Microtubule-Associated Proteins: Modifications in Disease. Amsterdam: Harwood Academic Publishers, 1997;185–240.

Series Preface

The *Blue Books of Practical Neurology* series is the new name for the *BIMR Neurology* series, which was itself the successor to the *Modern Trends in Neurology* series. As before, the volumes are intended for use by physicians who grapple with the problems of neurologic disorders on a daily basis, be they neurologists, neurologists in training, or those in related fields such as neurosurgery, internal medicine, psychiatry, and rehabilitation medicine.

Our purpose is to produce monographs on topics in clinical neurology in which progress through research has brought about new concepts of patient management. The subject of each monograph is selected by the Series Editors using two criteria: first, that there has been significant advance in knowledge in that area and, second, that such advances have been incorporated into new ways of managing patients with the disorders in question. This has been the guiding spirit behind each volume, and we expect it to continue. In effect, we emphasize research, both in the clinic and in the experimental laboratory, but principally to the extent that it changes our collective attitudes and practices in caring for those who are neurologically afflicted.

C. David Marsden
Arthur K. Asbury
Series Editors

Preface

Dementia is one of the most devasting symptoms of neurologic disease. Dementia is feared because it strikes the mind: Memory fails, language capacities deteriorate, judgment suffers, and personality disintegrates. Dementia is especially threatening because it affects those qualities that place humans on a par with the gods and that stamp each individual as unique.

> What a piece of work is a man! How noble in reason!
> How infinite in faculty! In form, in moving, how express and admirable!
> In action how like an angel! In apprehension how like a god!
> —Shakespeare, *Hamlet*, II, ii, 317

When the mental faculties fail, when apprehension and reason wither, humans lose their godlike status. The fall from perfection is especially hard because humanity's perch is so high. This fall is a personal tragedy for each demented individual, as well as for his or her family and friends. This book is dedicated to those with dementia and to those who care for them. We hope that the new information summarized here will improve current diagnosis and care of patients with dementia and spur further clinical and basic science research that will lead to prevention and cure of dementing illnesses.

Dementia is technically defined as cognitive impairments sufficiently pervasive and severe that they disrupt independent life. More than 50 medical, psychiatric, and neurologic conditions are associated with dementia. Alzheimer's disease (AD) is the most common neurodegenerative disease that causes dementia. The incidence of AD is linked to age and increases from five in 100,000 in the sixth decade of life to more than 1,500 in 100,000 by the tenth decade of life. Criteria for the clinical diagnosis of AD, its characteristic course of progression, and neuropathologic features have been extensively described. In the course of studying AD, clinical investigators have defined other neurodegenerative diseases distinct from AD and that must now be included in the differential diagnosis of dementia. The most common non-AD dementias are discussed in Part I,

Degenerative Diseases That Cause Dementia. Each of these can mimic AD, but each has unique features that can be recognized clinically and neuropathologically. Some of these conditions, such as Pick's disease and Parkinson's disease, are classic neurologic diseases, whereas others, such as frontal and frontotemporal lobe dementia and dementia with Lewy bodies, are still being defined. For each disease, the authors provide authoritative descriptions that aim to sharpen clinical diagnosis and improve patient care. Human prion diseases are included in this group because they cause dementia through a novel mixture of genetic, transmissable, and degenerative processes. Vascular dementia, long considered the second most common cause of dementia after AD, is not included in this section, but is discussed as a separate topic. The definition of vascular dementia has changed over the years; in fact, its very existence has been questioned. For these reasons, vascular dementia is included in Part IV, Questions and Controversies.

Much of the scientific research on dementia has been conducted under the umbrella of AD. The chapters in Part II, Scientific Advances in Understanding the Dementias, document the major advances since the late 1980s. In each instance, the chapter topics were chosen for their clinical relevance to the problems of dementia. Our criteria for selecting topics were the extent to which the discoveries improve understanding of processes that cause dementia and alter the way clinicians deal with demented patients. The first topic is molecular genetics. Chapter 6, Molecular Genetics of Alzheimer's Disease, discusses familial versus sporadic AD and describes the molecular bases of familial AD. Chapter 7, Apolipoprotein E and Alzheimer's Disease, discusses the biological mechanisms whereby the apolipoprotein E alleles affect the expression of AD. This chapter also provides guidelines for counseling families about the risks of developing AD based on apolipoprotein E genotypes. Two subsequent chapters deal with brain imaging techniques. Dementia is a brain disease and can best be evaluated through knowledge of anatomy and physiology. Assessing the anatomic structure of the brain is an integral part of the diagnostic examination of an individual with dementia. Chapter 8, Anatomic Neuroimaging in the Dementias, addresses the place of anatomic imaging in clinical practice, emphasizes volumetric measurements of specific brain regions relevant to dementia, and illustrates how anatomic imaging aids in the differential diagnosis of the dementias. Chapter 9, Functional Neuroimaging in Dementia, emphasizes positron emission tomography studies as a complement to anatomic neuroimaging; brain regions that appear morphologically normal often have metabolic abnormalities. Technological advances in both anatomic and functional imaging modalities enhance neurologic diagnosis and offer biological correlates of behavioral abnormalities. Two subsequent chapters deal with the molecular pathology of AD and focus on amyloid and neuronal cytoskeletal abnormalities, the chief histopathologic hallmarks of AD. It is hoped that identifying the mechanisms whereby amyloid fibrils are deposited in the brain and neurofibrillary tangles are formed will provide insight into the cause of AD dementia, as well as suggest targets for therapeutic intervention. As important as amyloid and tangles may be, dementia ultimately results from neuronal loss and decreases in synaptic contacts. These features of neuropathology are not seen directly, but are apparent only in comparison to what is present in brains of nondemented individuals. Chapter 12, Bioenergetics, Excitotoxicity, and Oxidative Injury in the Pathogenesis of Neurodegenerative Disease, considers theories of why cells die. The chapter describes the evidence for apoptosis as well as energy failure leading to oxidative stress and neurotoxicity.

Part III, Treatment of the Dementias, consists of two chapters. Chapter 13, Current Pharmacologic Treatments for Dementia, reviews drugs that have been developed to treat the cognitive impairments with an emphasis on acetylcholinesterase inhibitors. There is also a discussion of drugs proposed for treating the noncognitive behavioral abnormalities that often accompany dementia, with recommendations for their use. Chapter 14, The Future of Drug Therapy in Alzheimer's Disease, builds on the scientific advances reviewed in Part II and places them in a broad social context. Scientific leads point to new classes of drugs that could improve memory in the short term, interfere with neurodegenerative processes and thereby slow dementia progression in the intermediate term, and even prevent or cure AD in the long term.

Among unresolved issues in the dementia field, we have highlighted three topics in Part IV, Questions and Controversies. The first of these, the controversy regarding vascular dementia, is discussed in Chapter 15, Rethinking Vascular Dementia: Moving from Myth to Mechanism. The second controversy considers whether AD is the inevitable consequence of aging or a specific brain disease. The various arguments in this controvery are discussed in Chapter 16, Is Alzheimer's Disease Just Old Age? The final chapter, Controversies in the Classification of Focal Lobar Atrophies, addresses the confusing nomenclature and concepts that surround conditions such as Pick's disease, frontal lobe dementia, and frontotemporal dementia.

JHG
MNR

I

Degenerative Diseases that Cause Dementia

Introduction

Martin N. Rossor and John H. Growdon

Part I of this book is notable for the absence of a specific chapter on Alzheimer's disease (AD), which is the most common cause of dementia. The important advances in AD are covered amply in the chapters of Parts II and III, which, although they encompass many general topics, are inevitably dominated by the recent discoveries in AD. In this clinical section, however, the emphasis is on dementias other than AD. The choice of diseases selected reflects the frequency with which they present to the neurologist (dementia with Lewy bodies, extrapyramidal disorders), the nosologic challenge (Pick's disease, frontal and frontotemporal dementia), or advances in molecular pathology; the latter is exemplified by the prion diseases that have led to new concepts of pathogenesis. Prion disease also has the dubious distinction of potentially becoming a common cause of dementia in the young with the emergence in the United Kingdom of a new variant of Creutzfeldt-Jakob disease (CJD).

The syndromic term *dementia*, used to distinguish the patient with a generalized cognitive impairment from those patients with focal neuropsychological deficits or with confusional and delirious states, has been clinically and scientifically valuable. Refinement of the term to demand that it include impairment of event or episodic memory has inevitably focused attention on AD, in which memory impairment is the salient feature. The term is less well suited to the cognitively impaired patients who present with subcortical or frontal lobe pathology and in whom memory may be relatively preserved. The term *subcortical dementia* was coined to describe the marked mental slowing, or bradyphrenia, that can be seen in patients with subcorticofrontal disease [1]. This term has been criticized on semantic grounds, because the prototypic disorder of subcortical dementia, namely progressive supranuclear palsy, can be associated with cortical pathology, and similarly, the prototypic cortical dementia, AD, can have subcortical pathology. The clinical distinction, however, remains helpful, as slowed speed of mental processing variably coupled to specific cognitive deficits are frequent accompaniments of extrapyramidal disorders. These features may not only be clinically important in their own right, but the pattern of the cognitive impairment found with the motor disorder provides important diagnostic clues. Moreover, studies of such patients have provided valuable insights into cognitive processing. These aspects of the cognitive deficits are reviewed by Harvey J. Sagar in Chapter 4. Dementia with Lewy bodies has justified its own chapter: In Chapter 3, Graham G. Lennox reviews the clinical picture of dementia with Lewy bodies and provides helpful diagnostic guidelines. Neuropathologic and epidemiologic evidence indicates that diffuse Lewy body disease is an important and relatively common disorder, particularly in the elderly, although the extent of overlap with AD is still not clear.

The other major area in which the criteria for the dementia syndrome, if strictly applied, can be misleading is the group of disorders encompassed by the term *frontal lobe dementia* or the broader term *frontotemporal dementia* [2]. In both groups of patients, recall memory may be inefficient, but recognition memory is often remarkably normal. In contrast to the relative preservation of memory, failure of executive skills and behavioral changes can be pervasive and devastating.

The delineation and diagnosis of these disorders rests on the presence of a characteristic pattern of deficit that arises from the involvement of particular areas of the cerebral cortex. This reflects the selective vulnerability of specific brain regions to the underlying disease process—for example, the medial temporal lobe and hippocampus to AD and the anterior temporal and frontal lobes to Pick's disease. The difficulty for the clinician is that although particular diseases have predilections for particular areas, the relationship is not a constant one, and a particular constellation of cognitive cortical deficits may be found with a variety of underlying histopathologic changes. This difficulty also applies to the even more selective focal neuropsychological deficits that can occur on a degenerative basis and have acquired syndromic terms such as *primary progressive dysphasia*, *semantic dementia*, *primary progressive prosopagnosia*, and *primary progressive dyspraxia*. Each of these syndromes can be associated with a variety of histopathologies. (The difficulties of diagnosing specific clinicopathologic entities, as opposed to broad clinical syndromes, are carefully argued by David Neary and colleagues in Chapter 17.)

Is the clinician foolish in attempting to take the diagnosis of frontal and frontotemporal dementia further? It is hoped not. The editors recognize the limitations of a more specific diagnosis but take the view that delineation in clinicopathologic terms is an enterprise worth the effort. There is an immediate difficulty with this ambition because the histologic features themselves need not relate to a specific molecular pathology. One can only see what is visible, and although the horizon expands with the increasing array of immunohistochemical techniques, the specificity of a particular feature—Lewy bodies or neurofibrillary tangles, for example—is uncertain. Nevertheless, our current histopathologic classification is important in that it bears a closer relationship to the underlying molecular pathology than a classification based on clinical features alone. It is for this reason that there is a specific chapter on Pick's disease by Giuliano Binetti and colleagues (Chapter 1). The confusion that has arisen between the clinical syndrome and the underlying histopathologic entity is discussed. As the authors point out, the original description by Arnold Pick was a clinical one, albeit underpinned by the macroscopic pathology of selective regional atrophy. The term, in this chapter, is more precisely defined by the presence of Pick inclusion bodies and Pick cells within the setting of regional atrophy. The alternative view—namely, that retention of the term *Pick's disease* or *Pick complex* as a clinical as opposed to neuropathologic syndrome is preferable—has been argued by a number of authors [3]; the challenge now is to see whether more careful delineation of the pattern of neuropsychological deficits and neuroradiologic changes can lead to an in vivo–specific diagnosis of Pick's disease. Dr. Binetti and colleagues provide some useful clues, and a European Concerted Action on Pick's Disease Committee has also provided clinical criteria that are currently undergoing validation [4].

Although difficult to diagnose clinically, Pick's disease does at least have the advantage that identifiable inclusion bodies can be used for a pathologic diagnosis. The group of disorders with nonspecific histologic change, most commonly presenting with a frontal lobe or frontotemporal dementia, offers an even greater challenge. This group may be associated with Pick bodies or with anterior horn cell disease with spongiform change. Commonly, however, it is associated with nonspecific changes of frontal lobe degeneration. The florid clinical features that can occur in these cases are amply illustrated in the chapter by Morgan L. Levy and colleagues (Chapter 2). The difficulty the clinician has relating a cluster of neuropsychological deficits and behavioral change to a specific histopathologic description and discrete nosologic entity is a recurring theme.

Identifying the molecular pathology of a dementia clarifies phenotypic variations in disease more than clinical descriptions and neuropathologic subtleties. Prion diseases illustrate this new direction best. As John Collinge argues in Chapter 5, diseases such as Gerstmann-Sträussler-Scheinker syndrome and familial fatal insomnia can now be grouped with CJD under the broad rubric of prion disorders. Most important, the genetic determinants of this phenotypic variability are now being identified; considerable clinical heterogeneity can occur with a given prion protein gene mutation, but additional genetic determinants such as the PrP 129 genotype can determine the clinical expression as with PrP 178 mutations and familial fatal insomnia. The recognition of the latter disease as a prion disorder suggests that the clinical presentations of the prion disorders have not yet been fully explored, and other clinical entities may yet await identification. This may be particularly applicable to psychiatric disorders and new variant CJD, which can present with behavioral disturbance.

REFERENCES

1. Albert ML, Feldman RG, Willis AL. The "subcortical dementia" of progressive supranuclear palsy. J Neurol Neurosurg Psychiatry 1974;37:121–130.
2. Lund and Manchester Group. Clinical and neuropathological criteria for frontotemporal dementia. J Neurol Neurosurg Psychiatry 1994;37:416–418.
3. Kertesz A. Pick complex and Pick's disease: the nosology of frontal lobe dementia, primary progressive aphasia, and corticobasal ganglionic degeneration. Eur J Neurol 1996;3:280–282.
4. European Concerted Action on Pick's Disease Committee. Provisional clinical and neuroradiological criteria for the diagnosis of Pick's disease. Eur J Neurol 1998. (In press.)

1
Pick's Disease

Giuliano Binetti, John H. Growdon,
and Jean-Paul G. Vonsattel

HISTORICAL REVIEW

Between 1892 and 1906, Arnold Pick (Figure 1.1) published a series of reports on six patients (four women, two men) with unusual dementia, in an attempt to understand the relationship between topography and function of the brain [1–4]. Pick's original idea was to evaluate patients whose brains showed a relatively mild diffuse atrophy with superimposed circumscribed areas of intense atrophy in certain lobes or convolutions. At first, Pick was inclined to attribute the atrophy to vascular disturbances. Gradually, however, he supported the concept that this uneven, bizarre cerebral atrophy, including areas with severe parenchymal shrinkage or "circumscribed atrophy," was the result of neurodegeneration rather than cerebrovascular disorders [1,2]. Eventually, Pick claimed that, in some instances, "senile brain atrophy" was circumscribed, challenging the dogmatic belief (defended by Wernicke) that senile cerebral atrophy was a diffuse process [2,4]. To support his claim, Pick presented both clinical data and the gross findings of the neuropathologic evaluation performed by Chiari on the brains of August H., who died at age 71 years [1], and Josef Vlasak, who died at age 60 years [4]. Clinical onset of illness in August H. occurred approximately 2 years before death, with gradual mental weakness, aggressiveness, apathy, and speech difficulties. The neuropathologic hallmarks described included brain weight of 1,150 g (right

This work was supported in part by grants AG05134, National Institutes of Health grant NINCDS 31862 (Brain Tissue Resource Center) and NS16367 (Huntington's Disease Center without Walls), and by a grant from the Instituto di Ricovero e Cura a Carattere Scientifico, Centro San Giovanni di Dio, Sacro Cuore Fatebenefratelli Institute.

Special thanks are given to Giovanni B. Frisoni, M.D.; Wendy Hobbs; Kathy Newell, M.D.; and Larry Cherkas for advice and technical assistance. We owe an exceptional debt of gratitude to Edward P. Richardson, Jr., M.D., for his immense support, and for his special role in getting us interested in neurodegenerative diseases.

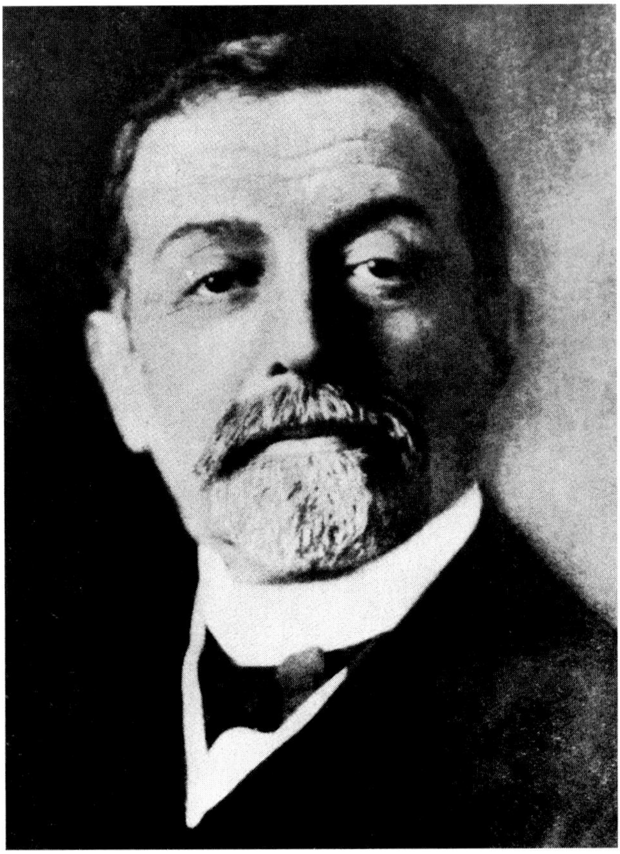

Figure 1.1 Arnold Pick (1851–1924).

hemisphere 500 g; left hemisphere 470 g) and diffuse atrophy of the brain, which was graded as marked except for the temporal lobe where it was severe and more conspicuous on the left side than on the right. No microscopic findings were provided [1]. Josef Vlasak's clinical hallmarks described by Pick that are relevant to the present understanding of the disease include family burden of mental illness involving at least a sister, "amnesic" aphasia with preserved ability to recite the months serially, memory loss, stereotypy, and apraxia. The neuropathologic hallmarks provided were brain weight of 1,105 g (right hemisphere 485 g; left hemisphere 460 g), severe atrophy involving the frontal lobes and left inferior parietal lobule, mild atrophy involving the right inferior parietal lobule and the bilateral temporal and occipital lobes, and no atrophy of the precentral gyri or superior parietal lobules. No microscopic evaluation was performed [4,5].

Definite, severe, circumscribed, asymmetric (left > right), frontal atrophy in a demented, 49-year-old woman was documented by Richter as early as 1918, corroborating Pick's observations [6]. These early publications emphasized that non-Alzheimer, nonvascular cerebral degeneration can be circumscribed and asymmetric; specific symptoms can be correlated with definite, regional cerebral atrophy; and the condition might be hereditary. Despite limited neuropathologic data, these data still constitute the solid basis of Pick's disease (PcD) as emphasized by Lüers and Spatz in 1957 [7] and by Tissot, Constantinidis, and Richard in 1975 [8].

The microscopic description of the intraneuronal inclusions—now called *Pick bodies*—and ballooned neurons, and their association with circumscribed atrophy was provided by Alzheimer [9]. He was puzzled that neuritic plaques and neurofibrillary tangles were absent in a demented patient (Therese Mühlich [10]). Furthermore, Alzheimer noticed that there was relative preservation of the superior temporal gyrus as compared to the severely atrophic middle and inferior temporal gyri [9]. Alzheimer's observations were confirmed and expanded by Altman, who described the detailed neuropathologic findings, including Pick bodies and ballooned neurons, in two patients [11]. Altman noticed that the superficial neocortical layers were more prone to degeneration than deep ones. He described the relative preservation of the hippocampus, which contrasted with the severe atrophy of the subiculum and nearby temporal gyri; atrophy of the medial thalamus and of the frontopontine fibers; and the abrupt transition between severely atrophic and relatively preserved regions of the cerebral hemispheres. Altman confirmed that the circumscribed atrophy could include the temporal lobes in addition to the frontal lobes. Richter illustrated ballooned neurons in his report on frontal, circumscribed atrophy; however, he did not mention the presence or absence of neuronal inclusions [6]. Gans referred to the frontal atrophy as *Pick atrophy* [12]. This restrictive, topographic designation was to become a source of confusion in categorizing brains with definite circumscribed atrophy. Whereas Arnold Pick saw a match between the circumscribed atrophy and the cerebral areas that are ontogenetically the latest to myelinate, Gans supported the hypothesis that the atrophic regions were phylogenetically recent. Gans referred to Edinger's school, which emphasized the frequent vulnerability of the phylogenetically newer parts of the brain in neurodegeneration, whereas Onari and Spatz reported that the atrophy often encroaches or includes phylogenetically old parts also, and they coined the term *Pick's disease* [10].

Stertz provided detailed clinical data in an attempt to characterize the distinct symptoms that result from predominantly frontal or predominantly temporal atrophy [13]. Stertz's report is especially interesting because the patients he described played a crucial role in the characterization of PcD: the brains of patients Bradt (no Pick bodies, no ballooned neurons) and Mühlich and Ruge (both with Pick bodies and ballooned neurons) were all extensively examined neuropathologically by Onari and Spatz [10]. Furthermore, the brain of patient Mühlich was studied by Alzheimer, which led him to the initial description of both Pick bodies and ballooned neurons [9]. Between 1922 and 1929, PcD gained acceptance as an entity characterized by gradual dementia that could be distinguished from presenile dementia by the presence of circumscribed atrophy and the absence or scarcity of plaques and tangles. This entity was referred to either as *Pick atrophy* [12,13], *Pick lobar sclerosis* [14], or *PcD* [10,14–16]. Bonfiglio scored the difficulty in categorizing brains with definite circumscribed atrophy. He reported the clinical and pathologic findings of a 35-year-old patient at onset of symptoms (gradual dementia, palilalia, logoclonia) and at death at age 45 years. The external surface of this brain showed slight, diffuse atrophy; however, there was "circumscribed atrophy" of the basal ganglia (head of caudate nucleus > putamen > globus pallidus; rostral > caudal), and there was no mention whether Pick bodies or ballooned neurons were present [17]. Bonfiglio pointed out that atrophy of the deep gray nuclei was often observed in PcD and that there may be instances in which the circumscribed atrophy could be centered in the basal ganglia. Although favoring the diagnosis of PcD, Bonfiglio preferred to categorize his patient as having "circumscribed atrophy of the basal ganglia." The atrophy of the striatum and substantia nigra in PcD was emphasized later by von Braunmühl, who reported the findings made in three patients with an akinetic-hypertonic syndrome [18]. His hypothesis was that the atrophy of the striatum and of the substantia nigra was a primary process and not secondary to the cortical degeneration [18], a claim supported later by Grünthal [19]. Schneider reported two patients with PcD and discussed the findings in patients Ruge and Mühlich (referred to as Mielich in this study), the same cases as originally evaluated by Alzheimer. Schneider claimed that Pick bodies, and especially ballooned neurons, were present in patients' brains with rapid course and absent or rare in those with chronic course [15,16].

The awareness of familial occurrences of PcD was greatly reinforced after the reports by von Braunmühl and Leonhard [20], Grünthal [19], and Schmitz and Meyer [21]. von Braunmühl and Leonhard described the findings of two sisters (29 and 31 years old at onset of symptoms and 32 and 35 years old at death, respectively), whose brains displayed circumscribed atrophy, Pick bodies, and ballooned neurons, and whose mother might have had PcD [20]. The circumscribed atrophy of the sister with the shorter disease course encompassed the frontal lobe, whereas the brain atrophy of the sister with the longer disease course included the frontal, temporal, and parietal lobes (especially on the left side). Severe atrophy of the striatum was noticed in both brains along with atrophy and pallor of the substantia nigra [20]. Grünthal further emphasized the familial occurrence of PcD by describing two demented brothers (42 and 45 years old at onset of symptoms and 45 and 50 years old at death), whose brains showed circumscribed atrophy including the orbital region, insula, temporal pole, hippocampal formation (with relative preservation of the Sommer sector), caudate nucleus, medial thalamus, and substantia nigra; Pick bodies and ballooned neurons were not present [19]. Schmitz and Meyer described a woman (52 years old at onset of symptoms and 56 years old at death) with gradual dementia and aphasia. Her brain showed severe circumscribed frontal atrophy, including striatum and ballooned neurons; there were no Pick bodies, tangles, or neuritic plaques. The father and two sisters of the patient had the same symptoms and clinical course; however, they were not evaluated pathologically [21]. Grünthal suggested that the circumscribed atrophy had a starting locus, referred to as the *primary shrinkage center*, from which the degenerative process gradually extended. The primary shrinkage center of the two brains in question was thought to be the frontal orbital region; however, Grünthal stated that this site could vary from brain to brain. Finally, he claimed that his findings supported von Braunmühl's hypothesis that the degeneration of the basal ganglia in PcD resulted from a degenerative process that spread from one or multiple centers. The joint occurrence of PcD and amyotrophic lateral sclerosis was first observed by von Braunmühl in 1932 [22]. Korbsch reported a family of 14 siblings, two of them with neurologic problems: a man with progressive dementia who died at age 42 years with circumscribed atrophy of the brain and ballooned neurons with neither Alzheimer pathology nor Pick bodies, and his 47-year-old sister with choreic movements that had started at age 14 years. The sister was diagnosed as having Huntington's disease although neither the father (described as healthy at 83 years) nor the mother (described as healthy until shortly before her death 10 years earlier) had movement disorders [14]. Remarkable summaries of the neuropathologic changes in PcD were provided by Schneider in 1927 and 1929 [15,16]. Schneider presented four new patients: patient Greppmager (no Pick bodies or ballooned neurons), patient Jatzel and patient Naumann (with ballooned neurons but without Pick bodies), and patient Moser (without reference to Pick bodies or ballooned neurons). Furthermore, Schneider reviewed reported patients including Ruge (with Pick bodies and ballooned neurons) and Mühlich, initially described by Alzheimer [9]. Recall that patients Ruge and Mühlich had circumscribed atrophy, Pick bodies, and ballooned neurons, and were both extensively studied by Onari and Spatz [10], with detailed clinical data provided by Stertz [13]. Schneider summarized patterns of cerebral atrophy in PcD: rostral > caudal and gyrus fusiformis, or parahippocampal gyrus > middle temporal gyrus > inferior temporal gyrus, or instances with the brunt of the atrophy in the poles of the superior and middle frontal gyri with relative preservation of the motor strip. Furthermore, he paid special attention to the ballooned neurons in PcD. He performed quantitative studies in the brains of patients Jatzel, Ruge, and Mühlich and concluded that the less marked the atrophy, the higher the number of ballooned neurons. Ballooned neurons were located mainly in the superficial cortical layers early in the course of the disease, and later they were also found in the deep cortical layers. Schneider noticed that Pick bodies were present in four of the six brains containing ballooned neurons (there is an apparent discrepancy between this statement and the neuropathologic descriptions) and remarked that they might be difficult to find; he claimed that their distribution matched that of the ballooned neurons [15]. Most of these reports, from Pick to Schneider, illustrate the efforts of investigators to establish detailed clinicopathologic correlation to understand the occurrence and course of the cerebral circumscribed atrophies, or PcD. These reports of detailed clinicopathological correlations indicate that Pick's disease has always been a clinical as well as pathological entity [23].

CLINICAL ASPECTS OF PICK'S DISEASE

Clinical Symptoms

The earliest symptoms of PcD are generally personality changes and behavioral abnormalities. Initial symptoms of Pick's original patient, August H., included agitation, aggressiveness, and loss of self-control [1]. Later in the course of his illness, he developed aphasia with paraphasic errors. Schneider identified three phases in the course of the disease [15]: Behavioral disturbances such as disinhibition, impulsivity, irritability, apathy, and impaired judgment characterized the

Table 1.1 Mean prevalence (%) of initial symptoms in Pick's disease patients or in Alzheimer's disease patients reported by caregivers

Symptoms or troubles involved	*Pick's disease (n = 34)*	*Alzheimer's disease (n = 78)*
Irritability/aggressiveness	11.8	3.9
Memory	61.8	93.6 ($P \leq .001$)
Personality	35.3	14.1 ($P = .07$)
Reasoning	5.9	6.5
Sense of direction	0.0	7.8
Socializing	2.9	2.6
Speech	29.4	9.1 ($P \leq .05$)
Temporal orientation	0.0	6.4
Use of objects	0.0	2.6
Vision	0.0	1.3
Writing	0.0	0.0

first phase or *preclinical phase*; dementia, with deficits in attention and language capacities, appeared during the second phase; finally, apathy, mutism, and myoclonus characterized the third phase. In a study of 32 PcD patients by Tissot and colleagues, behavioral abnormalities were noted as early symptoms: altered mood states, loss of ethical propriety, and neglect of daily routines [8]. In later stages of the disease, they noted aphasia often leading to mutism, difficulties in programming, and temporal disorientation.

Family and friends of patients with PcD are usually the only reliable source of information about the earliest symptoms. As part of a cross-sectional and longitudinal study of cognition [24] in PcD at the Massachusetts General Hospital, caregivers were asked to select from a set of 11 characteristics the one they first recalled as being abnormal. Their replies were compared with answers obtained from caregivers of Alzheimer disease (AD) patients (Table 1.1). After memory loss, personality change was the most common symptom, followed by aphasia. Gleaned from the literature, the types of personality changes include a wide range of symptoms: apathy, depression, irritability, jocularity, euphoria, disinhibition, obsessive and compulsive behavior, loss of social graces, diet disturbances or bulimia, hyperorality, wandering, and impaired judgment [15,16,25–30]. Three syndromes summarize clinical findings often observed in PcD: moriatic syndrome (or *moria*: foolishness or dullness of comprehension, frivolity, joviality, inability to take anything seriously), PES syndrome (*p*alilalia, *e*cholalia, *s*tereotypia), or PEMA syndrome (*p*alilalia, *e*cholalia, *m*utism, and *a*mimia) [8,31,32]. These manifestations reflect an early involvement of the frontal lobes in the PcD degenerative process as an explanation for the apathy and disinhibition syndromes. Damage to frontal lobes and subcortical areas such as the caudate nucleus may account for obsessive-compulsive behavior [33]. Some of the classic symptoms of the Klüver-Bucy syndrome may also occur early in the course of PcD [25,26,34]. For example, Cummings and Duchen reported two or more of these Klüver-Bucy components in their PcD patients: oral tendencies, emotional blunting, altered dietary habits, tendency to explore the environment, sensory agnosia, and hypersexuality [26]. When present early in a neurodegenerative disease, these features point toward bitemporal damage and raise the possibility of PcD.

Neuropsychological Examination

Initial Phase of Illness

Impairment in language function is the main neuropsychological deficit observed at the beginning of the disease. This deficit is classically described as *word-finding difficulty* or *anomia*. There is inability to retrieve words from lexical storage, as well as a tendency to use circumlocutions and supraordinate words [35]. Other aspects of communication are usually normal, including articulation of words, grammatical structure, comprehension, and the ability to copy a sentence and write spontaneously. Anomia probably stems from the underlying atrophy in frontal and temporal lobes that characterizes PcD [26,35,36].

Although aphasia is the most common finding, other cognitive impairments also occur in the early phases of PcD. For example, in a study of seven PcD patients with Pick bodies assessed with biopsy specimens or at postmortem examination, Knopman and colleagues reported marked although evanescent impairment of executive abilities, as measured by the Porteus maze test [37]. In our own studies, we found that PcD patients were impaired on a broad range of cognitive tests compared to normal control subjects. A set of tests were administered that assessed memory, language, visuospatial, and frontal lobe functions in 44 PcD patients (10 with autopsy confirmation) and 60 age- and education-matched nondemented control subjects. One hundred twenty-one AD patients (16 with autopsy confirmation) formed a comparison group [24]. Mean scores of the PcD patients were inferior to the normal control group's scores on all tests except on the Luria Mental Rotation test, which assesses visuospatial abilities. These results underscore the fact that PcD is a true dementia. Furthermore, PcD patients were as impaired as the AD patients except in two domains: mean scores for the PcD group were superior to the AD group scores on tests of explicit memory and visuospatial function. Our findings are consistent with prior reports that the ability to learn and recall new information and visuospatial skills is often relatively preserved in PcD [25,26,35,37]. Explicit memory depends to a great extent on medial temporal lobe structures, such as the entorhinal cortex and hippocampus, which participate in the initial encoding and storage of information [38–40]. Although these structures are affected in PcD [41], damage may occur later in the course of illness than it does in AD. At initial examination, memory was better in PcD than in AD but abnormal compared to control subjects. The perception and manipulation of spatial information is related to parietal and occipital lobe function [42], with the right hemisphere having a dominant role [43].

The preservation of these cognitive capacities may reflect the relative preservation of the posterior cortical regions in PcD [44]. These findings suggest that spared visuospatial skills in the early phase of a dementing illness may help discriminate PcD from AD, a suggestion consonant with a similar report by Pachana and colleagues [45]. Surprisingly, the PcD and AD groups did not differ at initial examination on tests of naming and on tests of verbal fluency in our study.

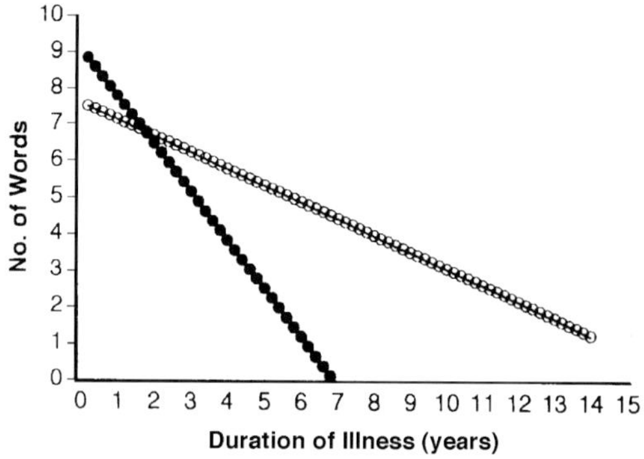

Figure 1.2 Maximum likelihood estimated model of score change on the Category Verbal Fluency Test. Solid circles denote Pick's disease (PcD) patients, and open circles represent Alzheimer's disease (AD) patients. PcD patients declined significantly faster than AD patients ($P < .0001$).

Evolution of Illness

There are declines in all areas of cognition as the disease evolves. Language functions bear the brunt of dissolution in PcD and decline at a faster rate than in AD. Anomia worsens, comprehension fails, echolalia and verbal stereotypes emerge, and mutism is common in the end stage of the disease. We followed the course of dementia in 44 PcD patients compared to 121 AD patients by annually repeating the set of cognitive tests administered at initial examination, and we found declines on all tests in both patient groups. Test scores of the control subjects remained relatively stable. Compared to AD, PcD patients deteriorated faster on tests of language, on a test of global cognitive function, and on activities of daily living measure. PcD patients declined more rapidly than AD patients in naming ability, as measured by the Boston Naming Test, and ease of retrieving words from the lexicon, as measured by the Category Verbal Fluency Test (Figure 1.2). These findings strengthen the diagnostic prominence of aphasia in PcD and emphasize rapid deterioration in expressive language as a marker of PcD. The Boston Naming Test and Category Verbal Fluency Test assess two aspects of language function with complex tasks that challenge multiple cognitive domains. Additional studies are needed to determine whether PcD patients differ from AD patients in other aspects of language function, such as types of semantic processing, as well as syntactic and phonologic processing. A further issue that requires study is whether the accelerated decline in PcD extends to language domains other than naming and lexical retrieval. Even though PcD patients were less impaired than AD patients on tests of explicit memory and visuospatial abilities at initial examination, the rates of decline were similar for both patient groups.

In summary, these neuropsychological observations help characterize the clinical course of PcD and identify differences from AD, the dementing illness most often confused in the clinical diagnosis. In the early phase of PcD, personality changes and language disturbances are prominent, along with variable degrees of

Table 1.2 Summary of the clinical criteria for Pick's disease: comparison between *The International Classification of Diseases* (10th ed) and the *Diagnostic and Statistical Manual of Mental Disorders* (4th ed)

The International Classification of Diseases *(10th ed)*	Diagnostic and Statistical Manual of Mental Disorders *(4th ed)*
Onset of dementia in Pick's disease: between 50 and 60 years The following features are prerequisites: Progressive dementia A predominance of frontal lobe features with euphoria, emotional blunting and coarsening of social behavior, disinhibition, and either apathy or restlessness Such behavioral manifestations commonly antedate frank memory impairment Frontal lobe features are more marked than temporal and parietal lobe features, unlike Alzheimer's disease Occasionally extrapyramidal phenomena are present Early-onset patients tend to exhibit a more malignant course than late-onset patients	Onset of dementia in Pick's disease: between 50 and 60 years or older Early clinical manifestations: personality changes, deterioration of social skills, emotional blunting, behavioral disinhibition, prominent language abnormalities Later in the course of the disease: difficulties in memory, apraxia, other features of dementia; prominent disinhibition, primitive reflexes (snout, suck, grasp) may be present Progression of the disease: apathy or extreme agitation; severe problems in language, attention, and behavior Structural brain imaging: prominent frontal or temporal (or both) atrophy Functional brain imaging: frontotemporal hypometabolism even in the absence of clear structural atrophy

memory loss, whereas impaired explicit memory alone dominates the initial symptoms of AD. PcD and AD patients are impaired in most cognitive domains compared to nondemented control subjects. PcD patients perform better than AD patients on tests of explicit memory and visuospatial function. Over time, test scores of both PcD and AD patients decline, but the rate of decline is faster in PcD for global measures of cognition and activities of daily living and for measures of language function.

Clinical Diagnostic Criteria of Pick's Disease

The clinical criteria for PcD summarized in *The International Classification of Diseases* (10th ed) (*ICD-10*) and the *Diagnostic and Statistical Manual of Mental Disorders* (4th ed) (Table 1.2) provide diagnostic guidelines. These clinical criteria do not specify levels of diagnostic certainty such as "possible" and "probable" that have been established for AD [46]. Further, the criteria lack the practical but subtle nuances obtained from history or seen on examination that clinicians appreciate. Some of these subtle symptoms and signs have been incorporated into the *Clinical and Neuropathological Criteria for Frontotemporal Dementia*, published in 1994, at the initiative of investigators in Lund, Sweden, and Manchester, England [47].

Although the nosology of frontotemporal dementia is in evolution (see Chapter 17), these investigators consider PcD a histologic variant of frontotemporal lobar degeneration; frontal lobe degeneration (see Chapter 2) is another variant. A strength of the proposed criteria is that they specify a large list of behavioral, affective, and cognitive symptoms that occur in the circumscribed lobar degenerations.

Instrumental Investigations in Pick's Disease

Electroencephalogram

The electroencephalogram (EEG) is usually normal in PcD during all phases of the illness. Gordon and Sim compared the EEGs of three PcD patients with the EEGs of 48 AD patients. The clinical diagnoses were confirmed by cerebral biopsies (pathologic criteria were not provided) [48]. They noted that the EEGs of two PcD patients were normal and that the EEG of one PcD patient was abnormal; all patients with AD had an abnormal EEG. Theta and delta slow wave activity can occur in the late stages of PcD, however. Tissot and colleagues obtained 21 EEGs from 10 PcD patients (four with Pick bodies and ballooned neurons, one with ballooned neurons only, and five with no Pick bodies or ballooned neurons). They observed abnormal EEGs in only two patients: in the one with ballooned neurons only and in one of the five who had no Pick bodies or ballooned neurons [8]. Groen and Endtz reported the EEG findings of 13 PcD patients; EEGs were normal in 11 instances, and there were some focal changes in two instances [49].

Computed Tomography and Magnetic Resonance Imaging

The reports on computed tomography (CT) and magnetic resonance imaging (MRI) brain scans in PcD are scant (see Chapter 8). In 1982, Groen and Endtz published the results of CT brain scans in three patients of the Schenk family who had familial PcD and eight nondemented offspring [49]. Of the three patients, two had symmetric atrophy limited to the frontal and temporal lobes, and one had generalized brain atrophy. Four of the nondemented subjects in the family had frontal atrophy, and one of them developed PcD symptoms 1 year later. This observation suggests that structural neuroimaging studies can disclose brain changes before the occurrence of detectable symptoms. Knopman and associates subsequently emphasized the value of CT scans in the differential diagnosis of PcD versus AD [37]. They described two CT patterns that are present early in the course of PcD. The first pattern consists of frontal atrophy with asymmetric or symmetric enlargement of the frontal horns of the lateral ventricles, atrophy of the head of the caudate nucleus, and thinning of the frontal cortex. The second pattern includes asymmetric or symmetric atrophy of the temporal poles with enlargement of the temporal horns of the lateral ventricles. These two patterns of circumscribed atrophy are distinctive neuroradiologic findings that differ from the diffuse atrophy commonly observed in AD. Studies with MRI confirmed the value of circumscribed atrophy in the diagnosis of PcD (Figure 1.3). For example, Frisoni and colleagues found greater atrophy in

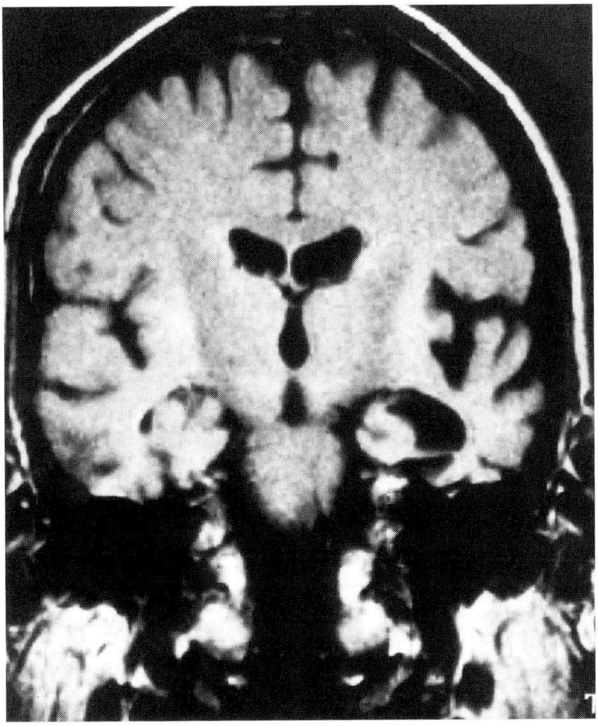

Figure 1.3 Magnetic resonance brain scan of a patient with a clinical diagnosis of Pick's disease. This coronal section shows characteristic focal atrophy of the left temporal lobe.

the anterior frontal lobe in patients with frontotemporal dementia (perhaps some with PcD) than in those with AD [50]. Suggested neuroimaging criteria for PcD are summarized in Table 1.3.

Single Photon Emission Computed Tomography and Positron Emission Tomography Neuroimaging Studies in Pick's Disease

Functional neuroimaging can complement CT and MRI morphologic findings and is especially valuable when lobar atrophy is not conspicuous (see Chapter 9). In general, the most characteristic finding is hypoperfusion or hypometabolism in the anterior portions of the brain [51–53] (Figure 1.4). In most of the recent reports, the designations *PcD* and *frontotemporal dementia* have been used interchangeably. Thus, Miller and associates found three different single photon emission computed tomography (SPECT) patterns in frontotemporal dementia (PcD) patients: (1) bilateral hypoperfusion in frontal and temporal lobes, (2) hypoperfusion limited to left frontal and temporal regions, and (3) hypoperfusion limited to right frontal and temporal regions [54]. In a SPECT study limited to PcD patients, Habert and colleagues found that the tracer technetium Tc 99m hexam-

Table 1.3 Suggested neuroimaging criteria for diagnosing Pick's disease

When the cerebral atrophy is severe, one of the following findings must be present*:
Cortical and subcortical anterior frontal atrophy with widening of the frontal horns of the lateral ventricles
Anterior temporal atrophy with widening of the temporal horns of the lateral ventricles
When the cerebral atrophy is marked or mild, both of the following findings must be present:
Perfusion SPECT or PET: asymmetric or symmetric anterior frontal and anterior temporal lobe deficits; rarely, isolated anterior frontal or anterior temporal deficit
MRI: "frontotemporal atrophy pattern"—that is, marked widening of the temporal horns of the lateral ventricles, marked increase of the bifrontal index, and normal minimum thickness of the medial temporal lobe

*Asymmetry of the atrophy is observed in 60% of patients with Pick's disease; usually the atrophy is more conspicuous on the left than on the right side.
SPECT = single photon emission computed tomography; PET = positron emission tomography; MRI = magnetic resonance imaging.

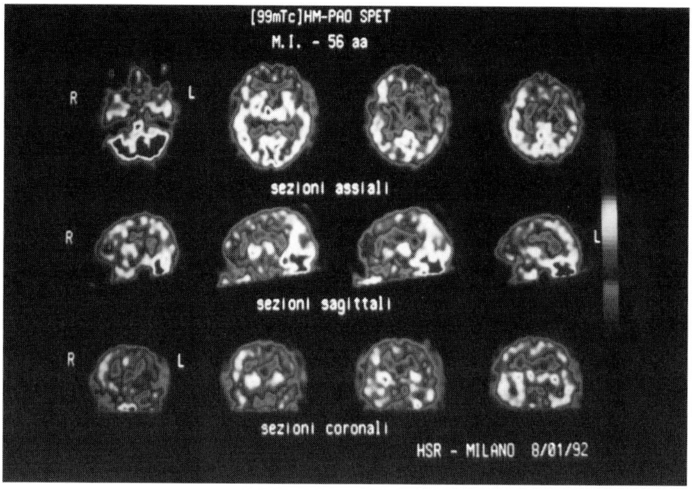

Figure 1.4 Single photon emission computed tomogram of a 56-year-old patient with a clinical diagnosis of Pick's disease. The axial (sezioni assiali), sagittal (sezioni sagittali), and coronal (sezioni coronali) views show frontotemporal hypoperfusion with greater reductions on the left than on the right. (Courtesy of Professor F. Fazio, S. Raffaele Hospital, University of Milan, Italy, and Professor S. Cappa, University of Brescia, Italy.)

ethyl propyleneamine oxime uptake was reduced in the superior and inferior temporal lobes [55].

Epidemiology of Pick's Disease

Reliable estimates of the incidence or prevalence of PcD cannot be determined because of the lack of universally accepted diagnostic criteria, possible clinical overlaps with AD and frontal lobe dementia, and uncertainties regarding the placement of PcD under the broad term *frontotemporal lobar degeneration*. Based on clinical evaluations, PcD has been reported to be three to five times less frequent than AD [56,57]. However, only 2% of all demented patients evaluated in the Memory Disorders Unit at the Massachusetts General Hospital between 1985 and 1996 had a diagnosis of PcD, whereas 63% were diagnosed with AD. The frequency of PcD in autopsy series ranged from 1.3% to 5.0% [57–59].

Onset of symptoms usually occurs during the fifth or sixth decades of life [7,8]; however, patients as young as 28 years [20,60,61] or older than 80 years at onset of symptoms have been reported [8,62]. In our series of 44 PcD patients, the mean age at onset was 63.6 (±9.4) years. Of these, 26 were men and 18 were women. Heston and colleagues reported that men were more at risk for PcD than women [63]. In other series, however, women were more frequently involved than men at a ratio of up to 2:1 [7,8,25,36,64–66]. In our postmortem series, there were 20 women and 15 men. Heston and associates estimated that the mean survival time for men was 6.3 years and for women 8.4 years [63]. The mean age of death in our neuropathologic series was 73.6 (±10.9) years.

Genetics of Pick's Disease

PcD may be sporadic or familial [7,8,19–21,49,64,67,68]. The two families (referred to as *W* and *D-G*) described by Löwenberg and colleagues [67] and Malamud and Waggoner [68] showed a dominant pattern of inheritance and a different but consistent age range of disease onset within each family. In the W family, the age of onset was between 25 and 26 years and the rate of decline was rapid, whereas in the D-G family, the disease started between 50 years and 65 years. The affected members of the W family showed abstract thinking impairments, space and time disorientation, difficulties in sequencing, and impaired language abilities with perservation and stereotypies. PcD in the D-G family was also characterized by a frontal lobe syndrome. Autopsies revealed severe atrophy involving the frontal, parietal, and temporal lobes with relative preservation of the superior temporal gyrus. Pick bodies and ballooned neurons were present.

In 1982, Groen and Endtz analyzed the data published on families with more than one PcD patient per generation and with at least one member with the disease confirmed neuropathologically [49]. They uncovered 26 families including the Dutch Schenk family. In these families, autosomal dominant transmission was the most likely mode of inheritance [64]. The Dutch Schenk family had 25 members with PcD across six generations. Of these 25 members, the diagnosis of PcD was confirmed neuropathologically in 14, although no Pick bodies were reported. The Schenk family continues to be evaluated and now includes 34 affected relatives across seven generations [69]. This family is one of three Dutch families (family II in the report by Heutink et al. [69]) linked to chromosome 17 and reported as *hereditary frontotemporal dementia* (HFTD). In these three families, the mean age of the patients at onset of symptoms was 51 years. Initial symptoms in the first two families were disinhibition, aggressiveness, stealing, jocularity, and obsessional behavior. In the third family, loss of initiative was the most prominent presenting feature [69].

Chromosome 17 has also been associated with other neurodegenerative dementing disorders, including disinhibition-dementia-parkinsonism-amyotrophy complex (DDPAC) [70,71], progressive subcortical gliosis (PSG) [72], and pallido-ponto-nigral degeneration (PPND) [73]. In addition to chromosome 17 linkage, all of these conditions share several features. Affected individuals in the DDPAC family first developed signs of illness in their 30s, with personality changes, disinhibition, hypersexuality, hyperreligiosity, depression, stereotyped and obsessive symptoms, and some aspects of the Klüver-Bucy syndrome [70]. Orientation and most language abilities were spared, but memory, naming, general knowledge, and construction were all impaired. Motor impairment included parkinsonism, bradykinesia, and amyotrophy. There was status spongiosus in the cortex, marked pallor of the substantia nigra pars compacta, and neuronal loss in the amygdala and ventral striatum. The hippocampal formation was relatively spared. Argyrophilic *tau*-negative neuronal inclusions were found in basal ganglia, brain stem nuclei, and hypothalamus [74]. Bird and associates described one family with non-AD dementia linked to chromosome 17 and one family with suggestive evidence for linkage to 17q. The initial symptoms were similar to those of DDPAC with an early occurrence of a schizophrenic-like psychosis and neurofibrillary tangles [75].

Personality changes, memory loss, and speech impairments beginning in the fourth to sixth decades were the chief symptoms of PSG, in which linkage to the same chromosome region (17q21–q22) as that in DDPAC was found. The histopathology of PSG was distinctive, however, with astrocytic gliosis at the cortex–white matter junction and mild atrophy of the substantia nigra [72].

The family with PPND consists of 300 members with 32 affected individuals [73]. The clinical features include gradual parkinsonism with dystonia, dementia, perseverative vocalizations, frontal lobe release signs, ocular motility abnormalities, pyramidal tract dysfunction, and urinary incontinence. The earliest symptoms were parkinsonism in 11 patients, behavioral disturbances in seven patients, dementia in five patients, and a mix of parkinsonism and behavioral abnormalities in three patients. There was severe neuronal loss and gliosis in the substantia nigra, pontine and mesencephalic tegmentum, and globus pallidus. These patients differed further from other dementias linked to chromosome 17 in that cortical pathology was mild to moderate.

There are no known causes of sporadic PcD. A single preliminary report [76] based on a small number of subjects suggested that the *ε4* allele of the apolipoprotein E gene (*APOE*) was overrepresented in PcD, as it is in AD. The *APOE-ε4* allele is three to four times more common in clinic populations of AD patients than in nondemented control subjects [77,78]. Among AD patients, having an *APOE-ε4* allele lowers the age of dementia onset but does not affect the overall rate of cognitive decline (see Chapter 7) [79,80]. Gómez-Isla and associates determined the *APOE* genotype in 31 PcD cases and found that the frequency of the *APOE-ε4* allele did not differ from the frequency in nondemented subjects [79]. These investigators concluded that *APOE-ε4* is not a risk factor for PcD.

NEUROPATHOLOGY

Gross Examination

On gross examination of the brain, PcD is characterized by definite, circumscribed atrophy, especially in the frontotemporal region, with relative preservation of the motor strip, caudal dorsal temporal lobe, and occipital lobe (Figures 1.5; 1.6; 1.7A; 1.8 A,B; and 1.9A–D). On microscopic examination, PcD is remarkable for neuronal loss, gliosis, and status spongiosus, principally involving the atrophic areas (see Figure 1.9F, and for comparison, see Figure 1.11, which shows normal cortex of same area). Neurons in cortical, limbic, and striatal regions may contain a single, round intracytoplasmic inclusion, argyrophilic inclusion, or Pick body (see Figures 1.7C and 1.8C–F); ballooned neurons or Pick cells are also common (Figure 1.10). Furthermore, neurofibrillary tangles of Alzheimer and neuritic plaques are rare or absent (see Figure 1.9E–G,I).

Brain Weight and Lateral Ventricular Volume

The average Pick brain weight reported is 900–1,000 g for women and 1,000–1,220 g for men [8,66]. In our postmortem series of 35 patients (20 women and 15 men; 23 with Pick bodies), the average brain weight and volume of one lateral ventricle are as follows: women, 955 ± 174 g, 26 ± 13 cc (normal 7–10 cc); men, 1,085 ± 172 g, 29 ± 15 cc [5].

Circumscribed Atrophy

PcD brains show circumscribed bilateral asymmetric or symmetric, panlaminar frontal, frontotemporal, or fronto-parieto-temporal atrophy, and may be with or without parietal involvement (see Figures 1.5; 1.6; 1.7A,B; 1.8A,B; and 1.9A–D). Unilateral parietal circumscribed atrophy with Pick bodies has been observed [81]. The atrophy is evidenced by widening of the sulci and narrowing of the gyri. It can be so severe that the gyri may resemble a knife edge, or *Nussrelief* (see Figures 1.5A and 1.6B) [82]. When more than one lobe is involved (at times referred to as *mixed atrophy*), the atrophy can be equally severe or predominant in any of them. The involvement can encompass the whole lobe or part of it (see Figures 1.7A and 1.8A); it might be more severe medially (see Figure 1.8B) than laterally, or vice versa. Approximately 60% of the PcD brains show more atrophy on one side than the other, most frequently on the left [66]. The transition between the atrophic and relatively preserved areas is abrupt (see Figures 1.5B and 1.6A), or when gradual, is usually confined over a narrow band (see Figures 1.7A and 1.8A). Often, the caudal third of the superior temporal gyrus is relatively preserved (see Figures 1.5A and 1.6B). Exceptionally, the atrophy also involves the occipital lobe [26] or is mainly confined to the parietal lobe on one side [81,83]. Spatz claimed that circumscribed atrophy is an essential diagnostic feature of PcD [82], a claim that gained acceptance [84].

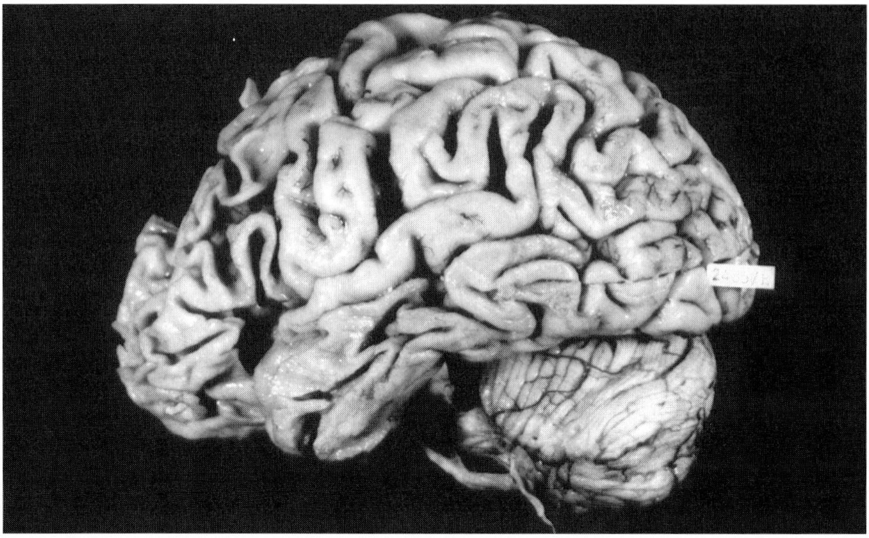

A

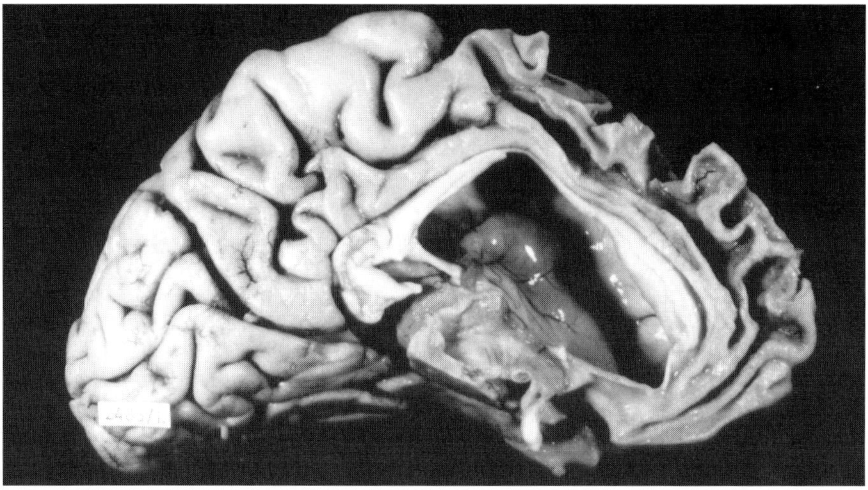

B

Figure 1.5 Pick's disease type A in a 71-year-old man. (A) Lateral aspect of the left half of the brain after removal of the leptomeninges. There is severe frontotemporal atrophy with relative preservation of the caudal two-thirds of the superior temporal gyrus, the parietal and occipital lobes, and the cerebellum. (B) Medial aspect of the left cerebral hemisphere showing frontal knife-edge atrophy (*Nussrelief*), abrupt demarcation between atrophic and preserved areas, and severe atrophy of the anterior portion of the corpus callosum and neostriatum. The paracentral lobule, caudal cingulate gyrus, precuneus, cuneus, occipital pole, and splenium corpori callosi are preserved.

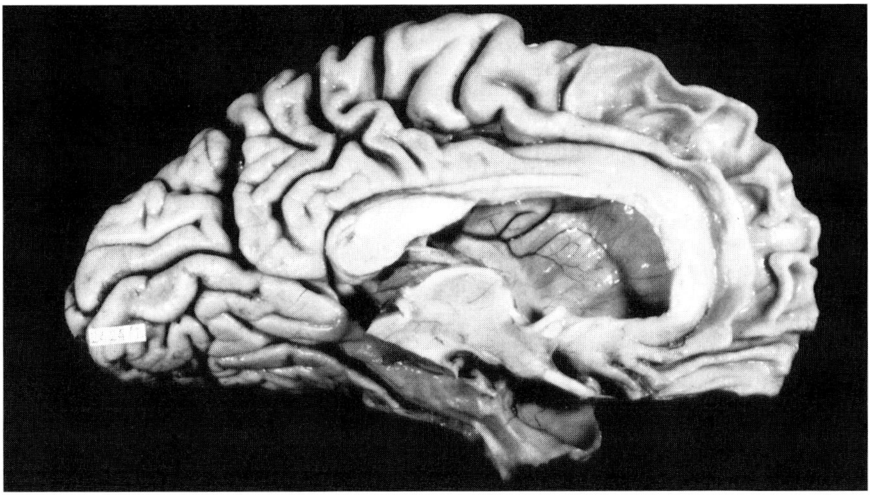

A

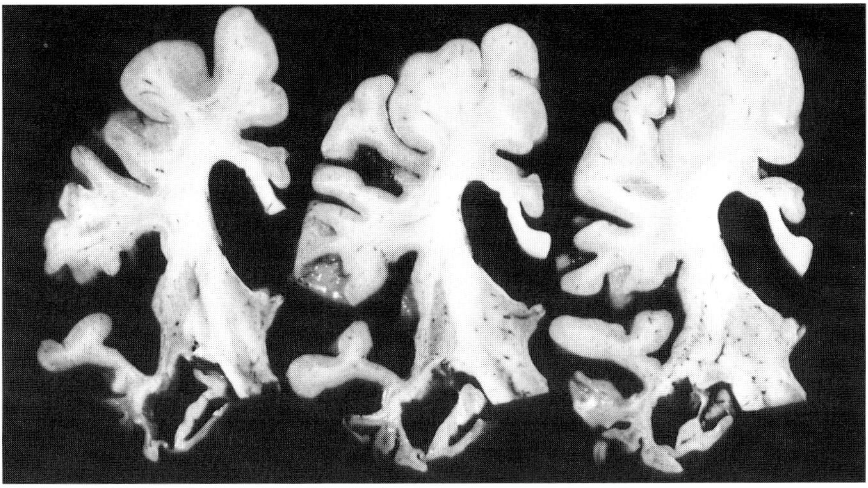

B

Figure 1.6 Pick's disease type A in a 71-year-old woman. (A) Medial aspect of the left cerebral hemisphere after removal of the leptomeninges. There is dilation of the lateral ventricle and knife-edge atrophy (*Nussrelief*) of the frontal and temporal gyri with abrupt transition between atrophic and relatively preserved parts. Note the atrophy of the rostral two-thirds of the corpus callosum and the apparently normal splenium corpori callosi. (B) Three coronal sections passing through the anterior thalamus (*left*), subthalamic nucleus (*middle*), and lateral geniculate body (*right*). The frontal atrophy gradually decreases in severity from rostral to caudal; there is very severe atrophy of the temporal lobe with relative preservation of the superior temporal gyrus. The dentate gyrus at the level of the lateral geniculate body is relatively preserved compared to the parahippocampal and occipitotemporal gyri. There is severe atrophy of the thalamus (rostral > caudal; medial > lateral) and of the body of the caudate nucleus. The substantia nigra is well pigmented (*middle coronal section*).

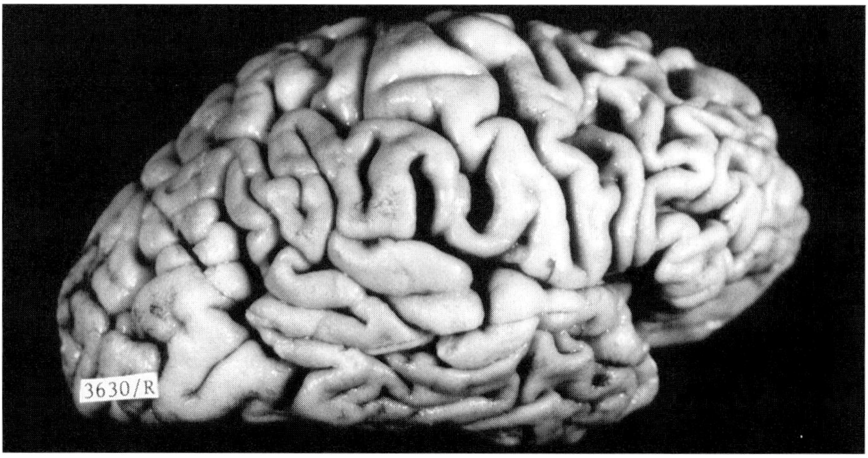

A

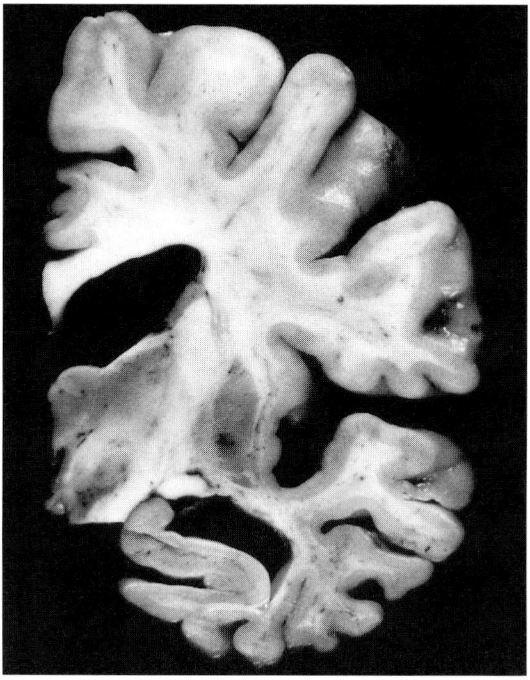

B

Figure 1.7 Pick's disease type A with rare Pick bodies in a 65-year-old woman (cf. Figure 1.8, also type A, but with abundant Pick bodies). Pick bodies were not identified initially in the Bielschowsky-stained sections; however, they were identified in sections processed with *tau* antibodies and then in repeated Bielschowsky-stained sections. (A) Lateral aspect of the right cerebral hemisphere after removal of the leptomeninges. There is definite circumscribed atrophy of the frontal lobe; the sulci of the inferior parietal lobule are wider than normal (cf. Figure 1.8A). (B) Coronal section passing through the subthalamic nucleus. The atrophy is obvious in the medial parts of the temporal lobe (cf. Figure 1.8B).

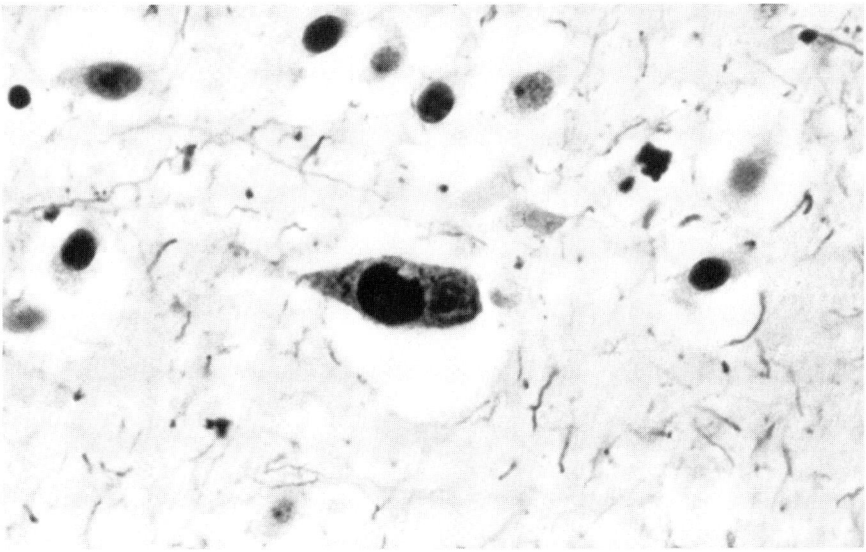

C

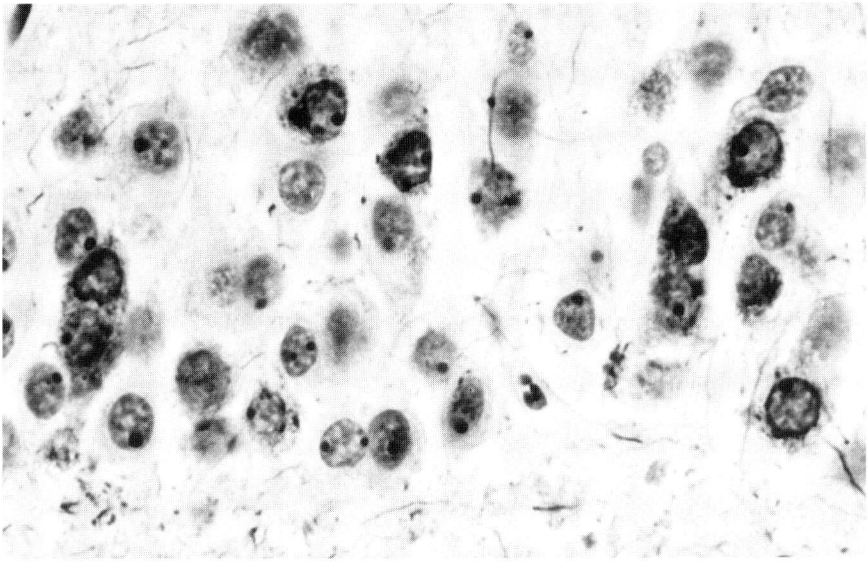

D

(C) Dorsal putamen with a neuron containing an argyrophilic inclusion indistinguishable from a Pick body (Bielschowsky stain [950×]). (D) Hippocampal dentate gyrus with occasional neurons containing small argyrophilic intracytoplasmic round inclusions, perinuclear argyrophilic rims, or both. Occasional argyrophilic intracytoplasmic inclusions are indistinguishable from those present in the dentate gyrus of Figure 1.8C (Bielschowsky stain [950×]).

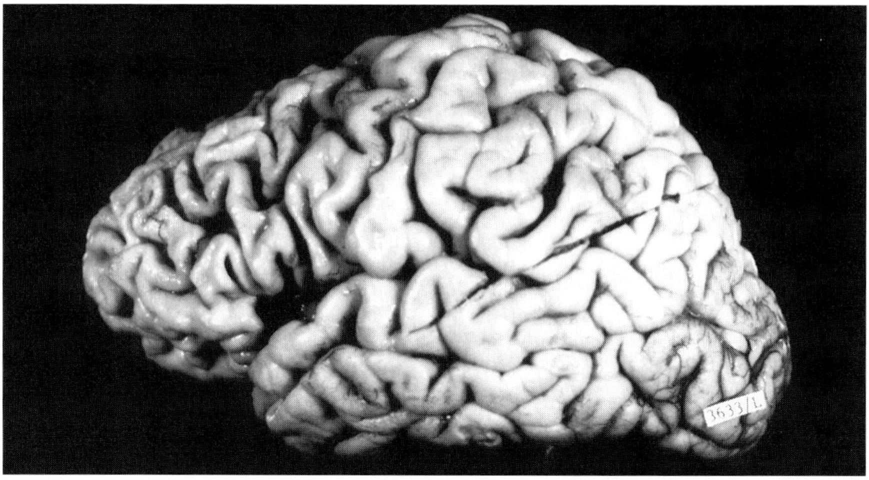

A

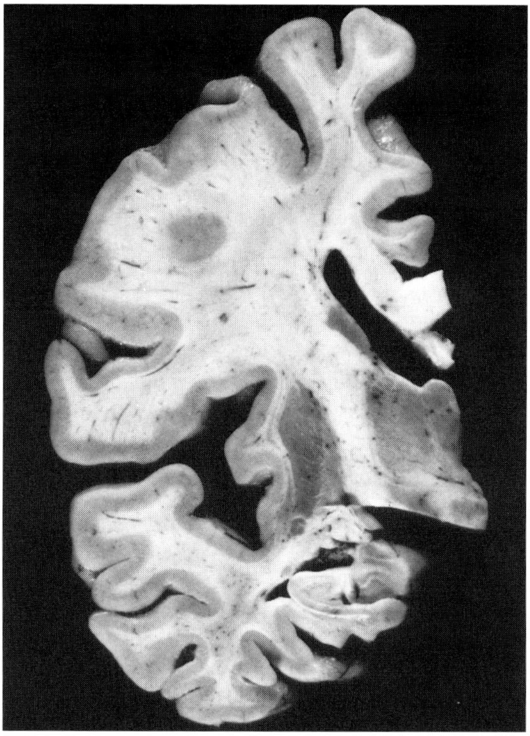

B

Figure 1.8 Pick's disease type A with abundant Pick bodies in an 82-year-old man (cf. Figure 1.7A–D, also type A, but with rare Pick bodies). (A) Lateral aspect of the left cerebral hemisphere. There is definite circumscribed atrophy of the frontal lobe; the sulci of the inferior parietal lobule are wider than normal (cf. Figure 1.7A). (B) Coronal section passing through the subthalamic nucleus. The atrophy is obvious in the medial parts of the frontal and temporal lobes (cf. Figure 1.7B).

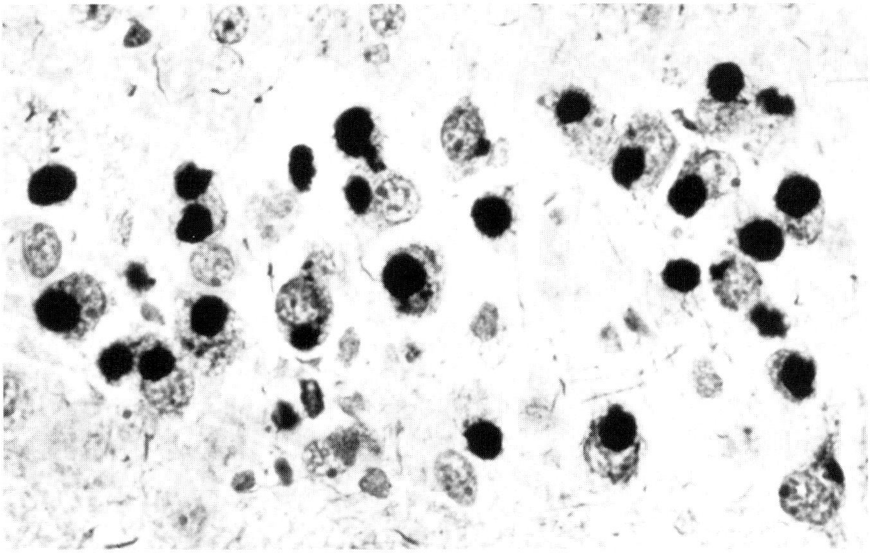

C

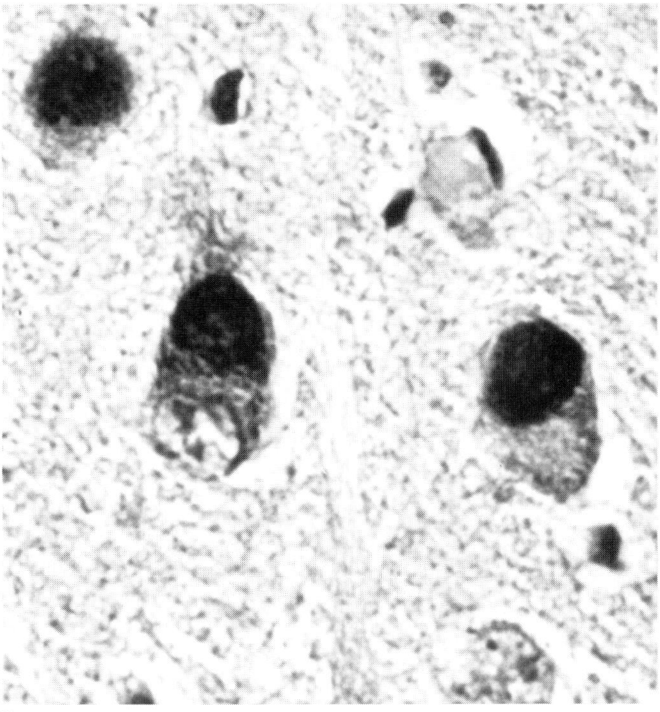

D

(C) Hippocampal dentate gyrus with neurons containing Pick bodies evident by reaction with antibodies recognizing abnormal *tau* (950×). (D) Sommer sector with neurons containing Pick bodies reacting with abnormal *tau* antibodies (950×).

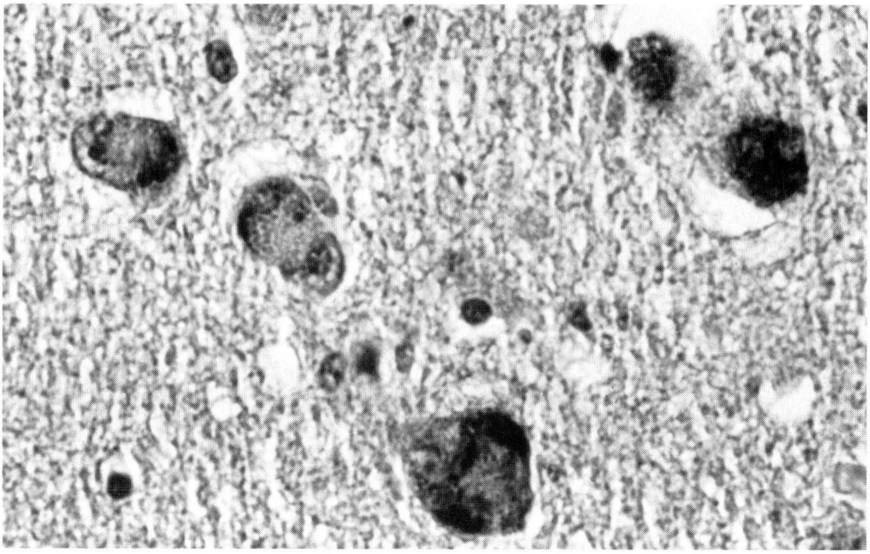

E

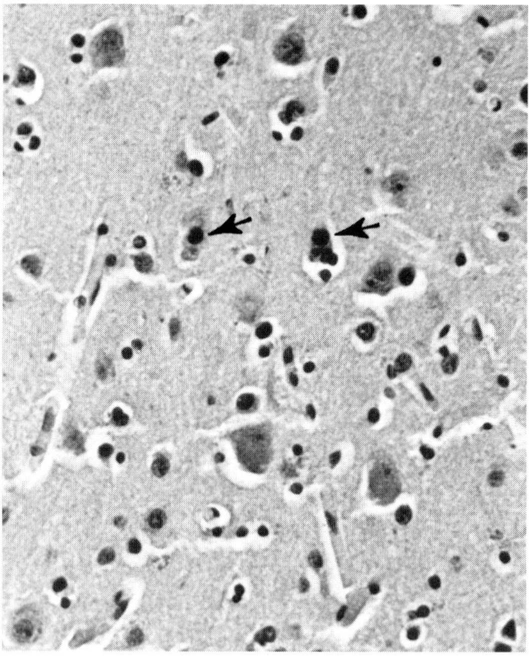

F

Figure 1.8 (continued) (E) Entorhinal cortex with three *tau*-positive "uneven" Pick bodies (as drawn by Alzheimer [9]) and one "typical" Pick body (*upper right corner*) (950×). (F) Cortex of superior parietal lobule. Two neurons (*arrows*) with Pick bodies in an otherwise normal cortex. Anti-*tau* (350×).

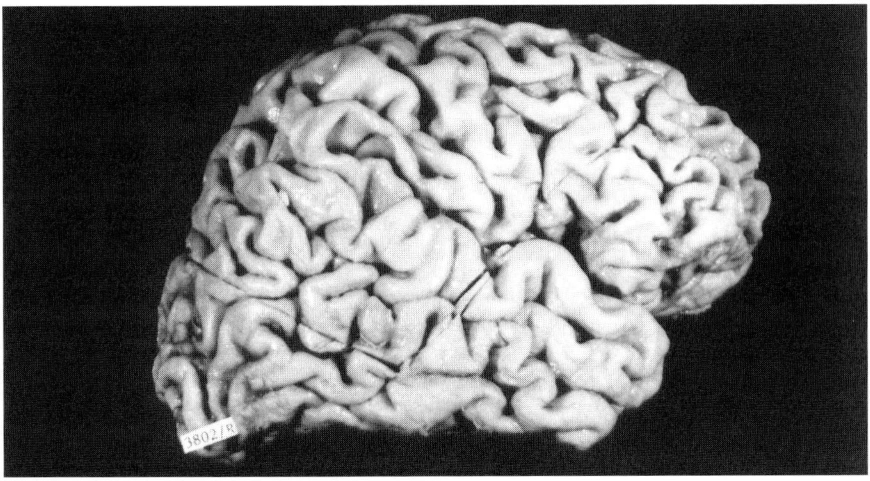

A

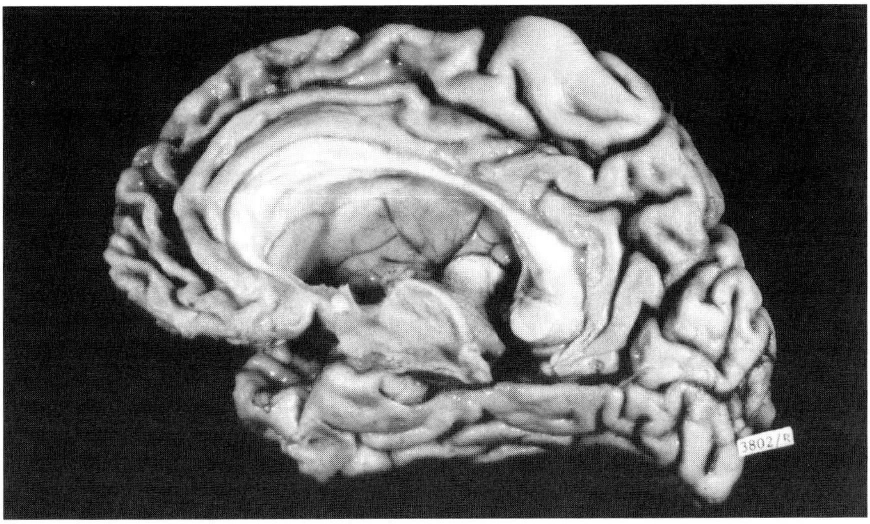

B

Figure 1.9 Pick's disease type C with abundant argyrophilic grains in a 60-year-old man. (A) Lateral aspect of the right cerebral hemisphere showing mild diffuse atrophy with severe superimposed atrophy of the anterior frontal lobe. (B) Medial aspect of the right cerebral hemisphere showing severe atrophy of the anterior frontal lobe and adjacent corpus callosum, neostriatum, and thalamus.

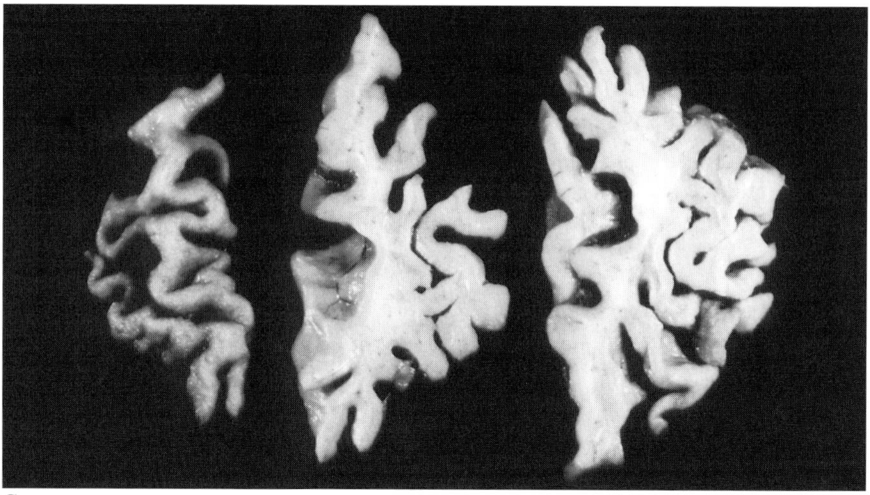

C

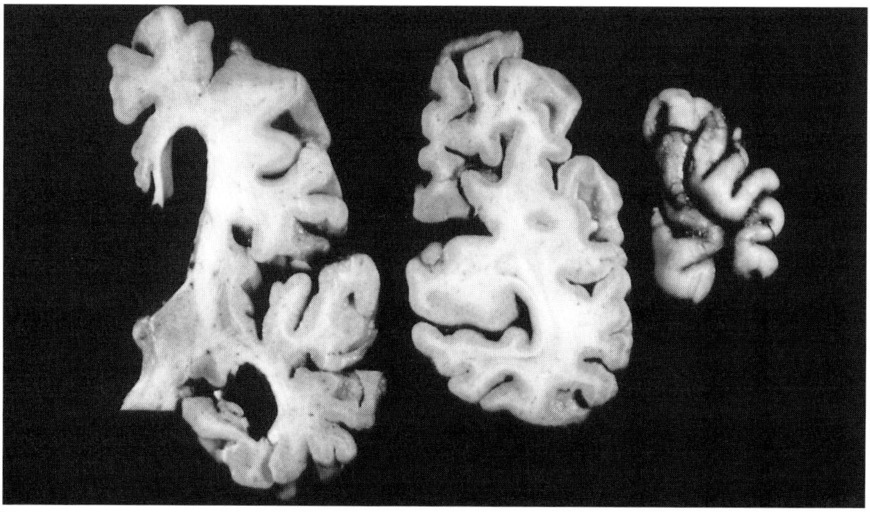

D

Figure 1.9 (continued) (C) Three coronal sections through the anterior frontal lobe showing severe cortical thinning and white matter loss. (D) Three coronal sections, one passing through the lateral geniculate body (*left*), one through the cuneus with precuneus (*middle*), and one including the occipital pole (*right*). The severity of the atrophy decreases in a rostrocaudal direction (cf. Figure 1.9C). The ventricular surface of the caudate nucleus is flat.

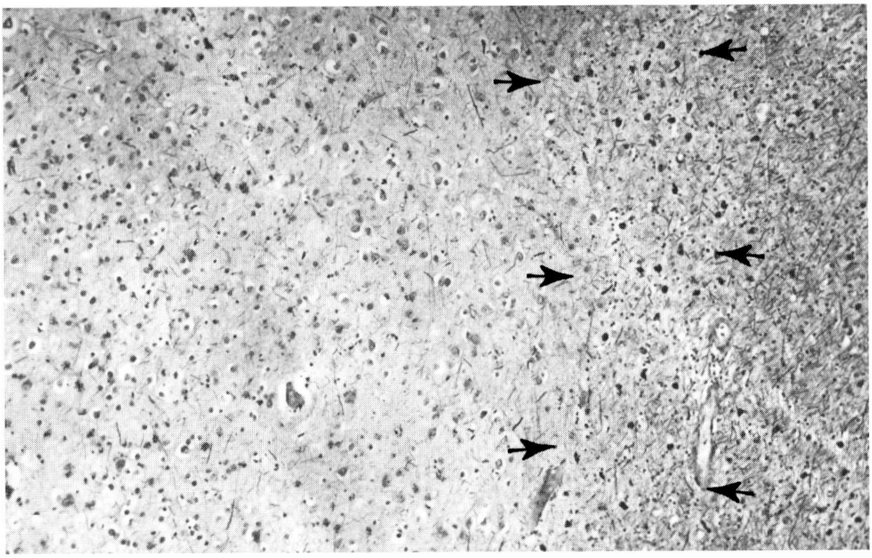

E

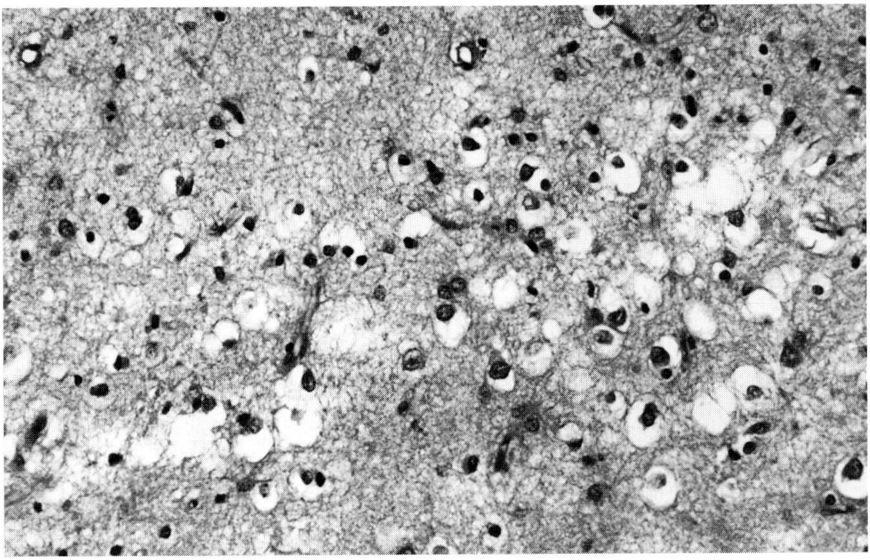

F

(E) Superior frontal gyrus (Brodmann area 9) with subcortical white matter on the right. There is severe neuronal loss. Note the absence of neuritic plaques, tangles, Pick bodies, and ballooned neurons. Argyrophilic grains are readily visible in a subcortical band (*between arrows*; cf. Figure 1.9H higher magnification) of white matter (*right*) and to a lesser extent in the upper cortical layers (*left*) (Bielschowsky stain [10×]). (F) Upper cortical layers of Brodmann area 9 showing optically empty vacuoles with reactive astrocytes (status spongiosus) and neuronal loss. Luxol fast blue counterstained with hematoxylin and eosin (cf. Figure 1.11, which depicts normal cortical microscopic features of Brodmann area 9 [350×]).

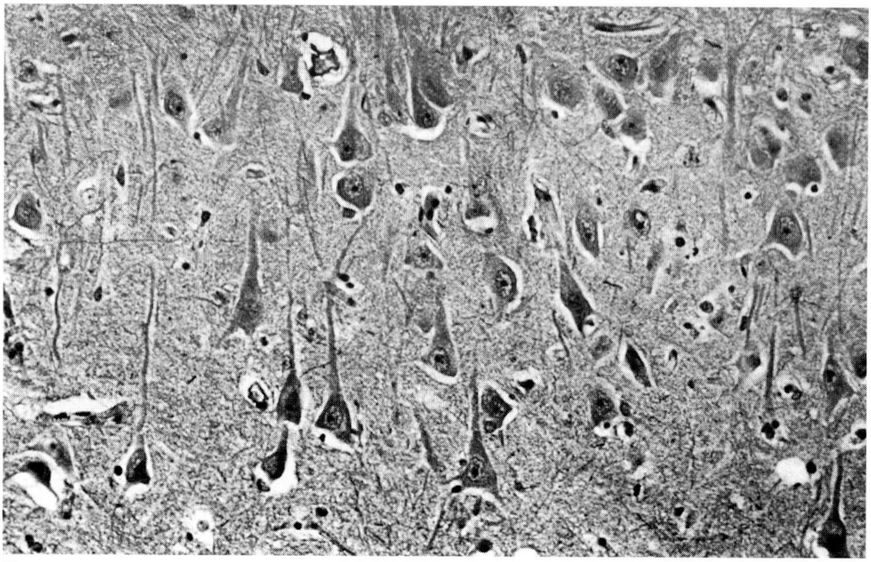

G

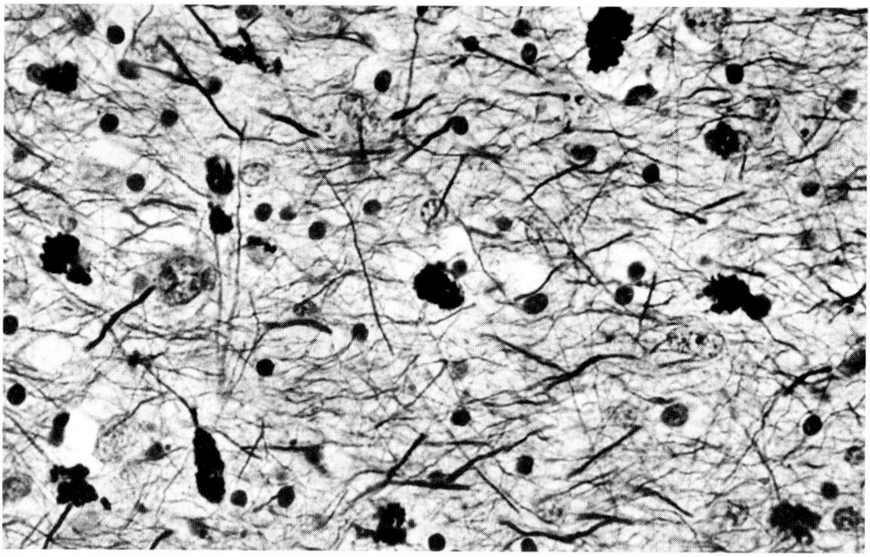

H

Figure 1.9 (continued) (G) Hippocampal formation: CA2–CA1. Neuronal density is within normal limits in contrast to subiculum (cf. Figure 1.9I). There are no argyrophilic inclusions, argyrophilic grains, or neuritic plaques (Bielschowsky stain [350×]). (H) Argyrophilic grains in the subcortical white matter of Brodmann area 9 (Bielschowsky stain [950×]). (I) Severe neuronal loss and argyrophilic grains in the subiculum. There are no Pick bodies, neurofibrillary tangles, or plaques (Bielschowsky stain [950×]).

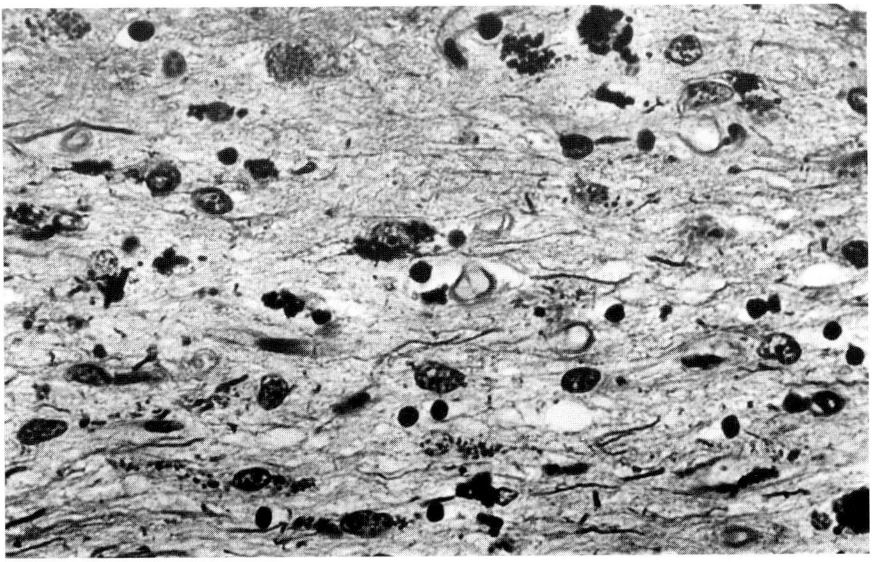

I

Panlaminar atrophy refers to the involvement of all the structures included in the circumscribed atrophic area. For example, if the lobar atrophy extends from the frontal pole to the precentral gyrus, including the temporal lobe, usually the pathologic changes will be conspicuous in the cortex, white matter, anterior portion of the striatum, and thalamus with mesencephalic extension, amygdala, and hippocampal formation (see Figures 1.6B and 1.9C). When involved, the thalamus is more atrophic rostrally than caudally; the dorsomedian and anterior nuclei usually are more prone to degeneration than the other nuclei (see Figure 1.6B) [11,18,85]. The same observations were made by Löwenberg and colleagues in a 27-year-old patient (with Pick bodies and ballooned neurons); however, they also found that the pulvinar was involved [67]. The substantia innominata is usually preserved [86]. Neuronal density of the substantia innominata appeared normal in 18 of our 35 postmortem series with PcD; the rest showed mild (n = 11) or marked (n = 6) decrease of the neuronal density. In contrast to the atrophy noted in Huntington's disease, the atrophy of the rostral portion of the neostriatum can be extreme while the caudal portion is relatively preserved [87]. Furthermore, the head of the caudate nucleus and the head of the nucleus accumbens are more atrophic than the nearby putamen, which shows more pathologic changes along the internal capsule than along the external capsule.

The Tissot and associates series (n = 32; 10 with Pick bodies) found atrophy of the caudate nucleus in 69%, of the globus pallidus in 56%, of the thalamus in 62%, and of the substantia nigra in 59% of the brains [8,36,65]. Kosaka and colleagues found striato-pallido-nigral degeneration in 78% of the 41 brains in their series (11 with Pick bodies) [88]. Hulette and Crain reported four patients with "Pick syndrome" but without movement disorder, whose brains showed severe circumscribed frontotemporal atrophy and marked atrophy of the caudate

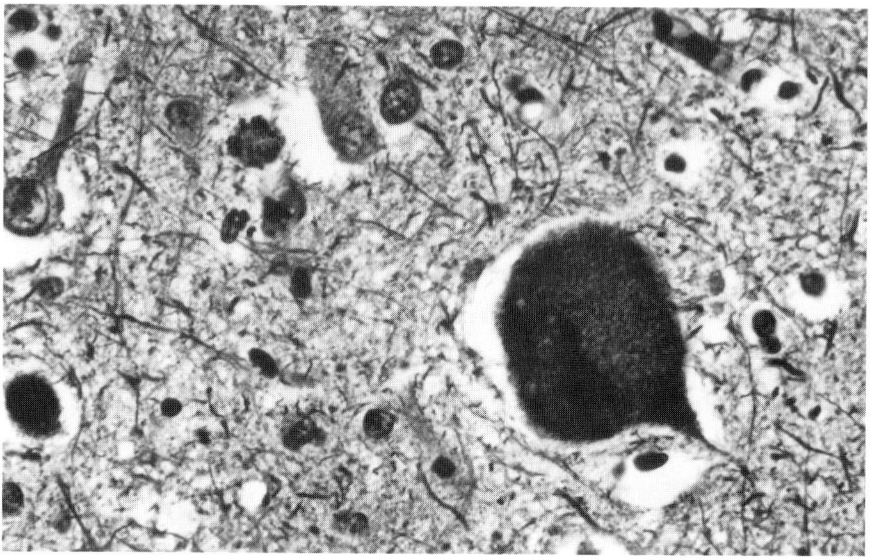

Figure 1.10 Microphotograph of the caudal cingulate gyrus at the transition zone between severely atrophic and relatively preserved areas showing an argyrophilic ballooned neuron; there were occasional nearby pyramidal neurons with Pick bodies (*not shown*) (Bielschowsky stain [350×]).

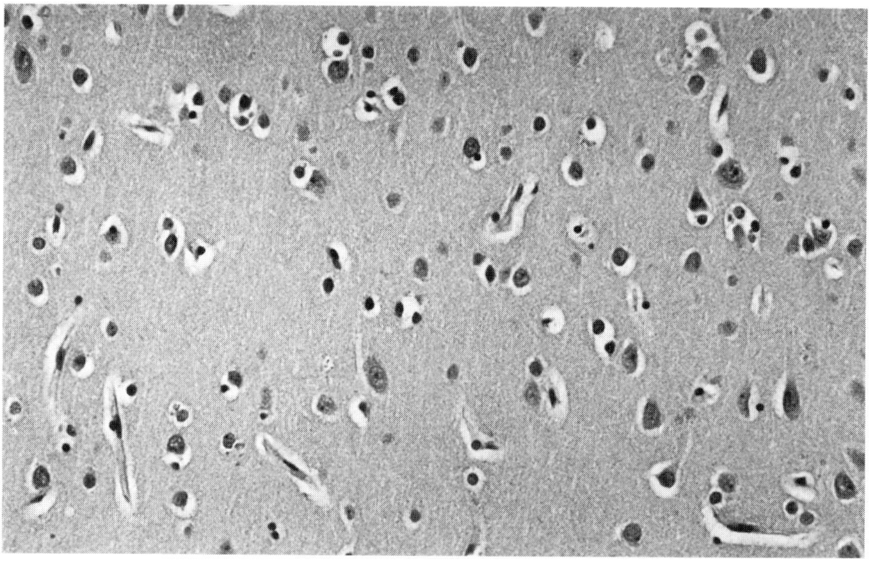

Figure 1.11 Upper cortical layers of Brodmann area 9 showing normal cortex for comparison with microscopic features of Pick's disease from same area (see Figure 1.9F) (Luxol fast blue counterstained with hematoxylin and eosin [350×]).

nucleus; no Pick bodies or ballooned neurons were found [89]. In addition to the nigral damage, two features may be obvious: fiber loss in the crus cerebri and atrophy of the inferior olivary nucleus [7,8,11].

Microscopic Examination

Neuronal loss, cortical status spongiosus (see the section, Status Spongiosus), myelin and axonal loss, and astrogliosis are obvious in the atrophic areas of gray and white matter (see Figure 1.9F and, for comparison, Figure 1.11, which shows normal cortex of same area). In "typical" PcD, scattered neurons are present with Pick bodies (see Pick Bodies below) (see Figure 1.8C–F) and ballooned neurons (see Figure 1.10).

The three outer cortical layers are more prone to degeneration than the inner layers (see Figure 1.9F and, for comparison, Figure 1.11, which shows normal cortex of same area). Proliferation of microglial cells was found to be conspicuous in both atrophic cortex and white matter using the microgliocyte marker KiM1P [90]. Scattered astrocytes and oligodendrocytes with *tau*-positive inclusions were observed [91–93]. The density of neurons, fibers, or myelin may be apparently normal in nonatrophic areas (see Figure 1.8F). In contrast to AD, in PcD the amygdala is diffusely damaged without apparent nuclear selectivity [26].

Cortical or cortical-subcortical argyrophilic grains are often present in neurodegenerative diseases, including PcD [94,95]. They consist of small, spindle-shaped argyrophilic grains loosely scattered in the neuropil. They may be interconnected by coiled bodies of silver-stained filaments and are accompanied by elongated argyrophilic glial cytoplasmic inclusions located especially in the subcortical white matter (see Figure 1.9E,H) and subiculum (see Figure 1.9I) [95]. Argyrophilic grains and coiled bodies contain dense accumulations of straight filaments with a diameter of approximately 9.0 nm [94].

Pick Bodies

Pick bodies were initially described by Alzheimer while evaluating brains with circumscribed atrophy from demented patients. Alzheimer's description is as follows:

> Sections prepared with Bielschowsky method show small pyramidal cells containing an argyrophilic, sometimes structureless ball near the nucleus, whose size varies from half to twice that of the nucleus. The inclusion is either above or below the nucleus, which is displaced accordingly downward or upward. Fibrillary changes are absent in the rest of the cell, the protoplasm and the axonal process are partially visible [9].

This description is accompanied by a figure illustrating five neuronal inclusions: four inclusions are round or slightly oval but differ by their size, and one inclusion is clearly oval, larger than the others, and contains optically empty vacuoles or pale foci. In addition to being argyrophilic, Pick bodies are weakly eosinophilic. Alzheimer's description of the Pick body is that of classic inclusion (see Figure 1.8C–D) corresponding to the appearance of the majority of the inclusions seen at postmortem examination. However, a minority of Pick bodies, or Pick body–like inclusions, are smaller (see Figure 1.7D) or larger than the usual ones with apparent uneven features, as depicted by Alzheimer in his original drawing of Pick bodies (see Figure 1.8E) [9]. The smaller Pick body–like inclusions tend to be present in the early stage of the disease or in the areas with little degenerative changes. They may be as small as the nucleolus and tend to abut the cytoplasmic aspect of the slightly argyrophilic nuclear membrane (see Figure 1.7D). At times, the cytoplasm of the neurons containing these small Pick body–like inclusions is weakly discolored a dirty gray with the Bielschowsky stain. The larger Pick body–like inclusions tend to occupy most of the neuronal cytoplasm; they may be lobulated and express variable argyrophilia or immunoreactivity (see Figure 1.8E). Argyrophilic Pick bodies that appear as basophilic spheroids containing an eosinophilic core in hematoxylin and eosin–stained sections are referred to as *compound Pick bodies* [96]. Ultrastructurally, the inclusions lack membranes and are composed of 15- to 18-nm-diameter straight filaments without sidearm or fuzzy material attached to them [44,97,98].

The sites of predilection for Pick bodies are the hippocampal formation (Sommer sector, subiculum, indusium griseum, and stratum granulosum of the dentate gyrus); entorhinal cortex; amygdala; septal nuclei; and in the second, third, and sixth cortical layers of the frontal, cingulate, and temporal neocortices [8,99–101]. Rare Pick bodies may be identified in otherwise normal cortical areas (see Figure 1.8F). Pick bodies that are apparently free in the neuropil are occasionally present in the cortical areas displaying extreme atrophy [8]. Pick bodies may be prominent in the anterior neostriatum (caudate nucleus, putamen, and nucleus accumbens) and hypothalamus [8,44] but are rarely found in the globus pallidus (personal observation). They have been observed in the nucleus coeruleus [102].

Pick bodies are stained with antibodies to ubiquitin, chromogranin A [103,104], phosphorylated neurofilament epitopes, or *tau* (see Figure 1.8D–E), or to A2B5, which recognizes neuronal surface ganglioside, indicating that membrane proteins may be incorporated into the inclusions [91,93,105]. They also react with the N-terminal and the intermediate segments of amyloid precursor protein [106]. However, Pick body immunocytochemical inconsistencies have been reported, such as lack of affinity with antibodies directed against ubiquitin [107,108].

In the classification of Tissot and colleagues, Pick bodies are found in 31% of brains with lobar atrophy [8] at about the same frequency as that reported previously [7]. We systematically evaluated 35 brains with circumscribed lobar atrophy; 22 of them had definite Pick bodies (many in 12, rare in 10) detected with Bielschowsky silver impregnation. However, using antibodies for *tau* and ubiquitin, scattered cortical or limbic Pick bodies, although rare, were detected in five of the 13 brains in which no Pick bodies could be found with the Bielschowsky method during the initial evaluation. These "Bielschowsky false-negative" brains were those with the most severe pathology. Pick bodies might fail to stain when silver impregnation is not optimal, and this false-negative finding may result from the lack of standardization of the silver staining techniques [8,92]. Furthermore, Pick bodies stain poorly with silver and with antibodies to neurofilaments or microtubules as well as straight filaments when the

Pick bodies contain granular material possibly derived from ribosomes [44]. Perhaps Pick bodies are hard to find when the pathology is extreme, similar to the way neurofibrillary tangles can be difficult to detect in brains of patients with very severe AD [109]. The presence of Pick bodies (and ballooned neurons) may be a transient event and only apparent in the early stages of the disease [15,20,66,110], although many Pick bodies may be observed even in severely involved areas in some brains, illustrating the heterogeneity of this degenerative disorder [20,101].

Immunoblot evaluation of brain samples containing Pick bodies revealed abnormally phosphorylated 55- and 64-kd *tau* protein doublets. This differs from the triplet *tau* profile (55, 64, and 69 kd) of the paired helical filaments in AD [111]. Buée-Scherrer and associates confirmed this particular *tau* profile in brains with Pick bodies but without neurofibrillary tangles of Alzheimer; however, they also demonstrated that the *tau* profile of brains containing both Pick bodies and neurofibrillary tangles of Alzheimer was similar to that of AD (55, 64, and 69 kd) [112]. In some instances, cortical Lewy bodies are strongly argyrophilic and therefore may be difficult to differentiate from Pick bodies by usual staining methods; hence, discrimination between cortical Lewy bodies and Pick bodies may require ultrastructural evaluation [98].

Ballooned Neurons

Ballooned neurons (see Figure 1.10) are swollen neurons with convex contours; homogeneous, glassy, pale eosinophilic cytoplasm; and eccentric nuclei. The cytoplasm is diffusely argyrophilic with variable intensity. At times, cytoplasmic vacuoles with or without a centrally located granule are present [15,31,66,113, 114]. Ultrastructurally, ballooned neurons have variable features; some are filled with straight filaments similar to those found in Pick bodies, whereas others contain normal elements with admixed straight filaments of variable density [44,66,97]. Ballooned neurons can be distinguished from swollen chromatolytic neurons, suggesting a different pathogenesis. Irregular dilatation of proximal neuronal processes and cytoplasmic vacuoles characterize ballooned neurons but not chromatolytic neurons [114]. Spatz hypothesized that the process of ballooned neuron formation in PcD is identical to that of the retrograde reaction of the cell body following axonal injury [82]. During chromatolysis, there is transient neuronal swelling in reaction to the axonal degeneration, which is thought to start at the periphery; this process is followed by shrinkage and disappearance of the neuron [7,82].

In the classification of Tissot and colleagues, ballooned neurons are found in 62% of brains with lobar atrophy [8,36]. They are scattered especially in the intermediary zones between the severely affected and the relatively preserved areas of the neocortex and entorhinal cortex. They are frequently observed in the anterior cingulate gyrus (see Figure 1.10), insular cortex, and claustrum. At times, they are found in the anterior neostriatum [8]. Ballooned neurons share most of the immunocytochemical characteristics of the filaments in Pick bodies [66,104,114]. Many ballooned neurons in PcD are positive with antibodies to αB-crystallin; they may or may not stain with antibodies to ubiquitin [92,115] or Alz-50 [116].

Status Spongiosus

In the atrophic areas, the parenchyma is severely gliotic with vacuoles that give a loose texture to the tissue under the microscope (see Figure 1.9F and, for comparison, Figure 1.11, which shows normal cortex of the same area). The outer cortical layers are especially involved. Status spongiosus is defined as "nonspecific, and characteristically is the manifestation of end-stage gliosis; it consists of irregular cavitation of the neuropil in the presence of a dense glial meshwork" [117]. Status spongiosus is to be distinguished from spongiform change, which is the presence of small round or ovoid vacuoles within the neuropil that are a feature of the spongiform encephalopathies [117,118]. To some extent, spongiform changes are also observed in diffuse Lewy body disease, AD Lewy body variant, and in some brains of AD patients [119–122].

Neuropathologic Diagnostic Criteria of Pick's Disease

As yet, there is no consensus on the neuropathologic diagnostic criteria for PcD. For some investigators, the presence of lobar atrophy, gliosis, and neuronal loss with mild or no AD pathology and with or without Pick bodies is the prerequisite for diagnosing PcD [5,7,8,25,31,36,58,62,65,66,76,82,88,108,115,116,123–125]. Others require that Pick bodies and ballooned neurons be present in addition to the circumscribed atrophy and that neuronal loss and neurofibrillary tangles of Alzheimer and neuritic plaques be absent or rare [44,63,92,100,101,104,111, 126–129]. For these investigators, the brains from demented patients with lobar atrophy but no Pick bodies are categorized in groups with the following designations: "atypical" PcD [130], frontotemporal degeneration [47], frontal lobe dementia [31,131], frontal lobe dementia of non-Alzheimer type [32,132], frontal lobe degeneration [115], dementia of frontal lobe type [131–133], primary progressive aphasia [134–136], or dementia lacking distinctive histopathology [130,137–139]. Of interest is that Pick bodies were found in at least one brain of a patient with hereditary frontotemporal dementia linked to chromosome 17 [69].

In the face of this confusing terminology (see Chapter 17), we prefer the classification scheme proposed by Tissot and colleagues [8,36]. This classification embraces three subgroups of non-Alzheimer dementia brains with lobar, or circumscribed, atrophy: (1) group A includes brains with Pick bodies and ballooned neurons, (2) group B includes brains with ballooned neurons and no Pick bodies, and (3) group C includes brains with no Pick bodies or ballooned neurons [8,36,65]. The *ICD-10* contains no reference to Pick bodies in the definition of PcD, and the neuropathologic picture is described as a selective atrophy of the frontal and temporal lobes without the occurrence of neuritic plaques and neurofibrillary tangles in excess of what is seen in normal aging. As pointed out, some patients' brains are clinically and pathologically indistinguishable from those categorized as "typical" PcD except for the absence of Pick bodies; according to Tissot and colleagues, these could be referred to as *"atypical" PcD* (*PcD without Pick bodies*), *PcD type B*, or *PcD type C* [8].

Munoz-Garcia and Ludwin proposed to subcategorize PcD brains into two groups (classic and generalized) on the basis of the involvement of the subcortical structures, including the distribution and histochemical, immunochemical, and ultrastructural characteristics of the Pick bodies [44]. According to this scheme, the "classic" group includes brains with predominantly cortical atrophy and with Pick bodies that stain with antibodies to neurofilament proteins and tubulin. The "generalized" group includes brains with subcortical and cortical atrophy and with weakly argyrophilic RNA-containing Pick bodies, which stain poorly with antibodies to neurofilaments or microtubules.

It is controversial whether Pick bodies must be present for diagnosing PcD, or conversely, whether the lack of Pick bodies rules out the diagnosis of PcD. From a practical neuropathologic point of view, the requirement of the presence of Pick bodies for the diagnosis of PcD is seductive yet perhaps too rigid. Such a requirement would undercut the clinical diagnosis during life [61,89]. It would disqualify Pick's original six patients, who were reported between 1892 and 1906, in which clinicopathologic correlation was based only on the gross examination of the brains without reference to neuronal inclusions [1–4]. Indeed, these inclusions were not identified until 1911. Furthermore, the original description of Pick bodies did not result from the evaluation of the brains of Pick's patients [9].

More recent diagnostic concepts on PcD are discussed by Baldwin and Förstl [126] and Jellinger [104]. According to these concepts, PcD should not be diagnosed on the basis of frontotemporal degeneration alone. The presence of ballooned neurons is not specific to PcD, as ballooned neurons are seen in many other neurodegenerative conditions [7,113], including corticobasal degeneration, AD, primary progressive aphasia, chromosome 17–linked dementia, Creutzfeldt-Jakob disease, and progressive supranuclear palsy [69,74,93,110,114,134,140–146]. However, special emphasis is given to the presence of Pick bodies for diagnosing typical PcD because Pick bodies are almost never identified in conditions other than those combining dementia and circumscribed cerebral atrophy. Pick body–like inclusions may, however, be encountered in AD or other neurodegenerative diseases [147–149]. Furthermore, Sparks and associates reported Pick bodies and ballooned neurons in the grossly normal brain of a nondemented patient, suggesting that neuropathologic features of PcD may precede the occurrence of symptoms [150].

The neuropathologic features that are usually accepted as being characteristic of PcD may be summarized as follows: circumscribed, asymmetric or symmetric, frontal, frontotemporal, or fronto-temporo-parietal atrophy (lobar atrophy often including the hippocampal formation, amygdala, and deep gray nuclei, especially in the anterior portion of the striatum, with relative preservation of the caudal third of the superior temporal gyrus); status spongiosus; reactive gliosis; and neuronal loss in the atrophic areas with or without the presence of Pick bodies or ballooned neurons and with rare or no neurofibrillary tangles of Alzheimer or neuritic plaques.

REFERENCES

1. Pick A. Über die Beziehungen der senilen Hirnatrophie zur Aphasie. Prager Med Wochenschr 1892; 16:165–167.
2. Pick A. Senile Hirnatrophie als Grundlage von Herderscheinungen. Wiener Klin Wochenschr 1901; 14:403–404.
3. Pick A. Zur Symptomatologie des linksseitigen Schläfenlappenatrophie. Monatsschr Psychiatr Neurol 1904;16:378–388.
4. Pick A. Über einen weiteren Symptomenkomplex im Rahmen der Dementia senilis, bedingt durch umschriebene stärkere Hirnatrophie (gemischte Aparxie). Monatsschr Psychiatr Neurol 1906;19:97–108.

5. Vonsattel JP, Binetti G, Kelley LM. Pick Disease. In W Wasco, RE Tanzi (eds), Molecular Mechanisms of Dementia. Totowa, NJ: Humana Press, 1997;253–269.
6. Richter H. Eine besondere Art von Stirnhirnschwund mit Verblödung. Z Neurol Psychiatr 1918;38: 127–160.
7. Lüers TH, Spatz H. Picksche Krankheit (Progressive umschriebene Grosshirnatrophie). In O Lubarsch, F Henke, R Rössle, W Scholz (eds), Handbuch der Speziellen Pathologischen Anatomie und Histologie (XIII/1 Bandteil A). Berlin: Springer Verlag, 1957;614–715.
8. Tissot R, Constantinidis J, Richard J. La maladie de Pick. Paris: Masson, 1975.
9. Alzheimer A. Über eigenartige Krankheitsfälle des späteren Alters. Z Neurol Psychiatr 1911;4:356–385.
10. Onari K, Spatz H. Anatomische Beiträge zur Lehre von der Pickschen umschriebenen Grosshirnrinden-Atrophie ("Picksche Krankheit"). Z Neurol Psychiatr 1926;101:470–511.
11. Altman E. Über die umschriebene Gehirnatrophie des späteren Alters. Z Neurol Psychiatr 1923;83: 610–643.
12. Gans A. Betrachtungen über Art und Ausbreitung des krankhaften Prozesses in einem Fall von Pickscher Atrophie des Stirnhirns. Z Neurol Psychiatr 1922;80:10–28.
13. Stertz G. Über die Picksche Atrophie. Z Neurol Psychiatr 1926;101:729–747.
14. Korbsch H. Picksche und Huntingtonsche Krankheit bei Geschwistern. Arch Psychiatr Nervenkrankheiten 1933;100:326–349.
15. Schneider C. Über Picksche Krankheit. Monatsschr Psychiatr Neurol 1927;65:230–275.
16. Schneider C. Weitere Beiträge zur Lehre von der Pickschen Krankheit. Z Neurol Psychiatr 1929;120:340–384.
17. Bonfiglio F. Die umschriebene Atrophie der Basalganglien. Z Neurol Psychiatr 1937;160:306–333.
18. von Braunmühl A. Über Stammganglienveränderungen bei Pickscher Krankheit. Z Neurol Psychiatr 1930;124:214–221.
19. Grünthal, E. Über ein Brüderpaar mit Pickscher Krankheit. Eine vergleichende Untersuchung, zugleich ein Beitrag zur Kenntnis der Verursachung und des Verlaufs der Erkrankung. Z Neurol Psychiatr 1930;129:350–375.
20. von Braunmühl A, Leonhard K. Über ein Schwesternpaar mit Pickscher Krankheit. Z Neurol Psychiatr 1934;150:209–241.
21. Schmitz HA, Meyer A. Über die Picksche Krankheit, mit besonderer Berücksichtigung der Erblichkeit. Arch Psychiatr Nervenkrankheiten 1933;99:747–761.
22. von Braunmühl A. Picksche Krankheit und amyotrophische Lateralsklerose. Allgemeine Z Psychiatr Psychischgerichtliche Med 1932;96:364–366.
23. Snowden JS, Neary D, Mann DMA. Fronto-Temporal Lobar Degeneration: Fronto-Temporal Dementia, Progressive Aphasia, Semantic Dementia. New York: Churchill Livingstone, 1996.
24. Binetti G, Locascio JJ, Corkin S, et al. Pick's disease: clinical presentation and rate of cognitive decline. Neurology 1998. (In press.)
25. Sjögren T, Sjögren H, Lindgren AGH. Morbus Alzheimer and morbus Pick: a genetic, clinical and patho-anatomical study. Acta Psychiatr Neurol Scand Suppl 1952;82:1–152.
26. Cummings JL, Duchen LW. Klüver-Bucy syndrome in Pick disease: clinical and pathologic correlations. Neurology 1981;31:1415–1422.
27. Binetti G, Bianchetti A, Padovani A, et al. Delusions in Alzheimer's disease and multi-infarct dementia. Acta Neurol Scand 1993;88:5–9.
28. Mendez MF, Selwood A, Mastri AR, Frey MH. Pick's disease versus Alzheimer's disease: a comparison of clinical characteristics. Neurology 1993;43:289–292.
29. Binetti G, Padovani A, Magni E, et al. Delusions and dementia: clinical and CT correlates. Acta Neurol Scand 1995;91:271–275.
30. Binetti G, Mega ME, Magni E, et al. Behavioral disorders in Alzheimer disease: a transcultural perspective. Arch Neurol 1998. (In press.)
31. Brion S, Plas J, Jeanneau A. La maladie de Pick. Point de vue anatomo-clinique. Rev Neurol 1991; 147:693–704.
32. Gustafson L, Brun A, Passant U. Frontal Lobe Degeneration of Non-Alzheimer Type. In MN Rossor (ed), Baillière's Clinical Neurology. International Practice and Research. Unusual Dementias. London: Baillière Tindall/Saunders, 1992;559–582.
33. Pénisson-Besnier I, Le Gall D, Dubas F. Comportement compulsif d'allure obsessionnelle (arythmomanie). Atrophie des noyaux caudés. Rev Neurol 1992;148:262–267.
34. Klüver H, Bucy PC. Preliminary analysis of functions of the temporal lobes in monkeys. Arch Neurol Psychiatry 1939;42:979–1000.
35. Graff-Radford NR, Damasio AR, Hyman BT, et al. Progressive aphasia in a patient with Pick's disease. Neurology 1990;40:620–626.

36. Tissot R, Constantinidis J, Richard J. Pick's Disease. In JAM Frederiks (ed), Handbook of Clinical Neurology: Neurobehavioural Disorders, vol 2. Amsterdam: Elsevier, 1985;233–246.
37. Knopman DS, Christensen KJ, Schut LJ, et al. The spectrum of imaging and neuropsychological findings in Pick's disease. Neurology 1989;39:362–368.
38. Bechara A, Tranel D, Damasio H, et al. Double dissociation of conditioning and declarative knowledge relative to the amygdala and hippocampus in humans. Science 1995;269:1115–1118.
39. Stern CE, Corkin S, González RG, et al. The hippocampal formation participates in novel picture encoding: evidence from functional magnetic resonance imaging. Proc Natl Acad Sci U S A 1996;93: 8660–8665.
40. Corkin S, Amaral DG, Gonzalez RG, et al. H.M.'s medial temporal-lobe lesion: findings from magnetic resonance imaging. J Neurosci 1997;17:3964–3979.
41. Spatz, H. Über die Bedeutung der basalen Rinde. Auf Grund von Beobachtungen bei Pickscher Krankheit und bei gedeckten Hirnverletzungen. Z Ges Neurol Psychiatr 1937;158:208–232.
42. Desimone R, Ungerleider LG. Neuronal Mechanisms of Visual Processing in Monkeys. In H Goodglass, AR Damasio (eds), Handbook of Neuropsychology. Amsterdam: Elsevier, 1989;267–300.
43. De Renzi E. Disorders of Space Exploration and Cognition. New York: Wiley, 1992.
44. Munoz-Garcia D, Ludwin SK. Classic and generalized variants of Pick's disease: a clinicopathological, ultrastructural, and immunocytochemical comparative study. Ann Neurol 1984;16:467–480.
45. Pachana NA., Brauer K, Boone BL, et al. Comparison of neuropsychological functioning in Alzheimer's disease and frontotemporal dementia. J Int Neuropsychol Soc 1996;2:505–510.
46. Mirra SS, Heyman A, McKeel D. The Consortium to Establish a Registry for Alzheimer's Disease (CERAD). Part II. Standardization of the neuropathologic assessment of Alzheimer's disease. Neurology 1991;41:479–486.
47. The Lund and Manchester Groups. Clinical and neuropathological criteria for frontotemporal dementia. J Neurol Neurosurg Psychiatry 1994;57:416–418.
48. Gordon EB, Sim M. The EEG in presenile dementia. J Neurol Neurosurg Psychiatry 1967;30:285–291.
49. Groen JJ, Endtz LJ. Hereditary Pick's disease second re-examination of a large family and discussion of other hereditary cases, with particular reference to electroencephalography and computerized tomography. Brain 1982;105:443–459.
50. Frisoni GB, Beltramello A, Geroldi C. Brain atrophy in frontotemporal dementia. J Neurol Neurosurg Psychiatry 1996;61:157–165.
51. Neary D, Snowden JS, Northen B, Goulding P. Dementia of frontal lobe type. J Neurol Neurosurg Psychiatry 1988;51:353–361.
52. Salmon E, Franck G. Positron emission tomographic study in Alzheimer's disease and Pick's disease. Arch Gerontol Geriatr 1989;1:241–247.
53. Goto I, Taniwaki T, Hosokawa S, et al. Positron emission tomographic (PET) studies in dementia. J Neurol Sci 1993;114:1–6.
54. Miller BL, Ikonte C, Ponton M, et al. A study of the Lund-Manchester research criteria for frontotemporal dementia: clinical and single-photon emission CT correlations. Neurology 1997;48: 937–942.
55. Habert MO, Spampinato U, Mas JL, et al. A comparative technetium 99m hexamethylpropylene amine oxime SPET study in different types of dementia. Eur J Nucl Med 1991;18:3–11.
56. Terry RD. Dementia. A brief and selective review. Arch Neurol 1976;33:1–4.
57. Heston LL. The clinical genetics of Pick's disease. Acta Psychiatr Scand 1978;57:202–206.
58. Gustafson L, Nilsson L. Differential diagnosis of presenile dementia on clinical grounds. Acta Psychiatr Scand 1982;65:194–209.
59. Heston LL, Mastri AR. Age at onset of Pick's and Alzheimer's dementia: implication for diagnosis and research. J Gerontol 1982;37:422–424.
60. Stewart JT, Ware MR, Bauer RM, et al. A case of early-onset Pick's disease. J Clin Psychiatry 1992;53:380.
61. Mowadat HR, Kerr EE, StClair D. Sporadic Pick's disease in a 28-year-old woman. Br J Psychiatry 1993;162:259–262.
62. Binns JK, Robertson, EE. Pick's disease in old age. J Mental Sci 1962;108:804–810.
63. Heston LL, White JA, Mastri AR. Pick's disease. Clinical genetics and natural history. Arch Gen Psychiatry 1987;44:409–411.
64. Schenk VWD. Re-examination of a family with Pick's disease. Ann Hum Genet 1959;23:325–333.
65. Constantinidis J. Pick dementia: anatomical correlations and pathophysiological considerations. Interdisc Topics Gerontol 1985;19:72–97.
66. Brown J. Pick's Disease. In MN Rossor (ed), Baillière's Clinical Neurology. International Practice and Research. Unusual Dementias. London: Baillière Tindall/Saunders, 1992;535–557.

67. Löwenberg K, Boyd DA, Salon DD. Occurrence of Pick's disease in early adult years. Arch Neurol Psychiatry 1939;41:1004–1020.
68. Malamud N, Waggoner RW. Genealogic and clinicopathologic study of Pick's disease. Arch Neurol Psychiatry 1943;50:288–303.
69. Heutink P, Stevens M, Rizzu P, et al. Hereditary frontotemporal dementia is linked to chromosome 17q21–q22: a genetic and clinicopathological study of three Dutch families. Ann Neurol 1997;41: 150–159.
70. Lynch T, Sano M, Marder KS, et al. Clinical characteristics of a family with chromosome 17–linked disinhibition-dementia-parkinsonism-amyotrophy complex. Neurology 1994;44:1878–1884.
71. Baker M, Kwok JBJ, Kucera S, et al. Localization of frontotemporal dementia with parkinsonism in an Australian kindred to chromosome 17q21–22. Ann Neurol 1997;42:794–798.
72. Petersen RB, Tabaton M, Chen SG, et al. Familial progressive subcortical gliosis: presence of prions and linkage to chromosome 17. Neurology 1995;45:1062–1067.
73. Wijker M, Wszoleck ZK, Wolters ECH, et al. Localization of the gene for rapidly progressive autosomal dominant parkinsonism and dementia with pallido-ponto-nigral degeneration to chromosome 17q21. Hum Mol Genet 1996;5:151–154.
74. Sima AAF, Defendini R, Keohane C, et al. The neuropathology of chromosome 17–linked dementia. Ann Neurol 1996;39:734–743.
75. Bird TD, Wijsman EM, Nochlin D, et al. Chromosome 17 and hereditary dementia: linkage studies in three non-Alzheimer families and kindreds with late-onset FAD. Neurology 1997;48:949–954.
76. Schneider JA, Gearing M, Robbins RS, et al. Apolipoprotein E genotype in diverse neurodegenerative disorders. Ann Neurol 1995;38:131–135.
77. Rebeck GW, Reiter JS, Strickland DK, Hyman BT. Apolipoprotein E in sporadic Alzheimer's disease: allelic variation and receptor interactions. Neuron 1993;11:575–580.
78. Myers RH, Schaefer EJ, Wilson PWF, et al. Apolipoprotein E ε4 association with dementia in a population-based study: the Framingham Study. Neurology 1996;46:673–677.
79. Gómez-Isla T, West HL, Rebeck GW, et al. Clinical and pathological correlates of apolipoprotein E ε4 in Alzheimer's disease. Ann Neurol 1996;39:62–70.
80. Growdon JH, Locascio JJ, Corkin S, et al. Apolipoprotein E genotype does not influence rates of cognitive decline in Alzheimer's disease. Neurology 1996;47:444–448.
81. Cambier J, Masson M, Dairou R, Henin D. Étude anatomo-clinique d'une forme pariétale de la maladie de Pick. Rev Neurol 1981;137:33–38.
82. Spatz H. La Maladie de Pick, les Atrophies Systématisées Progressives et la Sénescence Cérébrale Prématurée Localisée. In The Proceedings of the First International Congress of Neuropathology, vol 2. Torino, Italy: Rosenberg and Sellier, 1952;375–406.
83. Lang AE, Bergeron C, Pollanen MS, Ashby P. Parietal Pick's disease mimicking cortico-basal ganglionic degeneration. Neurology 1994;44:1436–1440.
84. Dickson DW. Pick's disease: a modern approach. Brain Pathol 1998;8:339–354.
85. Lüers TH. Über fronto-thalamische Syndrome bei der Pickschen Krankheit. Dtsch Z Nervenheilkunde 1950;164:179–198.
86. Tagliavini F, Pilleri G. Basal nucleus of Meynert. A neuropathological study in Alzheimer's disease, simple senile dementia, Pick's disease and Huntington's chorea. J Neurol Sci 1983;62:243–260.
87. Vonsattel JP, Myers RH, Stevens TJ. Neuropathological classification of Huntington's disease. J Neuropathol Exp Neurol 1985;44:559–577.
88. Kosaka K, Ikeda K, Kobayashi K, Mehraein P. Striatopallidonigral degeneration in Pick's disease: a clinicopathological study of 41 cases. J Neurol 1991;238:151–160.
89. Hulette CM, Crain BJ. Lobar atrophy without Pick bodies. Clin Neuropathol 1992;11:151–156.
90. Paulus W, Bancher C, Jellinger K. Microglial reaction in Pick's diseae. Neurosci Lett 1993;161:89–92.
91. Iwatsubo T, Hasegawa M, Ihara Y. Neuronal and glial *tau*-positive inclusions in diverse neurologic diseases share common phosphorylation characteristics. Acta Neuropathol 1994;88:129–136.
92. Dickson DW, Feany MB, Yen SH, et al. Cytoskeletal pathology in non-Alzheimer degenerative dementia: new lesions in diffuse Lewy body disease, Pick's disease, and corticobasal degeneration. J Neural Transm 1996;47(suppl):31–46.
93. Feany MB, Mattiace LA, Dickson DW. Neuropathologic overlap of progressive supranuclear palsy, Pick's disease and corticobasal degeneration. J Neuropathol Exp Neurol 1996;55:53–67.
94. Braak H, Braak E. Cortical and subcortical argyrophilic grains characterize a disease associated with adult onset dementia. Neuropathol Appl Neurobiol 1989;15:13–26.
95. Martinez-Lage P, Munoz DG. Prevalence and disease associations of argyrophilic grains of Braak. J Neuropathol Exp Neurol 1997;56:157–164.

96. Sam M, Gutmann L, Schochet SS, Doshi H. Pick's disease: a case clinically resembling amyotrophic lateral sclerosis. Neurology 1991;41:1831–1833.
97. Wisniewski HM, Coblentz JM, Terry RD. Pick's disease. A clinical and ultrastructural study. Arch Neurol 1972;26:97–108.
98. Tiller-Borcich JK, Forno LS. Parkinson's disease and dementia with neuronal inclusions in the cerebral cortex: Lewy bodies or Pick bodies. J Neuropathol Exp Neurol 1988;47:526–535.
99. Ball MJ. Topography of Pick inclusion bodies in hippocampi of demented patients. A quantitative study. J Neuropathol Exp Neurol 1979;38:614–620.
100. Hof PR, Bouras C, Perl DP, Morrison JH. Quantitative neuropathologic analysis of Pick's disease cases: cortical distribution of Pick bodies and coexistence with Alzheimer disease. Acta Neuropathol 1994;87:115–124.
101. Jellinger KA. Quantitative neuropathologic analysis of Pick's disease cases. Acta Neuropathol 1994;87:223–224.
102. Fukui T, Sugita K, Kawamura M, et al. Primary progressive apraxia in Pick's disease: a clinicopathologic study. Neurology 1996;47:467–473.
103. Dickson DW, Wertkin A, Kress Y. Ubiquitin immunoreactive structures in normal human brains. Distribution and developmental aspects. Lab Invest 1990;63:87–99.
104. Jellinger KA. Neuropathological Criteria for Pick's Disease and Frontotemporal Lobe Dementia. In FF Cruz-Sánchez, R Ravid, ML Cuzner (eds), Neuropathological Diagnostic Criteria for Brain Banking. Amsterdam: IOS, 1995;35–54.
105. Yasuhara O, Matsuo A, Tooyama I, et al. Pick's disease immunohistochemistry: new alterations and Alzheimer's disease comparisons. Acta Neuropathol 1995;89:322–330.
106. Yasuhara O, Aimi Y, McGeer EG, McGeer PL. Accumulation of amyloid precursor protein in brain lesions of patients with Pick disease. Neurosci Lett 1994;171:63–66.
107. Wechsler AF, Verity MA, Rosenschein S, et al. Pick's disease. A clinical, computed tomographic, and histologic study with Golgi impregnation observations. Arch Neurol 1982;39:287–290.
108. Yokoo H, Oyama T, Hirato J, et al. A case of Pick's disease with unusual neuronal inclusions. Acta Neuropathol 1994;88:267–272.
109. Khachaturian ZS. Diagnosis of Alzheimer's disease. Arch Neurol 1985;42:1097–1105.
110. Clark AW, Manz HJ, White CL III, et al. Cortical degeneration with swollen chromatolytic neurons: its relationship to Pick's disease. J Neuropathol Exp Neurol 1986;45:268–284.
111. Delacourte A, Robitaille Y, Sergeant N, et al. Specific pathological *tau* protein variants characterize Pick's disease. J Neuropathol Exp Neurol 1996;55:159–168.
112. Buée-Scherrer V, Hof PR, Buée L, et al. Hyperphosphorylated *tau* proteins differentiate corticobasal degeneration and Pick's disease. Acta Neuropathol 1996;91:351–359.
113. Williams HW. The peculiar cells of Pick's disease. Their pathogenesis and distribution in disease. Arch Neurol Psychiatry 1935;34:508–519.
114. Dickson DW, Yen SH, Suzuki KI, Davies P. Ballooned neurons in select neurodegenerative diseases contain phosphorylated neurofilament epitopes. Acta Neuropathol 1996;71:216–223.
115. Cooper PN, Jackson M, Lennox G. *tau*, ubiquitin, and αB-crystallin immunohistochemistry define the principal causes of degenerative frontotemporal dementia. Arch Neurol 1995;52:1011–1015.
116. Wood BT, McKee AC. Case records of the Massachusetts General Hospital. Case 6-1992. N Engl J Med 1992;326:397–405.
117. Masters CL, Richardson EP Jr. Subacute spongiform encephalopathy (Creutzfeldt-Jakob disease). The nature and progression of spongiform change. Brain 1978;101:333–344.
118. Collinge J, Palmer MS, Sidle KCL, et al. Familial Pick's disease and dementia in frontal lobe degeneration of non Alzheimer type are not variants of prion disease. J Neurol Neurosurg Psychiatry 1994;57:762.
119. Smith TW, Anwer U, DeGirolami U, Drachman DA. Vacuolar change in Alzheimer's disease. Arch Neurol 1987;44:1225–1228.
120. Hansen L, Salmon D, Galasko D. The Lewy body variant of Alzheimer's disease: a clinical and pathologic entity. Neurology 1990;40:1–8.
121. Lippa CF, Smith TW, Swearer JM. Alzheimer's disease and Lewy body disease: a comparative clinicopathological study. Ann Neurol 1994;35:81–88.
122. Kazee AM, Han LY. Cortical Lewy bodies in Alzheimer's disease. Arch Pathol Lab Med 1995;119: 448–453.
123. Neumann MA. Pick's disease. J Neuropathol Exp Neurol 1949;8:255–282.
124. Hansen LA, Crain B. Making the diagnosis of mixed and non-Alzheimer's disease. Arch Pathol Lab Med 1995;119:1023–1031.
125. Schenk VWD. Maladie de Pick. Étude anatomo-clinique de 8 cas. Ann Med Psychol 1951;109:574–587.

126. Baldwin B, Förstl H. "Pick's disease"—101 years on still there, but in need of reform. Br J Psychiatry 1993;163:100–104.
127. Litvan I, Hauw JJ, Bartko JJ, et al. Validity and reliability of the preliminary NINDS neuropathologic criteria for progressive supranuclear palsy and related disorders. J Neuropathol Exp Neurol 1996;55:97–105.
128. Litvan I, Agid Y, Sastrj N, et al. What are the obstacles for an accurate clinical diagnosis of Pick's disease? A clinicopathologic study. Neurology 1997;49:62–69.
129. Morrison JH, Hof PR. Life and death of neurons in the aging brain. Science 1997;278:412–419.
130. Giannakopoulos P, Hof PR, Bouras C. Dementia lacking distinctive histopathology: clinicopathological evaluation of 32 cases. Acta Neuropathol 1995;89:346–355.
131. Mann DMA, South PW, Snowden JS, Neary D. Dementia of frontal lobe type: neuropathology and immunohistochemistry. J Neurol Neurosurg Psychiatry 1993;56:605–614.
132. Neary D. Non-Alzheimer's disease forms of cerebral atrophy. J Neurol Neurosurg Psychiatry 1990;53:929–931.
133. Wightman G, Anderson VER, Martin J, et al. Hippocampal and neocortical ubiquitin-immunoreactive inclusions in amyotrophic lateral sclerosis with dementia. Neurosci Lett 1992;139:269–274.
134. Lippa CF, Cohen R, Smith TW, Drachman DA. Primary progressive aphasia with focal neuronal achromasia. Neurology 1991;41:882–886.
135. Mesulam MM, Weintraub S. Spectrum of Primary Progressive Aphasia. In MN Rossor (ed), Baillière's Clinical Neurology. International Practice and Research. Unusual Dementias. London: Baillière Tindall/Saunders, 1992;583–609.
136. Scheltens P, Ravid R, Kamphorst W. Pathologic findings in a case of primary progressive aphasia. Neurology 1994;44:279–282.
137. Knopman DS, Mastri AR, Frey WH, et al. Dementia lacking distinctive histologic features: a common non-Alzheimer degenerative dementia. Neurology 1990;40:251–256.
138. Jackson M, Lowe J. The new neuropathology of degenerative frontotemporal dementias. Acta Neuropathol 1996;91:127–134.
139. Turner RS, Kenyon LC, Trojanowski JQ, et al. Clinical, neuroimaging, and pathologic features of progressive nonfluent aphasia. Ann Neurol 1996;39:166–173.
140. Rebeiz JJ, Kolodny EH, Richardson EP Jr. Corticodentatonigral degeneration with neuronal achromasia. Arch Neurol 1968;18:20–33.
141. Gibb RG, Luthert PJ, Marsden CD. Corticobasal degeneration. Brain 1989;112:1171–1192.
142. Lippa CF, Smith TW, Fontneau N. Corticonigral degeneration with neuronal achromasia. A clinicopathologic study of two cases. J Neurol Sci 1990;98:301–310.
143. Budka H, Aguzzi A, Brown P, et al. Neuropathological diagnostic criteria for Creutzfeldt-Jakob disease (CJD) and other human spongiform encephalopathies (prion diseases). Brain Pathol 1995;5: 459–466.
144. Feany MB, Dickson DW. Widespread cytoskeletal pathology characterizes corticobasal degeneration. Am J Pathol 1995;146:1388–1396.
145. Mackenzie IRA, Hudson LP. Achromatic neurons in the cortex of progressive supranuclear palsy. Acta Neuropathol 1995;90:615–619.
146. Pillon B, Blin J, Vidailhet M, et al. The neuropsychological pattern of corticobasal degeneration: comparison with progressive supranuclear palsy and Alzheimer's disease. Neurology 1995;45:1477–1483.
147. Dickson DW, Ksiezak-Reding H, Liu WK, et al. Immunocytochemistry of neurofibrillary tangles with antibodies to subregions of tau protein: identification of hidden and cleaved *tau* epitopes and a new phosphorylation site. Acta Neuropathol 1992;84:596–605.
148. Jendroska K, Rossor MN, Mathias CJ, Daniel SE. Morphological overlap between corticobasal degeneration and Pick's disease: a clinicopathological report. Mov Disord 1995;10:111–114.
149. Feany MB, Dickson DW. Neurodegenerative disorders with extensive *tau* pathology: a comparative study and review. Ann Neurol 1996;40:139–148.
150. Sparks DL, Danner FW, Davis DG, et al. Neurochemical and histopathologic alterations characteristic of Pick's disease in a non-demented individual. J Neuropathol Exp Neurol 1994;53:37–42.

2
Frontal and Frontotemporal Dementia

Morgan L. Levy, Bruce L. Miller,
and Jeffrey L. Cummings

The frontotemporal dementias (FTDs) are a clinically heterogenous group of diseases that involve lobar atrophy of frontal and temporal cortex [1–4]. Frontal lobe dementia of non-Alzheimer type [5], or frontal lobe degeneration [6], is one of the most common and well characterized forms of FTD. Clinically, it is marked by early personality changes, such as apathy, sociopathy, disinhibition, and euphoria, and by behavioral disturbances, such as hyperorality, dietary change, and repetitive behaviors [7]. There is progressive impairment of language and executive function together with loss of insight and abstract thinking. Onset is usually between age 50 and 65 years and most patients survive 6–12 years. More than half of the cases are familial, and an autosomal dominant pattern of inheritance is common [7,8]. Frontal lobe degeneration shares many clinical features with other FTD categories such as Pick's disease and FTD with motor neuron disease. Frontal lobe degeneration is characterized by spongiform change without Pick bodies. FTD patients may exhibit diverse behavioral patterns and several different histopathologic subtypes have been identified. The etiologic significance of these subtypes is currently unknown.

This chapter describes the clinical and histopathologic subtypes of FTD and summarizes the differential diagnosis of disorders causing frontal lobe dysfunction. Clinical characteristics presented include psychiatric, behavioral, and cognitive abnormalities and their anatomic correlates. Neurodiagnostic tests, including psychiatric inventories, neuropsychological evaluations, and structural and functional neuroimaging, are reviewed. Finally, genetic studies linking some forms of FTD to chromosomes 17 and 3 are summarized.

This project was supported by a Department of Veterans Affairs Neuroscience Fellowship, a National Institute on Aging Alzheimer's Disease Center grant (AG10123), and the Sidell-Kagan Research Fund.

HISTORY

Arnold Pick was a late-nineteenth-century German neuropsychiatrist who published 280 scientific articles on topics such as aphasia, apraxia, agnosia, memory, consciousness, agrammatism, hysterical psychosis, and counseling for relatives of psychiatric patients [9]. In 1892, he reported a 71-year-old man with a 3-year history of progressive dementia marked by prominent aphasia who, at autopsy (performed by Chiari), was found to have lobar atrophy of the frontal and temporal cortex [10]. He published at least three more articles on frontal and temporal lobe atrophy, but it was Alzheimer [11] who described "ballooned cells, argentophilic globes, and spongicortico wasting." These changes were labeled "Pick cells" and "Pick bodies" by Newman in 1926 (see Chapter 1).

Pick-type histopathologic changes became synonymous with lobar atrophy, and disorders with these features were termed *Pick's disease* (PcD). PcD was considered a relatively rare form of dementia in the past. A renewal of interest in neuropsychiatric illnesses over the past two decades has led to the discovery that Pick-type histopathologic changes are present in a minority of patients with dementia and frontotemporal lobar atrophy [6]. Several additional histopathologies associated with lobar degeneration have been identified, and the concept of FTD has been broadened. Frontal lobe degeneration may comprise 10–15% of all dementias [5] and appears to be the most common cause of FTD. FTD patients are frequently misdiagnosed as having Alzheimer's disease (AD) during life. One recent study found that 18 of 21 autopsy-confirmed cases of PcD had been misdiagnosed as AD before death [12].

HISTOPATHOLOGIC CLASSIFICATION

Disorders producing a frontal lobe syndrome are listed in Table 2.1. In light of its history, *PcD* probably should refer to the gross pathologic changes of frontal and temporal lobe atrophy, but it is currently considered a subtype of FTD that is distinguished by the histopathologic appearance of widespread gliosis, loss of large cortical nerve cells, and severe astrocytosis with swollen neurons (Pick cells) and inclusions (Pick bodies) that are both *tau*- and ubiquitin-positive. There is minimal or no spongiform change or microvacuolation in the cortex (Figure 2.1) [13,14]. Atrophic changes may appear more marked in some cases of PcD compared to other forms of FTD. PcD is described in more detail in Chapter 1.

Frontal lobe degeneration is the second and most common subtype of FTD. Its clinical features and gross anatomy may be indistinguishable from PcD. The histologic appearance includes a spongiform degeneration or microvacuolation of the superficial neuropil (cortical layer II) with mild astrocytosis, loss of large cortical nerve cells, minimal gliosis, and no inclusions (Figure 2.2) [2,8,14].

FTD with amyotrophic lateral sclerosis (FTD-ALS) is the third major subtype of FTD. Several features of FTD-ALS are similar to frontal lobe degeneration and PcD, including neuropsychiatric symptoms, neuropsychological deficits, age at onset, and frontal and temporal lobe atrophy. Differences include a faster rate of decline, with a mean survival of approximately 3 years [15], and the presence of upper and lower motor neuron disease, which typically follows the appearance

Table 2.1 Primary degenerative disorders associated with frontal lobe dementia

Frontotemporal degenerations
Pick's disease
Frontal lobe degeneration
Frontotemporal dementia with amyotrophic lateral sclerosis
Progressive subcortical gliosis
Corticobasal degeneration
Chromosome 17–linked disorders
Disinhibition-dementia-parkinsonism-amyotrophy complex (DDPAC)
Hereditary dysphasic dementia
Tauopathy
Alzheimer's disease

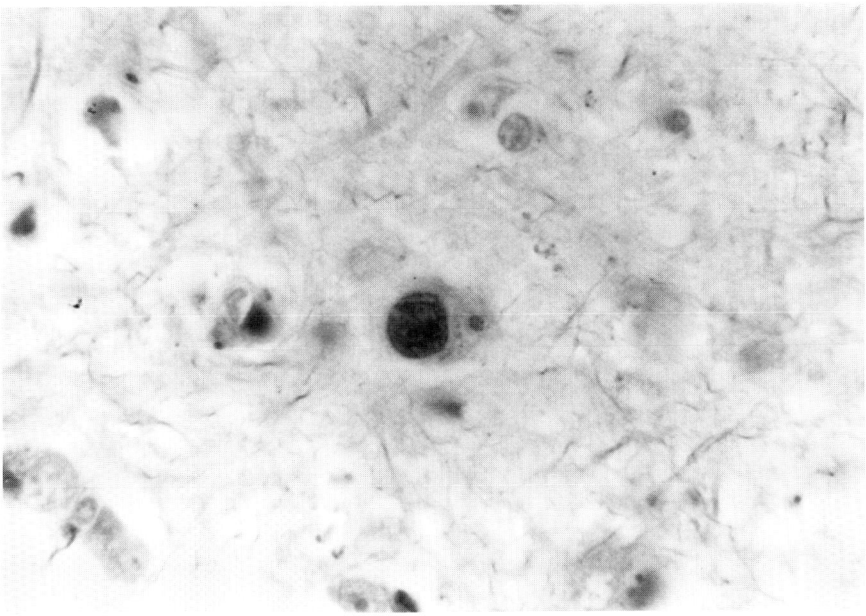

Figure 2.1 High magnification (1,000×) of a pyramidal neuron containing a Pick body (Bielschowsky silver stain). (Courtesy of Pier Luigi Di Patre, M.D., Department of Pathology, University of California at Los Angeles.)

of mental symptoms. The histologic changes seen in FTD-ALS share features of both frontal lobe dementia and PcD and include microvacuolation of the outer cortical laminae with mild astrocytosis, loss of large cortical nerve cells, and ubiquitinated but not *tau*-containing inclusions. Occasional cases have Pick-type inclusions. Histologic changes unique to FTD-ALS include loss of neurons and severe astrocytosis in the substantia nigra (with or without parkinsonism) and loss of anterior horn cells and motor neuron cells of trigeminal and hypoglossal nuclei [14].

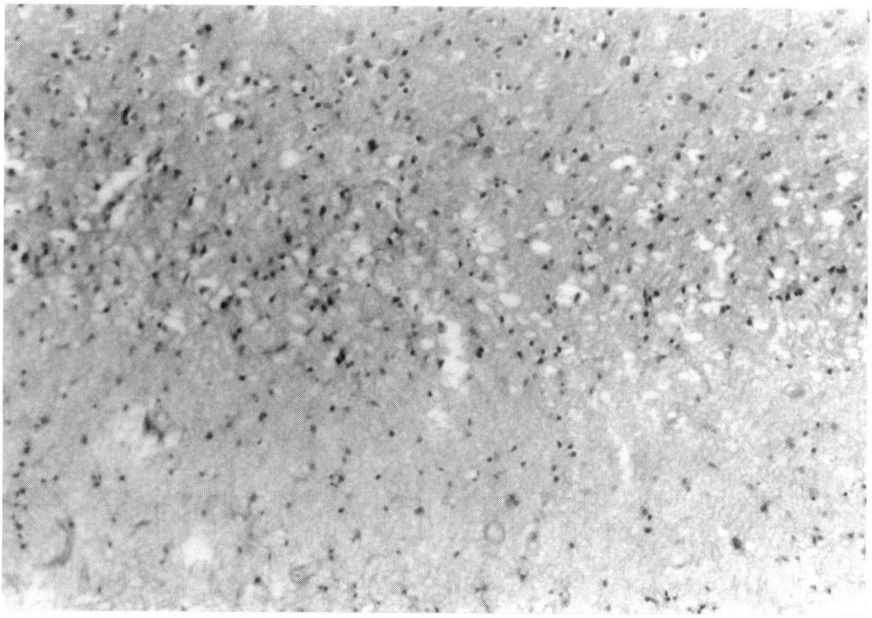

Figure 2.2 Frontal cortex of a patient with frontal lobe degeneration at 100× magnification. There is prominent vacuolization of the external pyramidal layer with astrocytosis of the molecular layer. No Pick bodies are present (hematoxylin and eosin stain). (Courtesy of Pier Luigi Di Patre, M.D., Department of Pathology, University of California at Los Angeles.)

Progressive subcortical gliosis is a rare cause of frontotemporal atrophy. In addition to disinhibition, poor judgment, and perseveration, memory impairment is common. Some patients develop muscle atrophy before death. Neuronal loss with reactive astrocytosis occurs in the cortex, but the distinguishing feature is extensive gliosis in subcortical areas, including frontal and temporal lobe white matter, thalamus, and olivary nuclei [16,17].

Corticobasal degeneration is a rare disorder that usually affects the basal ganglia and parietal cortex, producing extrapyramidal symptoms and symptoms of parietal lobe dysfunction similar to AD, but in some cases it involves the frontal lobes. A distinctive feature of many cases of corticobasal degeneration is the "alien hand" sign; a syndrome in which one hand performs involuntary but seemingly purposeful activities [18,19]. At autopsy, gliosis and swollen achromatic neurons are seen in the frontal lobes, basal ganglia, rostral brain stem, and thalamus. Occasional cases have had Pick bodies within affected neurons.

Hereditary dysphasic dementia is a rare autosomal dominant disease with prominent language abnormalities. Postmortem examination reveals frontotemporal atrophy, neuronal loss, conspicuous spongiform changes in the outer layers of the cortex, intracellular argyrophilic cytoplasmic fibrillary material, and subcortical Lewy body formation [20]. This disorder has been linked to chromosome 17 in a study of three Dutch families [21].

FTD and parkinsonism linked to chromosome 17 have been found in eight kindreds with progressive neurologic disorders presenting at ages younger than 65 years. There is considerable clinical variation, but patients typically manifest many of the psychiatric and cognitive symptoms described in FTD. In addition, they commonly have levodopa-resistant parkinsonism early or late in the course and corticospinal disturbances such as hyperreflexia, clonus, and extensor plantar responses. Histopathologic changes consist of neuronal loss and gliosis in frontotemporal cortices and substantia nigra, and in four of the kindreds there was involvement of motor cortex and motor neurons of the brain stem and spinal cord. Argyrophilic inclusions, *tau*-positive inclusions, or both may also be found along with neuropil vacuolation and white matter gliosis [22]. At least two families have this phenotypic picture without linkage to chromosome 17, and one of these families has been linked to chromosome 3 [23].

AD generally does not produce marked frontal atrophy until late in its course. Nevertheless, it must be recognized that AD can sometimes have an atypical presentation with frontal lobe features.

Primary progressive aphasia refers to a progressive nonfluent aphasia associated with degeneration localized in the left frontotemporal cortex [24]. These patients may develop the typical cognitive deficits and neuropsychiatric symptoms associated with FTD late in the course. The histologic appearance is usually that of frontal lobe degeneration with spongiform degeneration and cell loss [14], but some cases have had Pick-type histopathology, whereas others have had Alzheimer-type changes.

A syndrome of right-sided atrophy also has been described. Miller and colleagues [25] described five cases of right frontotemporal dysfunction diagnosed clinically and with single photon emission computer tomography (SPECT). The patients demonstrated dramatic changes in personality, including remote affect, severe behavioral disinhibition, agitation, hyperreligiosity, impaired judgment, and profound disruption of social conduct. They had difficulty recognizing familiar faces and voices and some had a semantic anomia. Language problems were less severe compared to patients with primarily left frontotemporal involvement.

Semantic dementia is a rare clinical syndrome characterized by fluent dysphasia with severe anomia, reduced vocabulary, and prominent impairment of single-word comprehension. It can progress to a stage of virtually complete dissolution of the semantic components of language. Phonology and grammar are largely preserved. Episodic memory, nonverbal memory, and perceptual and visuospatial abilities also are strikingly preserved. Behavioral changes such as Klüver-Bucy symptoms may occur, and there is focal atrophy in the dominant temporal lobe [26]. It is currently unknown whether semantic dementia and primary progressive aphasia are independent disease states or whether they represent highly focal examples of degeneration affecting primarily the anterior temporal or dorsolateral cortex, respectively.

Other CNS diseases with frontal lobe involvement are summarized in Table 2.2. Many disorders commonly disrupt frontal lobe function. Extensive connections exist between the frontal cortex and subcortical structures such as the striatum, basal ganglia, and thalamus; frontal lobe function is dependent on the integrity of these pathways. Pathology in these structures or in the white matter

Table 2.2 Secondary causes of "frontal lobe" syndromes

Degenerative	
	Parkinson's disease
	Progressive supranuclear palsy
	Huntington's disease
Vascular	
	Frontal lobe aneurysm or infarct
	Binswanger's disease
	Lacunar state
Cerebral autosomal dominant arteriopathy with subcortical infarcts and leukoencephalopathy (CADASIL)	
White matter disease	
	Multiple sclerosis
	Metachromatic leukodystrophy
	Marchiafava-Bignami disease
Infectious and transmissible	
	Human immunodeficiency virus
	Progressive multifocal leukoencephalopathy
	Syphilis
	Creutzfeldt-Jakob disease
Neoplasm	
Trauma	
Hydrocephalus	

tracts connecting them to the frontal cortex can cause symptoms similar to a frontal lobe syndrome. Degenerative causes may be separated into a cortical and a subcortical group [27]. Trauma frequently affects the frontal lobes due to their size and position, and both the frontal and temporal lobes are susceptible to trauma from closed head injury because they rest in enclosed, irregular bony fossae. Also, the basal forebrain receives projections from the brain stem and is involved in arousal and attention. Therefore, toxic, metabolic, or other conditions that alter consciousness may cause frontal signs and symptoms.

CLINICAL FEATURES

When affected by disease, different anatomic regions produce distinct behavioral syndromes frequently seen in FTD (Table 2.3). Pathology is generally simultaneously present in several of these areas, producing a combination of symptoms. Dysfunction of the dorsolateral prefrontal cortex produces perseveration, poor judgment, and other abnormalities of executive function [28]. Orbitofrontal damage is associated with disinhibition or socially inappropriate behavior [28], and anterior cingulate damage is related to apathy or loss of motivation [28]. Involvement of the anterior temporal lobes can produce aspects of the Klüver-Bucy syndrome, including hyperorality and placidity. Throughout the clinical examination there may be contributions from several of these anatomic regions, or one or two regions may predominate. Clinicopathologic correlates are not yet available in

Table 2.3 Clinical characteristics of frontotemporal syndromes

Region	*Characteristic abnormalities*
Dorsolateral prefrontal	Perseveration
	Difficulty shifting set
	Reduced verbal fluency
	Reduced nonverbal fluency
	Impaired abstraction
	Poor judgment
	Poor planning
	Poor response inhibition
	Reduced spontaneous recall
Orbitofrontal	Disinhibition
	Impulsivity
	Sociopathy
	Euphoria
	Socially inappropriate behavior
Anterior cingulate	Apathy
	Reduced motivation
	Loss of interest
Anterior temporal	Hyperorality
	Weight gain
	Placidity
	Bizarre and remote affect
	Hyperreligiosity
	Hypermetamorphosis (over-attention to external stimuli)
	Semantic anomia

large numbers of patients, and differences in the behavioral syndromes of frontal lobe degeneration, PcD, and FTD-ALS have not been fully explored.

Frontal lobe degeneration usually begins with psychiatric symptoms, such as loss of motivation or disengagement from usual activities, and patients typically present for clinical assessment after the disease has been present for several years. Before being diagnosed, patients may receive treatment for depression, and several patients have undergone electroconvulsive therapy. Bizarre ideas and a remote affect may be present. Compulsive collecting or stealing of ordinary objects may occur, and this symptom may be partially responsive to selective serotonin reuptake inhibitors [29]. Patients may become anxious when performing tasks that they used to do with ease and are increasingly dependent on their spouse. Retirement may be hastened due to seemingly inexplicable mistakes in job performance such as poor planning, poor judgment, or simple but important oversights. Memory problems are sometimes reported as the initial symptom, but true memory or visuospatial problems are rarely present in early disease. More frequently, problems with naming, word-finding, or lack of interest and poor motivation are perceived as memory problems. In addition, patients usually lack insight into their deficits.

Psychiatric symptoms usually persist as the disease progresses. Disinhibition is prominent and sociopathic behaviors may occur [30]. Patients may be arrested for shoplifting or making sexual advances toward strangers. They may repeatedly steal small items that they do not need or they may disrobe or urinate in public places. Angry outbursts are not uncommon, and they may shout inappropriately at a caregiver or at a total stranger. Casual conversation can be punctuated by tactless phrases such as "My house is bigger" or "That's a nice body." Their affect may become detached or remote, which adds to the bizarre nature of their spontaneous comments and outbursts. Approximately one-third of patients develop an affect that can be described as euphoric but which may be unaccompanied by genuine emotion. Their affect may change quickly from inappropriate jocularity to passivity or anger, but anger is rarely sustained. Patients are impulsive, responding immediately and unpredictably to changing environmental circumstances. They lack conscientiousness and fail to complete assigned tasks. Orbitofrontal damage is likely responsible for the symptoms of disinhibition, irritability, euphoria, and sociopathy.

Apathy is almost always present and may become severe as the disease progresses. Decreased motivation, loss of interest, lack of follow-through, poor initiation of activities, and emotional disengagement are frequent descriptions of patients. In addition, they lose concern about the consequences of their actions or inaction. The emotional state of these patients may be best characterized by an absence of emotions rather than the presence of negative emotions. One man described the intimate interactions with his affected wife by saying, "It's like making love to a robot." Anterior cingulate cortex is the anatomic region that is most commonly associated with apathy.

Repetitive behaviors are common [31,32], such as compulsive checking of trash cans, collecting and stacking antacid wafers, watering small areas of the lawn one section at a time, and spending several hours a day putting random letters in a crossword puzzle.

The anterior temporal lobes are involved as the pathology of frontal lobe degeneration extends (hence the clinical term *frontotemporal dementia*) and dysfunction in this region is likely responsible for several of the most unusual symptoms of this disorder. Klüver-Bucy syndrome was described in Macaque monkeys after the anterior temporal lobes and amygdalae were removed [33]. These monkeys developed hyperorality, hypersexuality, visual hypermetamorphosis, placidity, and sensory agnosia. Patients often manifest hyperorality by excessive gum chewing, smoking, drinking, or eating, and the majority have weight gain, with some patients gaining as much as 80 pounds [31,34]. In severe cases, patients may place nonfood objects in their mouths. Placidity is common and patients may become drawn to stimuli in the environment (hypermetamorphosis). Often they have utilization behavior in which they may repeatedly use objects in the environment such as a telephone, door knob, or drinking glass simply because they are there and not because they really need to call someone, leave the room, or drink water. They sometimes follow their spouse and copy his or her behavior (imitation behavior). These symptoms are further examples of the human Klüver-Bucy syndrome.

On neuropsychological examination, executive function impairment is the most prominent finding if the patient is seen within 2–3 years of disease onset. Patients often perseverate on mental tasks. For example, it may be difficult to get them "in set" to start a new test, and then it may be difficult to get them to stop one test and "shift set" to another test. When instructed to draw a round clock and

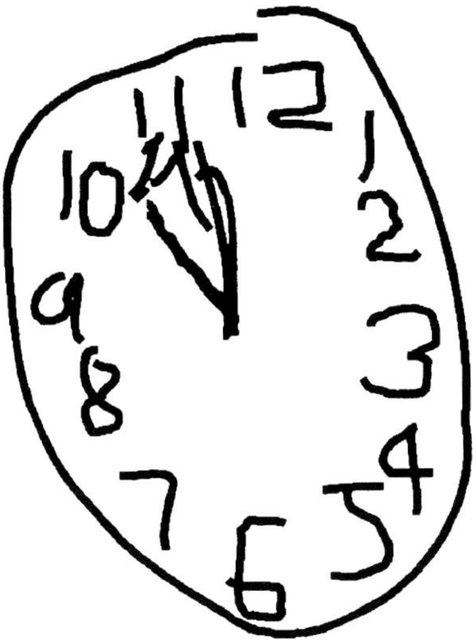

Figure 2.3 The draw-a-clock task performed by a stimulus-bound patient with frontotemporal dementia. Instructions: Draw a round clock and set the time at ten after eleven.

make the time read 10 past 11, the stimulus-bound patient places one hand on the 11 and the other hand on the 10 (Figure 2.3). Poor planning strategies may also be seen with more complex constructions such as the Rey-Osterrieth and Taylor complex figures. The patient may begin by drawing the details or the internal lines instead of drawing the overall shape first and then adding the details in an orderly fashion. They may be unable to inhibit a response to a cue even when it directs them to a clearly wrong answer. For example, the Stroop test requires the patient to name the color red when the word *green* is written in red ink and the patient cannot inhibit reading the written word *green*. Spontaneous memory recall may be impaired, and yet the patient produces correct responses when cues are provided. Patients may also give concrete responses when asked to explain similarities and proverbs and may display poor judgment when given a simple problem-solving task. They may be generally awake and alert, but they are easily distracted and sustained attention is often impaired. Executive dysfunction is associated with damage to the dorsolateral prefrontal cortex.

Motor perseveration is the inability to stop or change tasks [35] and can be seen when drawing multiple loops or alternating programs (Figure 2.4). Motor perseveration also may be demonstrated by motor programming tasks such as the Luria hand sequence task in which the patient must perform three consecutive hand positions (e.g., fist, palm, side). Patients may be pulled to a stimulus and may "copy" a figure by drawing directly on top of the lines of the original figure. Dorsolateral prefrontal cortex also is responsible for motor programming.

Language may be normal in the early stages of frontal lobe dementia, but spontaneous verbal output is frequently reduced and responses are often brief. Empty speech, word-finding difficulties, circumlocution, impaired confrontation naming, and reduced verbal fluency may occur early in the course. Verbal fluency is

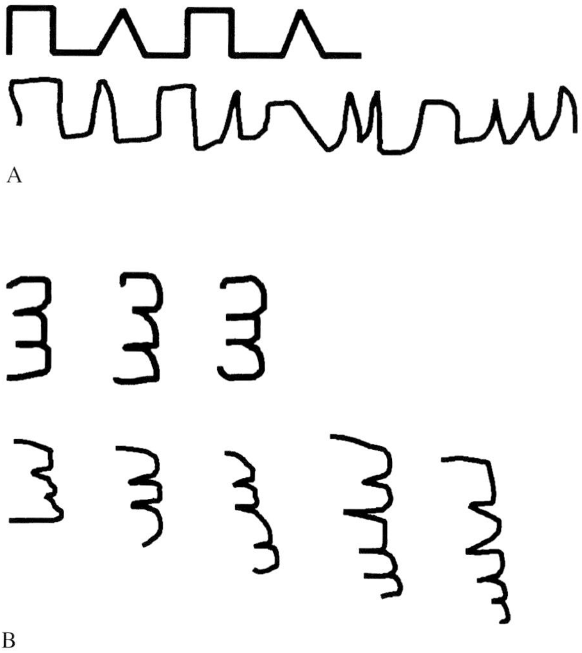

Figure 2.4 Perseveration in a patient with frontotemporal dementia as demonstrated by (A) alternating programs and (B) multiple loops.

a function of left dorsolateral prefrontal cortex and is impaired if the patient produces fewer than 12 animal names when asked to name as many animals as possible in 1 minute. Nonverbal fluency is a function of right prefrontal cortex and is impaired if the patient produces fewer than eight figures in 1 minute (four lines of equal length and each line must touch at least one other line). Occasional paraphasic errors can occur, and generic names such as "thing" may be used to indicate a variety of objects.

Some patients develop a semantic anomia. They may fail to accurately name a pen or a watch and when given the name in a multiple-choice list they may fail to recognize it. Comprehension may also be reduced due to auditory agnosia or "pure word deafness." These symptoms are rare in other brain diseases and are likely related to anterior temporal dysfunction.

Perseverative speech output is common and probably indicates significant involvement of dorsolateral prefrontal cortex. Initially, patients may repeat the same story or anecdote over and over. As the disease progresses, they may repeat a stereotyped phrase such as "I've got too damn many kids." They may reproduce this phrase in response to any question. A common stereotyped phrase is "Let's go . . . gotta go . . . let's go." This phrase is usually associated with anxiety in those patients who say it, and they begin repeating it soon after they arrive at a new location. Echolalia can develop with patients repeating phrases or words that are said to them. Apathy, aspontaneity, inattention, and concrete thinking may also affect patients' language ability, and it may be difficult to determine whether a true aphasia exists. Most patients with frontal lobe degeneration become mute in the final stages, and some may become mute before other cognitive functions are significantly impaired.

Premotor and motor cortex is generally spared in the course of frontal lobe degeneration but may be more prominently involved in other diseases that affect the frontal lobes. The neurologic examination is usually unremarkable except for the presence of primitive reflexes such as snout, suck, and grasp. These reflexes can become dramatic during the moderate to severe stages of the disease. Left-sided dysfunction is typically associated with reduced fluency, poverty of speech output, and brief replies. Right-sided dysfunction may be associated with affective aprosody, which is an inability to add emotional content to speech through the tone and inflection of voice. Supplementary motor area dysfunction may produce akinesia and bradykinesia. Later in the course there may be paralysis, spasticity, hyperreflexia, and left-sided apraxia. Urinary and fecal incontinence occur in the final stages. Subcortical involvement can cause parkinsonism in some patients, and dysfunction of the frontal eye fields can cause abnormalities of saccadic eye movements.

NEURODIAGNOSTIC ASSESSMENT

The Neuropsychiatric Inventory (NPI) is a 10-item caregiver-rated instrument designed to assess neuropsychiatric symptoms in dementia [36]. The profile of symptoms in 22 patients with FTD is illustrated in Figure 2.5. In this group, 21 patients had apathy and nine had depression; the severity of apathy was not correlated with severity of depression. Apathy was also present in 14 of the 15 patients who had disinhibition, but the disinhibited patients had significantly less

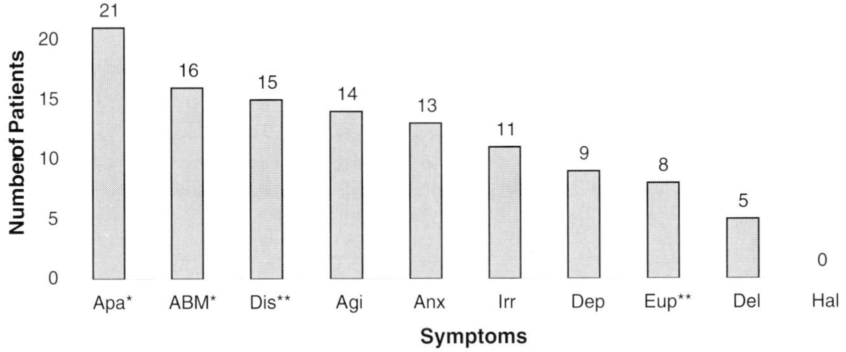

Figure 2.5 Neuropsychiatric symptom profile for the frontotemporal dementias (n = 22). (*Significantly more severe than in Alzheimer's disease (AD); **significantly more frequent and severe than in AD; Apa = apathy; AMB = aberrant motor behavior; Dis = disinhibition; Eup = euphoria; Hal = hallucinations; Del = delusions; Dep = depression; Irr = irritability; Anx = anxiety; Agi = agitation.)

Table 2.4 Neuropsychological tests of frontal lobe function

Test	*Function*
Naming (letter or category)	Verbal fluency
Design fluency	Nonverbal fluency
Wisconsin Card Sort	Set shifting
Trails B	Set shifting
Stroop color-word interference	Response inhibition
Similarities and differences	Abstraction
Proverbs	Abstraction
Cognitive estimates	Abstraction
Evaluation of insight and plans	Judgment
Rey auditory verbal learning test	Spontaneous recall
California verbal learning test	Spontaneous recall and memory organization
Rey-Osterrieth complex figure	Drawing strategies
Taylor complex figure	Drawing strategies
Draw-a-clock	Drawing strategies and stimulus boundedness
Consonant trigrams	Divided attention
Cancellation tests	Sustained attention
Alternating programs	Motor perseveration
Reciprocal programs	Motor perseveration
Multiple loops	Motor perseveration
Serial hand sequence	Motor perseveration

apathy compared to those without disinhibition. Euphoria is a rare symptom in AD but was present in 36% of FTD patients (see Figure 2.5). The NPI accurately assigned 77% of 22 FTD patients and 77% of 30 AD patients in this study to the correct diagnostic group. Patients with FTD had significantly more disinhibition and apathy and relatively less depression for their level of apathy [37]. Lopez and associates [38] used the Hamilton Depression Rating Scale [39] and found that eight of 20 FTD patients had depressed mood, whereas more than 70% had loss of interest, reduced motivation, social withdrawal, and anergia.

Barber and colleagues [40] developed a retrospective caregiver-based questionnaire that differentiates between AD and FTD. The instrument is designed for use in family history studies of dementia and has demonstrated the ability to separate autopsy-proved AD from FTD. Few other instruments include features helpful in distinguishing FTD and AD.

Neuropsychological tests reveal selective impairment of executive skills early in the course of FTD. Perseveration, set-shifting difficulties, and impairments in verbal fluency, attention, and response inhibition can be assessed with a variety of instruments (Table 2.4). Memory, calculation, and visuospatial skills are generally spared relative to executive function at mild to moderate levels of disease severity [34]; more global cognitive dysfunction is seen in more advanced stages of disease [41].

Several studies compared neuropsychological tests of AD and FTD patients. Johanson and Hagberg [42] found that FTD patients have greater dysfunction of expressive speech. Frisoni and colleagues [43] reported higher nonverbal learning scores in FTD patients and equal performance on verbal learning tasks, sug-

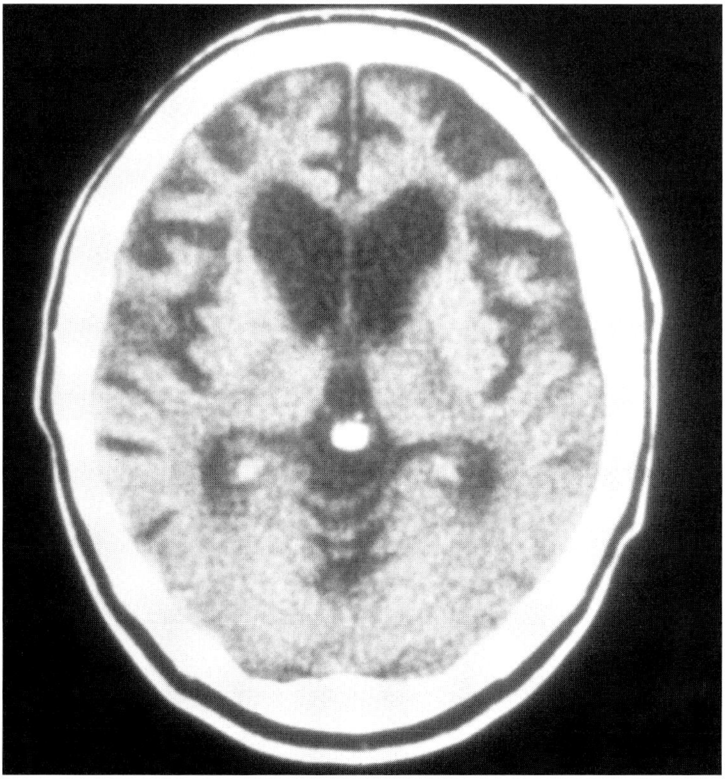

Figure 2.6 Magnetic resonance imaging scan of a patient with severe frontotemporal atrophy.

gesting that FTD patients may have a superior ability to learn despite having poor verbal fluency. Mendez and associates [44] found that FTD patients performed better on constructions and calculations than did AD patients with comparable global impairment. Pachana and coworkers [45] found that FTD patients exhibited greater impairment on executive tasks than on memory tasks, whereas AD patients had the reverse pattern, performing worse on memory than executive function tasks. Several smaller studies have reported conflicting results [34,46,47]. It should be noted that AD patients can have frontal dysfunction, especially patients with moderate to severe AD, and FTD patients can perform poorly on tests of posterior cortical function due to executive impairment.

Structural imaging, including computed tomography (CT) and magnetic resonance imaging (MRI), usually appear normal in the early stages of frontal lobe degeneration [6]. With progression there may be either generalized atrophy or frontotemporal lobar atrophy (Figure 2.6) [34]. The degree to which frontotemporal areas are disproportionately affected can vary considerably, and symmetry within the affected areas also can be variable. An abrupt transition is sometimes evident between involved and uninvolved areas, and coronal sections reveal deep sulci and knife-edged gyri, although these changes are more fre-

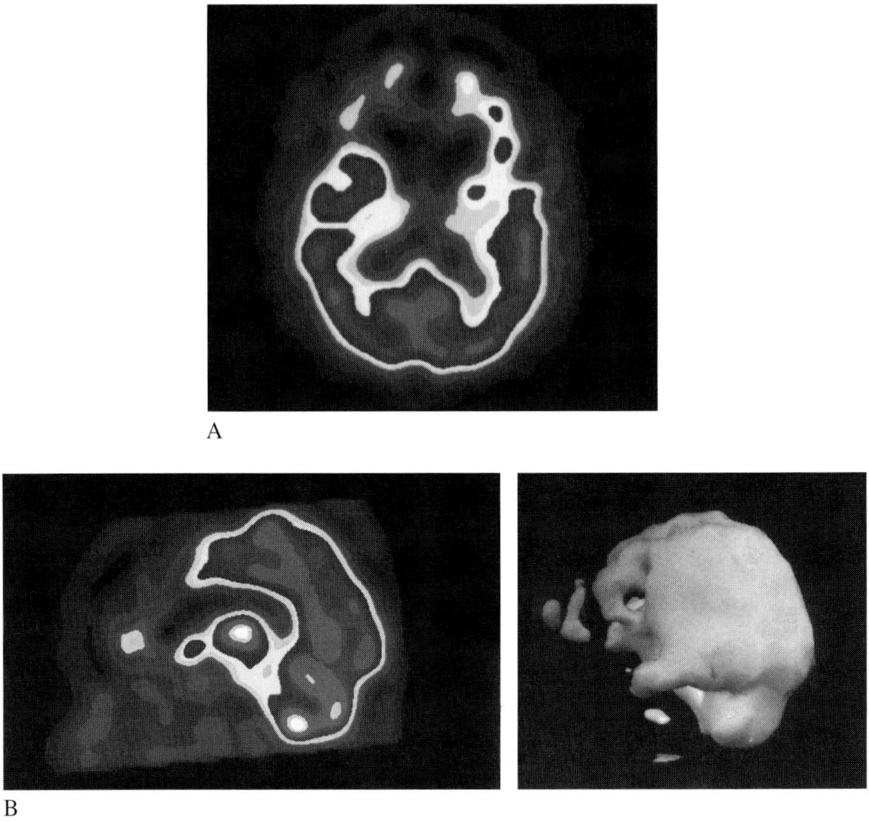

Figure 2.7 (A) Transverse cut of the brain from a patient with frontal lobe dementia imaged by hexamethyl propyleneamine oxime single photon emission computer tomography (SPECT) showing frontal hypoperfusion. (B) Sagittal sections from the left side of the brain of the same patient as in Figure 2.7A. On the left is a two-dimensional image and on the right is a computer-constructed three-dimensional image derived from multiple SPECT slices. (Courtesy of Dr. Fred Mishkin, Harbor-UCLA Medical Center, Torrance, CA.)

quent in PcD. The temporal horns of the lateral ventricles may be disproportionately dilated.

Functional imaging, including positron emission tomography (PET) and SPECT, show frontotemporal hypometabolism and hypoperfusion in patients with FTD (Figure 2.7) [34,43,46,48,49]. With xenon 133 SPECT measurements, frontal perfusion usually is less than 30 ml per 100 g tissue per minute, whereas parietal and occipital perfusion is between 35 to 45 ml per 100 g tissue per minute [34]. In patients with advanced disease, hypoperfusion appears posteriorly, although the frontal areas continue to show more severe abnormalities. Frontal abnormalities may be seen on functional imaging in a variety of other conditions, including chronic alcoholism [50], schizophrenia [51,52], depression [53], and progressive supranuclear palsy [54]. Vascular dementia and AD do not typically cause predominantly frontotemporal abnormalities, but occasionally patients have disproportionate frontal involvement that may be difficult to distinguish from FTD. Risberg and colleagues [55] reported four patients diagnosed clinically as having FTD. These patients all had reduced frontal blood flow based on xenon 133 SPECT. At autopsy, three had AD, and one had frontal lobe infarction.

Neuropsychological and psychiatric abnormalities in frontal lobe degeneration may be associated with dysfunction specific to frontal regions, although this area has received little investigation. Starkstein and associates [56] studied 16 mildly demented patients, eight with AD and eight with a frontal lobe dementia, using technetium Tc 99m hexamethyl propyleneamine oxime. They found that the latter patients with disinhibited behavior had more hypoperfusion in the orbitofrontal and anterior temporal cortex compared with AD patients without disinhibited behavior.

Quantitative electroencephalography (qEEG), also called *computed electroencephalography*, is a functional brain-mapping technique in which electroencephalogram tracings from various brain regions are subjected to computerized analysis. Power is a measure of energy based on the amplitude and frequency, and coherence is a measure of the degree to which waveforms are synchronized. Coherence may be a measure of functional connections among different brain regions. This technology is only recently being perfected and there are few studies comparing dementing illnesses. Yener and colleagues [57] found that qEEG could be used to differentiate among FTD, AD, and age-matched controls. They found that the qEEG measures that best separated FTD and AD were in the temporal and parietal regions. Mean left temporal beta-2 and left parietal theta band relative power were higher in AD than FTD, whereas mean right parietal beta-2 and right parietal alpha were lower in AD than FTD. These results were consistent with the only other published study of FTD and qEEG [58].

DIAGNOSTIC CLASSIFICATION

Dementia due to other general medical conditions appears in the *Diagnostic and Statistical Manual of Mental Disorders* (4th ed) (*DSM-IV*) [59] and subsumes dementias not due to AD or cerebrovascular disease (Table 2.5). The essential points of the definition are that memory and other cognitive deficits develop gradually over time, impair function, and are the direct physiologic consequence of the general medical condition, and that delirium does not explain the dysfunction. A list of other general medical conditions is provided that includes PcD but should presumably also include other types of FTD. The features of PcD are described as changes in personality early in the course, deterioration of social skills, emotional blunting, behavioral disinhibition, and prominent language abnormalities.

The International Classification of Diseases (10th ed) (*ICD-10*) [60] specifies several criteria that must exist for a dementia to be present, including a decline in memory and other cognitive abilities. A decline in emotional control or motivation or a change in social behavior must be present and the patient must have a clear sensorium with symptoms present for at least 6 months (Table 2.6). The *ICD-10* further specifies dementia in Pick's disease under the categorical heading of Dementia

Table 2.5 Diagnostic criteria for Dementia Due to Other General Medical Conditions* from the *Diagnostic and Statistical Manual of Mental Disorders* (4th ed)

A. Both of the following:
   (1) Memory impairment
   (2) One or more of the following:
      (a) Aphasia
      (b) Apraxia
      (c) Agnosia
      (d) Disturbance in executive functioning
B. Significant impairment in social or occupational functioning and significant decline from previous level of functioning
C. Disturbance is the direct physiologic consequence of a general medical condition
D. Deficits do not occur exclusively during the course of a delirium

*Pick's disease may be specified as the general medical condition, and the manual provides a paragraph with a general description of the syndrome.

Source: Reprinted from American Psychiatric Association. Diagnostic and Statistical Manual of Mental Disorders (4th ed). Washington, DC: American Psychiatric Association, 1994.

Table 2.6 Diagnostic criteria for dementia from *The International Classification of Diseases* (10th ed)

Dementia

G1. Both of the following:
   (1) Decline in memory
   (2) Decline in other cognitive abilities
G2. Absence of clouding of consciousness
G3. Decline in emotional control, motivation, or social behavior:
   (1) Emotional lability
   (2) Irritability
   (3) Apathy
   (4) Coarsening of social behavior
G4. Symptoms present for at least 6 months

Dementia in Pick's disease

A. General criteria for dementia (G1–G4) must be met
B. Onset is slow with steady deterioration
C. Two or more of the following:
   (1) Emotional blunting
   (2) Coarsening of social behavior
   (3) Disinhibition
   (4) Apathy or restlessness
   (5) Aphasia
D. In the early stages, memory and parietal lobe functions are relatively preserved

Source: Reprinted from World Health Organization. Classification of Mental and Behavioral Disorders: Clinical Descriptions and Diagnostic Guidelines. In The International Classification of Diseases (10th ed). Geneva: World Health Organization, 1992.

Table 2.7 Core clinical diagnostic features of frontotemporal dementia

Behavioral disorder	
	Insidious onset and slow progression
	Early loss of personal awareness
	Early loss of social awareness
	Early signs of disinhibition
	Mental rigidity and inflexibility
	Hyperorality
	Stereotyped and perseverative behavior
	Utilization behavior
	Distractibility, impulsivity, and impersistence
Affective symptoms	
	Depression, anxiety, excessive sentimentality, suicidal ideation, delusion
	Hypochondriasis, bizarre somatic preoccupation
	Emotional unconcern
	Amimia (aspontaneity)
Speech disorder	
	Progressive reduction of speech
	Stereotypy of speech
	Echolalia and perseveration
	Late mutism
Spatial orientation and praxis preserved	
Physical signs	
	Early primitive reflexes
	Early incontinence
	Late akinesia, rigidity, tremor
	Low and labile blood pressure
Investigations	
	Electroencephalogram: normal
	Brain imaging: frontal or anterior temporal changes
	Neuropsychological tests: fail frontal lobe tests

Source: Adapted from A Brun, B Englund, L Gustafson, et al. Consensus statement: clinical and neuropathological criteria for frontotemporal dementia; the Lund and Manchester Groups. J Neurol Neurosurg Psychiatry 1994;57:416.

in Other Diseases Elsewhere Classified. The critical elements are a slow, steady deterioration, predominance of frontal lobe involvement, and relatively preserved memory and parietal lobe functions early in the course. The major difference between the *ICD-10* and the *DSM-IV* criteria is that the *DSM-IV* requires a functional impairment whereas the *ICD-10* requires merely a change in social behavior.

Clinical and neuropathological criteria for FTD were published in the form of a consensus statement by the Lund and Manchester groups [2] (Table 2.7). The main clinical features include insidious onset, early behavioral and affective changes, speech disorder, primitive reflexes, and relatively preserved spatial orientation and praxis. Features supportive of the diagnosis include onset before age 65 years, predominantly frontal abnormalities on structural or functional imaging, and profound failure on neuropsychological tests of frontal lobe function in the absence of severe amnesia, aphasia, or perceptual spatial disorder. Miller and colleagues [61] tested the clinical criteria in Table 2.7 and found that loss of personal awareness, hyperorality, stereotyped and perseverative behavior, progressive reduction of speech, and preservation of spatial orientation and praxis differentiated 100% of 30 FTD and 30 AD subjects. The Lund-Manchester criteria also describe neuropathologic features of FTD, dividing them into three categories: frontal lobe degeneration, Pick-type, and motor neuron disease–type.

CLINICAL DIAGNOSIS

In practice, the diagnosis of FTD begins by taking a careful longitudinal history. Symptoms of frontal lobe dysfunction should not immediately lead to the diagnosis of FTD. Other medical conditions should be excluded if the onset is acute, subacute, or fluctuating; if the time course is stepwise; or if the patient is inattentive or delirious. A dementing illness may be suspected if the onset is insidious over several years and the patient is in the presenium or senium. Laboratory tests that may be used for initial screening include a complete blood count; urinalysis; analysis of electrolytes and calcium, liver functions, blood urea nitrogen and creatinine, thyroid functions (thyroid-stimulating hormone, free thyroxine index), and serum B_{12}; and a fluorescent treponemal antibody absorption test. A structural image such as a CT or MRI scan should be obtained to rule out tumors, subdural hematomas, or hydrocephalus. Functional imaging is not clinically necessary but may help differentiate dementia syndromes in ambiguous cases and aid in distinguishing FTD from AD (see Chapter 9). It does not help in differentiating different types of FTD.

A diagnosis of FTD is suggested by early changes in personality including disinhibition, sociopathy, hyperorality, euphoria, reduced speech output, and severe apathy with executive function impairment, such as perseveration and poor judgment. Relative preservation of memory and visuospatial function supports the diagnosis, and patients may also have primitive reflexes such as snout, suck, and grasp. Fasciculations or other evidence of motor neuron disease may be associated with FTD-ALS. Neuropsychological testing may provide additional information that can further differentiate the specific dementia syndrome. Clinical features do not distinguish frontal lobe degeneration and PcD.

A personal or family history of affective illness or the presence of sadness, anhedonia, guilt, or hopelessness may indicate a depressive disorder. An early movement disorder such as parkinsonism or chorea may indicate the presence of a subcortical dementia syndrome. Early memory and visuospatial difficulty suggests AD, and focal neurologic symptoms, such as paresis or hyperreflexia, may be associated with vascular causes of brain injury.

GENETICS

FTD may be familial in 60% of cases [7], and in 1994 a variant of FTD with dementia, disinhibition, parkinsonism, and amyotrophy was linked to chromosome 17 [62]. Subsequently, eight kindreds have been definitely linked to the q21–22 region on chromosome 17 and five more kindreds are probably linked. Twelve other kindreds have been found to have similar clinical and neuropathologic features, but linkage has yet to be shown. In at least two families, the q21–22 region has been excluded, and one of these families has been linked to chromosome 3 [23].

Chromosome 17–linked disorders are phenotypically heterogenous even within the same kindred, but there are many clinical and neuropathologic features that appear consistently. The age of onset; clinical course; imaging findings; and cognitive, psychiatric, and behavioral symptoms are the same as those described for FTD except that there is more prominent and earlier involvement of the pyramidal and extrapyramidal motor systems. Parkinsonism without resting tremor is a common finding; corticospinal disturbances, muscle wasting, and fasciculations are also common. Among the names that have been given to these chromosome 17–linked dementia syndromes are *hereditary dysphasic disinhibition dementia*, *pallido-ponto-nigral degeneration*, *familial multiple system tauopathy with presenile dementia*, *familial progressive subcortical gliosis*, and *familial frontal lobe degeneration of the non-Alzheimer type*.

SUMMARY

Frontotemporal dementia is a clinical syndrome of unknown etiology marked by early personality changes such as apathy, sociopathy, disinhibition, and euphoria, and by behavioral disturbances such as hyperorality, dietary change, and repetitive behaviors. There is progressive impairment of executive function and language, but memory and visuospatial skills are relatively well preserved until late in the course. There are several histopathologic subtypes including PcD, frontal lobe degeneration, and FTD-ALS. A variety of disorders may produce symptoms of frontal lobe dysfunction and need to be assessed before the diagnosis of FTD can be confirmed. Neurodiagnostic tests such as psychiatric inventories, neuropsychological evaluations, and structural and functional neuroimaging enable more accurate differentiation from other dementia syndromes. Finally, genetic linkages to chromosomes 3 and 17 may offer new hope for understanding the basic pathophysiology of these unusual and devastating conditions.

REFERENCES

1. Frisoni GB, Beltramello A, Geroldi C. Brain atrophy in frontotemporal dementia. J Neurol Neurosurg Psychiatry 1996;61:157–165.
2. Brun A, Englund B, Gustafson L, et al. Consensus statement: clinical and neuropathological criteria for frontotemporal dementia; the Lund and Manchester Groups. J Neurol Neurosurg Psychiatry 1994;57:416–418.
3. Miller BL, Chang L, Oropilla G, et al. Alzheimer's Disease and Frontal Lobe Dementias. In CE Coffey, JL Cummings (eds), American Psychiatric Press Textbook of Geriatric Neuropsychiatry. Washington, DC: American Psychological Association, 1994;389–404.
4. Neary D, Snowden J. Fronto-temporal dementia: nosology, neuropsychology, and neuropathology. Brain Cogn 1996;31:176–187.
5. Gustafson L, Brun A, Risberg J. Frontal lobe dementia of non-Alzheimer type. Adv Neurol 1990; 51:65–71.
6. Brun A. Frontal lobe degeneration of non-Alzheimer type. I. Neuropathology. Arch Gerontol Geriatr 1987;6:193–208.

7. Gustafson L. Clinical picture of frontal lobe degeneration of non-Alzheimer type. Dementia 1993; 4:143–148.
8. Knopman DS, Mastri AR, Frey WH. Dementia lacking distinctive histologic features: a common non-Alzheimer degenerative dementia. Neurology 1990;40:251–256.
9. Kertesz A, Kalvach P. Arnold Pick and German neuropsychiatry in Prague. Arch Neurol 1996;53: 935–938.
10. Pick A. On the Relation between Aphasia and Senile Atrophy of the Brain (1892). WC Schoene (trans). In DA Rottenberg, FH Hochberg (eds), Neurological Classics in Modern Translation. New York: Hafner, 1977;35–40.
11. Alzheimer A. Über eigenartige Krankheitsfalle des spateren Alters. Z Ges Neurol Psychiatr 1911; 4:356–385.
12. Mendez MF, Selwood A, Mastri AR, et al. Pick's disease versus Alzheimer's disease: a comparison of clinical characteristics. Neurology 1993;43:289–292.
13. Jackson M, Lowe J. The new neuropathology of degenerative frontotemporal dementias. Acta Neuropathol 1996;91:127–134.
14. Mann DMA, Neary D, Testa H. Color Atlas and Text of Adult Dementias. New York: Mosby–Wolfe, 1994;71–95.
15. Morita K, Kaiya H, Ikeda T, et al. Presenile dementia combined with amyotrophy: a review of 34 Japanese cases. Arch Gerontol Geriatr 1987;6:263–277.
16. Neumann MA, Cohn R. Progressive subcortical gliosis; a rare form of presenile dementia. Brain 1967;90:405–418.
17. Verity MA, Wechsler AF. Progressive subcortical gliosis of Neumann: a clinicopathologic study of two cases with review. Arch Gerontol Geriatr 1987;6:245–261.
18. Gibb WRG, Luthert PT, Marsden CD. Corticobasal degeneration. Brain 1989;112:1171–1192.
19. Rebeiz JJ, Kolodny EH, Richardson EP Jr. Corticodentatonigral degeneration with neuronal achromasia. Arch Neurol 1968;18:20–33.
20. Morris JC, Cole M, Banker BQ, et al. Hereditary dysphasic dementia and the Pick-Alzheimer spectrum. Ann Neurol 1984;16:455–466.
21. Heutink P, Stevens M, Rizzu P, et al. Hereditary frontotemporal dementia is linked to chromosome 17q21–q22: a genetic and clinicopathological study of three Dutch families. Ann Neurol 1997;41: 150–159.
22. Foster NL, Wilhelmsen K, Sima AA, et al. Frontotemporal dementia and parkinsonism linked to chromosome 17: a consensus statement. Ann Neurol 1997;41:706–715.
23. Brown J, Ashworth A, Gydesen S, et al. Familial non-specific dementia maps to chromosome 3. Hum Mol Genet 1995;4:1625–1628.
24. Mesulam MM. Slowly progressive aphasia without generalized dementia. Ann Neurol 1982;11: 592–598.
25. Miller BL, Chang L, Mena I, et al. Progressive right frontotemporal degeneration: clinical, neuropsychological and SPECT characteristics. Dementia 1993;4:204–213.
26. Hodges JR, Patterson K, Oxbury S, et al. Semantic dementia. Progressive fluent aphasia with temporal lobe atrophy. Brain 1992;115:1783–1806.
27. Benson DF. Progressive frontal dysfunction. Dementia 1993;4:149–153.
28. Cummings JL. Fronto-subcortical circuits and human behavior. Arch Neurol 1993;50:873–880.
29. Swartz JR, Miller BL, Lesser IM, et al. Frontotemporal dementia: treatment response to serotonin selective reuptake inhibitors. J Clin Psychiatry 1997;58:212–216.
30. Miller BL, Darby A, Benson DF, et al. Aggressive, socially disruptive and antisocial behaviour associated with fronto-temporal dementia. Br J Psychiatry 1997;170:150–154.
31. Miller BL, Darby AL, Swartz JR, et al. Dietary changes, compulsions and sexual behavior in frontotemporal degeneration. Dementia 1995;6:195–199.
32. Ames D, Cummings JL, Wirshing WC, et al. Repetitive and compulsive behavior in frontal lobe degenerations. J Neuropsychiatry Clin Neurosci 1994;6:100–113.
33. Klüver H, Bucy PC. Preliminary analysis of functions of the temporal lobes in monkeys. Arch Neurol Psychiatry 1939;42:979–1000.
34. Miller BL, Cummings JL, Villanueva-Meyer J, et al. Frontal lobe degeneration: clinical, neuropsychological, and SPECT characteristics. Neurology 1991;41:1374–1382.
35. Luria AR. Two kinds of motor perseveration in massive injury to the frontal lobes. Brain 1965; 88:1–10.
36. Cummings JL, Mega M, Gray K, et al. The Neuropsychiatric Inventory: comprehensive assessment of psychopathology in dementia. Neurology 1994;44:2308–2314.

37. Levy ML, Miller BL, Cummings JL, et al. Alzheimer disease and frontotemporal dementias: behavioral distinctions. Arch Neurol 1996;53:687–690.
38. Lopez OL, Gonzalez MP, Becker JT. Symptoms of depression and psychosis in Alzheimer's disease and frontotemporal dementia: exploration of underlying mechanisms. Neuropsychiatry Neuropsychol Behav Neurol 1996;9:154–161.
39. Hamilton M. Development of a rating scale for primary depressive illness. Br J Soc Psychol 1967;44: 929–932.
40. Barber R, Snowden JS, Craufurd D. Frontotemporal dementia and Alzheimer's disease: retrospective differentiation using information from informants. J Neurol Neurosurg Psychiatry 1995;59:61–70.
41. Elfgren C, Passant U, Risberg J. Neuropsychological findings in frontal lobe dementia. Dementia 1993;4:214–219.
42. Johanson A, Hagberg B. Psychometric characteristics in patients with frontal lobe degeneration of non-Alzheimer type. Arch Gerontol Geriatr 1989;8:129–137.
43. Frisoni GB, Pizzolato G, Geroldi C, et al. Dementia of the frontal type: neuropsychological and [^{99}Tc]-HM-PAO SPET features. J Geriatr Psychiatry Neurol 1995;8:42–48.
44. Mendez MF, Cherrier M, Perryman KM, et al. Frontotemporal dementia versus Alzheimer's disease: differential cognitive features. Neurology 1996;47:1189–1194.
45. Pachana NA, Boone KB, Miller BL, et al. Comparison of neuropsychological functioning in Alzheimer's disease and frontotemporal dementia. J Int Neuropsychol Soc 1996;2:505–510.
46. Jagust WJ, Reed BR, Scab JP, et al. Clinical-physiologic correlates of Alzheimer's disease and frontal lobe dementia. Am J Physiol Imaging 1989;4:89–96.
47. Neary D, Snowden JS, Bowen DM, et al. Neuropsychological syndromes in presenile dementia due to cerebral atrophy. J Neurol Neurosurg Psychiatry 1986;49:163–174.
48. Herholz K. FDG PET and differential diagnosis of dementia. Alzheimer Dis Assoc Disord 1995;9: 6–16.
49. Neary D, Snowden JS, Shields RA, et al. Single photon emission tomography using ^{99m}Tc-HM-PAO in the investigation of dementia. J Neurol Neurosurg Psychiatry 1987;50:1101–1109.
50. Volkow ND, Hitzemann R, Wang GJ, et al. Decreased brain metabolism in neurologically intact healthy alcoholics. Am J Psychiatry 1992;149:1016–1022.
51. Buchsbaum MS, Haier RJ, Potkin SG, et al. Frontostriatal disorder of cerebral metabolism in never-medicated schizophrenics. Arch Gen Psychiatry 1992;49:935–942.
52. Wolkin A, Sanfilipo M, Wolf AP, et al. Negative symptoms and hypofrontality in chronic schizophrenia. Arch Gen Psychiatry 1992;49:959–965.
53. Baxter LR Jr, Schwartz JM, Phelps ME, et al. Reduction of prefrontal cortex glucose metabolism common to three types of depression. Arch Gen Psychiatry 1989;46:243–250.
54. Blin J, Baron JC, Dubois B, et al. Positron emission tomography study in progressive-supranuclear-palsy—brain hypometabolic pattern and clinicometabolic correlations. Arch Neurol 1990;47:747–752.
55. Risberg J, Passant U, Warkentin S, et al. Regional cerebral blood flow in frontal lobe dementia of non-Alzheimer type. Dementia 1993;4:186–187.
56. Starkstein SE, Migliorelli R, Teson A, et al. Specificity of changes in cerebral blood flow in patients with frontal lobe dementia. J Neurol Neurosurg Psychiatry 1994;57:790–796.
57. Yener GG, Leuchter AF, Jenden D, et al. Quantitative EEG in frontotemporal dementia. Clin Electroencephalogr 1996;27:61–68.
58. Stigsby B, Johannesson G, Ingvar DH. Regional EEG analysis and regional cerebral blood flow in Alzheimer's and Pick's diseases. Electroencephalogr Clin Neurophysiol 1981;51:537–547.
59. American Psychiatric Association. Diagnostic and Statistical Manual of Mental Disorders (4th ed). Washington, DC: American Psychiatric Association, 1994.
60. World Health Organization. Classification of Mental and Behavioral Disorders: Clinical Descriptions and Diagnostic Guidelines. In The International Classification of Diseases (10th ed). Geneva: World Health Organization, 1992.
61. Miller BL, Ikonte C, Ponton M, et al. A study of the Lund-Manchester research criteria for frontotemporal dementia. Neurology 1997;48:937–942.
62. Wilhelmsen KC, Lynch T, Pavlou E, et al. Localization of disinhibition-dementia-parkinsonism-amyotrophy complex to 17q21–22. Am J Hum Genet 1994;55:1159–1165.

3
Dementia with Lewy Bodies

Graham G. Lennox

Dementia with Lewy bodies (DLB) is currently the recommended term for a condition that has been described under a bewildering variety of rubrics, including *diffuse* or *cortical Lewy body disease* [1], *Lewy body dementia* [2], *senile dementia of Lewy body type* [3], and the *Lewy body variant of Alzheimer's disease* (AD) [4]. The earliest descriptions of DLB have recently been rediscovered in the seminal German literature of the early twentieth century, but the first detailed reports of cases appeared in an American journal in 1961 [5]. A stream of subsequent reports from Japan [6,7] led to the description of cases with large series since the late 1980s [8–10]. A reasonably coherent picture of the clinical features of DLB has emerged from these studies [11].

This chapter focuses on the clinical aspects of DLB, aiming to outline both the typical clinical picture and the range of atypical presentations that may give rise to difficulties in diagnosis, and to provide a pragmatic guide to diagnosis and treatment. The clinicopathologic studies, however, have not yet answered some of the most fundamental questions about DLB, such as the pathologic basis of the dementia itself, the relationship between DLB and AD, and the etiology of DLB. Molecular studies are starting to shed some light on these issues, and this chapter briefly reviews some of these scientific advances.

EPIDEMIOLOGY

DLB is defined as a disorder with the core clinical feature of dementia and the characteristic pathology of Lewy bodies within cortical neurons. Several autopsy series have shown that approximately 15–25% of demented patients fit this definition of DLB [3,9,12–19]. In hospital series, DLB is the second most common pathologic finding after AD. It is also a common pathologic finding in patients who have been diagnosed as having AD on the basis of the currently accepted diagnostic criteria [4,15]. Most cases are elderly, although young-onset cases do occur. There may be a slight preponderance of men.

Attempts to study the prevalence of DLB in clinical populations have been limited by the lack of a specific test for the disorder and the fact that a consensus on clinical diagnostic criteria has only recently emerged. Studies using a range of clinical diagnostic criteria have, however, produced similar estimates of prevalence (10–26%) in both community and hospital samples of elderly people with dementia [20–23]. DLB is a common disorder and accounts for a significant proportion of the workload of psychiatrists treating elderly patients.

PATHOLOGY

Cortical Lewy bodies are pale hyaline eosinophilic inclusions that can be identified with experience using conventional hematoxylin and eosin stains but which are perhaps more readily quantified using special stains such as ubiquitin immunohistochemistry [24,25]. They are almost invariably associated with the classic core-and-halo Lewy bodies in pigmented brain stem nuclei that are the pathologic hallmark of Parkinson's disease (PD). Indeed, the brain stem pathology in most cases of DLB is indistinguishable from that of PD [13]. For this reason, it has been suggested that PD and DLB may have a close nosologic relationship as different parts of a single spectrum of Lewy body disorders.

Both PD and DLB share a second and probably related pathologic feature, the dystrophic neurite. These swollen processes have a similar immunohistochemical profile to that of Lewy bodies and are again best identified using ubiquitin stains. They are typically found in the CA2–3 region of the hippocampus, although they occur elsewhere in subcortical nuclei and the cerebral cortex in a distribution that mirrors that of the Lewy bodies [26].

Complicating matters is the observation that most elderly cases of DLB also have senile pathology such as senile plaques, and many also have neurofibrillary tangles [2]. The plaques are of a kind that Dickson and colleagues [27] have described as indicative of pathologic aging rather than AD, taking the form of diffuse amyloid deposits and lacking a *tau*-immunoreactive neuritic component [14]; their density correlates with that of the cortical Lewy bodies [13]. It is probably legitimate to regard such plaques as part of the pathology of DLB rather than indicative of a second diagnosis of AD.

The presence of neurofibrillary tangles and neuropil threads in approximately 50% of DLB cases, however, does raise the question of a nosologic relationship with AD. Qualitative and quantitative differences between DLB and AD usually are present in the distribution of these pathologies—for example, tangles commonly spare the hippocampus in DLB but almost invariably affect it severely in AD [14,28]. There are two main hypotheses to explain this pathologic overlap: (1) chance coincidence of two common pathologic processes and (2) shared genetic risk factors. The latter hypothesis is discussed in more detail in a later section, Genetics.

The neurochemical pathology of DLB reflects the histologic picture. The damage to the substantia nigra causes a reduction in caudate dopamine levels, whereas damage in the nucleus basalis leads to a severe reduction in cholinergic markers such as choline acetyltransferase (ChAT) in the cerebral cortex [29]. In fact, the ChAT reductions are more severe than those found in AD except in the hippocampus, which generally is spared [29,30]. The cholinergic deficits are particularly severe in patients who experience hallucinations; conversely, reductions in 5-hydroxytryptamine markers tend to be more severe in those who do not [31] have hallucinations. The relative selectivity of these neurochemical deficits allows some optimism regarding drug treatment.

CLINICAL FEATURES

The central clinical feature of DLB is a progressive dementia. This is typically slowly progressive and leads to a global dementia over a period of several years. In most established cases, there is a temporoparietal pattern of cognitive deficits, with impairment of memory, language, and visuospatial skills. At this stage, DLB often appears to be similar to AD. Some important psychometric differences between the two conditions have been noted, however, especially in the first 2–3 years of the illness [4,32–34].

First, in the early stages of illness, patients with DLB may have either no memory deficit or a selective deficit of memory retrieval, which differs from the deficit in memory acquisition and consolidation of AD. Although these differences were demonstrated using detailed psychometry, they are often discernible on simple bedside tests of memory (such as recall of a list of items or a name and address) [34]. DLB patients often recall nothing at first but with judicious prompting suddenly remember all the items correctly. In this respect, DLB patients often behave more like patients with frontotemporal dementia than patients with AD.

Second, other manifestations of frontal lobe dysfunction may be more prominent in DLB than in AD in the early stages of illness. Again, these were demonstrated using psychometric tests of executive function such as the Wisconsin Card Sorting Test and the Trail-Making Test. It is harder to translate these into simple bedside tests, particularly as most tests of executive function are sensitive to the confounding effects of premorbid intelligence, but disproportionate difficulty with tests of verbal fluency for letters and categories may provide a useful pointer toward DLB. Perhaps the most useful guide comes from behavioral observations: Patients with DLB often have a greater degree of disinhibition or apathy and less insight into their disabilities than AD patients with a similar overall level of cognitive impairment. They also tend to be more inattentive.

Third, the early loss of visuospatial skills tends to be more severe in DLB than in AD. This is revealed, for example, by the block design subtest of the Wechsler Adult Intelligence Scale and on bedside tests such as clock drawing and figure copying. Clinicians who are used to visuospatial skills deteriorating in line with the overall level of dementia in AD may be startled to find mildly demented patients with DLB who are completely unable to arrange the numbers on a clock.

The pattern of language disturbance in DLB is not greatly different from that found in AD, although DLB patients may show the phenomenon of speech block (which is also seen in PD) early in the course of their illness. This progresses to word-finding difficulty and then frank dysphasia.

Table 3.1 Early cognitive impairments in dementia with Lewy bodies and Alzheimer's disease

	Dementia with Lewy bodies	*Alzheimer's disease*
Memory	± (normal or retrieval defect)	++ (acquisition defect)
Executive functions	++	±
Visuospatial functions	++	+
Language	+	+
Fluctuations	+++	±

± = absent or mild; + = mild; ++ = moderate; +++ = severe.

These differences in the pattern of early cognitive deficit are summarized in Table 3.1. But perhaps the most striking difference between DLB and AD is not in the nature of the cognitive deficits but in the fluctuation in their severity [3,8]. All patients with dementia experience some variation in their abilities, which tend to deteriorate toward the end of the day or when they are anxious or in unfamiliar surroundings. Most patients with DLB have much greater swings in their abilities, which cannot be explained by exogenous factors. In the early stages, patients may have periods of cognitive impairment that alternate with periods of normality or near normality. Attention and alertness are often affected during the periods of impairment, giving the impression of a recurring confusional state. Such patients are often repeatedly subjected to a search for intercurrent infection or are erroneously diagnosed as suffering from cerebrovascular disease. Persistent cognitive impairment eventually emerges and it becomes clear that these episodes were the first manifestation of DLB.

Fluctuation often persists, however, with even moderately demented patients experiencing occasional "good days" of lucidity and markedly improved functioning. Some patients have more rapid fluctuations, lasting only minutes or hours; caregivers will report that these patients have "blank spells." Such episodes may give rise to concern over the possibility of epilepsy, but they are not associated with paroxysmal changes in the surface electroencephalogram (EEG) and are probably related to changes in the frontal-subcortical systems that control attention. A few patients have slower changes occurring over weeks or months. Again, caregivers will usually draw attention to these swings, but they are also apparent on serial interviews or psychometric assessments.

The range of different types of fluctuation causes difficulty in devising simple operational criteria that can robustly distinguish them from the minor variations seen in all dementing illnesses. It is clear, however, that fluctuations are very common in DLB and, to an experienced physician, are an important clinical pointer to the diagnosis [11].

Another important pointer is the development of visual hallucinations. Again, a range of interrelated perceptual disorders occurs [35]. Many patients experience true visual hallucinations, seeing complex and detailed images in the absence of a triggering external stimulus. The images are typically of people or animals that may be familiar to the patient, and they often move and make noises and are occasionally distorted in size or shape. These hallucinations tend to be more common and prolonged (but less detailed) in patients with pre-existing visual impairment due to ocular disease [36], suggesting a contribution from the Charles-Bonnet phenomenon (in which blind people see complex images, often following the onset of additional brain disease). Sometimes the hallucinations can be relieved by improving visual function (with new glasses or better lighting) or by providing a more stimulating general environment.

In some cases the images arise out of misperception of external stimuli: For example, the patient may see figures or writing in a wallpaper pattern. These patients often have evidence of visual agnosia on bedside testing. Often hallucination and misperception coexist. If these perceptual disturbances occur in isolation, they may be surprisingly well tolerated by the patient, who may react to them with relatively little distress. Some patients come to realize that the images are unreal (i.e., so-called *pseudohallucinations*) and are actually amused by them.

In approximately 50% of cases, however, the visual hallucinations are accompanied by delusions, usually with an unpleasant persecutory theme. Delusional misidentification of people, the patient's own mirror image, and pictures also occurs in many patients, usually transiently [37]. Although many patients report that they can hear their hallucinatory figures talking, they often find it hard to make out the words and clear third-person auditory hallucinations are rare, as are auditory hallucinations in the absence of visual ones. Olfactory or sensory hallucinations are very rare.

Visual hallucinations carry considerable diagnostic weight. Persistent visual hallucinations occur in approximately 80% of patients with DLB; they are much less common in other dementing illnesses, including AD. When visual hallucinations do occur in AD, they are often transient and are frequently part of a delirium provoked by intercurrent illness. Visual hallucinations in AD are also usually silent.

Another feature of diagnostic value is the spontaneous development of the motor manifestations of parkinsonism. In patients whose first symptoms have been cognitive, the parkinsonism is often mild and typically takes the form of a stooped posture, shuffling gait, and mild rigidity and bradykinesia in the upper limbs. Hypomimia and hypophonia are also common. The classic resting tremor of PD is the least common motor feature, although many patients do develop a mild and atypical tremor with a substantial postural or action component. Another difference from PD is that the parkinsonism is very rarely unilateral, or even markedly asymmetric, in patients who have presented with dementia. The parkinsonism in some but not all cases is responsive to levodopa [38].

The parkinsonism tends to progress, and by the late stages of DLB it may become a significant source of disability in its own right, causing frequent falls, immobility, and feeding problems.

The presence of parkinsonism is of diagnostic value when it occurs early in the course of DLB [39,40]. Parkinsonism is, however, a relatively common feature of almost all dementing illnesses in their late stages, including AD, frontotemporal dementias, vascular dementias, and Creutzfeldt-Jakob disease (CJD). Parkinsonism can also occur as an early feature in AD (due to neuronal loss and tangle formation within the substantia nigra), but this appears to be rare [9,41].

It is much harder to interpret the significance of parkinsonism that develops after exposure to neuroleptic drugs. Severe rigidity and obtundation, particularly if it persists after the drug is withdrawn, do raise the possibility of underlying Lewy body disease [42]. Milder and short-lived forms of drug-induced parkinsonism are much less specific, although even here a suspicion may be raised if

Table 3.2 Clinical features in favor of a diagnosis of dementia with Lewy bodies

Features strongly associated with dementia with Lewy bodies:
Cognitive fluctuation
Visual hallucinations (with or without hallucinations in other modalities)
Spontaneous parkinsonism
Features with less firmly established strength of association:
Repeated falls
Blackouts
Sensitivity to adverse effects of neuroleptics

the parkinsonism seems out of proportion to the dose and potency of the neuroleptic used (Table 3.2).

Other movement disorders occur in DLB, particularly myoclonus [38]. This is usually mild, spontaneous, and multifocal. A few patients develop very prominent myoclonus. Chorea occasionally occurs, often early in the disease, as does dystonia, usually in the later stages. A combination of alien limb phenomena and apraxia resembling corticobasal degeneration has also been described [43].

Autonomic dysfunction occurs in DLB, although relatively little systematic work has been done to establish its prevalence. It may be one cause of episodes of apparent syncope that are quite common in patients with established dementia due to DLB. Upgaze palsy is common in established DLB but very nonspecific [44,45]. Orofacial dyskinesia can occur, even without exposure to neuroleptics [46]. Pyramidal signs, such as spasticity and extensor plantar responses, tend to occur late in the disease.

CLINICAL DIAGNOSTIC CRITERIA

These features have been used as the basis for clinical diagnostic criteria, devised with the primary intention of facilitating diagnosis in the group of patients who present with dementia. A consortium meeting consolidated two early sets of criteria from Nottingham and Newcastle [47,48]. The revised criteria [11] have the central requirement of a progressive cognitive decline of sufficient magnitude to interfere with normal social or occupational function, in which memory impairment may not necessarily occur in the early stages but is usually evident with progression, and deficits on tests of attention and frontal-subcortical skills and visuospatial ability may be especially prominent. In addition to this, two of the three features of fluctuations, visual hallucinations, and spontaneous parkinsonism are required for a diagnosis of probable DLB, or one of these three features is required for a diagnosis of possible DLB.

Additional features, such as repeated falls, syncope, or transient loss of consciousness; neuroleptic sensitivity; and systematized delusions and hallucinations in other modalities, are regarded as supporting the diagnosis. Finally, the diagnosis is regarded as less likely in the presence of evidence of stroke or other organic disorders that could explain the clinical picture.

These studies await detailed validation. A small study by Mega and colleagues [49] assessed the probable DLB criteria against an autopsy diagnosis based on finding "many" cortical Lewy bodies. This study revealed a sensitivity of 75% and a specificity of 79%, although the latter could be improved if parkinsonism was made a requirement for the diagnosis.

Unusual Presentations

Most patients with DLB present with the syndrome as already described and are relatively easy to diagnose. In such cases, the only major pitfall for the unwary is the temptation to invoke cerebral vascular disease as the basis for cognitive fluctuations. In fact, fluctuations are rare in both small-vessel vascular dementia (e.g., Binswanger's disease) and medium- and large-vessel disease (e.g., multi-infarct dementia); both of these conditions give rise to neurologic signs, such as pyramidal deficits, that are rare in early DLB. A few clinical scenarios create much greater diagnostic difficulty.

The first concerns the small minority of DLB patients who present with a rapidly progressive dementia that becomes severe within a matter of weeks or months. These patients often have myoclonus and a gait disorder, raising concerns about CJD. Cerebellar signs such as nystagmus have not been described in patients with DLB (although there have been isolated pathologic reports of occasional Lewy bodies in the cerebellum), and this distinguishes rapid-onset DLB from the classic form of CJD (but not necessarily from the variant form of CJD in younger patients). Rapid-onset DLB cases often stabilize and survive for a few months in a severely demented state, unlike classic CJD cases, in which patients continue to deteriorate and die within 1 year of the onset of symptoms. The EEG is not helpful in distinguishing between the two diseases: In both conditions it may show either nonspecific slowing or periodic complexes.

The second difficult clinical scenario is the pure psychiatric presentation of DLB. Depression may be the first harbinger of a wide range of dementing illnesses (including DLB), but DLB has an apparently unique tendency to cause an isolated late-onset psychotic illness [36], usually in middle-aged or elderly patients who present with delusions and hallucinations who may go on to develop dementia and parkinsonism more than 10 years later. No reliable way of distinguishing such cases from paraphrenia has been reported, although these patients may be more susceptible to the adverse effects of neuroleptic drugs. The diagnosis is usually established only at autopsy.

A third area of difficulty relates to dementia in patients with established PD.

Dementia in Parkinson's Disease

PD is the prototypic Lewy body disease, and it has long been accepted that it is characterized pathologically by the presence of Lewy bodies in the substantia nigra and various other brain stem nuclei. When DLB was first delineated, it was suggested (by this author and others) that DLB would provide a parsimonious explanation for the fact that approximately one-third of patients with PD go on to develop dementia. The suggestion was that the pathology spread from the brain stem to the cerebral cortex, thus giving rise first to PD and then to dementia.

The suggestion that cortical Lewy bodies contribute to the dementia of PD (or are a marker for a related pathologic process that does so) is supported by two studies that have shown a correlation between the density of cortical Lewy bodies and the severity of dementia [13,50]. In the study by Lennox and colleagues [13], this correlation was seen regardless of the mode of presentation (i.e., whether patients had presented with PD or dementia, or both).

Nonetheless it appears to be an oversimplification. It has now been established that most if not all patients with PD also have some cortical Lewy bodies [51]. Indeed, these may be present in large numbers, even in brains from patients with PD who were not apparently demented in life. There does not appear to be any clear threshold for cortical Lewy body density, either globally or in any given region, that absolutely distinguishes between nondemented and demented PD. Presumably this means that other pathologic processes are important in determining whether an individual patient with a given density of cortical Lewy bodies manifests dementia. Such processes might be related to the Lewy body pathology (e.g., Lewy body–related neurite formation or cell loss and Lewy body formation in subcortical structures like the nucleus basalis) or might be unrelated (e.g., neurofibrillary tangle formation and associated synapse loss). The study of Hughes and colleagues [51] suggested that Alzheimer pathology made a major contribution to the development of dementia in PD, but no definite pathologic basis for dementia was found in 55% of their cases.

From a clinical point of view, the phenomenology of dementia in PD is very similar to that in DLB. Older patients with PD typically are affected, and they initially develop mental inflexibility and other mild defects of executive function accompanied by visual hallucinations [52]. These are often attributed to PD medication and may improve or resolve with the withdrawal of anticholinergic and dopamine agonist drugs. Very often they return again after a few months or years with more definite global cognitive impairment, often with prominent "frontal" and visuospatial deficits. Fluctuations are common.

It remains to be seen whether any particular clinical features will allow an accurate distinction between those PD patients whose dementia is associated with numerous cortical Lewy bodies and those with cortical Alzheimer changes but few cortical Lewy bodies. In view of these difficulties, the recent consortium meeting proposed that patients who have PD for a period of at least 1 year before the onset of dementia should receive a descriptive diagnosis of *PD with dementia* until a pathologic diagnosis becomes available [11].

A number of other conditions can present with parkinsonism and go on to cause dementia, but these rarely give rise to diagnostic confusion. Many of the degenerative disorders causing parkinsonism are associated with a relatively restricted frontotemporal pattern of cognitive defects without significant visuospatial problems. Examples include multiple system atrophy, progressive supranuclear palsy, corticobasal degeneration, and Huntington's disease, all of which characteristically lead to additional neurologic problems. Similarly, the cognitive impairment in hydrocephalus and dementia pugilistica is often mainly frontotemporal. Vascular disease rarely presents with pure parkinsonism; a gait apraxia with pyramidal deficits is more common. The differential diagnosis is more difficult in young patients, in which unusual metabolic conditions including Wilson's disease and Hallervorden-Spatz disease must be considered.

INVESTIGATIONS

Routine blood tests are normal in DLB. Structural brain imaging with computed tomography or magnetic resonance imaging may show generalized cerebral atrophy, sometimes with a discernible frontal predominance, and subcortical signal changes that are thought to be due to secondary white matter degeneration; these changes are very hard to distinguish from the leukoariosis of small-vessel disease and again contribute to the tendency to overdiagnose vascular dementia in cases of DLB.

The EEG is usually nonspecifically abnormal; it is occasionally of value in confirming the presence of cortical disease in patients with mainly psychiatric presentations and to distinguish cases of predominantly "frontal" DLB from the frontotemporal dementias (in which the EEG usually remains normal).

Most studies of functional brain imaging have been hampered by a lack of pathologic confirmation, but Albin and colleagues [53] studied cerebral metabolism in six confirmed cases using positron emission tomography. They not only identified the expected hypometabolism in temporal, parietal, and frontal regions with relative sparing of primary sensory and motor areas, but they also found hypometabolism in the occipital lobes, involving both primary visual and association areas, in a manner that may distinguish DLB from AD. The occipital lobes usually contain relatively little Lewy body pathology, but this functional impairment may contribute to the visual hallucinations in DLB. Brain biopsy is not routinely justified in suspected cases of DLB in the absence of curative or even protective therapy.

TREATMENT

DLB causes many problems for disease management because of the conflicting requirements of the neuropsychiatric disturbance and parkinsonism. In general, treatments for hallucinations, delusions, and behavioral disturbance tend to aggravate the movement disorder and vice versa. Small-scale studies, however, have shown that the newer atypical neuroleptics such as clozapine and olanzapine may be able to suppress psychotic symptoms without precipitating excessive parkinsonism [54]. Several more such agents are in development. Olanzapine is the most convenient of the drugs currently available (because it does not require hematologic monitoring), but its anticholinergic effects can precipitate confusion (and it is not licensed for use in DLB).

These drugs are sometimes successful in treating hallucinations and delusions in patients with PD who are becoming demented, allowing antiparkinsonian treatment to be continued or even increased. Such treatment is a significant improvement on the traditional approach of withdrawing antiparkinsonian medication, leaving the patient lucid but immobile. It is still reasonable to try to simplify antiparkinsonian medication as a first step, particularly withdrawing drugs of lower potency (and particular tendency to cause confusion), such as anticholinergics and selegiline. When possible, dopamine agonists should also be withdrawn, leaving most patients on levodopa alone.

The cognitive impairment of DLB may, by virtue of the more prominent role of attentional deficits and because of its neurochemical differences, be more amenable to drug therapy than that of AD. Existing clinical diagnostic criteria for AD have enabled many patients with DLB to enter Alzheimer drug trials, and anecdotal experience from these studies suggests that cholinergic drugs such as tacrine and donepezil may be of some benefit in DLB. The author's experience suggests that this benefit derives mainly from an increase in attention, but other cognitive improvements, a reduction in psychotic phenomena, and behavioral improvement may all occur. Large prospective trials in DLB are now under way, assessing both cholinergic therapies and other novel drugs that are thought to have cognitive effects.

GENETICS

Genetic studies are making rapid progress in elucidating the matrix of causative factors in DLB. These factors appear to be complex but may explain the relationship of DLB to the other primary Lewy body disorders (including PD) as well as the association with AD. It remains to be seen whether genetic testing will be sufficiently simple to help in clinical diagnosis.

So far two genes have been identified that predispose to Lewy body formation (if one excludes conditions such as ataxia-telangiectasia and superoxide dismutase-1–related motor neuron disease in which Lewy bodies are a rare and inconstant pathologic finding). Polymeropoulos and colleagues [55] have shown that the large Italian-American Contursi kindred, who suffer from autosomal dominant Lewy body PD with a variable degree of dementia, and two unrelated Greek families with PD have mutations in the alpha-synuclein gene. This is particularly interesting because alpha-synuclein is known to be expressed in normal neuronal synapses and is a component of both Lewy bodies [56] and amyloid plaques [57]. Alpha-synuclein mutations have not, however, been identified in several other European families with PD in which other genes must be involved. Mutant alleles of the cytochrome P-450 gene *CYP2D6* (or a closely linked gene) may act as a relatively weak risk factor for brain stem Lewy body formation [58]; this may also apply to cortical Lewy body formation [59].

It is possible that other genetic factors such as apolipoprotein E gene (*APOE*) polymorphisms influence whether the pathology is predominantly subcortical or cortical. The *APOE-ε4* genotype is more frequent in patients with Lewy body dementia (particularly those with plaques and tangles) than in nondemented PD patients or normal controls [60–63]. Presumably the *ε4* allele is acting as a risk factor for cortical plaque or tangle formation, or both in Lewy body disease, just as it does in AD.

A further overlap with the genetics of AD comes from the finding of both cortical Lewy bodies and classic Alzheimer pathology in some but not all cases of autosomal dominant dementia due to a missense mutation at codon 717 of the amyloid precursor protein gene (*APP*) [64,65]. Although this finding clearly demonstrates that *APP* mutations can give rise to cortical Lewy body formation, its wider significance is unclear because Lewy bodies are no more common in patients with a range of different *APP* mutations than in patients with sporadic AD. It remains to be seen whether other genes that are involved in AD, such as the presenilins, are also involved in DLB.

CONCLUSION

DLB is one manifestation of the spectrum of primary Lewy body disorders. It has characteristic clinical features that allow many cases to be recognized in life. Pathologically, it is defined by the formation of both brain stem and cortical Lewy bodies. Senile plaques are common in older patients but are usually diffuse rather than neuritic. Neurofibrillary pathology is usually sparse or absent. This finding, and the severity of the cholinergic deficit (together with the presence of the Lewy bodies themselves), distinguish DLB from AD. The overlap of Lewy body and Alzheimer pathology may be due to common genetic risk factors such as *APOE* genotype. Genes that predispose to Lewy body formation are now being located. As they are cloned and we come to understand their function, we are likely to develop a far greater understanding of the pathogenesis and nosology of DLB. We must hope that this in turn will lead to improvements in the management of this common cause of dementia.

REFERENCES

1. Yoshimura M. Cortical changes in the Parkinsonian brain: a contribution to the delineation of "diffuse Lewy body disease." J Neurol 1983;229:17–32.
2. Gibb WRG, Esiri MM, Lees AJ. Clinical and pathological features of diffuse cortical Lewy body disease (Lewy body dementia). Brain 1987;110:1131–1153.
3. Perry RH, Irving D, Blessed G, et al. Senile dementia of Lewy body type. A clinically and neuropathologically distinct type of Lewy body dementia in the elderly. J Neurol Sci 1990;95:119–139.
4. Hansen LA, Salmon D, Galasko D, et al. The Lewy body variant of Alzheimer's disease: a clinical pathological entity. Neurology 1990;40:1–8.
5. Okazaki H, Lipkin LE, Aronson SM. Diffuse intracytoplasmic ganglionic inclusions (Lewy type) associated with progressive dementia and quadriparesis in flexion. J Neuropathol Exp Neurol 1961; 20:237–244.
6. Kosaka K, Matsushita M, Oyanagi S, et al. A clinicopathological study of "Lewy body disease." Psychiatry Neurol 1980;82:292–311.
7. Kosaka K. Diffuse Lewy body disease in Japan. J Neurol 1990;237:197–204.
8. Byrne EJ, Lennox G, Lowe J, Godwin-Austen RB. Diffuse Lewy body disease: clinical features in 15 cases. J Neurol Neurosurg Psychiatry 1989;52:709–717.
9. Forstl H, Burns A, Luthert P, et al. The Lewy body variant of Alzheimer's disease: clinical and pathological findings. Br J Psychiatry 1993;162:385–392.
10. Kosaka K, Iseki E, Odawara T, Yamamoto T. Cerebral type of Lewy body disease. Neuropathol 1996; 16:32–35.
11. McKeith IG, Galasko D, Kosaka K, et al. Clinical and pathological diagnosis of dementia with Lewy bodies (DLB): report of the CDLB international workshop. Neurology 1996;47:1113–1124.
12. Forno LS, Langston JW. The amygdala-parahippocampal region: a predilection site for Lewy bodies [abstract]. J Neuropathol Exp Neurol 1988;47:354.

13. Lennox G, Lowe J, Landon M, et al. Diffuse Lewy body disease: correlative neuropathology using anti-ubiquitin immunocytochemistry. J Neurol Neurosurg Psychiatry 1989;52:1236–1247.
14. Dickson DW, Crystal H, Mattiace LA, et al. Diffuse Lewy body disease: light and electron microscopic immunocytochemistry of senile plaques. Acta Neuropathol 1989;78:572–584.
15. Hansen LA, Masliah E, Galasko D, Terry RD. Plaque-only Alzheimer disease is usually the Lewy body variant, and vice versa. J Neuropathol Exp Neurol 1993;52:648–654.
16. Galasko D, Hansen LA, Katzman R, et al. Clinical-neuropathological correlations in Alzheimer's disease and related dementias. Arch Neurol 1994;51:888–895.
17. Victoroff J, Mack WJ, Lyness SA, Chui HC. Multicentre clinicopathological correlation in dementia. Am J Psychiatry 1995;152:1476–1484.
18. Ince PG, McArthur FK, Bjertness E, et al. Neuropathological diagnoses in elderly patients in Oslo: Alzheimer's disease, Lewy body disease, vascular lesions. Dementia 1995;6:162–168.
19. Kalra S, Bergeron C, Lang AE. Lewy body disease and dementia. Arch Int Med 1996;156:487–493.
20. Ballard CG, Mohan RNC, Patel A, Bannister C. Idiopathic clouding of consciousness—do these patients have cortical Lewy body disease? Int J Geriatr Psychiatry 1993;8:571–576.
21. Ballard CG, Saad K, Patel A, et al. The prevalence and phenomenology of psychotic symptoms in dementia sufferers. Int J Geriatr Psychiatry 1995;10:477–485.
22. Shergill S, Mullan E, Dath P, Katona C. What is the clinical prevalence of Lewy body dementia? Int J Geriatr Psychiatry 1994;9:907–912.
23. Collerton D, Davies C, Thompson P. Lewy Body Dementia in Clinical Practice: Experience in Gateshead. In RH Perry, IG McKeith, EK Perry (eds), Dementia with Lewy Bodies. Cambridge, England: Cambridge University Press, 1996;171–186.
24. Lennox G, Lowe J, Morrell K, et al. Anti-ubiquitin immunocytochemistry is more sensitive than conventional techniques in the detection of diffuse Lewy body disease. J Neurol Neurosurg Psychiatry 1989;52:67–71.
25. Lowe J. Lewy Bodies. In DB Calne (ed), Neurodegenerative Diseases. Philadelphia: Saunders, 1994;51–69.
26. Dickson DW, Schmidt ML, Lee VM, et al. Immunoreactivity profile of hippocampal CA2–3 neurites in diffuse Lewy body disease. Acta Neuropathol 1994;87:269–276.
27. Dickson DW, Crystal HA, Mattiace LA, et al. Identification of normal and pathological aging in prospectively studied nondemented elderly humans. Neurobiol Aging 1992;13:179–189.
28. Ince PG, Irving D, McArthur F, Perry RH. Quantitative neuropathological study of Alzheimer-type pathology in the hippocampus: comparison of senile dementia of Alzheimer type, of senile dementia of Lewy type, Parkinson's disease and nodemented elderly control patients. J Neurol Sci 1991; 106:142–152.
29. Perry EK, Marshall E, Smith CJ, et al. Cholinergic and dopaminergic activities in senile dementia of the Lewy body type. Alzheimer Dis Assoc Disord 1990;4:87–95.
30. Dickson DW, Davies P, Mayeux R, et al. Diffuse Lewy body disease. Neuropathological and biochemical studies of six patients. Acta Neuropathol 1987;75:8–15.
31. Perry EK, Marshall E, Thompson P, et al. Monoaminergic activities in Lewy body dementia: relation to hallucinosis and extrapyramidal features. J Neural Transm Park Dis Dement Sect 1993;6:167–177.
32. Sahgal A, Galloway PH, McKeith IG, et al. A comparative study of attentional deficits in senile dementias of Alzheimer and Lewy body types. Dementia 1990;3:350–354.
33. Salmon DP, Galasko D. Neuropsychological Aspects of Lewy Body Dementia. In RH Perry, IG McKeith, EK Perry (eds), Dementia with Lewy Bodies. New York: Cambridge University Press, 1996;99–113.
34. Walker Z, Allen RL, Shergill S, Katona CLE. Neuropsychological performance in Lewy body dementia and Alzheimer's disease. Br J Psychiatry 1997;170:156–158.
35. Klatka LA, Louis ED, Schiffer RB. Psychiatric features in diffuse Lewy body disease. Neurology 1996;47:1148–1152.
36. McShane R, Gedling K, Reading M, et al. Prospective study of relations between cortical Lewy bodies, poor eyesight and hallucinations in Alzheimer's disease. J Neurol Neurosurg Psychiatry 1995;59:185–188.
37. Baldwin RC, Snowden JS, Mann DMA. Delusional misidentification in association with cortical Lewy body disease. Int J Geriatr Psychiatry 1995;10:893–898.
38. Louis ED, Klatka LA, Liu Y, Fahn S. Comparison of the extrapyramidal features in 31 pathologically confirmed cases of diffuse Lewy body disease and 34 pathologically confirmed cases of Parkinson's disease. Neurology 1997;48:376–380.
39. Burkhardt CR, Filley CM, Kleinschmidt-DeMasters BK, et al. Diffuse Lewy body disease and progressive dementia. Neurology 1988;38:1520–1528.
40. Crystal HA, Dickson DW, Lizardi JE, et al. Antemortem diagnosis of diffuse Lewy body disease. Neurology 1990;40:1523–1528.

41. Daniel SE, Lees AJ. Neuropathological features of Alzheimer's disease in non-demented parkinsonian patients. J Neurol Neurosurg Psychiatry 1991;54:972–975.
42. McKeith I, Fairbairn A, Perry R, et al. Neuroleptic sensitivity in patients with senile dementia of Lewy body type. BMJ 1992;305:673–678.
43. Santacruz P, Torner L, Cruz-Sanchez F, et al. Corticobasal degeneration syndrome: a case of Lewy body variant of Alzheimer's disease. Int J Geriatr Psychiatry 1996;11:559–564.
44. Mori H, Yoshimura M, Tomonaga M, Yamanouchi H. Progressive supranuclear palsy with Lewy bodies. Acta Neuropathol 1986;71:344–346.
45. Fearnley JM, Revesz T, Brooks DJ, et al. Diffuse Lewy body disease presenting with a supranuclear gaze palsy. J Neurol Neurosurg Psychiatry 1991;54:159–161.
46. Mark MH, Sage JI, Dickson DW, et al. Meige syndrome in the spectrum of Lewy body disease. Neurology 1994;44:1432–1436.
47. Byrne EJ, Lennox G, Godwin-Austen RB, et al. Diagnostic criteria for dementia associated with cortical Lewy bodies. Dementia 1991;2:283–284.
48. McKeith IG, Perry RH, Fairbairn AF, et al. Operational criteria for senile dementia of Lewy body type (SDLT). Psychol Med 1992;22:911–922.
49. Mega MS, Masterman DL, Benson DF, et al. Dementia with Lewy bodies: reliability and validity of clinical and pathologic criteria. Neurology 1996;47:1403–1409.
50. Samuel W, Galasko D, Masliah E, Hansen LA. Neocortical Lewy body counts correlate with dementia in the Lewy body variant of Alzheimer's disease. J Neuropathol Exp Neurol 1996;55:44–52.
51. Hughes AJ, Daniel SE, Blankson S, Lees AJ. A clinicopathologic study of 100 cases of Parkinson's disease. Arch Neurol 1993;50:140–148.
52. Sanchez-Ramos JR, Ortoll R, Paulson GW. Visual hallucinations associated with Parkinson disease. Arch Neurol 1996;53:1265–1268.
53. Albin RL, Minoshima S, D'Amato CJ, et al. Fluoro-deoxyglucose positron emission tomography in diffuse Lewy body disease. Neurology 1996;47:462–466.
54. Wolters EC, Jansen ENH, Tuynman-Qua HG, Bergmans PLM. Olanzapine in the treatment of dopaminomimetic psychosis in patients with Parkinson's disease. Neurology 1996;47:1085–1087.
55. Polymeropoulos MH, Lavedan C, Leroy E, et al. Mutation in the alpha-synuclein gene identified in families with Parkinson's disease. Science 1997;276:2045–2047.
56. Spillantini MG, Schmidt ML, Lee VMY, et al. Alpha-synuclein in Lewy bodies. Nature 1997; 388:839–840.
57. Irizarry MC, Kim TW, McNamara M, et al. Characterization of the precursor protein of the non-Abeta component of senile plaques (NACP) in the human central nervous system. J Neuropathol Exp Neurol 1996;55:889–895.
58. Rempfer R, Crook R, Houlden H, et al. Parkinson's disease, but not Alzheimer's disease, Lewy body variant associated with mutant alleles at cytochrome P450 gene. Lancet 1994;344:815.
59. Saitoh T, Xia Y, Chen X, et al. The CYP2D6B mutant allelle is over-represented in the Lewy body variant of Alzheimer's disease. Ann Neurol 1995;37:110–112.
60. Benjamin R, Leake A, Edwardson JA, et al. Apolipoprotein E genes in Lewy body and Parkinson's disease. Lancet 1994;343:1565.
61. Galasko D, Saitoh T, Xia Y, et al. The apolipoprotein E allelle ε4 is overrepresented in patients with the Lewy body variant of Alzheimer's disease. Neurology 1994;44:1950–1951.
62. Harrington CR, Louwagie J, Rossau R, et al. Influence of apolipoprotein E genotype on senile dementia of the Alzheimer and Lewy body types: significance for etiological theories of Alzheimer's disease. Am J Pathol 1994;145:1472–1484.
63. Lippa CF, Smith TW, Saunders AM, et al. Apolipoprotein E genotype and Lewy body disease. Neurology 1995;45:97–103.
64. Mann DMA, Jones D, Snowden JS, et al. Pathological changes in the brain of a patient with familial Alzheimer's disease having a missense mutation at codon 717 in the amyloid precursor protein gene. Neurosci Lett 1992;137:225–228.
65. Lantos PL, Ovenstone IMK, Johnson J, et al. Lewy bodies in the brain of two members of a family with the 717 (Val to Ile) mutation of the amyloid precursor protein gene. Neurosci Lett 1994;172:77–79.

4
Parkinsonian Syndromes Associated with Dementia

Harvey J. Sagar

Cognitive impairment is a common feature of many neurologic disorders and is increasingly recognized as a particular accompaniment of movement disorders because the structures serving motor control also play a role in cognitive function. Some movement disorders are associated with frank clinical dementia, but in other cases, more subtle deficits are detected on neuropsychological tests, commonly those sensitive to frontal lobe function. Although not reaching the criteria for clinical dementia, these deficits may nevertheless combine with the motor disability to impair activities of daily living. This chapter focuses particularly on cognitive disorders associated with parkinsonism, but cognitive deficits, particularly of the frontal lobe type, are also associated with other movement disorders.

Although strict diagnostic criteria are used for the clinical diagnosis of idiopathic Parkinson's disease (IPD) [1], the term *parkinsonism* is often used more loosely in clinical contexts. For the purposes of this chapter, *parkinsonism* is defined as a clinical syndrome with predominant akinesia and muscular rigidity, with or without tremor. Many of the conditions are also accompanied by postural instability. Dysfunction in nonextrapyramidal systems accompanies the parkinsonism in multiple system disorders. In general, few specific laboratory tests exist for the diagnosis of most of these conditions, and the diagnosis depends on clinical evaluation. Clinical diagnoses in this sphere of neurology, however, are notoriously unreliable. For example, in one autopsy study of IPD diagnosed in life, the diagnosis was changed in approximately 20% of cases, usually to one of multiple system atrophy (MSA) [2].

IDIOPATHIC PARKINSON'S DISEASE

IPD affects between 1 in 500 and 1 in 1,000 of the general population. The mean age of presentation is approximately 60 years, but the true prevalence increases with age, reaching a prevalence of approximately 1 in 50 older than age 80 years

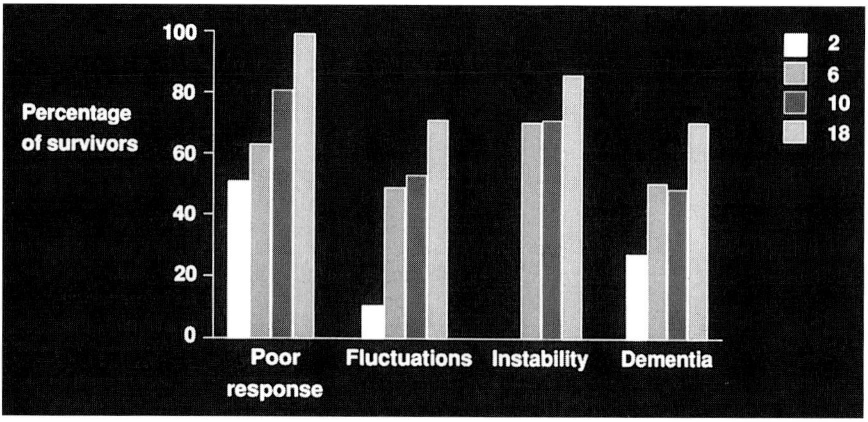

Figure 4.1 Chronic complications of idiopathic Parkinson's disease related to disease duration (years).

[3]. Due to the increasing frequency of multiple pathology in older people, however, the frequency of inaccurate diagnosis also increases with age.

IPD is a progressive motor disorder comprising akinesia plus rigidity, tremor, or postural instability with no evidence of other causes of parkinsonism (Parkinson's Disease Society of the United Kingdom research criteria) [1]. Akinesia is universal, but the classic rest tremor is absent in approximately 20–25% of cases [4]. The condition typically develops unilaterally in the upper limbs but progresses to become bilateral and later involves postural instability and gait disorder. Later complications include response fluctuations, declining levodopa response, and dyskinesia [5] (Figure 4.1).

In addition to the primitive motor deficits, IPD includes dysfunction of higher-order motor control. Thus, patients with IPD show disproportionate impairment in their capacity to carry out motor acts sequentially, to perform two motor acts simultaneously, to sequence movements into a coordinated motor plan, and to perform predictive movements in the absence of visual feedback [6–8]. Many of these motor disorders have parallels in the cognitive domain and probably reflect common mechanisms in the genesis of some cognitive and motor dysfunction.

Although James Parkinson said in his original description of the disorder that the "senses and intellect are uninjured" [9], behavioral change in the disease was recognized in the late nineteenth and early twentieth century [10]. Clinical dementia is now recognized in IPD and is associated with a higher mortality [11,12]. The overall prevalence, according to the *Diagnostic and Statistical Manual of Mental Disorders* (4th ed) (*DSM-IV*) criteria, is approximately 20–30% in large series of white populations [13], representing a 10–15% excess over that of an age-matched population [14]. The prevalence of dementia increases with disease duration reaching, in one series, approximately 50% after 12 or more years of disease progression [15] (see Figure 4.1). The early development of severe dementia, however, is recognized in pathologically proved IPD [16]. The tremor-predominant form of IPD has a lower risk of development of dementia [11].

Table 4.1 Distinguishing characteristics of cortical and subcortical dementia

	Cortical	*Subcortical*
Language	Aphasia	Dysarthria
Memory	Long-term deficits	Registration deficits
	Rapid forgetting	Working memory deficits
Other cognitive deficits	Agnosia	Executive deficits
	Acalculia	
	Apraxia	
Processing speed	Proportional to error	Disproportionately slow
Mood	Normal	Depressed
		Athymic
Motor disability	Minor	Prominent

Source: Adapted from JL Cummings, DF Benson. Subcortical dementia. Review of an emerging concept. Arch Neurol 1984;41:874–879.

Early clinical studies of the characteristics of dementia associated with progressive supranuclear palsy (PSP) highlighted differences from the classic syndrome associated with Alzheimer's disease (AD) [17]. These observations led to a distinction between cortical dementia (such as AD) and subcortical dementia (such as PSP) [18]. The term *subcortical dementia* has since been applied to other movement disorders characterized by basal ganglia pathology, including IPD. Although the classification is probably an inaccurate reflection of the underlying pathology, it remains useful in considering differences in the pattern of cognitive deficit between different dementing disorders [19] (Table 4.1).

Unlike cortical dementia, which is characterized by memory loss (including rapid forgetting), aphasia, apraxia, acalculia, and agnosia, the principal features of subcortical dementia are forgetfulness, slow cognitive processing speed, depression, and impaired ability to manipulate acquired knowledge in addition to the motor disability. The clinical observations of slow cognitive processing speed in subcortical dementia led to application of the term *bradyphrenia* [20] to indicate a cognitive analogy with the slowness of movement, bradykinesia. The concept of bradyphrenia, distinct from other manifestations of cognitive impairment, has subsequently been challenged by formal neuropsychological studies. A key component of bradyphrenia as a specific disorder is the notion that, given sufficient time, patients perform accurately in cognitive tasks, unlike patients with cortical dementias, who may take longer to complete a task but make frequent errors, regardless of the time available. Some studies support this [21–23]; others do not [24–26].

Mood disturbance is a common feature of IPD. Depression sufficient to reach the diagnostic criteria of major depression occurs in up to 40% of patients at some stage of the disease [27] and occurs more commonly than in AD [28,29]. Many other patients show degrees of mood disturbance insufficient to reach those diagnostic criteria but manifest as psychomotoretardation or athymia [30]. Some studies have drawn attention to the higher than expected incidence of psychiatric disorder before the development of clinical signs of IPD [30]. These observations have been used to suggest that the pathology of IPD begins many years before the onset of motor dysfunction and is manifest as behavioral disturbance.

The relationship between depression, motor disability, and cognitive impairment is unclear and probably depends on the disease stage. In some studies, depression is related to cognitive impairment in the later stages of the disease and has been attributed to common pathology [30]. In the early stages, however, depression appears to be more of a reactive nature, secondary to the diagnosis of a progressive neurologic disorder [31]. Major depression is characterized by impaired cognitive processing efficiency, and some studies of IPD have attributed bradyphrenia and depression to common pathophysiologic mechanisms [22]. Although cognitive deficits may be more marked in the presence of depression [32], however, the differences are not great, and qualitatively similar cognitive impairment certainly occurs in nondepressed patients [33]. Some studies have highlighted associations between depression and motor disability [34], whereas others fail to find any relationship between depression and either cognitive impairment or motor disability [35].

The lack of consistency in these observations is probably due to the multifaceted nature of both depression and cognitive impairment. The distinction between cortical and subcortical dementia highlights the conclusion that not all dementias are the same, and we now recognize many differences in the behavior patterns of various dementing disorders attributable to differences in the nature of the cerebral pathology. Similarly, cognitive dysfunction and motor disability in IPD are not unitary phenomena. Thus, whether or not a relationship between "depression" and cognitive or motor disability is recognized depends on patient selection and the definition of the behavioral disorders [36]. IPD is a markedly heterogeneous condition, clinically and pathologically; the evaluation of whether cognitive, motor, and affective disorders are based on common pathology will depend on a more precise evaluation of clinicopathologic relationships.

Some studies from our department have attempted to dissect the behavioral syndrome of depression in IPD, to compare the characteristics with those of primary major depression, and to explore the neuroanatomic basis of components of the depressive disorder using magnetic resonance imaging (MRI) and single photon emission computed tomography [37]. These studies have supported the notion that empirically defined components of the depressive syndrome in IPD are related to dysfunction in different brain areas that relate to each other as components of distinct functionally related networks.

Early observations on clinical differences between dementias of different etiology have been followed by an extensive series of psychological studies characterizing more specifically the concept of subcortical dementia, the nature and origin of the cognitive deficits in IPD, and the ways IPD differs from other neurodegenerative disorders [19,38]. One problem in interpreting the results of these studies is in matching patient groups for the overall severity of cognitive impairment [36]. Cognitive deficits may be found in one disorder not necessarily because they are specific to that disease but because the pathology is overall less advanced than in other disorders used for comparison (Figure 4.2). If the characteristics of the cognitive disability differ between conditions, however, it is difficult to know on what criteria the groups should be matched. Many studies have used the criteria of the *DSM-IV* for the selection of patients with clinical dementia. These criteria were developed principally for the diagnosis of demen-

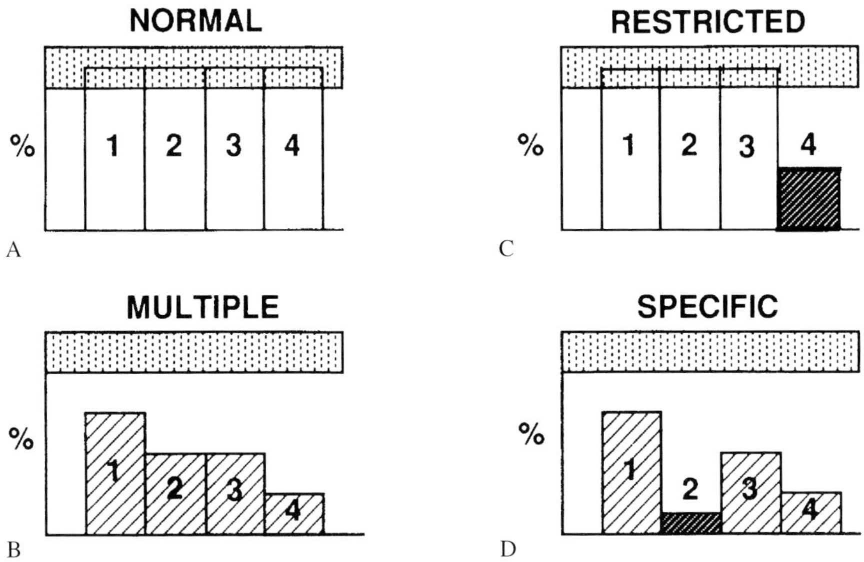

Figure 4.2 Potential errors in the use of neuropsychological tests to define selective cognitive deficits in neurodegenerative disease. Performance on four cognitive tests (1–4) shows significantly different cognitive profiles in four conditions (e.g., disease or drug effects), A–D. (A) Normal: normal and possibly equal performance on all tests. (B) Multiple cognitive impairments ("dementia"): impaired on several tests. Performance on some tests (e.g., 4) more impaired because of (1) different test sensitivities or (2) differences between cognitive processes in the extent of involvement by disease or drug. (C) Restricted: impairment on some tests (e.g., 4) but not others because of (1) different test sensitivities or (2) selectivity of the disease to certain cognitive processes. (D) Specific: similar to B for tests 1, 3, and 4 but worse for test 2. Selective impairment on process 2 compared with B indicates specific cognitive deficit despite impairment on multiple cognitive tests.

tia in AD, however, and it is not clear, given probable behavioral differences between the diseases, that the same criteria can be applied meaningfully to IPD. Moreover, *DSM-IV* criteria incorporate a quantitative inclusion criterion ("of sufficient severity"). The classification of patients into demented and nondemented may be useful for clinical purposes but does not necessarily assist the understanding of clinicopathologic relationships. Cognitive deficits that are detected in nondemented patients may be due to the same but milder pathology that causes clinical dementia and indeed may be a harbinger of dementia in a later stage of the disease.

Early studies highlighted the impairment of IPD patients on tests sensitive to frontal lobe function, particularly the Wisconsin Card Sorting Test and tests of verbal fluency [39]. The Wisconsin Card Sorting Test is a measure of ability to change cognitive attitude in response to changing environmental demands (set-shifting) which, according to some views, lies at the foundation of many of the other task failures highlighted in the disease [40]. Others have highlighted specific deficits in intentional or effortful memory [35,41]. Automatic memory, such as skill-learning and performance on implicit memory tasks, is variable, but a role for

Table 4.2 Causes of cognitive impairment in idiopathic Parkinson's disease

Alzheimer histopathology
Cortical Lewy body disease
Chronic levodopa therapy
Dopamine deficiency
Acute dopaminergic effects
Cholinergic, noradrenergic, serotonergic deficits
Anticholinergic drugs
Depression

the basal ganglia in skill-learning, and a deficit in skill-learning in IPD, have been proposed. Learning and memory processes in IPD and other movement disorders and their relationship to underlying neuropathology and current theories of memory are reviewed in detail elsewhere [42].

The precise pattern of dysfunction on neuropsychological tests shown by PD patients is generally inconsistent across studies, almost certainly depending on the disease stage of the study subjects, degree of interference in cognitive test results by motor impairment, coexistent depression, and the deleterious effects of medication [36] (Table 4.2). One way to avoid these confounds is to examine patients early in the disease and naive of medication. A detailed study of a large group of such patients demonstrated deficits on tasks sensitive (although not specific) to frontal lobe function, including immediate recall, set formation, working memory, and sequencing and verbal fluency [33]. The pattern of impairment was unlike that seen in AD, which typically includes major deficits in memory, particularly recall after a delay. Similar results have been shown in other studies, particularly those that compare PD with other dementing disorders, such as AD [43–46].

Attempts have been made to relate the pattern of neuropsychological test performance in PD to a single cognitive processing deficit [47,48]. One current view is that most of the cognitive impairment in early PD can be explained by attention deficits and, more specifically, impairment in components of working memory systems [49]. Thus, the most sensitive tests for detection of impairment, even in early PD, are those that tap working memory, such as the Digit Ordering Test, in which subjects are presented with a string of digits (e.g., 2, 3, 1, 9, 7) and are required to represent them in ascending order (in this example, 1, 2, 3, 7, 9) [33]. These conclusions provide experimental support for the early clinical observations that patients with PD show "impaired ability to manipulate acquired knowledge" [17], essentially a working memory function. Given the multifaceted nature of the pathology, however, it would be surprising if all cognitive dysfunction in PD could be explained by a single processing deficit, and caution should be exercised in attributing all impairments in PD to dysfunction of working memory.

The relationship between early neuropsychological deficits and the later development of clinical dementia is incompletely explored. However, a number of studies have attempted to identify factors that are predictors of incident dementia (Table 4.3). The most powerful studies for identification of these risk factors are prospective. Most studies identify older age, high levels of motor disability (particularly akinesia and rigidity), depression, and possibly lack of education as

Table 4.3 Early risk factors for dementia in idiopathic Parkinson's disease

Older age
Short duration of symptoms
Greater motor disability
Less tremor
Working memory deficits
Poor verbal fluency
Depression

the major risk factors [50–57]. Among cognitive measures, poor verbal fluency [58] and impaired working memory capacity at diagnosis [57] have been implicated as early risk factors for later clinical dementia. The severity of cognitive impairment, however, does not necessarily correlate with motor disability or severity of depression in cross-sectional studies. These apparent contradictions are explained by the heterogeneity of the disease in that a subgroup of patients shows more aggressive disease progression encompassing not only motor control but also cognitive function and affect [59,60].

Disease heterogeneity probably accounts for much of the controversy in the literature on the relationship among cognitive, motor, and affective disability. One of our studies [59] addressed this question through a cluster analysis of the results of cognitive, motor, and affective tests in a community-based cohort of 176 patients who fulfilled the Parkinson's Disease Society of the United Kingdom Brain Bank criteria for the diagnosis of IPD [1]. Cluster analysis identified five subgroups of patients: three of short duration, and two of long duration. Two of the short-duration groups were probably forerunners of the long-duration groups. Thus, three subgroups were identified when disease duration was controlled (Figure 4.3). One group was characterized by motor disability but no cognitive impairment; the second consisted of patients with motor disability and selective cognitive deficits, particularly those sensitive to frontal lobe function; and the third had a particularly malignant course with rapid onset of motor complications and dementia. None of the differences between subgroups could be accounted for by differences in medication, severity of depression, or demographic measures apart from age. The rapidly progressive group had an older age at disease onset. The pathologic basis for these subgroups remains unknown at present, but the findings provide strong support for the concept of clinicopathologic heterogeneity in PD, including cognitive dysfunction. One explanation for the results is that the pure motor group is characterized by pure nigrostriatal pathology, the "frontostriatal" group by additional neurochemical pathology, and the rapidly progressive group by diffuse Lewy body disease.

One major problem in the clinical management of advanced IPD is the development of drug-induced psychosis, characterized by episodic confusion, hallucinations, and delusions. The hallucinations are typically visual, but sometimes auditory hallucinations also occur and occasionally are the only form. Anticholinergic drugs produce marked impairment in memory and confusion, particularly in elderly subjects [61], but the more classic psychosis is a typical result of treatment with drugs that modulate the dopaminergic system. Dopamine agonists have more psychotic side effects than does levodopa [62]. However, the

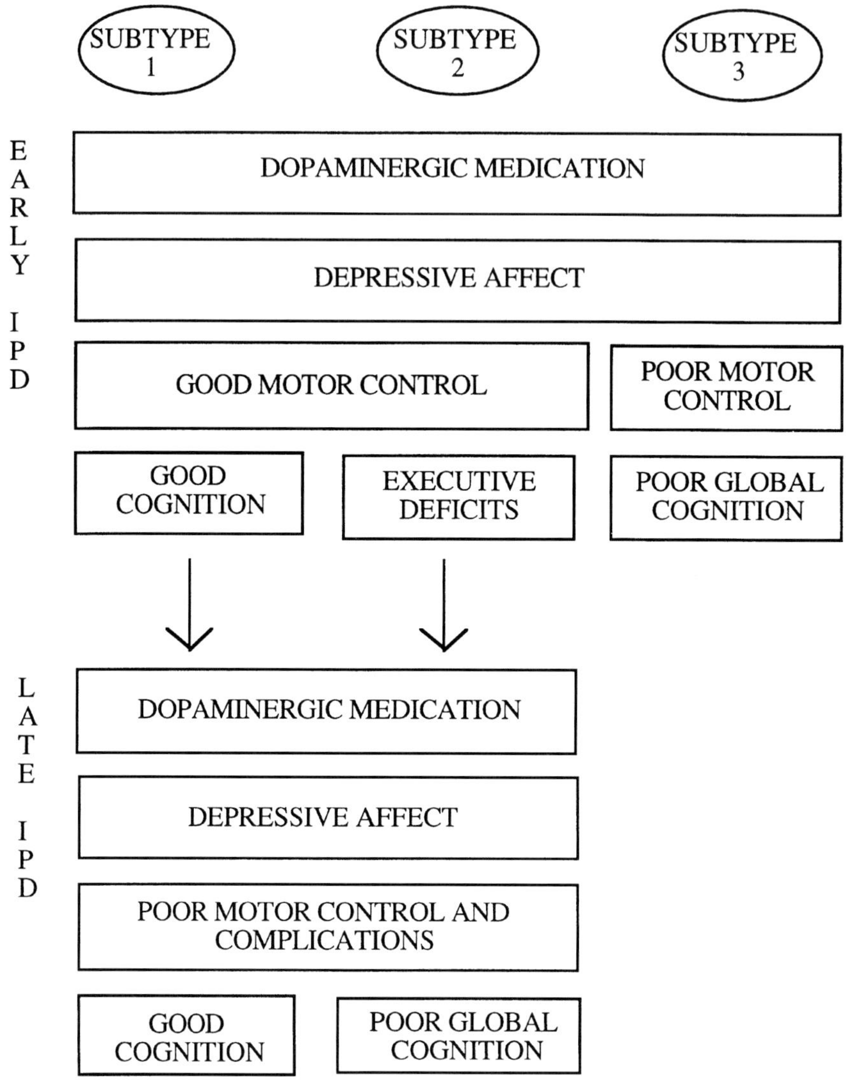

Figure 4.3 The heterogeneity of idiopathic Parkinson's disease (IPD).

pathophysiology of psychosis is undoubtedly more complex. Most studies show that psychosis develops particularly in older, cognitively impaired patients [63] and is related to the dose of dopaminergic agents. Psychosis is a particular problem of advanced disease due to the greater prevalence of dementia and the higher dose of drugs used to treat the motor disorder.

Hallucinations also occur in disease of short duration and may have a different origin. In one study [64], the frequency distribution of first hallucination related to disease duration was bimodal, comprising the well-recognized increased frequency with long disease duration and a second peak of first hallucination within the first 5 years of the disease. Patients with early hallucinations had a shorter time to onset and greater prevalence of motor complications but no major cognitive impairment, whereas the late hallucinators were cognitively impaired and had no more motor complications than their nonhallucinating counterparts. Dopamine receptor supersensitivity in mesolimbic circuits may contribute to hallucinations in early disease, whereas late hallucinations probably result from nondopaminergic pathology, particularly involvement of the cerebral cortex with Lewy bodies. Similar psychotic features are now well recognized in diffuse Lewy body disease with or without IPD [65]. Dopaminergic agents, particularly dopamine agonists, act as an additional complication to these underlying pathophysiologic mechanisms.

Other nonmotor features of IPD include autonomic failure, probably due to involvement of the lateral columns with Lewy bodies [66,67]. Features of autonomic failure, particularly postural hypotension, are more frequent in rapidly progressive disease with early dementia. In clinical practice, management of severe disease is complicated by the added effects of dopaminergic agents on the postural hypotension as well as the behavioral disorder.

Etiology and Pathogenesis

Loss of dopamine projections from the substantia nigra to the putamen causes the fundamental motor disorder of IPD, particularly akinesia and rigidity [5]. Thus, attention has focused on the substantia nigra to elucidate the etiology of IPD. The most popular current theory of etiology is a combination of genetic predisposition plus exposure to an environmental toxin. Two sets of observations have prompted this theory: First, IPD populations show a greater prevalence of the slow metabolizer phenotype than do normal subjects, which corresponds to a higher frequency of the CYP2D6B variant of the polymorphic allele [68]. Thus, IPD patients may have genetically poor detoxification processes. Second, exposure to 1-methyl-4-phenyl-1,2,3,6-tetrahydropyridine (MPTP), a by-product of the illicit synthesis of narcotics, leads to a syndrome indistinguishable from IPD and accompanied by nigral cell death [69]. Thus, similar environmental toxins may be involved in the cell death of IPD. Epidemiologic studies show that patients with IPD have a greater than normal frequency of exposure to potentially toxic substances, including heavy metals, organic solvents, wood preservatives, and well water [70]. Moreover, certain compounds, such as tetrahydroisoquinolones, are widespread in food and are chemically similar to MPTP [71]. Molecular biology studies have suggested that nigral cell death in IPD occurs through oxidative stress and genesis of free radicals, partially because of weak neuroprotective mechanisms, such as low levels of nigral glutathione [72]. These abnormalities appear to be specific to the substantia nigra and are a plausible mechanism for nigral cell death in IPD.

Application of these pathogenic mechanisms to the pathology underlying cognitive impairment in PD is less acceptable. Dopamine deficiency underlies some but not all of the cognitive disability in the disease. Studies of dopamine modulation, either by drug treatment of de novo subjects [73] or drug withdrawal in chronically medicated patients [74], indicate that some impairments, notably in working memory, planning, and set-shifting, are sensitive to dopamine modula-

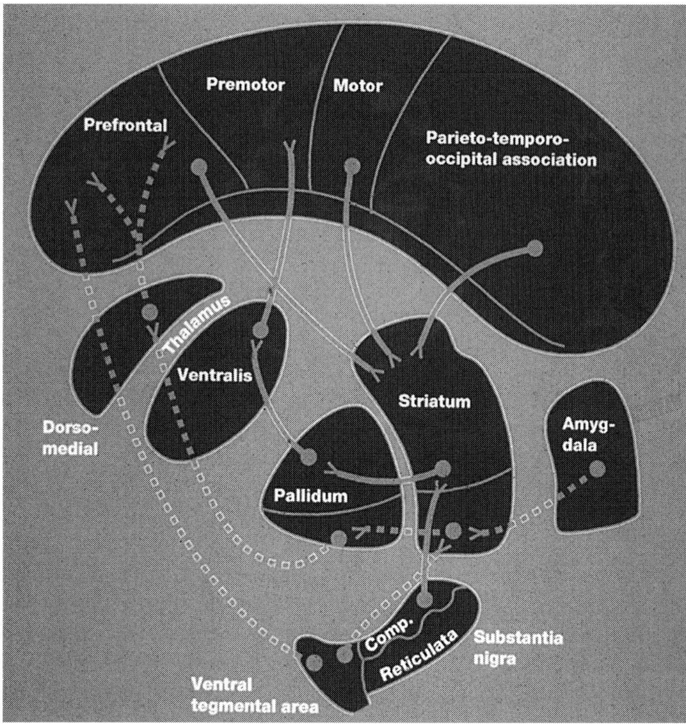

Figure 4.4 Subcortical-cortical dopamine circuits involved in cognition.

tion. The most likely mechanism to account for these findings is disruption of dopamine circuits either between the caudate nucleus and the prefrontal cortex or in the mesocortical loops between the ventral tegmental area and the prefrontal cortex [75] (Figure 4.4). Frontal lobe hypometabolism occurs in PD and is correlated with impairment on working memory tasks [76].

By contrast, much of the cognitive impairment in IPD, even in early disease, is insensitive to dopamine modulation, and the dopamine-sensitive deficits are incompletely corrected by dopamine replacement, suggesting nondopaminergic and possibly nonfrontal pathology in the genesis of the impairment [77]. In one of our studies [78], comparison of subgroups of IPD patients with either selective memory deficits or selective depression using positron emission tomography (PET) functional flow imaging demonstrated that prefrontal dysfunction was the major correlate of both the cognitive and the affective disorder. When the two groups were compared directly, however, depressed patients were distinguished from cognitively impaired patients in the extent of prefrontal hypometabolism. By contrast, cognitively impaired patients were distinguished from depressed patients not in prefrontal metabolism but in dysfunction of the middle and superior temporal cortex (Figure 4.5).

PD with dementia in life can be distinguished from PD without dementia by the presence of multiple subcortical and cortical pathologies at autopsy [79]. Non-

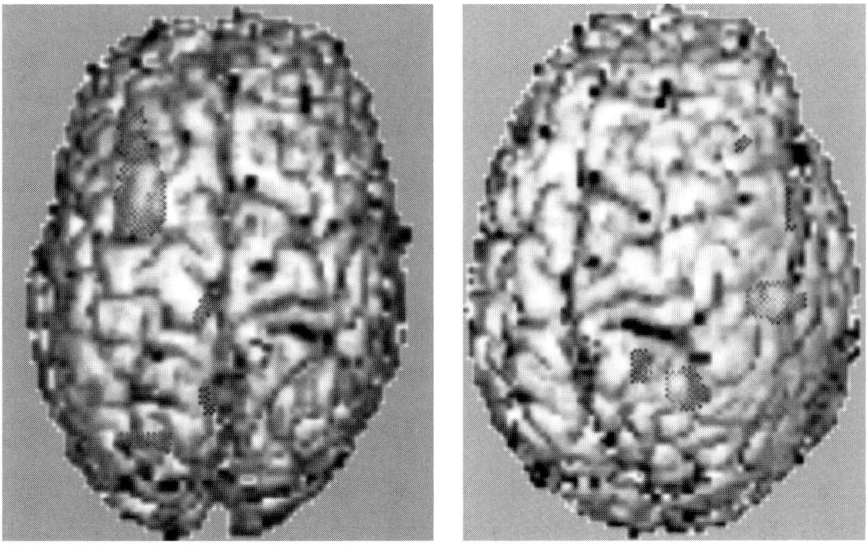

A B

Figure 4.5 Areas of hypometabolism that distinguish depressed (A) from cognitively impaired (B) patients with idiopathic Parkinson's disease on ^{15}O positron emission tomography scanning using a cognitive choice reaction time challenge task.

dopaminergic neurochemical systems, particularly the noradrenergic, cholinergic, and serotonergic systems, are known to be involved in cognitive dysfunction in other conditions and in experimental animals and are deficient in PD. In IPD, cerebrospinal fluid (CSF) levels of 5-hydroxytryptamine (5-HT) metabolites have been correlated with severity of depression [80] and levels of noradrenergic metabolites have been correlated with other cognitive deficits [81]; cholinergic deficiency has been correlated with lower scores on a mini-mental test [82]. These neurochemical changes are associated with more cell loss from the locus coeruleus, ventral tegmental area, and nucleus basalis (possibly affecting particularly a monoamine oxidase [MAD] A subset [83]) in demented compared with nondemented patients with IPD [84].

Intrinsic cortical pathology also occurs in IPD. Cortical Lewy body disease is a well-recognized cause of clinical dementia in IPD (see Chapter 3), and cortical Lewy bodies are recognized in small numbers, even in early disease [4]. Moreover, diffuse Lewy body disease may present with asymmetric rest tremor and levodopa response indistinguishable from IPD and later incorporating dementia. However, cortical Lewy body disease does not account for a large proportion of demented cases of pathologically proven IPD [4]. AD-type histologic changes are found in some demented patients with PD and have been considered to be more relevant to the cognitive changes than are cortical Lewy bodies [85]. A rise in CSF somatostatin in nondemented IPD, especially with memory deficits, has been attributed to early degeneration of cortical neurons [86].

Taken together, this evidence strongly suggests that cognitive deficits of IPD, even in early disease, have a multifactorial origin, including deficiency of dopamine and nondopaminergic neurochemical transmitters and intrinsic cortical pathology. However, the distribution of cortical pathology may not be identical across diseases with common pathology: Reports of abnormal *tau* protein, typical of AD, in the cortex and CSF of PD patients are controversial; however, when detected, abnormal *tau* protein accumulated in higher levels in the prefrontal cortex of patients with PD than in patients with AD [87,88], suggesting that different etiologic factors operate to produce shared pathology in different diseases. Dopaminergic deafferentation of the frontal cortex may, for example, predispose to neuronal loss in that region [89].

Further evidence of clinicopathologic relationships in the cognitive impairment of IPD is derived from neuroimaging studies [90–94]. Demented patients differ from nondemented patients in showing lower fluorodeoxyglucose (FDG) uptake in parietal cortex, temporal cortex, and striatum on PET [95]; posterior changes similar to those in AD on flow single photon emission tomography (SPET) [96–101] and FDG-PET [102,103]; lower densities of presynaptic cholinergic terminal densities throughout the cerebral cortex on iodobenzovesamicol-SPET [104]; hippocampal atrophy on volumetric MRI [105]; and increased occipital lactate–*N*-acetyl aspartate ratio on proton magnetic resonance spectroscopy [106]. Similar but milder changes are seen in nondemented cases compared to controls [99,104], supporting the concept that demented and nondemented cases of PD represent a spectrum of pathologies in multiple systems important to cognitive function. Neuroimaging studies also support the notion that some abnormalities are relatively specific to IPD, notably hypometabolism in the frontal cortex [96,107–109].

Neurophysiologic changes, in general, mirror the cognitive disability. Thus, compared to nondemented patients, demented IPD patients show decreased alpha amplitude on the electroencephalogram (EEG) [110], longer P100 latencies on visual evoked potentials (VEPs) [111,112], and prolonged P300 event-related potential latencies [113]. These methods are very useful for investigation of the temporal relationships of cognitive processes and, in principle, as an aid to diagnosis and study of the effects of medication. The sensitivity and specificity for the delineation of specific syndromes, however, is not yet evaluated. As yet, the methods provide limited information on clinicopathologic relationships owing to the lack of knowledge of the neural origins of most of the potentials.

Not all motor disability in IPD is sensitive to dopamine. Axial disability, notably posture, gait, speech, and swallowing, are resistant to standard treatments. Neuroimaging studies of higher-order motor disability (clinical apraxia) in IPD have implicated cortical dysfunction in the origin of these impairments [114]. Some studies have compared cognitive function with motor disability on and off dopaminergic therapy. Residual motor disability, resistant to dopaminergic treatment, has been found to correlate with cognitive function better than motor disability does in the untreated state [73,115]. Because resistant motor disability is arguably nondopaminergic in origin, axial motor disability and cognitive dysfunction may be based on common pathology, probably within the cerebral cortex.

The etiology of these nondopaminergic changes is unknown. Genes coding for apolipoprotein E ε4 (*APOE-ε4*) have been strongly implicated in the pathogenesis of AD and in cortical Lewy body disease in which AD changes are also present (Lewy body variant of AD). Most studies, however, fail to show an increase in

APOE-ε4 genotype in either pure cortical Lewy body disease or idiopathic PD with or without dementia [116–122], especially when coexistent AD changes have been confidently excluded. Undoubtedly some of the dementia of IPD is related to coexistent Alzheimer changes, although whether these occur more frequently than expected for age remains controversial. *APOE-ε4* may predispose to amyloid beta-protein accumulation in IPD but does not seem responsible for Lewy body density or abnormal *tau* accumulation in diffuse Lewy body disease, AD, or IPD [122,123]. On present evidence, it seems unlikely that *APOE-ε4* or any of the other gene mutations associated with AD can account for other non-dopaminergic causes of cognitive failure in IPD. The pathogenic mechanism, however, is likely to be different from that underlying nigral cell death. Multiple pathogenic mechanisms exist in IPD and underlie the marked clinical heterogeneity of the disorder.

Treatment

The mainstay of treatment of the motor disorder of IPD is levodopa with a dopa-decarboxylase inhibitor (benserazide-levodopa, carbidopa-levodopa, cobeneldopa, cocareldopa), dopamine agonists (apomorphine, bromocriptine, cabergoline, pergolide, pramipexole, ropinirole), MAO inhibitors (selegiline), catechol *O*-methyltransferase inhibitors (entacapone, tolcapone), and neurosurgical procedures (fetal nigral grafts; stereotactic surgery, notably pallidotomy; and deep brain stimulation) [5]. In clinical practice, and from experimental observations, none of these treatments has clinically significant benefit to the cognitive dysfunction. Indeed, the main difference between treatments is the extent to which they precipitate or exacerbate behavioral disorder.

Few specific treatments other than adjusting dopaminergic drug dosages for the cognitive disorder have been investigated in IPD. However, recognition of cholinergic, noradrenergic, and serotonergic deficits paves the way for manipulation of these systems to benefit the milder cognitive impairments that may contribute to disability, even in early disease. Depression in IPD responds to selective serotonin reuptake inhibitors (SSRIs), although the effect on cognition has been little investigated. If bradyphrenia is linked to affective disorder, SSRIs should benefit this aspect of behavioral dysfunction. Beneficial effects of fluvoxamine have been obtained in alcohol-induced memory disorder and cholinergic and noradrenergic manipulation have been beneficial in several conditions. For example, manipulation of the cholinergic system is well known to aid aspects of attention and memory in AD, and noradrenergic manipulation by clonidine or guanfacine provides benefit to the memory disorder of Korsakoff's syndrome. Noradrenergic enhancement by idazoxan has produced beneficial effects in frontal lobe dementia [77]. In principle, similar therapies could aid the cognitive impairment of IPD. Small but significant improvements in frontal cognitive function were obtained in one study of guanfacine treatment in IPD, supporting the potential use of noradrenergic modulation for cognitive therapy [77]. One problem with cholinergic manipulation is that stimulation of muscarinic receptors in the striatum is likely to impede motor control. Potential exists, however, for the use of nicotine because the striatum contains few nicotinic receptors in higher-order mammals [124].

Table 4.4 Organic psychosis in Parkinson's disease: therapeutic strategy

Exclude coincidental conditions
Stabilize environment and medication
Stop anticholinergics, amantadine, and selegiline
Change dopamine agonist
Reduce dopaminergic load
Benzodiazepines
Neuroleptics
Electroconvulsive therapy

Treatment of Psychosis

In principle, management of hallucinations and delusions in IPD involves reduction of dopaminergic stimulation in the mesolimbic and mesocortical circuits. This concept is currently of limited practical value, however, because selective reduction of such activity without impairing dopaminergic transmission in nigrostriatal circuits that govern motor control is scarcely possible using existing drugs. Other practical methods have to be used (Table 4.4). Patients with psychotic behavior are easily disturbed by changes in environmental circumstances, so frequent changes of their environment should be avoided. Coincidental medical conditions should be excluded. Drugs that have relatively weak therapeutic benefit to motor control compared to their behavioral side effects should be discontinued, notably anticholinergic drugs, amantadine, and selegiline; selegiline in particular produces agitation and nocturnal wakefulness due to its amphetamine-like effects [125]. If possible, the dose of dopamine agonists should be reduced relative to levodopa or changed to one, such as pergolide, which is said to have fewer neuropsychiatric side effects [126]. Apomorphine, which can currently only be given subcutaneously, has relatively fewer neuropsychiatric side effects relative to its efficacy compared to oral dopamine agonists [127]. Thus, a change from oral treatments to parenteral apomorphine therapy may be beneficial. Despite the reported benefit of some dopamine agonists over others, individual patients may benefit less predictably from one dopamine agonist compared to another. Thus, a simple change in the oral dopamine agonist may produce beneficial effects that are not predicted from published group studies.

The majority of neuroleptic drugs are dopamine (D) antagonists and have powerful extrapyramidal side effects due to blockade of D_2 receptors. Patients with IPD are especially vulnerable to these drugs. Even the newer generation of neuroleptics have powerful deleterious effects on motor control in IPD that are not seen when such treatments are given to schizophrenic patients [128]. If neuroleptics have to be used, they should be given in very low doses with careful monitoring of motor disability. The atypical neuroleptic clozapine is of particular benefit in IPD [129] because its major action is against the D_4 receptor with relatively less binding at D_2. Clozapine is associated with a significant risk of agranulocytosis, however, so regular blood monitoring is necessary. The new neuroleptic olanzapine has a similar profile of action to that of clozapine and may be similarly beneficial. In our own experience, the drug is useful but undoubtedly exacerbates motor disability except at low doses (1–5 mg daily)

[130]. The antiemetic ondansetron, a 5-HT_3 antagonist, has antipsychotic actions at low doses and is beneficial in the treatment of drug-induced psychosis of IPD in a double-blind trial [131]. General sedation with benzodiazepines may help agitation. Electroconvulsive therapy has been reported to be useful [132].

When all these measures fail, as they often do, the only resort is to reduce the dopaminergic load. In patients with both psychosis and dyskinesia, reduction in treatment may assist both behavior and motor disability. Often, however, control of the psychosis by reduction in total dose of medication has to be achieved at the expense of increased motor disability. The aim is to provide a dose of medication that provides the optimal balance for control of activities of daily living between the behavioral and motor disabilities. The ease of provision of nursing care to severely disabled patients is an important consideration in this optimization of treatment.

IPD is a multifaceted clinical disorder that may require input from a number of subspecialties, including neurology, psychiatry, physiotherapy, occupational therapy, speech therapy, and social work. When behavioral disturbance also exists, the need for a multidisciplinary team becomes even more important. A nurse practitioner or specialist PD liaison nurse operating between primary care and specialist services can facilitate monitoring of patients, anticipatory management, avoidance of emergency crises, and rapid access to specialist services, according to need.

PROGRESSIVE SUPRANUCLEAR PALSY

PSP was recognized as a distinct clinical syndrome by Steele and colleagues [133], hence its eponym *Steele-Richardson-Olszewski syndrome*. The main early descriptions of this disorder included a supranuclear ophthalmoparesis, pseudobulbar palsy, dysarthria, dystonic rigidity of the neck and trunk, and other cerebellar and pyramidal features. The condition was recognized to be gradually progressive. The features of the syndrome have since been amplified [134–138] and attempts made to reach a consensus on the clinicopathologic criteria required to establish the diagnosis. However, the syndrome is now recognized to be quite diverse in its clinical manifestations, which overlap substantially with those of other movement and cognitive disorders. Important clinical features for diagnosis highlighted in later descriptions are parkinsonism, paroxysmal disequilibrium, early falling, and progressive dementia.

The classic pathology of PSP is degeneration involving the pons, midbrain, dentate and subthalamic nuclei, globus pallidus, and nucleus basalis. More widespread atrophy is present in later stages. Histologic studies show neurofibrillary tangles and gliosis but not plaques [133,135,138].

Difficulties in establishing the diagnosis clinically and the relative paucity of pathologic confirmation renders epidemiologic data of questionable precision. However, published series describe prevalence ratios of approximately 1.4 per 100,000, with a male preponderance of approximately 66%. The incidence is estimated at 4.7 new cases per million per year [139]. A review of 178 autopsy-confirmed cases published since 1979 showed a mean age of onset of 61 years (range, 43–74 years), broadly comparable with clinical series [140]. The mean survival from diagnosis is 5.6 years. PSP appears to be equally common among all races. The cause is unknown, but tantalizing associations have been made in small series with greater education, previous urban residence, and exposure to organic solvents and hydrocarbons [139]. A familial form has been suggested in small studies, but most cases appear to be sporadic [139,141].

The "pure" form of PSP is easy to recognize, but atypical forms occur and may be easily confused with other neurodegenerative conditions. In the early stages, the classic supranuclear ophthalmoparesis, initially particularly affecting downward gaze but later spreading to all eye movements, may be completely absent. Some patients show atypical ocular signs, suggesting myasthenia gravis. Other patients present with a condition similar to amyotrophic lateral sclerosis. Some cases show pure akinetic rigid syndromes or pure akinesia. When parkinsonism is prominent, the differential diagnosis includes IPD, MSA, corticobasal ganglionic degeneration, the rigid form of Huntington's disease, and rarer conditions of the basal ganglia, including Wilson's disease. When dementia is prominent, the disorder is easily confused with other neurodegenerative dementias, particularly those accompanied by prominent frontal lobe signs. The combination of parkinsonism and dementia may suggest particularly IPD, corticobasal ganglionic degeneration (CBGD), Creutzfeldt-Jakob disease (CJD), and diffuse Lewy body disease. The early involvement of gait, particularly in combination with prominent dementia, may suggest normal pressure hydrocephalus (NPH). Diffuse vascular disease commonly masquerades as PSP when there is brain stem ischemia, producing ophthalmoparesis and spasticity, and widespread involvement of small cerebral vasculature, producing parkinsonism and dementia [142,143].

Classic descriptions of the parkinsonian features of PSP allow a distinction from those of IPD. Unlike IPD, PSP presents with symmetric onset, early gait disturbance, frequent and early falls, erect posture, late loss of arm swing, a "surprised" facial expression, rare rest tremor, and marked axial rigidity as opposed to limb rigidity. Loss of ocular upgaze is recognized in IPD (although many of these patients may be misdiagnosed cases of PSP or MSA), but the initial gaze palsy in PSP usually affects downward gaze. Florid supranuclear gaze palsies do not occur in IPD and are a more common feature of CBGD. The features of CBGD also include axial rigidity, postural instability, and limb dystonia [144–146]. Limb apraxia and the "alien hand" [147], however, which are common in CBGD [148], are not typical features of PSP. Clinical dementia occurs relatively early in PSP but late in IPD. When a tremor does occur in PSP, it is more often postural and of higher frequency than that in IPD.

Other clinical features described in PSP are spasticity, focal dystonia, disturbed sleep rhythm, depression, action myoclonus, autonomic dysfunction, psychosis, chorea, rest tremor, muscle atrophy, and paroxysmal kinesogenic dystonia [149]. Severe autonomic failure does not occur in PSP, and autonomic disturbances of any severity tend to be late, unlike in MSA in which they may be early and severe.

Urethral and anal sphincter electromyography has been proposed as a sensitive and specific test for the diagnosis of MSA and its distinction from IPD [150]. Similar degrees of denervation of the external anal sphincter, however, qualitatively indistinguishable from that seen in MSA, have been described in PSP [149].

Neuroimaging is of little value in the diagnosis of PSP. In advanced disease, midbrain and pontine atrophy may be present. In the early stages, however, routine neuroimaging is usually normal. Neuroimaging may help to exclude other conditions with more typical positive findings, such as MSA of the olivo-ponto-cerebellar type and some conditions that show abnormal signal intensities within the basal ganglia, such as Leigh disease, Hallevorden-Spatz disease, Wilson's disease, and cerebrovascular disease [151].

The supranuclear nature of the ophthalmoparesis can be demonstrated by preserved reflex movements in the presence of markedly impaired volitional, saccadic movements. Reflex movements can be elicited clinically by passive movement of the head with the eyes fixated and by relative preservation of pursuit movements, which are partially reflex in origin, compared to voluntary eye movements. More formal examination by vestibulo-ocular reflex testing and electronystagmography may be helpful in subclinical cases.

The concept of subcortical dementia, comprising cognitive slowing, forgetfulness, depression, and impairment of executive functions, was based initially on clinical evaluation of patients with PSP [17]. Dubois and colleagues examined some of these concepts using a reaction time paradigm that controlled for movement time and concluded that the concept of bradyphrenia in PSP was supported: Cognitive processing time became disproportionately long with increasing complexity of the task [152]. Patients with PSP are also impaired in "frontal" cognitive tests, including verbal and nonverbal fluency, the Wisconsin Card Sorting Test of set-shifting (in which change in response selection based on previous experience is required by altered environmental demands), Trail-Making Test, picture arrangement subtest of the Wechsler Adult Intelligence Scale, motor sequencing, and other tasks that tap problem solving and abstract thinking. PSP patients are also impaired in immediate and delayed verbal and nonverbal recall and show poor learning and rapid forgetting. When learning and recall are manipulated, however, the pattern of memory impairment in PSP is different from that of AD and related, albeit more severely, to that of IPD. Cognitive slowing and impairment on executive tasks are closely associated in PSP. Which of these two represents the primary deficit is unclear, but it is probably loss of frontally mediated executive control. Thus, most of the deficits in PSP can be explained by pathology in the striatopallidal complex and its projections to the frontal lobes.

The frontal lobe disorder is more severe than that of IPD and is usually of clinical significance. Cognitive features of "cortical dementia," however, including apraxia, aphasia, and agnosia, do not occur in uncomplicated PSP. Some patients with PSP have been shown to have coincidental Alzheimer pathology, which may be responsible for any impairment in these cognitive domains [153].

There is no specific treatment for PSP. Lack of response to levodopa or dopaminergic drugs may help in distinguishing the condition from IPD. Moreover, dyskinesias and response fluctuations that complicate later stages of IPD do not occur in PSP. Some beneficial effect to the motor disorder has been provided by idazoxan [154]. No specific treatment exists for the cognitive disorder, although the effects of idazoxan have not been evaluated in detail. Postural tremor may be helped by propranolol but is rarely troublesome. The mainstay of treatment is supportive using physiotherapy, occupational therapy, speech therapy, and social support. The behavioral disorder does not generally have positive features of agitation or delirium but adds to the nursing burden.

There is no specific test for the diagnosis of PSP. A number of clinical diagnostic criteria have been proposed that differ in their emphasis on sensitivity or specificity. One classification is aimed to provide high specificity with few false-positives at the expense of missing some less typical cases [149]. These criteria are listed in Table 4.5.

CORTICOBASAL GANGLIONIC DEGENERATION

Isolated examples of CBGD were recognized in the mid-1960s and described as cortico-dentato-nigral degeneration with neuronal achromasia [155]. The condition has been increasingly recognized since then, although data on pathogenesis, cognitive features, and clinicopathologic relationships are meager compared with other parkinsonian dementing disorders [144–146,148]. CBGD is a degenerative disorder that seems to be sporadic, with no particular ethnic or geographic clustering, no familial tendency, and no evidence of toxic etiologic factors. Age of onset is usually greater than 60 years, and sex incidence is equal.

CBGD comprises an akinetic-rigid parkinsonian syndrome. A key distinguishing feature from most other parkinsonian conditions apart from IPD is its asymmetric onset. Although the akinesia and rigidity may be similar in the affected upper limb, rest tremor is usually absent; a postural tremor may occur. A key diagnostic feature of the unilateral extrapyramidal disorder in the early stages is the alien hand, usually accompanied by apraxia and cortical sensory impairment [147,148]. Spread to the contralateral upper limb usually occurs within 1–3 years and is accompanied by progressive axial involvement with disturbance of gait and posture and hypophonic dysarthria. The condition usually progresses to a state of profound rigidity and immobility within 5–7 years when the alien limb may have progressed to develop a flexed, dystonic posturing, particularly affecting distal joints. Myoclonus is another useful diagnostic feature. It is commonly precipitated by posture and action and is stimulus sensitive. As the condition progresses, the clinical syndrome incorporates bilateral pyramidal signs, supranuclear gaze palsies, choreoathetosis, blepharospasm, and cerebellar ataxia. Other focal dystonias may occur.

Cognitive studies of CBGD are few. Although from a clinical perspective cognition may appear to be intact in the early stages, clinically evident cognitive dysfunction develops progressively over the first few years. Unlike IPD and PSP, the dementia of CBGD includes aphasia and marked disturbances of memory and other intellectual functions. The development of dementia is accompanied by primitive reflexes, including grasp and palmomental reflexes. The cortical sensory impairments of astereognosis and dysgraphesthesia become more prominent in concert with increasing apraxia. By the most advanced stages, the patient is immobile and communication ceases due to a combination of severe monotonous dysarthria and aphasia.

The diagnosis is principally made on clinical grounds. The asymmetric onset and presence of apraxia and cortical sensory loss, sometimes with extensor plantar responses, provide important diagnostic clues to differentiate the condition from other parkinsonian syndromes such as PSP, MSA, atypical IPD, the disinhibition-dementia-parkinsonism-amyotrophy complex (DDPAC) [156], and other rare causes of parkinsonism with dementia discussed in this chapter. Like

Table 4.5 NINDS-SPSP clinical criteria for the diagnosis of progressive supranuclear palsy

Progressive supranuclear palsy (PSP)	*Mandatory inclusion criteria*	*Mandatory exclusion criteria*	*Supportive criteria*
Possible	Gradually progressive disorder Onset at age 40 or later Either vertical (upward or downward gaze) supranuclear palsy or both slowing of vertical saccades and prominent postural instability with falls in the first year of disease onset No evidence of other diseases that could explain the foregoing features, as indicated by mandatory exclusion criteria	Recent history of encephalitis Alien limb syndrome, cortical sensory deficits, focal frontal or temporoparietal atrophy Hallucinations or delusions unrelated to dopaminergic therapy Cortical dementia of Alzheimer's type (severe amnesia and aphasia or agnosia, according to NINCDS-ADRDA criteria) Prominent, early cerebellar symptoms or prominent, early unexplained dysautonomia (marked hypotension and urinary disturbances)	Symmetric akinesia or rigidity, proximal more than distal Abnormal neck posture, especially retrocollis Poor or absent response of parkinsonism to levodopa therapy Early dysphagia and dysarthria Early onset of cognitive impairment including at least two of the following: apathy, impairment in abstract thought, decreased verbal fluency, utilization or imitation behavior, or frontal release signs
Probable	Gradually progressive disorder Onset at age 40 or later Vertical (upward or downward gaze) supranuclear palsy and prominent postural instability with falls in the first year of disease onset No evidence of other diseases that could explain the foregoing features, as indicated by mandatory exclusion criteria	Severe, asymmetric parkinsonian signs (i.e., bradykinesia) Neuroradiologic evidence of relevant structural abnormality (i.e., basal ganglia or brain stem infarcts, lobar atrophy) Whipple's disease, confirmed by polymerase chain reaction if indicated	
Definite	Clinically probable or possible PSP and histopathologic evidence of typical PSP		

NINDS = National Institute of Neurologic Diseases and Stroke; SPSP = Society for Progressive Supra-nuclear Palsy; ADRDA = Alzheimer's Disease and Related Disorders Association.

most other non-IPD causes of parkinsonism, the condition is not responsive to dopaminergic modulation. The alien hand provides a particularly useful early diagnostic pointer.

In cases of diagnostic doubt, neuroimaging may be helpful [146]. Although computed tomography (CT) and MRI are commonly normal in the early stages, the development of asymmetric atrophy, reflecting the clinical asymmetry, helps to distinguish the condition from other causes of parkinsonism. Structural imaging shows asymmetric atrophy in the frontal and parietal areas, which spreads as the clinical condition advances and becomes bilateral and is often accompanied by abnormalities in the subcortex. EEG slow wave abnormalities usually mirror the neuroimaging findings, with asymmetric slowing in the early stages progressing to bilateral abnormalities later. Some patients show abnormalities of somatosensory evoked potentials and prolonged P100 latencies on pattern VEPs.

PET studies of blood flow and metabolism show patterns that generally conform to those of the clinical features and the distribution of neuropathology. Thus, hypometabolism and reduced flow have been demonstrated, particularly in frontal, temporal, and parietal cortex asymmetrically. Fluorodopa studies have shown reduced striatal fluorodopa uptake indicative of nigrostriatal dopamine deficiency.

The classic microscopic pathology of CBGD is asymmetric atrophy affecting particularly the frontal cortex and, to a lesser extent, the temporal and parietal cortex. Histologically, the atrophy is accompanied by severe loss of medium to large pyramidal neurons that, at an earlier stage of degeneration, show a typical appearance of cytoplasmic swelling and pallor on standard histologic stains (achromasia). Similar histologic changes occur to a lesser extent in subcortical, brain stem, and cerebellar nuclei. Neuronal loss is accompanied by marked gliosis and degeneration of descending tracts in the white matter. Severe neuronal loss and gliosis also occur in the lateral and middle portions of the pars compacta of the substantia nigra but without the typical Lewy bodies of IPD. Achromatic neurons may occur, albeit to a much milder degree, in basal ganglia and limbic nuclei, including the striatum, pallidum, amygdala, and thalamus; in brain stem nuclei, including the noradrenergic locus coeruleus, serotonergic raphe nuclei, and the ocular motor nuclei; and in cerebellar nuclei. The nucleus basalis, which is affected in IPD and PSP, is largely spared. The abnormal neurons stain positively with antibodies to ubiquitin and phosphorylated neurofilament protein but not *tau*. This staining pattern is in contrast to that of AD tangles and Pick cells (despite being histologically similar to achromatic neurons), which stain positively to *tau*.

The distribution of pathology accounts for the typical clinical signs: Involvement of the motor and sensory cortices accounts for the early features of apraxia, cortical sensory loss, and loss of voluntary, saccadic eye movements. Involvement of the substantia nigra accounts for parkinsonian features, whereas involvement of other basal ganglia nuclei probably produces other extrapyramidal features, such as dystonia. Degeneration of ocular motor nuclei occurs later and is responsible for the progression of the ocular motor abnormalities to involve reflex as well as saccadic eye movements.

The relationship of the underlying neuropathology to the behavioral disorder is largely unknown, owing to the paucity of behavioral studies of CBGD. The aphasia and apraxia, however, clearly correspond to the pattern of focal cortical degeneration. The influence of involvement of subcortical neurotransmitter systems remains unknown but, in theory, degeneration of the 5-HT and noradrenergic systems may have specific effects. In contrast to AD and IPD, in CBGD, the cholinergic system seems to be relatively spared and may lead to relative preservation of memory functions. This subcortical neurochemical pathology occurs late, however, and is relatively minor compared to the overwhelming cortical pathology. Therefore, attempts to influence cognitive function by pharmacologic means are unlikely to be successful.

The condition is largely untreatable. Specifically, there is no beneficial response to antiparkinsonian therapies. As with all movement disorders, propranolol may help the action tremor and clonazepam may help rigidity and myoclonus. The most important management, however, as with other parkinsonian syndromes unresponsive to dopamine modulation, is supportive, particularly in the later stages in which severe disability supervenes.

NORMAL PRESSURE HYDROCEPHALUS

NPH is a clinical triad encompassing gait disturbance, dementia, and loss of sphincter control that was first described as a sequel to subarachnoid hemorrhage but later recognized in an idiopathic form [157]. The condition arises as a communicating hydrocephalus in which the ventricular and extracerebral CSF spaces are in free communication, although a similar syndrome may occur in obstructive hydrocephalus in which there is gradual rise in CSF pressure, such as that occurring in decompensating aqueduct stenosis and slow-growing third and fourth ventricular tumors [158]. Communicating hydrocephalus arises from blockage of CSF uptake in the arachnoid villi of the higher cerebral convexities and thus may follow arachnoiditis and bacterial meningitis. The term *NPH* has been used because single measurements of CSF pressure are commonly normal. Continuous CSF pressure monitoring, however, reveals abnormal intermittent elevations or more or less sustained low levels of CSF pressure in the ventricular system [159], which has led to ostensibly more accurate terms such as *intermittent-* and *low-pressure hydrocephalus*. The transmantle pressure, rather than the absolute ventricular pressure, may be the key pathogenic variable. By tradition, the term *NPH* has been applied particularly to this pathology arising without identifiable cause. The clinical features of this idiopathic variety are not clearly different from those of secondary causes, more often termed *communicating hydrocephalus*, but relevant pathology is often not identified.

NPH is most common in the seventh decade of life and is more common in males (2:1). It may account for as many as 5.5% of dementias. Approximately 48% of patients present with the complete triad of dementia, gait disturbance, and incontinence, but 13% of cases present monosymptomatically [160]. However, NPH is a progressive disorder and usually ultimately encompasses the other clinical features. The typical sphincter disturbance is urgency and later unwitting incontinence. The dementia syndrome has been poorly characterized, but clinical observations suggest prominent memory disturbance as a key feature. The cognitive deficits are usually milder than those of AD, and cortical deficits of aphasia, agnosia, and limb apraxia are uncommon. The gait disorder is often termed *gait apraxia*, manifest as a wide-based gait with difficulty in the normal bipedal coordination, gait initiation, and changing of direction [161]. Attempts to walk are accompanied by cocontraction of agonist and antagonist muscle groups. Antigravity muscles show increased tone in response to foot pressure against the floor, and patients show difficulty in the normal sequence of contraction and relaxation necessary for normal gait. Patients with this syndrome do not, however, show the typical flexed posture of IPD nor the paroxysmal disequilibrium of PSP. There is no festination or retropulsion, and pyramidal signs are absent. The general clinical impression of patients with gait apraxia is that they have "forgotten how to walk."

Few studies have evaluated clinicopathologic relationships. The prominent memory disorder, however, is likely to result from dilatation of the third ventricle and involvement of medial temporal lobe and diencephalic structures critical to memory function. Equally, the pathophysiology of the gait disturbance is unclear, but distortion of descending fibers from the precentral gyrus and association areas has been proposed as an etiologic mechanism. Unwitting urinary incontinence is a recognized clinical result of frontal lobe lesions and, in NPH, is likely to result from interruption of inhibitory descending influences from the prefrontal cortex [160]. In general, ventricular size correlates with the extent of the clinical disability [162].

The mainstay of treatment is ventricular shunting, although the predictors of outcome are unclear [160,163]. Gait disorder, particularly when it occurs early or in isolation, responds best [164], whereas a long history of dementia has a poor prognosis from such treatment. The presence of periventricular low densities on CT scanning, absence of cortical atrophy, and dilatation of the temporal horns have been proposed as good predictors of outcome. Significant, albeit temporary, clinical improvement after lumbar puncture, frequent spontaneous increases in CSF pressure (B waves) on continuous intracranial pressure monitoring, and resistance to CSF outflow (CSF infusion test) have also been claimed as good predictors of outcome from shunting.

CEREBROVASCULAR DISEASE

Cerebral vascular injury produces a pattern of cognitive impairment that depends critically on the locus of infarction or hemorrhage. Highly selective deficits, such as amnesia, aphasia, and prosopagnosia follow discrete damage, usually from infarction, in areas critical to those functions, such as the dorsomedial nucleus of the thalamus bilaterally in the case of amnesia [165]. Dementia, defined as a syndrome of multiple cognitive deficits, follows multifocal damage (multi-infarct dementia [MID] [166]). Cerebral ischemia may lead to vascular parkinsonism [167], which coexists with the dementia syndrome, but more commonly the motor disorder is distinct from that of IPD.

MID may result from the combination of deficits from several large-vessel infarctions (or more rarely hemorrhages) or bilateral watershed ischemia; each event is usually symptomatic. More commonly, however, particularly when part of a parkinsonian syndrome, dementia occurs as a consequence of multiple lacunar infarcts. Single lacunar infarcts in this context are often silent, and the cognitive failure constitutes the presenting symptom resulting from the sum of deficits of the multiple lesions.

Binswanger's disease, or subcortical ischemic encephalopathy (SIE), is probably a variety of a multiple lacunar state, but controversy persists about whether it is a discrete pathologic entity. The disorder is characterized by "diffuse incomplete demyelination" of the periventricular white matter, with diffuse scattered cystic subcortical lacunae. The vessels are affected by thickening and hyalinization of the long penetrating arteries, usually without occlusion. Neuroimaging by CT reveals periventricular low-density areas that may be difficult to differentiate from those of NPH. MRI is much more sensitive in detection of these lesions, which show a high signal intensity on T1-weighted images [168].

The mean age of onset of SIE is 57 years (range, 40–78 years). The sexes are equally affected. The prevalence in the population aged older than 50 years is 3.8–6.7% [169]. The clinical syndrome of SIE comprises a triad of dementia, gait disturbance, and urinary incontinence, similar to NPH, although the latter two components are less prominent in SIE [170]. The typical motor disturbance of Binswanger's disease is a gait apraxia (see the previous section, Normal Pressure Hydrocephalus). In less specific clinical syndromes of diffuse subcortical ischemia, parkinsonism may occur when the ischemia extends more preferentially to the basal ganglia region [167], but the role of basal ganglia ischemia in the genesis of parkinsonism has probably been overestimated. Axial disturbances, particularly of gait, remain prominent and have been variously termed *lower-body parkinsonism* [171], *parkinsonian ataxia* [172], and *gait apraxia*. Similar to the gait apraxia of NPH, the patient has particular difficulty in initiation of gait. This seems to occur due to a reflex provoked by pressure of the foot against the floor, because leg movements are relatively preserved in a non–weight-bearing position, such as lying on the bed. Stride length is reduced, so-called marche à petits pas, but with an appearance different from that of IPD. Parkinsonian features are often impure and accompanied by a variable constellation of atypical tremors and other involuntary movements that may be difficult to classify. Rest tremor is rare. A parkinsonian gait and posture are often compounded with spasticity and gait apraxia. Brain stem involvement may produce additional features of pseudobulbar palsy and disordered eye movements suggestive of PSP [142,143].

The cognitive disorder conforms approximately to that of other "subcortical dementias," notably in the absence of aphasia and limb apraxia and the presence of psychomotor slowing. Mood disturbances, psychosis with paranoid delusions, and irritability may occur. Memory deficits are mild. The features of the dementia, however, may be quite variable, depending on the distribution of the ischemia, and cortical deficits of neglect and aphasia develop in patients with combined subcortical and cortical ischemia [165].

The course is often said to be typically stepwise or fluctuating, distinct from the gradually progressive course of other neurodegenerative conditions. However, chronic progression without clear episodes of acute deterioration is relatively common [168].

Chronic hypertension is the main risk factor for these small-vessel syndromes, although some patients have increased blood viscosity and fibrinogen levels [169]. The mainstay of treatment is control of blood pressure and other vascular risk factors. Individuals with higher hematocrits, even still within the normal range, have lower cerebral blood flow [173] and poorer performance on attentional tests [174] compared to those with low-normal hematocrits. Venesection may improve cognitive performance, although formal evaluation of this treatment has not been undertaken. Standard antiparkinsonian therapies are usually ineffective.

RARE SYNDROMES

This chapter outlines the features of the main conditions in clinical practice that produce dementia and parkinsonism. The main distinguishing characteristics are given in Table 4.6. It must be stressed, however, that few of these signs are absolute owing to considerable overlap of the clinical features of these disorders, particularly at different stages of the diseases.

Several other conditions that are not discussed in detail in this chapter may produce prominent parkinsonism and behavioral change, usually as part of a wider clinical spectrum. Reviews of these conditions are available elsewhere [19,175–177]. Recent definitions of MSA do not include dementia within the clinical spectrum [150]; although earlier descriptions have done so, many of these cases may, in retrospect, have had diffuse Lewy body disease. Juvenile Huntington's disease, unlike the adult variety, presents in children with an akinetic-rigid syndrome. Postencephalitic parkinsonism is characterized by parkinsonism, dementia, and oculogyric crises but is no longer a significant clinical problem. Repeated minor head injury, as in boxing (dementia pugilistica), produces varying degrees of an akinetic-rigid syndrome, usually without tremor, and cognitive impairment. Wilson's disease is due to a congenital deficiency of ceruloplasmin, which leads to impaired copper binding and copper accumulation in the basal ganglia and liver. Although the syndrome usually includes other extrapyramidal features, such as choreoathetosis and dystonia, pure parkinsonism may occur. The behavioral disorder has been characterized but is nonspecific. CJD may present with insidious parkinsonism, dementia, and visual hallucinations, leading rapidly to severe physical incapacity, dementia, anarthria, and visual hallucinations (see Chapter 5). The recently described new variant of CJD, possibly associated with transmission of bovine spongiform encephalopathy to humans, has different clinical features, including early onset with anxiety and depression, and affects younger people than those of traditional CJD [178]. AD is often accompanied by extrapyramidal features, which in early studies were considered to be proportional to the severity of dementia. Recent neuropathologic studies, however, demand revision of these observations in light of the unexpected findings of high prevalence of cortical Lewy body disease in conditions diagnosed as clinical AD and the different clinical syndromes that may result from the combined pathology of cortical Alzheimer changes and Lewy body disease. The parkinsonism-dementia complex of Guam is of theoretical interest in the etiology of parkinsonian conditions but is of little clinical relevance in other countries. In children, rare disorders such as Hallervorden-Spatz disease (due to iron accumulation in the basal ganglia), lipofuscinosis, and Leigh disease (which may present in adults) are rare causes of parkinsonism and dementia [151]. The familial complex of DDPAC has been mapped to chromosome 17 [179]. Certain accumulations or chronic exposure to toxins and heavy metals, including manganese, alcohol, carbon monoxide, disulfide, and certain drugs, may present as a syndrome of parkinsonian motor disorder and behavioral disturbance. Hypoparathyroidism has been described as a cause of parkinsonism and behavior

Table 4.6 Clinical differentiation of idiopathic Parkinson's disease, progressive supranuclear palsy, corticobasal ganglionic degeneration, normal pressure hydrocephalus, and subcortical ischemic encephalopathy

	Idiopathic Parkinson's disease	*Progressive supranuclear palsy*	*Corticobasal ganglionic degeneration*	*Normal pressure hydrocephalus*	*Subcortical ischemic encephalopathy*
Early motor signs					
Key sign	Rest tremor	Falls	Alien hand	Gait apraxia	Marche à petits pas
Limb or axial	Limb	Axial	Limb	Axial	Axial
Symmetry	No	Yes	No	Yes	Yes
Flexed or erect	Flexed	Erect	Flexed	Erect	Erect
Gait	Parkinsonian	Parkinsonian	Parkinsonian	Apraxic	Apraxic
Falls	No	Yes	No	No	No
Lost arm swing	Prominent	Yes	Yes	No	No
Other significant motor signs					
Pyramidal/cerebellar	No	Yes	Yes	No	Yes
Myoclonus	Infrequent	Yes	Prominent	No	No
Dystonia	Yes	Yes	Marked	No	No
Supranuclear gaze palsy	No	Prominent	Yes	No	Infrequent
Early cognitive features					
Key sign	Normal	Frontal	Aphasia	Memory	Dementia
Limb apraxia/cortical sensory loss	No	No	Yes	No	Sometimes
Aphasia	No	No	Yes	No	Sometimes
Mood and psychosis	Yes	Yes	No	No	Yes
Other early features					
Incontinence	No	No	No	Prominent	Yes
Hypertension	No	No	No	No	Yes

change due to calcium accumulation in the basal ganglia. The toxin MPTP, which was ingested by recreational drug abusers as a by-product of illicitly synthesized narcotics, produces a syndrome indistinguishable from clinical IPD [69]. Neuropsychological studies have shown features similar to those of early IPD [180], probably secondary to dopamine deficiency, but extensive Lewy body involvement and clinical dementia does not occur. Cerebral tumors rarely present as a combination of parkinsonism and behavioral disturbance, particularly when the frontal lobes are involved, but the syndrome is usually distinguishable clinically from other causes of parkinsonism and dementia. The behavioral disturbance in these conditions is prominent, and the motor disturbance is usually either frontal lobe apraxia or psychomotor retardation. Other conditions, such as neuroacanthocytosis, may produce extrapyramidal behavioral disturbances, but the motor disorder is usually one of dystonia rather than parkinsonism.

CONCLUSION

The pathology of clinical syndromes producing combined dementia and parkinsonism is multiple and varied. Clinical phenotypes of single disease categories are markedly heterogeneous. Diagnosis of traditional clinical syndromes is difficult owing to considerable overlap in the clinical features and the general absence of specific diagnostic tests. Clinically defined syndromes usually incorporate overlapping pathologies. The etiology and pathogenesis of most of these diagnostic categories are unknown. Treatment is closely linked to an understanding of the underlying pathologic mechanisms. Thus, the way forward for effective therapy of these conditions is to abandon traditional diagnostic categories and to address questions of pathogenesis and treatment to components of the overlapping pathologies.

REFERENCES

1. Gibb WRG, Lees A. The relevance of the Lewy body to the pathogenesis of idiopathic Parkinson's disease. J Neurol Neurosurg Psychiatry 1988;51:745–752.
2. Hughes AJ, Ben-Schlomo Y, Daniel SE, Lees AJ. What features improve the accuracy of clinical diagnosis in Parkinson's disease: a clinicopathologic study. Neurology 1992;42:1142–1146.
3. Marttila RJ. Epidemiology. In WC Koller (ed), Handbook of Parkinson's Disease. New York: Marcel Dekker, 1987;35–50.
4. Hughes AJ, Daniel SE, Blankson S, Lees AJ. A clinicopathologic study of 100 cases of Parkinson's disease. Arch Neurol 1993;50:140–148.
5. Oertel WH, Quinn NP. Parkinsonism. In T Brandt, LR Caplan, J Dishgans, et al. (eds), Neurological Disorders: Course and Treatment. San Diego: Academic, 1996;715–772.
6. Benecke R, Rothwell JC, Dick JPR. Disturbance of sequential movement in patients with Parkinson's disease. Brain 1987;110:361–379.
7. Marsden D. The mysterious motor function of the basal ganglia: the Robert Wartenberg Lecture. Neurology 1982;32:514–539.
8. Stern Y, Mayeux R, Rosen J, Ilson J. Perceptual motor dysfunction in Parkinson's disease: a deficit in sequential and predictive voluntary movement. J Neurol Neurosurg Psychiatry 1983;46:145–151.
9. Parkinson J. An Essay on the Shaking Palsy. London: Sherwood, Neely and Jones, 1817.
10. Reviewed by Tyler KL. A History of Parkinson's Disease. In WC Koller (ed), Handbook of Parkinson's Disease. New York: Marcel Dekker, 1987.

11. Roos RA, Jongen JC, van der Velda EA. Clinical course of patients with idiopathic Parkinson's disease. Mov Disord 1996;11:236–242.
12. Piccirilli M, D'Alessandro P, Finali G, Piccinin GL. Neuropsychological follow-up of parkinsonian patients with and without cognitive impairment. Dementia 1994;5:17–22.
13. Mortimer JA, Christensen KJ, Webster DD. Parkinsonian Dementia. In PJ Vinken, GW Bruyn, HL Klawans, Handbook of Clinical Neurology. New York: Wiley, 1985;46;2.
14. Brown RG, Marsden CD. How common is dementia in Parkinson's disease? Lancet 1984;2:1262–1265.
15. Markham CH, Diamond SG. Long-term follow-up of early dopa treatment in Parkinson's disease. Ann Neurol 1986;19:365–372.
16. Hughes AJ, Daniel SE, Blankson S, Lees AJ. A clinicopathologic study of 100 cases of Parkinson's disease. Arch Neurol 1993;50:140–148.
17. Albert ML, Feldman RG, Willis AL. The "subcortical dementia" of progressive supranuclear palsy. J Neurol Neurosurg Psychiatry 1974;37:121–130.
18. Cummings JL, Benson DF. Subcortical dementia. Review of an emerging concept. Arch Neurol 1984;41:874–879.
19. Cummings JL (ed). Subcortical Dementia. Oxford: Oxford University Press, 1990.
20. Naville F. Etudes sur les complications et les sequelles mentales de l'encephalite epidemique: la bradyphrenie. Encephale 1922;17:336–369.
21. Cooper JC, Sagar HJ, Tidswell P, Jordan NJ. Slowed central processing in simple and go–no-go reaction time tasks in Parkinson's disease. Brain 1994;117:517–529.
22. Rogers D, Lees AJ, Smith E, et al. Bradyphrenia in Parkinson's disease and psychomotor retardation in depressive illness. Brain 1987;110:761–776.
23. Pate DS, Margolin DI. Cognitive slowing in Parkinson's and Alzheimer's patients: distinguishing bradyphrenia from dementia. Neurology 1994;44:669–674.
24. Daum I, Quinn N. Reaction times and visuospatial processing in Parkinson's disease. J Clin Exp Neuropsychol 1991;13:972–982.
25. Duncombe ME, Bradshaw JL, Iansek R, Phillips JG. Parkinsonian patients without dementia or depression do not suffer from bradyphrenia as indexed by performance in mental rotation tasks with and without advance information. Neuropsychologia 1994;32:1383–1396.
26. Howard LA, Binks MG, Moore AP, Playfer JR. How convincing is the evidence for cognitive slowing in Parkinson's disease? Cortex 1994;30:431–442.
27. Mayeux R, Stern Y, Rosen J, Leventhal J. Depression, intellectual impairment and Parkinson's disease. Neurology 1981;31:645–650.
28. Starkstein SE, Sabe L, Petracca G, et al. Neuropsychological and psychiatric differences between Alzheimer's disease and Parkinson's disease with dementia. J Neurol Neurosurg Psychiatry 1996;61:381–387.
29. Glosser G, Wolfe N, Kliner Krenzel L, Albert ML. Cross-cultural cognitive examination performance in patients with Parkinson's disease and Alzheimer's disease. J Nerv Ment Dis 1994;182:432–436.
30. Reviewed by Mayeux R. Mental State. In WC Koller (ed), Handbook of Parkinson's Disease. New York: Marcel Dekker, 1987.
31. Taylor AE, Saint-Cyr JA, Lang AE, Kenny FT. Parkinson's disease and depression. Brain 1986;109: 279–292.
32. Troster AI, Stalp LD, Paolo AM, et al. Neuropsychological impairment in Parkinson's disease with and without depression. Arch Neurol 1995;52:1164–1169.
33. Cooper J, Sagar HJ, Jordan N, et al. Cognitive impairment in early, untreated Parkinson's disease and its relationship to motor disability. Brain 1991;114:2095–2122.
34. Chia LG, Cheng LJ, Chuo LJ, et al. Studies of dementia, depression, electrophysiology and cerebrospinal fluid monoamine metabolites in patients with Parkinson's disease. J Neurol Sci 1995;133:73–78.
35. Elwan OH, Baradah OH, Madkour O, et al. Parkinson's disease, cognition and aging. Clinical, neuropsychological, electrophysiological and cranial computerized tomographic assessment. J Neurol Sci 1996;143:64–71.
36. Sagar HJ. Specificity of cognitive impairment in neurological disease: a methodological critique of Parkinson's disease. Behav Neurol 1991;4:89–102.
37. Doherty SM, Barber D, Hunt E, et al. Clinical correlates of resting state cerebral blood flow abnormalities in depressed patients with Parkinson's disease. A 99m-Tc-HMPAO SPECT study. Neurology 1997;48:A352.
38. Brown RG, Marsden CD. "Subcortical dementia": the neuropsychological evidence. Neuroscience 1988;25:363–387.

39. Lees AJ, Smith E. Cognitive deficits in the early stages of Parkinson's disease. Brain 1983;106: 257–270.
40. Cronin-Golomb A, Corkin S, Growdon JH. Impaired problem solving in Parkinson's disease: impact of a set-shifting deficit. Neuropsychologia 1994;32:579–593.
41. Appollonio I, Grafman J, Clark K, et al. Implicit and explicit memory in patients with Parkinson's disease with and without dementia. Arch Neurol 1994;51:359–367.
42. Sagar HJ, Tooth C. Learning and Memory. In R Brown, M Jahanshani (eds), Neuropsychology of Movement Disorders. (In press.)
43. Pillon R, Dubois R, l'Hermitte F, Agid Y. Heterogeneity of cognitive impairment in progressive supranuclear palsy, Parkinson's disease and Alzheimer's disease. Neurology 1986;36:1179–1185.
44. Stern Y, Richards M, Sano M, Mayeux R. Comparison of cognitive changes in patients with Alzheimer's and Parkinson's disease. Arch Neurol 1993;50:1040–1045.
45. Rothlind JC, Brandt J. A brief assessment of frontal and subcortical functions in dementia. J Neuropsychiatry Clin Neurosci 1993;5:73–77.
46. Paolo AM, Troster AI, Glatt SL, et al. Differentiation of the dementias of Alzheimer's and Parkinson's disease with the dementia rating scale. J Geriatr Psychiatry Neurol 1995;8:184–188.
47. Brown RG, Marsden CD. Internal versus external cues and the control of attention in Parkinson's disease. Brain 1988;111:363–387.
48. Downes JJ, Sharp HM, Costall RM, et al. Alternating fluency in Parkinson's disease: an evaluation of the attentional control theory of cognitive impairment. Brain 1993;116:887–902.
49. Cooper JA, Sagar HJ, Sullivan EV. Short-term memory and temporal ordering in early Parkinson's disease: effects of disease chronicity and medication. Neuropsychologia 1993;31:933–949.
50. Hely MA, Morris JG, Reid WG, et al. Age at onset: the major determinant of outcome in Parkinson's disease. Acta Neurol Scand 1995;92:455–463.
51. Friedman A, Barcikowska M. Dementia in Parkinson's disease. Dementia 1994;5:12–16.
52. Stern Y, Marder K, Tang MX, Mayeux R. Antecedent clinical features associated with dementia in Parkinson's disease. Neurology 1993;43:1690–1692.
53. Glatt SL, Hubble JP, Lyons K, et al. Risk factors for dementia in Parkinson's disease: effect of education. Neuroepidemiology 1996;15:20–25.
54. Ott A, Breteler MM, van Harskamp F, et al. Prevalence of Alzheimer's disease and vascular dementia: association with education. The Rotterdam study. BMJ 1995;310:970–973.
55. Marder K, Tang MX, Cote L, et al. The frequency and associated risk factors for dementia in patients with Parkinson's disease. Arch Neurol 1995;52:695–701.
56. Ross HF, Hughes TA, Boyd JL, et al. The Evolution and Profile of Dementia in Parkinson's Disease. In L Battistin, G Scarlato, T Saraceni, S Ruggieri (eds), Advances in Neurology, vol 69. Philadelphia: Lippincott–Raven, 1996.
57. Mason DL, Sagar HJ. The effect of initial treatment on the development of motor and cognitive complications in Parkinson's disease: a randomised, longitudinal comparison of levodopa, dopamine agonists and anti-cholinergic drugs. Neurology 1997;48(suppl 2):A369–A370.
58. Jacobs DM, Marder K, Cote LJ, et al. Neuropsychological characteristics of preclinical dementia in Parkinson's disease. Neurology 1995;45:1691–1696.
59. Graham JM, Sagar HJ. A data-driven approach to the study of heterogeneity in idiopathic Parkinson's disease: identification of three distinct subtypes. (In press.)
60. Li K, Ito H, Tanaka K, Hirano A. Pathology of clusters: immunocytochemical co-localization of the proteasome in ubiquitinated structures in neurodegenerative diseases and the elderly. J Neuropathol Exp Neurol 1997;56:125–131.
61. De Smet Y, Ruberg M, Serdaru M, et al. Confusion, dementia and anticholinergics in Parkinson's disease. J Neurol Neurosurg Psychiatry 1982;45:1161–1164.
62. Liberman A. Dopamine Agonists in Parkinson's Disease. In WC Koller, G Paulson (eds), Therapy of Parkinson's Disease (2nd ed). New York: Marcel Dekker, 1995.
63. Sanchez-Ramos JR, Ortoll R, Paulson GW. Visual hallucinations associated with Parkinson's disease. Arch Neurol 1996;53:1265–1268.
64. Graham JM, Grünewald RA, Sagar HJ. Hallucinosis in idiopathic Parkinson's disease. J Neurol Neurosurg Psychiatry 1997;63:434–440.
65. McKeith LG, Galasko D, Kosaka K, et al. Consensus guidelines for the clinical and pathologic diagnosis of dementia with Lewy bodies (DLB): report of the consortium on DLB international workshop. Neurology 1996;47:1113–1124.
66. den Hartog Jager WA, Bethlem J. The distribution of the Lewy bodies in the central and autonomic nervous system in idiopathic paralysis agitans. J Neurol Neurosurg Psychiatry 1969;23: 283–290.

67. Gibb WRG, Lees AJ. Pathological Clues to the Cause of Parkinson's Disease. In CD Marsden, S Fahn (eds), Movement Disorders III. Boston: Butterworth–Heinemann, 1994.
68. Landi NT, Ceroni M, Martignoni E, et al. Environment Interaction in Parkinson's Disease: The Case of CYP2D6 Gene Polymorphism. In L Battistin, G Scarlato, T Saraceni, S Ruggieri (eds), Advances in Neurology, vol 69. Philadelphia: Lippincott–Raven, 1996.
69. Langston JW, Ballard PA, Tetrud JW, Irwin I. Chronic parkinsonism in humans due to a product of meperidine analogue synthesis. Science 1983;219:979–980.
70. Seidler A, Heelenbrand W, Robra BP, et al. Possible environmental, occupational and other etiologic factors for Parkinson's disease: a case-control study in Germany. Neurology 1996;46:1275–1284.
71. Suzuki K, Mizuno Y, Yoshida M. Selective inhibition of complex I of the brain electron transport system by tetrahydroisoquinolone. Biochem Biophys Res Commun 1989;162:1541–1545.
72. Jenner P, Dexter DT, Sian J, et al. Oxidative stress as a cause of nigral cell death in Parkinson's disease and incidental Lewy body disease. Ann Neurol 1992;32:S82–S87.
73. Cooper JC, Sagar HJ, Doherty SM, et al. Different effects of dopaminergic and anticholinergic therapies on cognitive and motor function in Parkinson's disease: a follow-up study of untreated patients. Brain 1992;115:1701–1725.
74. Lange KW, Robbins TW, Marsden CD, et al. L-Dopa withdrawal in Parkinson's disease selectively impairs cognitive performance in tests sensitive to frontal lobe dysfunction. Psychopharmacology (Berl) 1992;107:394–404.
75. Flaherty AW, Graybiel AM. Anatomy of the Basal Ganglia. In CD Marsden, S Fahn (eds), Movement Disorders III. Boston: Butterworth–Heinemann, 1994.
76. Mason DL, Tindale WB, Hunt E, Sagar HJ. The pathophysiological basis of cognitive impairment in early, untreated Parkinson's disease: an investigation with 99m Tc HMPAO SPECT. (In press.)
77. Sagar HJ. Psychopharmacology of Cognitive Impairment in Parkinson's Disease. In E Perry, I McKeith (eds), Proceedings of the International Conference on Lewy Body Dementia. Cambridge: Cambridge University Press, 1995.
78. Berry EL, Sagar HJ, Nicolson RI, Brooks D. Investigation of the pathological relationship between affective and cognitive disturbance in Parkinson's disease by functional neuroimaging. J Neurol Neurosurg Psychiatry 1996.
79. Jellinger KA, Paulus W. Clinicopathological correlations in Parkinson's disease. Clin Neurol Neurosurg 1992;94:S86–S88.
80. Mayeux R. The "serotonin hypothesis" for depression in Parkinson's disease. Adv Neurol 1990;53: 163–166.
81. Stern Y, Mayeux R, Cote L. Reaction time and vigilance in Parkinson's disease: possible role of altered norepinephrine metabolism. Arch Neurol 1984;41:1086–1089.
82. Perry EK, Curtis M, Dick DJ, et al. Cholinergic correlates of cognitive impairment in Parkinson's disease: comparison with Alzheimer's disease. J Neurol Neurosurg Psychiatry 1985;48:413–421.
83. Chan-Palay V, Hochli M, Savaskan E, Hungerecker G. Calbindin D28k and monoamine oxidase A immunoreactive neurons in the nucleus basalis of Meynert in senile dementia of the Alzheimer type and Parkinson's disease. Dementia 1993;4:1–15.
84. Zweig RM, Cardillo JE, Cohen M, et al. The locus ceruleus and dementia in Parkinson's disease. Neurology 1993;43:986–991.
85. de Vos RA, Jansen EN, Stam FC, et al. Lewy body disease: clinicopathological correlation in 18 consecutive cases of Parkinson's disease with and without dementia. Clin Neurol Neurosurg 1995;97:13–22.
86. Espino A, Calopa M, Ambrosio S, et al. CSF somatostatin increase in patients with early parkinsonian syndrome. J Neural Transm Park Dis Dement Sect 1995;9:189–196.
87. Vermersch P, Delacourte A, Javoy-Agid F, et al. Dementia in Parkinson's disease: biochemical evidence for cortical involvement using the immunodetection of abnormal Tau proteins. Ann Neurol 1993;33:445–450.
88. Delacourte A. Pathological Tau proteins of Alzheimer's disease as a biochemical marker of neurofibrillary degeneration. Biomed Pharmacother 1994;48:287–295.
89. Double KL, Halliday GM, McRitchie DA, et al. Regional brain atrophy in idiopathic Parkinson's disease and diffuse Lewy body disease. Dementia 1996;7:304–313.
90. Drayer BP. Degenerative disorders of the central nervous system: an integrated approach to the differential diagnosis. Neuroimaging Clin North Am 1995;5:135–153.
91. Krausz Y, Bonne O, Marciano R, et al. Brain SPECT imaging of neuropsychiatric disorders. Eur J Radiol 1996;21:183–187.
92. Saha GB, MacIntyre WJ, Go RT. Radiopharmaceuticals for brain imaging. Semin Nucl Med 1994; 24:324–349.
93. Davis PC, Mirra SS, Alazraki N. The brain in older persons with and without dementia: findings on MR, PET, and SPECT images. AJR Am J Roentgenol 1994;162:1267–1278.

94. Mazziotta JC, Frackowiak RS, Phelps ME. The use of positron emission tomography in the clinical assessment of dementia. Semin Nucl Med 1992;2:233–246.
95. Piert M, Koeppe RA, Giordani B, et al. Determination of regional rate constants from dynamic FDG-PET studies in Parkinson's disease. J Nucl Med 1996;37:115–122.
96. Tarczy M, Szirmai L. Failure of dopamine metabolism: borderlines of parkinsonism and dementia. Acta Biomed Ateneo Parmense 1995;66(3–4):93–97.
97. Jagust WJ, Johnson KA, Holman BL. SPECT perfusion imaging in the diagnosis of dementia. J Neuroimaging 1995;5:S45–S52.
98. Tachibana H, Tomino Y, Kawabata K, et al. Twelve-month follow-up study of regional cerebral blood flow in Parkinson's disease. Dementia 1995;6:89–93.
99. Tachibana H, Kawabata K, Tomino Y, et al. Three-dimensional surface display of brain perfusion with 1231-IMP in Parkinson's disease. Neuroradiology 1994;36:276–280.
100. Tachibana H, Kawabata K, Tomino Y, et al. Brain perfusion imaging in Parkinson's disease and Alzheimer's disease demonstrated by three-dimensional surface display with 1231-iodoamphetamine. Dementia 1993;4:334–341.
101. Liu RS, Lin KN, Wang SJ, et al. Cognition and 99Tcm-HMPAO SPECT in Parkinson's disease. Nucl Med Commun 1992;13:744–748.
102. Eberling JL, Richardson BC, Reed BR, et al. Cortical glucose metabolism in Parkinson's disease without dementia. Neurobiol Aging 1994;15:329–335.
103. Peppard RF, Martin WR, Carr GD, et al. Cerebral glucose metabolism in Parkinson's disease with and without dementia. Arch Neurol 1992;49:1262–1268.
104. Kuhl DE, Minoshima S, Fessler JA, et al. In vivo mapping of cholinergic terminals in normal aging, Alzheimer's disease, and Parkinson's disease. Ann Neurol 1996;40:399–410.
105. Laakso MP, Partanen K, Riekkinen P, et al. The hippocampal volumes in Alzheimer's disease, Parkinson's disease with and without dementia, and in vascular dementia: an MRI study. Neurology 1996;46:678–681.
106. Bowen BC, Block RE, Sanchez Ramos J, et al. Proton MR spectroscopy of the brain in 14 patients with Parkinson's disease. Am J Neuroradiol 1995;16:61–68.
107. Kumar A. Functional brain imaging in late-life depression and dementia. J Clin Psychiatry 1993;54: S21–S25.
108. Wang SJ, Liu RS, Liu HC, et al. Technetium-99m hemamethylpropylene amine oxime single photon emission tomography of the brain in early Parkinson's disease: correlation with dementia and lateralization. Eur J Nucl Med 1993;20:339–344.
109. Sawada H, Udaka F, Kameyama M, et al. SPECT findings in Parkinson's disease associated with dementia. J Neurol Neurosurg Psychiatry 1992;55:960–963.
110. Neufeld MY, Blumen S, Aitkin I, et al. EEG frequency analysis in demented and nondemented parkinsonian patients. Dementia 1994;5:23–28.
111. Okuda B, Tachibana H, Takeda M, et al. Visual and somatosensory evoked potentials in Parkinson's and Binswanger's disease. Dementia 1996;7:E53–E58.
112. Okuda B, Tachibana H, Kawabata K, et al. Visual evoked potentials (VEPs) in Parkinson's disease: correlation of pattern VEPs abnormality with dementia. Alzheimer Dis Assoc Disord 1995;9:68–72.
113. Toda K, Tachibana H, Sugita M, Konishi K. P300 and reaction time in Parkinson's disease. J Geriatr Psychiatry Neurol 1993;6:131–136.
114. Leiguarda RC, Pramstaller PP, Merello M, et al. Apraxia in Parkinson's disease, progressive supranuclear palsy, multiple system atrophy and neuroleptic-induced parkinsonism. Brain 1997;120:75–90.
115. Pillon R, Dubois R, Cusimano G, et al. Does cognitive impairment in Parkinson's disease result from non-dopaminergic lesions? J Neurol Neurosurg Psychiatry 1989;52:201–206.
116. Whitehead AS, Bertrandy S, Finnan F, et al. Frequency of the apolipoprotein E epsilon 4 allele in a case-control study of early onset Parkinson's disease. J Neurol Neurosurg Psychiatry 1996;61:347–351.
117. Ibarreta D, Gomez-Isla T, Portera Sanchez A, et al. Apolipoprotein E genotype in Spanish patients of Alzheimer's or Parkinson's disease. J Neurol Sci 1995;134:146–149.
118. Katzman R, Galasko D, Saitoh T, et al. Genetic evidence that the Lewy body variant is indeed a phenotypic variant of Alzheimer's disease. Brain Cogn 1995;28:259–265.
119. Koller WC, Glatt SL, Hubble JP, et al. Apolipoprotein E genotypes in Parkinson's disease with and without dementia. Ann Neurol 1995;37:242–245.
120. Hardy J, Crook R, Prihar G, et al. Senile dementia of the Lewy body type has an apolipoprotein E epsilon 4 allele frequency intermediate between controls and Alzheimer's disease. Neurosci Lett 1994;182:1–2.
121. Marder K, Maestre G, Cote L, et al. The apolipoprotein epsilon 4 allele in Parkinson's disease with and without dementia. Neurology 1994;44:1330–1331.

122. Harrington CR, Louwagie J, Rossau R, et al. Influence of apolipoprotein E genotype on senile dementia of the Alzheimer and Lewy body types: significance for etiological theories of Alzheimer's disease. Am J Pathol 1994;145:1472–1484.
123. Benjamin R, Leake A, Ince PG, et al. Effects of apolipoprotein E genotype on cortical neuropathology in senile dementia of the Lewy body and Alzheimer's disease. Neurodegeneration 1995;4:443–448.
124. Stolerman IP. Psychopharmacology of Nicotine: Stimulus Effects and Receptor Mechanisms. In LL Iversen, SD Iversen, SH Snyder (eds), Handbook of Psychopharmacology, vol 19. New York: Plenum, 1987.
125. Reynolds GP, Elsworth JD, Blau K, et al. Deprenyl is metabolised to methamphetamine and amphetamine in man. Br J Clin Pharmacol 1978;6:542–544.
126. Lieberman A, et al. D-1 and D-2 agonists in Parkinson's disease. Can J Neurol Sci 1987;14:466–473.
127. Gancher ST. Dopamine Agonists Under Investigation Including Apomorphine. In WC Koller, G Paulson (eds), Therapy of Parkinson's Disease (2nd ed). New York: Marcel Dekker, 1995;273–286.
128. Wolters EC, Kuiper MA, Zwaan WA, et al. Dopaminomimetic Psychosis: Therapeutic Strategies. In EC Wolters, P Scheltens (eds), Mental Dysfunction in Parkinson's Disease. Dordrecht, Netherlands: ICG Publications, 1994;285–295.
129. Musser WS, Akil M. Clozapine as a treatment for psychosis in Parkinson's disease: a review. J Neuropsychiatry Clin Neurosci 1996;8:1–9.
130. Graham JM, Sussman JD, Ford KS, Sagar HJ. Olanzapine in the treatment of psychosis in idiopathic Parkinson's disease: a cautionary note. J Neurol Neurosurg Psychiatry. (In press.)
131. Zoldan J, Friedberg G, Weizman A, Melamed E. Ondansetron. A 5-HT_3 Antagonist for Visual Hallucinations and Paranoid Delusional Disorder Associated with Chronic L-DOPA Therapy in Advanced Parkinson's Disease. In L Battistin, G Scarlato, T Caraceni, S Ruggieri (eds), Advances in Neurology, vol 69. Philadelphia: Lippincott–Raven, 1996;541–544.
132. Zwil AS, Pelchat RJ. ECT in the treatment of patients with neurological and somatic disease. Int J Psychiatry Med 1994;24:1–29.
133. Steele JC, Richardson JC, Olszewski J. Progressive supranuclear palsy: a heterogeneous degeneration involving the brain stem, basal ganglia and cerebellum with vertical gaze and pseudobulbar palsy, nuchal dystonia and dementia. Arch Neurol 1964;10:333–358.
134. Maher ER, Lees AJ. The clinical features and natural history of the Steele-Richardson-Olszewski syndrome (progressive supranuclear palsy). Neurology 1986;36:1005–1008.
135. Litvan I, Mangone CA, McKee A, et al. The national history of progressive supranuclear palsy (Steele-Richardson-Olszewski syndrome) and clinical predictors of survival: a clinicopathological study. J Neurol Neurosurg Psychiatry 1996;60:615–620.
136. Vallderiola F, Tolosa E, Valls-Sole J. Differential diagnosis and clinical diagnostic criteria of progressive supranuclear palsy. Adv Neurol 1996;69:405–412.
137. Litvan I, Hauw JJ, Bartko JJ, et al. Validity and reliability of the preliminary NINDS neuropathologic criteria for progressive supranuclear palsy and related disorders. J Neuropathol Exp Neurol 1996;55:97–105.
138. Lees AJ. The Steele-Richardson-Olszewski Syndrome (Progressive Supranuclear Palsy). In CD Marsden, S Fahn (eds), Movement Disorders II. London: Butterworth–Heinemann, 1987;272–287.
139. Golbe LI. The Epidemiology of Progressive Supranuclear Palsy. In L Battistin, G Scarlato, T Saraceni, S Ruggieri (eds), Advances in Neurology (vol. 69). Philadelphia: Lippincott–Raven, 1996;25–31.
140. Brusa A, Peloso PF. An Introduction of Progressive Supranuclear Palsy. New York: John Libby, 1993.
141. Gazeley S, Maguire JA. Familial progressive supranuclear palsy. Clin Neuropathol 1996;15: 215–220.
142. Dubinsky RM, Jankowic J. Progressive supranuclear palsy and a multi-infarct state. Neurology 1987; 37:570–576.
143. Arnold G, Tatsch K, Oertel WH, et al. Clinical progressive supranuclear palsy: differential diagnosis by IBZM-SPECT and MRI. J Neur Trans 1994:S111–S118.
144. Feifel E, Brenner M, Teiwes R, et al. Corticobasal degeneration: the significance of clinical criteria for establishing the diagnosis. Nervenarzt 1994;65:653–659.
145. Rinne JO, Lee MS, Thompson PD, Marsden CD. Corticobasal degeneration: a clinical study of 36 cases. Brain 1994;117:1183–1196.
146. Thompson PD, Marsden CD. Corticobasal degeneration. Baillieres Clin Neurol 1992;1:677–686.
147. Levine DN. The Alien Hand. In AB Joseph, RR Young (eds), Movement Disorders in Neurology and Neuropsychiatry. Boston: Blackwell, 1992;691–695.
148. Watts RL, Mirra SS, Richardson EP. Cortico-Basal Ganglionic Degeneration. In CD Marsden, S Fahn (eds), Movement Disorders III. Boston: Butterworth–Heinemann, 1994;282–299.

149. Valldeoriola F, Tolosa E, Valls-Sole J. Differential Diagnosis and Clinical Diagnostic Criteria of Progressive Supranuclear Palsy. In CD Marsden, S Fahn (eds), Movement Disorders III. Boston: Butterworth–Heinemann, 1994;405–412.
150. Quinn N. Multiple System Atrophy. In CD Marsden, S Fahn (eds), Movement Disorders III. Boston: Butterworth–Heinemann, 1994;262–281.
151. Moxley RT. Hereditary Metabolic Disorders in Infancy and Childhood. In M Swash, J Oxbury (eds), Clinical Neurology. New York: Churchill Livingstone, 1991;1632–1653.
152. Dubois B, Deweer B, Pillon B. The Cognitive Syndrome of Progressive Supranuclear Palsy. In L Battistin, G Scarlato, T Saraceni, S Ruggieri (eds), Advances in Neurology, vol 69. Philadelphia: Lippincott–Raven, 1996;399–403.
153. Braak H, Braak E, Bohl JTI. Staging of Alzheimer-related cortical destruction. Eur Neurol 1993;33: 403–408.
154. Cole DG, Growdon JH. Therapy for progressive supranuclear palsy: past and future. J Neur Trans 1994;42:S283–S290.
155. Rebeiz JJ, Kolodny EH, Richardson EP. Corticodentatonigral degeneration with neuronal achromasia. Arch Neurol 1968;18:20–33.
156. Lynch T, Sano M, Marder KS, et al. Clinical characteristics of a family with chromosome 17–linked disinhibition-dementia-parkinsonism-amyotrophy complex. Neurology 1994;44:1878–1884.
157. Hakim S, Adams RD. The special clinical problem of symptomatic hydrocephalus with normal cerebrospinal fluid pressure: observation on cerebrospinal fluid hydrodynamics. J Neurol Sci 1965;2:307–327.
158. Watson CP. Spastic gait and acquired aqueductal stenosis in an adult. Arch Neurol 1980;37:116.
159. Symon L, Dorsch NWC, Stephens RJ. Pressure waves in so-called low pressure hydrocephalus. Lancet 1972;2:1291–1292.
160. Gerloff C, Pickard JD. Normal Pressure Hydrocephalus. In T Brandt, LR Caplan, J Dishgans (eds), Neurological Disorders: Course and Treatment. San Diego: Academic, 1996.
161. Black P McL. The Gait Disorder in Normal Pressure Hydrocephalus. In AB Joseph, RR Young (eds), Movement Disorders in Neurology and Psychiatry. Boston: Blackwell, 1992.
162. Fisher CM. Hydrocephalus as a cause of disturbances of gait in the elderly. Neurology 1982;32: 1358–1363.
163. Vanneste J, Augustijn P, Dirven C, et al. Shunting normal pressure hydrocephalus: the predictive value of combined clinical and CT data. J Neurol Neurosurg Psychiatry 1993;56:251–256.
164. Graff-Radford NR, Godersky JC. Normal pressure hydrocephalus: onset of gait abnormalities before dementia predicts good surgical outcome. Arch Neurol 1986;43:940–942.
165. Stuss D, Cummings JL. Subcortical Vascular Dementias. In JL Cummings (ed), Subcortical Dementia. Oxford: Oxford University Press, 1990;145–163.
166. Hachinski VC, Lassen NA, Marshall J. Multi-infarct dementia: a cause of mental deterioration in the elderly. Lancet 1974;2:207–209.
167. Critchley M. Arteriosclerotic parkinsonism. Brain 1929;52:23–83.
168. Caplan LR, Diener HCD. Cerebral Ischemia. In T Brandt, LR Caplan, J Dishgans (eds), Neurological Disorders: Course and Treatment. San Diego: Academic, 1996.
169. Caplan LR. Binswanger's disease revisited. Neurology 1995:45;626–633.
170. Gallassi R, Morreale A, Montagna P, et al. Binswanger's disease and normal pressure hydrocephalus: clinical and neuropsychological comparison. Arch Neurol 1991;48:1156–1159.
171. Jankovic J. Lower body (vascular) parkinsonism. Arch Neurol 1990;47:728.
172. Thompson PD, Marsden CD. Gait disorder of subcortical arteriosclerotic encephalopathy: Binswanger's disease. Mov Disord 1987;2:1–8.
173. Meyer JS, Judd BW, Tawaklna T, et al. Improved cognition after control of risk factors for multi-infarct dementia. JAMA 1986;256:2203–2209.
174. Willison JR, Thomas DJ, du Boulay GH, et al. Effect of high haematocrit on alertness. Lancet 1980; 1:846–848.
175. Brandt T, Caplan LR, Dishgans J, et al. (eds). Neurological Disorders: Course and Treatment. San Diego: Academic, 1996.
176. Swash M, Oxbury J (eds). Clinical Neurology. New York: Churchill Livingstone, 1991.
177. Joseph AB, Young RR (eds). Movement Disorders in Neurology and Psychiatry. Boston: Blackwell, 1992.
178. Will RG, Ironside JW, Zeidler M, et al. A new variant of Creutzfeldt-Jakob disease in the UK. Lancet 1996;347:921–925.
179. Wijker M, Wszolek ZK, Wolters EC, et al. Localization of the gene for rapidly progressive autosomal dominant parkinsonism and dementia with pallido-ponto-nigral degeneration to chromosome 17q21. Hum Mol Genet 1996;5:151–154.
180. Stern Y, Tetrud JW, Martin WR, et al. Cognitive change following MPTP exposure. Neurology 1990; 40:261–264.

5
Human Prion Diseases: Etiology and Clinical Features

John Collinge

The human prion diseases, also known as the *subacute spongiform encephalopathies*, have been traditionally classified into Creutzfeldt-Jakob disease (CJD), Gerstmann-Sträussler syndrome (GSS) (also known as *Gerstmann-Sträussler-Scheinker disease*), and kuru. Although these are rare neurodegenerative disorders affecting about 1 person per million worldwide each year, remarkable attention has been recently focused on these diseases. This is because of the unique biology of the transmissible agent, or prion, and also because of the fears that an epidemic of a newly recognized bovine prion disease, bovine spongiform encephalopathy (BSE), could pose a threat to public health through dietary exposure to infected tissues.

The transmissibility of the human diseases was demonstrated with the transmission, by intracerebral inoculation with brain homogenates into chimpanzees, of first kuru and then CJD in 1966 and 1968, respectively [1,2]. Transmission of GSS followed in 1981 [3]. The prototypic prion disease is scrapie, a naturally occurring disease of sheep and goats, which has been recognized in Europe for over 200 years [4] and is present in the sheep flocks of many countries. Scrapie was demonstrated to be transmissible by inoculation in 1936 [5], and it was the recognition that kuru and CJD resembled scrapie in their histopathologic appearances that led to the suggestion that these diseases may also be transmissible [6,7]. Kuru is a neurodegenerative condition characterized principally by a progressive cerebellar ataxia that reached epidemic proportions among the Fore linguistic group in the eastern highlands of Papua New Guinea and was transmitted by ritual cannibalism. Since the cessation of cannibalism in the 1950s, the disease has declined, but a few cases still occur as a result of the long incubation periods in this condition [8]. The term *Creutzfeldt-Jakob disease* was introduced by Spielmeyer in 1922 [9], bringing together the case reports published by Creutzfeldt [10] and Jakob [11–13]. Several of these cases would not meet modern diagnostic criteria for CJD, and indeed, it was not until the demonstration of transmissibility enabled diagnostic criteria to be reassessed and refined that a clear diagnostic entity developed. All these diseases share common histopathologic features; the classic triad of spongiform vacuolation (affecting any part of the cerebral gray matter), astrocytic proliferation, and neuronal loss may be accompanied by the deposition of amyloid plaques [14].

Many of the key advances in understanding the pathogenesis of the prion diseases have come from study of the various forms of human prion disease. In particular, the recognition that the familial forms of the human diseases are autosomal dominant inherited conditions associated with coding mutations in the prion protein gene and transmissible to laboratory animals by inoculation strongly supported the contention that the transmissible agent, or prion, was composed principally of an abnormal isoform of prion protein. The epidemiology of the human prion diseases encompasses the three etiologic types of prion disease: inherited, sporadic, and acquired. Inherited cases constitute approximately 15% of cases, whereas acquired cases are rare and include iatrogenic CJD and kuru. Most human cases are sporadic, however, and their precise etiology is still unclear. The advances in understanding the molecular biology of these diseases, in particular the availability of molecular genetic diagnostic markers, has allowed appreciation of the remarkable phenotypic diversity of these diseases at both the clinical and the histopathologic levels and has extended the recognized disease spectrum beyond the classically recognized syndromes of CJD, GSS, and kuru to what can now be defined as the *human prion diseases*.

ETIOLOGY

The transmissible agent, or prion, consists principally of an abnormal isoform of a host-encoded protein, the prion protein (PrP), designated PrP^{Sc}. PrP^{Sc} is derived from the cellular isoform, PrP^{C}, by a post-translational mechanism [15] that appears to involve a conformational rather than covalent modification [16,17] (Figure 5.1). Whereas PrP^{C} is fully sensitive to proteolysis, PrP^{Sc}, which accumulates in the brain in disease (and which may form amyloid), is partially protease resistant. The human PrP gene (*PRNP*) is a single-copy gene located on the short arm of chromosome 20 [18] in a region syntenic with the murine PrP gene (*Prn-p*) on chromosome 2; it spans 16 kb and contains two exons [19,20]. The complete open reading frame of 759 nucleotides is contained within the larger second exon that comprises the majority of the 2.4-kb mRNA. Clearly the PrP gene was an obvious candidate for genetic linkage studies in the familial forms of CJD and GSS, both of which showed an autosomal dominant pattern of disease segregation. A turning point in understanding the human prion diseases was the identification of mutations in *PRNP* in familial CJD and GSS in 1989. The first mutation to be identified in *PRNP* was in a family with CJD and constituted a 144–base pair (bp) insertion into the coding sequence [21]. A second mutation was reported in two families with GSS, and genetic linkage was confirmed between this missense variant at codon 102 and GSS, confirming that GSS was an autosomal dominant mendelian disorder [22]. This genetic variant was not present in the normal population but was rapidly identified in numerous other unrelated GSS kindreds [23–28]. On statistical grounds, therefore, it seemed likely that this mutation was causal for GSS in these families. Uniquely, these diseases are therefore both inherited and transmissible. A whole family of PrP

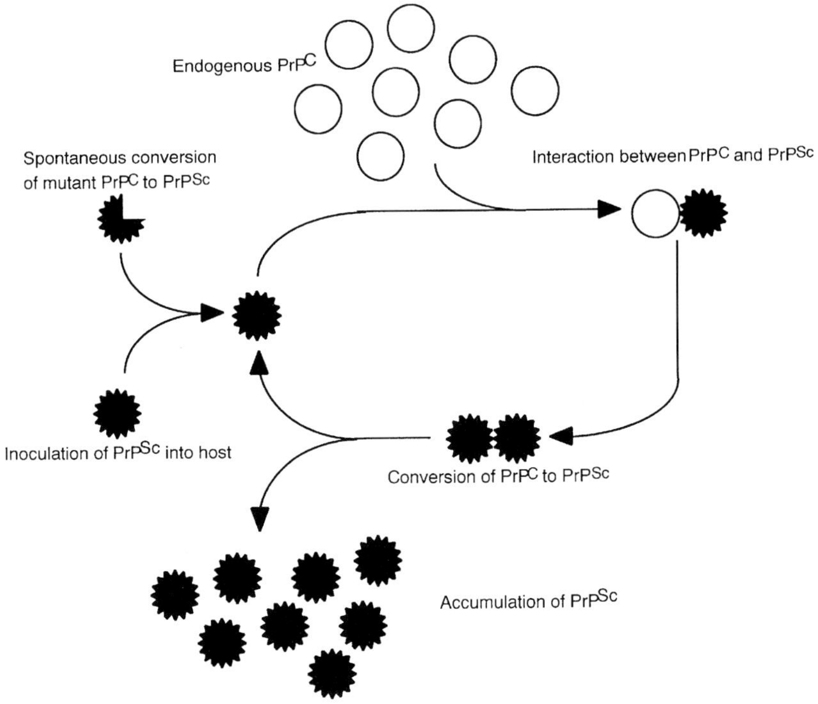

Figure 5.1 A model of prion propagation. The normal isoform of prion protein, PrP^C (open circles), interacts with the disease-associated form, PrP^{Sc} (shaded objects), which promotes its conversion to further PrP^{Sc} by an undefined mechanism. PrP^{Sc} is introduced by inoculation; alternatively, in inherited cases, mutant PrP^C may spontaneously convert to PrP^{Sc}.

mutations was rapidly described (Figure 5.2). The availability of such direct gene markers enabled molecular diagnosis of cases and the identification of cases expressing phenotypes that differed markedly from the classic ones of CJD and GSS [29,30]. Indeed CJD- and GSS-like syndromes could coexist in the same family, and it was appreciated that they form part of a more extensive disease spectrum better referred to as *inherited prion disease* [31].

Experimental confirmation of the pathogenicity of the codon 102 mutation was provided in 1990 by the demonstration that transgenic mice that overexpressed a murine PrP encoding an analogous mutation spontaneously developed spongiform neurodegeneration [32]. Further, brain tissue from such spontaneously sick transgenic animals appears to be able to transmit the disease to wild-type hamsters and transgenic mice with lower copy numbers of the same mutant transgene [33].

Current evidence suggests that approximately 15% of prion diseases are inherited, and at least 18 coding mutations in *PRNP* are now recognized. With the exception of the rare iatrogenic CJD cases mentioned above, most prion disease occurs as sporadic CJD. Although by definition there is no family history in sporadic cases, mutations are seen in occasional apparently sporadic cases, because in a late-onset disease, the family history may not be apparent or nonpaternity may

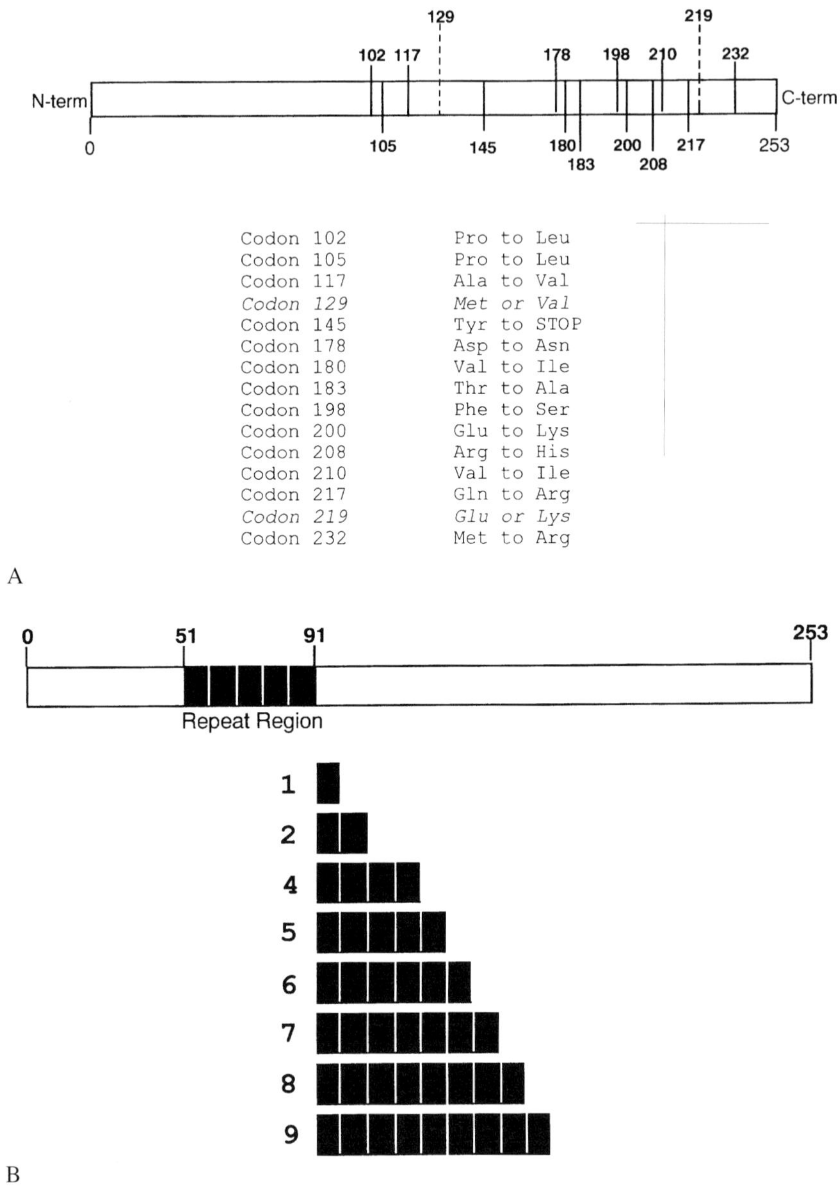

Figure 5.2 (A) Diagram of human prion protein gene coding mutations seen in prion diseases. Polymorphisms present in the normal population are shown with dotted lines and italicized text. (B) Diagram of the pathogenic repeat insertion mutations in the human PrP gene.

occur. In the majority of sporadic CJD cases, however, there is neither a coding mutation nor a history of iatrogenic exposure. Human prion diseases can therefore be subdivided into inherited, sporadic, and acquired forms.

Genetic predisposition, however, is highly relevant to the etiology of both acquired and sporadic CJD. A study of seven human pituitary hormone–related CJD cases revealed a significant excess of a valine 129 homozygous genotype [33]. There are two common forms of PrP in humans with either methionine or valine encoded at codon 129. In whites, approximately 51% are heterozygotes whereas 38% are methionine homozygotes; the least common genotype is valine homozygous, with approximately 11% of the population falling into this category. Four of the seven cases studied were valine homozygotes. This frequency suggested that this genotype may render an individual more susceptible to prion disease on challenge with the transmissible agent. Although the original study was based on a small series (although including all reported U.K. cases at the time of study), this finding has now been replicated in larger studies in the United States [34] and France [35].

A study of 22 clearly defined sporadic CJD cases with respect to this common protein polymorphism revealed that all but one case was a homozygote either to methionine or valine [36]. Although 51% of the white population are heterozygous with respect to this polymorphism, it seems that the vast majority of individuals that develop classic sporadic CJD are homozygotes. This finding has been borne out in other studies [35,37] and in a larger U.K. study [38].

In 1990, it was demonstrated that the species barrier to transmission of prion disease from hamsters to mice could be overcome by overexpressing normal hamster PrP in transgenic mice [39]. Although prion diseases can be transmitted between mammalian species by inoculation, in practice it is difficult to do so, and transmission typically occurs in only a small proportion of inoculated animals and then only after prolonged incubation periods. When such transgenic mice were challenged with mouse-derived prions, the infectivity they produced was fully pathogenic for mice but not hamsters, whereas on challenge with hamster-derived prions they produced prions fully pathogenic to hamsters but not mice. The interpretation of this finding is that a direct interaction between PrP molecules occurs at some stage in the process of prion propagation and that such interaction occurs most easily if the interacting PrP molecules are identical. Because there are a number of amino acid differences between murine and hamster PrP, interaction between the two forms is less favored. Such work has led to the idea that replication of prions may occur by the abnormal PrP isoform, PrP^{Sc}, interacting directly with the normal cellular isoform, PrP^{C}, and catalyzing the conversion of PrP^{C} to PrP^{Sc} [39,40]. Such an effect could lead to a chain reaction of conversion leading to the progressive conversion of increasing amounts of PrP^{C} to PrP^{Sc}. This could then produce disease either by progressive loss of PrP function or by cellular damage resulting from accumulation of PrP^{Sc}. Clearly, the implication is that the pathogenic mutations in the PrP result in the production of a protein that may convert spontaneously to PrP^{Sc} in individuals with inherited prion diseases. Once produced, PrP^{Sc} will then produce the same catalytic chain reaction as hypothesized in cases where PrP^{Sc} is inoculated. Such a model provides an explanation of how a disease can be simultaneously inherited and transmissible (see Figure 5.1). The finding that nearly all sporadic CJD occurs in homozygotes with respect to a common and apparently innocent protein polymorphism lends strong support to such a mechanism [36]. Again, PrP interaction would occur most favorably in individuals with two identical copies of the PrP. Heterozygotes, producing two different proteins, would be somewhat protected, as if by an internal "species barrier." It is possible that the occasional individuals heterozygous at codon 129 who do develop sporadic CJD have a more prolonged and atypical illness, although more detailed studies are required to investigate this further [41]. Additional evidence for this model is provided by the observation that in one of the inherited prion diseases, age at onset of the disease occurs one to two decades later in individuals heterozygous at codon 129 [42]. This effect has now also been reported in another inherited prion disease kindred with a different *PRNP* mutation [43].

PrP valine 129 and PrP methionine 129 would be expected to differ slightly in their propensity to convert to PrP^{Sc}. The excess of PrP valine 129 homozygotes among human pituitary hormone–related cases suggests that PrP valine 129 may be more susceptible to conversion [44].

It is of particular interest that mice heterozygous for a PrP null allele, which produces approximately 50% of the normal amount of PrP, have very prolonged incubation periods and then develop a much more slowly progressing illness than wild-type mice [45,46]. This finding may be relevant to the homozygosity issue in sporadic CJD in which having two different PrPs, in the case of heterozygotes at codon 129, may result in a similar situation, the disease process occurring only between homologous molecules present at 50% of the normal level.

The etiology of sporadic CJD remains unclear. It has been speculated that these cases might arise from somatic mutation of *PRNP* or spontaneous conversion of PrP^{C} to PrP^{Sc} as a rare stochastic event. The alternative hypothesis, that such cases arise as a result of exposure to an environmental source of either human or animal prions, is not supported by epidemiologic evidence [47]. Because transgenic mice expressing extremely high levels of wild-type hamster or murine PrP develop a spontaneous neuromuscular disease [48], it has also been suggested that some cases of sporadic CJD may arise as a result of PrP overexpression.

HUMAN PRION STRAINS

A major problem for the "protein-only" hypothesis of prion propagation has been how to explain the existence of multiple isolates or strains of prions. Such strains are distinguished by their biological properties: They produce distinct incubation periods and patterns of neuropathologic targeting in inbred mouse lines. Because these strains can be serially propagated in inbred mice with the same *Prn-p* genotype, they are not encoded by differences in PrP primary structure. Furthermore, strains can be re-isolated in mice after passage in intermediate species with different PrP primary structures [49]. Understanding how a protein-only infectious agent could encode such phenotypic information has been of considerable biological interest.

Support for the contention that strain specificity is encoded by PrP alone is provided by study of two distinct strains of transmissible mink encephalopathy prions that can be serially propagated in hamsters, designated *hyper* (HY) and *drowsy* (DY) [50]. These strains can be distinguished by differing physiochemical properties of the accumulated PrP^{Sc} in the brains of affected hamsters [51]. After limited proteolysis, strain-specific migration patterns of PrP^{Sc} on polyacrylamide gels can be seen. DY PrP^{Sc} appears to be more protease sensitive than HY PrP^{Sc}, producing a different banding pattern of PrP^{Sc} on Western blots after proteinase K treatment. This pattern relates to different N-terminal ends of HY and DY PrP^{Sc} after protease treatment and implies differing conformations of HY and DY PrP^{Sc} [52]. Furthermore, the demonstration that these strain-specific physiochemical properties can be maintained during in vitro production of protease-resistant PrP when PrP^{C} is mixed with HY or DY hamster PrP^{Sc} further supports the concept that prion strains involve different PrP conformers [53].

Several human PrP^{Sc} types have been identified that are associated with different phenotypes of CJD [54,55]. The different fragment sizes seen on Western blots after treatment with proteinase K suggest that there are several different human PrP^{Sc} conformations. To fulfill the criteria of strains, however, these patterns must be transmissible to animals both in the same and in different species. Remarkably, this is the case, with both PrP^{Sc} fragment sizes and the ratios of the three PrP glycoforms (diglycosylated, monoglycosylated, and unglycosylated PrP) maintained on passage in transgenic mice expressing human PrP [55]. Transmission of human and bovine prions to wild-type mice results in murine PrP^{Sc} with fragment sizes and glycoform ratios that correspond to the original inoculum [55]. New variant CJD is associated with PrP^{Sc} glycoform ratios that are distinct from those seen in classic CJD. Similar ratios are seen in BSE in cattle and BSE when transmitted to several other species [55]. These data strongly support the protein-only hypothesis of infectivity and suggest that strain variation is encoded by a combination of PrP conformation and glycosylation. Because PrP glycosylation is thought to be a cotranslational process, the different glycoform ratios may represent selection of particular PrP^{C} glycoforms by PrP^{Sc} of different conformations. According to such a hypothesis, PrP conformation would be the primary determinant of strain type, with glycosylation being involved as a secondary process. However, because it is known that different cell types may glycosylate proteins differently, PrP^{Sc} glycosylation patterns may provide a substrate for the neuropathologic targeting that distinguishes different prion strains. Particular PrP^{Sc} glycoforms may replicate most favorably in neuronal populations with a similar PrP glycoform expressed on the cell surface. Such targeting could also explain the different incubation periods that also discriminate strains, targeting more critical brain regions or regions with higher levels of PrP expression and producing shorter incubation periods.

Such studies may allow a new molecular classification of human prion diseases; it is likely that additional PrP^{Sc} types or strains will be identified, which may well open new avenues of epidemiologic investigation and offer insights into causes of "sporadic" CJD. In addition, PrP^{Sc} typing can be applied to other species; it is already apparent that PrP glycoform analysis alone can distinguish a number of mouse-passaged scrapie strains [56]. The combination of fragment size and glycoform analysis should enable better resolution and might be applied, for instance, to study whether BSE has transmitted to other species involved in the human diet, such as sheep. It will be necessary to study the full range of sheep strains to determine whether these can all be distinguished at a molecular level from BSE, and it is possible that more refined molecular techniques may be necessary [57]. Classic strain typing involving mouse transmissions takes 1–2 years

Table 5.1 Human prion diseases

Type	*Clinical syndromes*	*Etiology*
Acquired	Kuru	Exposure to human prions during cannibalistic feasts
	Iatrogenic CJD	Accidental inoculation with human prions
	New variant CJD	Exposure to BSE-like prion strain
Sporadic	CJD Atypical CJD	Somatic *PRNP* mutation or spontaneous conversion of PrP^C to PrP^{Sc} (?)
Inherited	Familial CJD GSS FFI Various atypical dementias	Germline *PRNP* mutation

CJD = Creutzfeldt-Jakob disease; BSE = bovine spongiform encephalopathy; GSS = Gerstmann-Sträussler-Scheinker disease; FFI = fatal familial insomnia; *PRNP* = human prion protein gene; PrP = prion protein.

and can only be applied to limited numbers of cases. Molecular strain typing takes days and allows large-scale screening.

The ability of a protein to encode a disease phenotype has important implications in biology, as it represents a nonmendelian form of transmission. It would be surprising, and also intriguing, if evolution had not used this mechanism for other proteins in a range of species. The recent identification of prion-like mechanisms in yeast is particularly interesting in this regard [58,59].

CLINICAL SYNDROMES OF HUMAN PRION DISEASE

The human prion diseases have been classically divided into CJD, GSS, and kuru. With the advances in our understanding of the etiology of these conditions, it now seems more appropriate to divide the human prion diseases into inherited, sporadic, and acquired forms (Table 5.1), with CJD, GSS, and kuru now seen as clinicopathologic syndromes within a wider spectrum of disease. Kindreds with inherited prion disease have been described with phenotypes of classic CJD, GSS, and other neurodegenerative syndromes, including fatal familial insomnia (FFI) [60]. Some kindreds show remarkable phenotypic variability that can encompass both CJD- and GSS-like cases as well as other cases that do not conform to either CJD or GSS phenotypes [31]. Cases diagnosed by PrP gene analysis have been reported that are not only clinically atypical but also lack the classic histologic features entirely [29]. Significant clinical overlap exists with familial Alzheimer's disease (AD), Pick's disease, frontal lobe degeneration of non-Alzheimer type, and amyotrophic lateral sclerosis (ALS) with dementia. Although classic GSS is described in the section on Inherited Prion Diseases, below, it now seems more sensible to designate the familial illnesses as inherited prion diseases and then subclassify these according to mutation (see Figure 5.2).

Acquired prion diseases include iatrogenic CJD, kuru, and now new variant CJD. Sporadic prion diseases at present consist of CJD and atypical variants of CJD. Cases lacking the characteristic histologic features of CJD have been transmitted. Because there are at present no equivalent etiological diagnostic markers for sporadic prion diseases to those for the inherited diseases, it cannot yet be excluded that more diverse phenotypic variants of sporadic prion disease exist that may not be as easily transmissible to primates as cases with classic spongiform encephalopathy.

Sporadic Prion Disease

Creutzfeldt-Jakob Disease

Epidemiology

Extensive epidemiologic studies of CJD have been performed in a number of countries and all have obtained broadly similar results [47]. The overall annual incidence in most studies was approximately 0.5–1.0 case per million. No significant case clustering is present other than with respect to familial clusters. Cases are distributed apparently at random with a frequency related only to local population density. In particular, there is no evidence for case-to-case spread (other than with respect to iatrogenic foci, which are discussed in the section on Iatrogenic Creutzfeldt-Jakob Disease) and no evidence of an association with local scrapie prevalence. For instance, CJD is as common in Australia and New Zealand, which have been scrapie-free for many years, as in the United Kingdom, where scrapie is endemic. Numerous case-control studies have failed to show consistent associations with particular occupational groups or dietary components. The BSE epidemic, however, has led to renewed interest in this area, and since 1990, an attempt has been made to monitor all suspected cases of CJD in the United Kingdom [61]. Parallel studies have commenced in a number of other European countries, some of which have recently reported BSE cases in their cattle population, and a coordinated study of CJD epidemiology in the European Union is in progress [47]. Although these large-scale prospective studies have generated an enormous body of experience of this rare disease, overall incidence figures do not appear to have risen in the United Kingdom compared with countries that do not have BSE. An overall increase in incidence is noted in most of these surveillance programs, but this is thought to be due to increased case ascertainment, as so much attention is now being focused on these diseases. Increased ascertainment may be particularly relevant to the increased incidence noted in the elderly, in which other dementing illnesses are common. Although occasional weak statistical associations with particular foodstuffs are reported, these have tended to disappear over subsequent years of the study and no consistent new risk factors have emerged. Recent concern has been focused on the occurrence of CJD in a number of dairy farmers in the United Kingdom [62,63] and in the occurrence of sporadic CJD in two teenagers [64,65] and a 28-year-old woman [66]. Whereas the dairy farmers had a typical clinicopathologic picture of sporadic CJD, the young patients had clinical and pathologic features that were unusual and in some respects reminiscent of kuru. Further epidemiologic

Table 5.2 Special investigations in prion disease

PrP gene analysis (pathogenic mutations and codon 129 genotype)
Cerebrospinal fluid assay of 14-3-3 protein, neuron-specific enolase, and S-100 proteins
Demonstration of PrP^{Sc} by tonsil biopsy

PrP = prion protein.

surveillance revealed additional young-onset cases early in 1996, and it was recognized that these cases shared a previously unrecognized pattern of neuropathology [67], raising the possibility that these cases were linked to BSE. This newly recognized variant of human prion disease will be discussed later (see New Variant of Human Prion Disease).

Clinical Features

The core clinical syndrome of classic CJD is of a rapidly progressive dementia, usually with myoclonus. The onset is usually between 45 and 75 years, with peak onset between 60 and 65 years. The clinical progression is typically over weeks, progressing to akinetic mutism and death often in 2–3 months. Approximately 70% of patients die in less than 6 months. Prodromal features, present in approximately one-third of cases, include fatigue, insomnia, depression, weight loss, headaches, general malaise, and ill-defined pain sensations. In addition to mental deterioration and myoclonus, frequent additional neurologic features include extrapyramidal signs, cerebellar ataxia, pyramidal signs, and cortical blindness. Approximately 10% of patients present initially with cerebellar ataxia.

Investigations

Routine hematologic and biochemical investigations are normal, although occasional cases have been noted to have raised serum transaminases or alkaline phosphatase. There are no immunologic markers and acute phase proteins are not elevated. Examination of the cerebrospinal fluid (CSF) is normal, but raised neuron-specific enolase and S-100 have both been proposed as useful markers, although it is clear that they are not specific for CJD and presumably represent markers of neuronal injury [68–70]. A promising CSF marker is estimation of 14-3-3 protein, which, although not a specific disease marker, appears to be a useful adjunct to diagnosis in the appropriate clinical context [71,72]. It is also positive in recent cerebral infarction or hemorrhage and in viral encephalitis, although these conditions do not usually present diagnostic confusion with CJD (Table 5.2). Neuroimaging with computed tomography or magnetic resonance imaging (MRI) is useful to exclude other causes of subacute neurologic illness, but there are no diagnostic features; cerebral and cerebellar atrophy may be present. The electroencephalogram (EEG) may, however, show characteristic pseudoperiodic sharp wave activity that is helpful in diagnosis but present only in approximately 70% of cases. To some extent, demonstration of a typical EEG is dependent on the number of EEGs performed, and serial EEG is indicated to try to demonstrate this appearance.

Prospective epidemiologic studies have demonstrated that cases with a progressive dementia and two or more of the following features nearly always turn out to be confirmed as histologically definite CJD if neuropathologic examination is performed: myoclonus; cortical blindness; pyramidal, cerebellar, or extrapyramidal signs; or akinetic mutism in the setting of a typical EEG.

Neuropathologic confirmation of CJD is by demonstration of spongiform change, neuronal loss, and astrocytosis. PrP amyloid plaques are usually not present in CJD, although PrP immunohistochemistry using appropriate pretreatments [73,74] will nearly always be positive. Protease-resistant PrP, seen in all the recognized prion diseases, can be demonstrated by immunoblotting of brain homogenates. *PRNP* analysis is important to exclude pathogenic mutations. Genetic susceptibility to CJD has been demonstrated in that most cases of classic CJD are homozygous with respect to the common 129 polymorphism of PrP (see Etiology, earlier).

Atypical Forms of Creutzfeldt-Jakob Disease

Atypical forms of CJD are well recognized. Approximately 10% of CJD cases have a much more prolonged clinical course with a disease duration of longer than 2 years [75]. These cases may represent the occasional occurrence of CJD in individuals heterozygous for PrP polymorphisms [76]. Approximately 10% of CJD cases present with cerebellar ataxia rather than cognitive impairment, so-called ataxic CJD [77]. Heidenhain's variant of CJD refers to cases in which cortical blindness predominates with severe involvement of the occipital lobes. The panencephalopathic type of CJD refers to cases with extensive degeneration of the cerebral white matter in addition to spongiform vacuolation of the gray matter and has been predominately reported from Japan [77].

Amyotrophic variants of CJD have been described with prominent early muscle wasting. However, most cases of dementia with amyotrophy are not experimentally transmissible [78], and their relationship with CJD is unclear. Most cases are probably variants of motor neuron disease with associated dementia. Amyotrophic features in CJD usually are seen in late disease when other features are well established.

Acquired Prion Diseases

Although human prion diseases can be transmitted to experimental animals by inoculation, they are not contagious in humans. Documented case-to-case spread has only occurred during ritual cannibalistic practices (kuru) or after accidental inoculation with prions during medical or surgical procedures (iatrogenic CJD).

Kuru

Although now nearly extinct, kuru remains of immense importance to an understanding of prion diseases. In particular, the kuru epidemic provides by far the most extensive clinical experience of an acquired prion disease in humans. The epidemiology of kuru illustrates the infectious but noncontagious properties of prions and suggests that vertical transmission from pregnant woman to child is either exceedingly rare or does not occur.

Epidemiology

Kuru reached epidemic proportions among a defined population living in the eastern highlands of Papua New Guinea. The earliest cases are thought to date back to the early part of the twentieth century [79]. Kuru affected the people of the Fore linguistic group and their neighbors, with whom they intermarried. The disease began in the northwestern part of the region among the Keiagana people, spread into the North Fore, and moved slowly further north and more dramatically into the South Fore, where it evolved into an epidemic [8]. The highlands were unknown to the outside world until 1930. Recognition of kuru followed formal administrative contacts with this region in the 1950s, and epidemiologic surveillance was started in 1957 [80].

At this stage, the annual mortality was approximately 200 people, affecting predominantly women and children (of both sexes), with only 2% of cases in adult males [8]. Kuru was the most common cause of death among women in affected villages. There was also occasional clustering of cases with four or five clan members in a village developing kuru within several months of each other. Approximately 10 years after the first contacts, although the overall kuru incidence had fallen only slightly, the disease, which had previously affected children as young as 5 years, had now disappeared in children under the age of 10 years [81]. This decline continued in the younger age groups with no new cases in those born after 1956. The government had established direct contact with these communities at this time and was discouraging ritual endocannibalism, the practice of engaging in consumption of dead relatives as a mark of respect and mourning. Women and children predominantly ate the brain and internal organs, which is thought to explain the differential age and sex incidence. Preparation of the cadaver for consumption was performed by the women and children such that other routes of exposure may also have been relevant. Liquefying brain tissue was scooped by hand into bamboo cylinders and would have been accompanied by scratching of ubiquitous itching scabies, insect bites, and sores. As well as wiping their eyes and noses, the women ate with their bare hands without washing, so oral, intradermal, and (possibly) conjunctival exposure to tissues would have been common.

The original slow progression of the disease from a single point was consistent with cannibalism as the mode of transmission. Such cannibalistic practices were not, however, confined to those living in the kuru region. It is thought that the epidemic related to a single sporadic CJD case occurring in the region some decades earlier. The clusters of cases within a particular clan could also be explained by this route of transmission as the same extended family would participate in a particular feast, thereby contracting kuru at the same time but at different ages. Clusters occurring during the later stages of the epidemic, which stood out against the low overall prevalence, could be related to the last, well remembered cannibalistic feast in the community [82].

Epidemiologic studies provided no evidence for vertical transmission, because most of the children born after 1956 and all of those born after 1959 of mothers affected with or incubating kuru were unaffected [8]. From the age of the youngest affected patient, the shortest incubation period is estimated as 4.5 years but may have been shorter because time of infection was usually unknown. Currently, four to six cases are occurring annually, all in individuals aged 40 years or older, which is consistent with exposure before 1956, indicating that incubation periods can be 40 years or more (Alpers, personal communication, 1997).

Clinical Features

Kuru affects both sexes, and onset of disease has ranged from age 5 years to older than 60 years. The mean clinical duration of illness is 12 months, with a range of 3 months to 3 years; the course tends to be shorter in children. The central clinical feature is progressive cerebellar ataxia. In sharp contrast to CJD, dementia is usually absent in kuru, even in the latter stages, although in the terminal stages many patients have their faculties obtunded [8]. The occasional case in which gross dementia occurs is in marked contrast to the clinical norm. Detailed clinical descriptions have been given by a number of observers, and the disease does not appear to have changed in features at different stages of the epidemic [79,83–87]. A prodrome and three clinical stages are recognized.

Prodromal Stage

Kuru typically begins with prodromal symptoms consisting of headache, aching of limbs, and joint pains that can last for several months.

Ambulatory Stage

Kuru was frequently self-diagnosed by patients at the earliest onset of unsteadiness in standing or walking or of dysarthria or diplopia. At this stage, there may be no objective signs of disease. Gait ataxia, however, worsens, and patients develop a broad-based gait, truncal instability, and titubation. A coarse postural tremor is usually present and accentuated by movement; patients characteristically hold their hands together in the midline to suppress this. Standing with feet together reveals clawing of toes to maintain posture. This marked clawing response is regarded as pathognomonic of kuru. Signs at this stage are, therefore, those of midline truncal ataxia. This is presumably due to paleocerebellar disease, reflected pathologically by the only clear macroscopic brain abnormality seen in kuru: atrophy of the cerebellar vermis.

Patients often become withdrawn at this stage and occasionally develop a severe reactive depression. Prodromal symptoms tend to disappear. Astasia and gait ataxia worsen, and the patient requires a stick for walking. Signs of neocerebellar disease such as intention tremor, dysmetria, hypotonia, and dysdiadochokinesis develop. Although eye movements are ataxic and jerky, nystagmus is rarely seen. Strabismus, usually convergent, may occur, particularly in children.

This strabismus does not appear to be concomitant or paralytic and may fluctuate in both extent and type, sometimes disappearing later in the clinical course. Photophobia is common and there may be an abnormal cold sensitivity with shivering and piloerection even in a warm environment. Tendon reflexes are reduced or normal, and plantar responses are flexor. Dysarthria usually occurs. As ataxia progresses, the patient passes from the first (ambulatory) stage to the second (sedentary) stage. The mean clinical duration of the first stage is approximately 8 months and correlates closely with total duration [88].

Sedentary Stage

At the sedentary stage, patients are able to sit unsupported but cannot walk. Attempted walking with support leads to a high steppage, wide-based gait with reeling instability, and flinging arm movements in an attempt to maintain posture. Hyperreflexia is seen, but plantar responses usually remain flexor with intact abdominal reflexes. Clonus is characteristically short lived. Athetoid and choreiform movements and parkinsonian tremors may occur. There is no paralysis, although muscle power is reduced. Obesity is common at this stage but may be present in early disease associated with bulimia. Characteristically, there is emotional lability and bizarre uncontrollable laughter, which has led to the disease being referred to as "laughing death." There is no sensory impairment. In sharp contrast to CJD, myoclonic jerking is rarely seen. EEG is usually normal or may show nonspecific changes [89]. This stage lasts approximately 2–3 months. When truncal ataxia reaches the point at which the patient is unable to sit unsupported, the third, or tertiary, stage is reached.

Tertiary Stage

In the tertiary stage, hypotonia and hyporeflexia develop and the terminal state is marked by flaccid muscle weakness. Plantar responses remain flexor with intact abdominal reflexes. Progressive dysphagia occurs and patients become incontinent of urine and feces. Inanition and emaciation develop. Transient conjugate eye signs and dementia may occur. Primitive reflexes develop in occasional cases. Brain stem involvement and both bulbar and pseudobulbar signs occur. Respiratory failure and bronchopneumonia eventually lead to death. The tertiary stage lasts 1–2 months.

Iatrogenic Creutzfeldt-Jakob Disease

Iatrogenic prion disease is usually referred to as CJD even though cases arising as a result of peripheral (as compared to intracerebral) inoculation with prions usually have a clinical picture more reminiscent of kuru, with a prominent cerebellar syndrome. Transmission of CJD from case to case has occurred by a number of routes involving accidental inoculation with human prions as a result of medical procedures. Such iatrogenic routes include the use of inadequately sterilized neurosurgical instruments, dura mater, and corneal grafting, and use of human cadaveric pituitary–derived growth hormone or gonadotrophin. The first recognized case of iatrogenic CJD occurred in 1974 in a 55-year-old woman who had received a corneal transplant 18 months earlier from a donor who was subsequently found to have died of CJD [90]. A second corneal transplantation–related case has also been reported [91]. Transmission through neurosurgical procedures has probably occurred for some time [92]. The first documented cases of transmission through neurosurgical instruments arose in 1977 when CJD was reported in two patients who had received stereotactic EEG depth recordings for epileptic conditions 16 and 20 months earlier [93]. The same electrodes had previously been used for stereotactic exploration of a CJD patient and had been sterilized with 70% alcohol and formaldehyde vapor. Although this procedure is sufficient to destroy conventional agents, it is ineffective against prions, and one of the electrodes was found still capable of transmitting disease to chimpanzees after implantation in the cerebral cortex. Homograft transmission by implantation of cadaveric dura mater has resulted in an increasing number of cases during the mid-1980s from the United States, Europe, New Zealand, and Japan [94–110].

The first case of CJD in a recipient of human cadaveric pituitary–derived growth hormone was in a 20-year-old man with idiopathic hypopituitarism. The first clinical use of human growth hormone was described in 1958 and adopted in a number of countries. In the United Kingdom, 1,908 people received this treatment, and in the United States there were approximately 10,000 recipients. Acetone-dried powdered pituitary tissue was subjected to repeated organic solvent extraction and acid-base precipitations, and the final hormone preparation contained many impurities. After 1975, the extraction method was modified to incorporate isoelectric precipitation and chromatography from frozen glands. Each batch of growth hormone was derived from pooled pituitaries and up to 2,000 glands were used per batch, with the remnants of some batches being mixed with new batches. Thus, there is the potential for even a single gland to contaminate many vials of hormone. Many additional cases have now been recorded in the United States, United Kingdom, and particularly in France, with approximately 100 cases now recorded internationally. In addition to the human growth hormone cases, there have been four cases of iatrogenic CJD among recipients of human cadaveric pituitary–derived gonadotrophin [111–112]. So far, all cases appear to have arisen in patients treated in Australia.

It is of considerable interest that cases arising from intracerebral or optic inoculation manifest clinically as classic CJD, with a rapidly progressive dementia, whereas those resulting from peripheral inoculation, most notably after pituitary-derived growth hormone exposure, typically present with a progressive ataxic syndrome and are in that respect somewhat reminiscent of kuru. Not surprisingly, the incubation period in intracerebral cases is short (19–46 months for dura mater grafts) as compared to peripheral cases (typically 15 years or more).

There is evidence for genetic susceptibility to iatrogenic CJD with an excess of codon 129 homozygotes, in particular valine 129 homozygotes, in iatrogenic cases arising from pituitary hormone therapy. This finding was reported initially in a study of seven U.K. cases [44] and has subsequently been confirmed in the larger U.S. and French series [34,35]. The separate origin of the contaminated growth hormone used in the three countries makes it unlikely that this effect is due to contamination of the batches of hormone with CJD material from individuals homozygous for valine at polymorphic residue 129, as this is the least common genotype. It has been argued that valine 129 PrP may be more susceptible to undergoing the conversion to the disease-related isoform than is methionine 129 PrP and, therefore, that valine 129 homozygotes may be particularly susceptible to acquired prion diseases [44].

Epidemiologic studies have not shown increased risks of particular occupations that may be exposed to human or animal prions, although individual CJD cases in two histopathology technicians, a neuropathologist, and a neurosurgeon have been documented.

Although there have been concerns that CJD may be transmissible by blood transfusion, extensive epidemiologic analysis in the United Kingdom has found that the frequency of blood transfusion and donation was no different in over 200 cases of CJD and a matched control population [113]. Recipients of blood transfusions who developed CJD had clinical presentations similar to those of sporadic CJD patients and not to the more kuru-like iatrogenic cases arising from peripheral exposure to human prions. Furthermore, experimental transmission studies have shown only weak evidence for infectivity in blood [114], even when inoculation occurs via the most efficient (intracerebral) route. It cannot be assumed that the same picture will hold for new variant CJD, as this is caused by a prion strain [55] distinct from those causing classic CJD and could have a different peripheral pathogenesis. It is also conceivable that many individuals could currently be incubating this disease.

New Variant of Human Prion Disease

In late 1995, two cases of sporadic CJD were reported in the United Kingdom in teenagers [64,65]. Only four cases of sporadic CJD had previously been recorded in the literature in teenagers, and none of these cases occurred in the United Kingdom. In addition, both cases were unusual in having kuru-type plaques, a finding seen only in approximately 5% of CJD cases. Soon afterward, a third very young sporadic CJD case occurred [66]. These cases caused considerable concern, and the possibility was raised that they might suggest a link with BSE. It was clearly of some importance to determine if any further such extraordinarily rare cases occurred in the United Kingdom. By March 1996, further extremely young-onset cases were apparent, and review of the histology of these cases showed a remarkably consistent and unique pattern. These cases were named *new variant CJD*, although it was clear that they were also rather atypical in their clinical presentation; in fact, most cases did not meet the accepted clinical diagnostic criteria for probable CJD. Extensive studies of archival cases of CJD or other prion diseases failed to show this picture, and it seemed likely to represent the arrival of a new form of prion disease in the United Kingdom. The statistical probability of such cases occurring by chance was vanishingly small, and ascertainment bias seemed most unlikely as an explanation. It was clear that a new risk factor for CJD had emerged and appeared to be specific to the United Kingdom. The U.K. government advisory committee on spongiform encephalopathy concluded that, although there was no direct evidence for a link with BSE, exposure to specified bovine offal before the ban on its inclusion in human foodstuffs in 1989 was the most likely explanation. Another case of the new variant CJD was soon reported in France [115].

The clinical presentation is with behavioral and psychiatric disturbances and, in some cases, with sensory disturbance [67]. Initial referral is usually to a psychiatrist, and the most prominent feature is depression, but anxiety, withdrawal, and behavioral change is also frequent [116]. Suicidal ideation is infrequent, and response to antidepressants poor. Delusions, which are complex and unsustained, are common. Other features include emotional lability, aggression, insomnia, and auditory and visual hallucinations. A prominent early feature in some was dysesthesia, pain in the limbs or face, or pain that was persistent rather than intermittent and unrelated to anxiety levels. A minority of cases have been noted to have forgetfulness or mild gait ataxia from an early stage, but in most cases overt neurologic features are not apparent until some months into the clinical course [117]. In most patients, a progressive cerebellar syndrome develops with gait and limb ataxia. Dementia usually develops later in the clinical course, with progression to akinetic mutism in the majority of cases. Myoclonus was seen in most patients, in some cases preceded by chorea. Cortical blindness develops in a minority of patients in the late stages of disease. Upgaze paresis, an uncommon feature of classic CJD, has been noted in some patients [117]. The age at onset in the initial 14 cases reported ranged from 16 to 48 years (mean = 29 years), and the clinical course was unusually prolonged (9–35 months; median = 14 months). The EEG was atypical, however, without the pseudoperiodic pattern seen in most sporadic CJD cases. Neuroimaging was normal or showed only mild atrophy. A high signal in the posterior thalamus on T2-weighted MRI, however, has been reported in a number of patients [117]. PrP gene analysis showed that all cases available for study were homozygous for methionine at codon 129. No known or novel pathogenic mutations were found in the coding sequence [117,118].

The neuropathologic appearances were striking and consistent. Although there was widespread spongiform change, gliosis, and neuronal loss most severe in the basal ganglia and thalamus, the most remarkable feature was the abundant PrP amyloid plaques in cerebral and cerebellar cortex. These consisted of kuru-like, "florid" (surrounded by spongiform vacuoles), and multicentric plaque types. The florid plaques, seen previously only in scrapie, were a particularly unusual but highly consistent feature. There was also abundant pericellular PrP deposition in the cerebral and cerebellar cortex. A further highly unusual feature was the extensive PrP deposition in the molecular layer of the cerebellum.

Some of the features of this syndrome are reminiscent of kuru, in which behavioral changes and progressive ataxia predominate. In addition, peripheral sensory disturbances are well recognized in the kuru prodrome. Kuru plaques are seen in approximately 70% of cases and are especially abundant in younger kuru patients. The observation that iatrogenic prion disease related to peripheral exposure to human prions has a more kuru-like than CJD-like clinical picture, which is discussed in detail earlier in this section, may well be relevant and could perhaps suggest that new variant CJD cases were also acquired via peripheral exposure to prions.

Direct experimental evidence that new variant CJD may be caused by BSE was provided by molecular analysis of human prion strains (PrP^{Sc} typing) (see Etiology, earlier). The identification of a biochemical marker that distinguished new variant CJD from previously recognized forms of sporadic and iatrogenic CJD confirmed that this was a novel variant and implied that it was caused by exposure to a single novel prion strain type [55]. The lack of any history of iatrogenic exposure to humans in these patients suggested that this was a novel animal prion. The molecular strain characteristics of new variant CJD closely resembled those seen in BSE itself and BSE transmitted to mice, domestic cats, and macaques, consistent with BSE being the origin of new variant CJD [55]. Such PrP^{Sc} markers are detectable in tonsil tissue [119], which may allow premortem diagnosis of new variant CJD without brain biopsy and may potentially allow earlier diagnosis. Transmission studies of new variant CJD into both transgenic and wild-type mice have been performed to further investigate a link with BSE. Remarkably, the transmission characteristics of new variant CJD are quite distinct from those of all other forms of sporadic and acquired CJD but closely resemble those of BSE. The PrP^{Sc} types produced on transmission of new variant CJD and BSE into wild-type mice were indistinguishable. These experiments confirmed that new variant CJD and BSE were caused by the same prion strain [120]. Classic strain-typing studies using a panel of inbred conventional mice and studies of both incubation period and patterns of neuropathologic targeting reached the same conclusion [121].

Although it is now clear that new variant CJD is human BSE, it is unclear why this particular age group should be affected and why none of these cases had a pattern of unusual occupational or dietary exposure to BSE. Very little is known, however, about which foodstuffs contained high-titer bovine offal. It is possible that certain foods containing particularly high titers were eaten predominately by younger people. It cannot be excluded at present, however, that young people have an inherently higher intrinsic susceptibility to the BSE agent after dietary exposure or that they simply have shorter incubation periods. It is important to appreciate that BSE-contaminated feed was given to sheep, pigs, and poultry and that although we have no evidence of natural transmission to these species, it would be prudent to remain open-minded about other dietary exposure to novel animal prions.

Inherited Prion Diseases

Gerstmann-Sträussler-Scheinker Syndrome

The first case of GSS was described by Gerstmann in 1928 and was followed by a more detailed report on seven other affected members of the same family in 1936 [122,123] as a "peculiar heredo-familial disease of the central nervous system." A detailed clinicopathologic report of this family was presented in 1962 by Seitelberger [124]. The classic presentation of GSS is a chronic cerebellar ataxia accompanied by pyramidal features, with dementia occurring later in a much more prolonged clinical course than that seen in CJD. The mean duration is approximately 5 years, with onset usually in either the third or fourth decades. Histologically, the hallmark is the presence of multicentric amyloid plaques. Spongiform change, neuronal loss, astrocytosis, and white matter loss are also usually present. Numerous GSS kindreds from several countries (including the original Austrian family described by Gerstmann, Sträussler, and Scheinker in 1936) have now been demonstrated to have mutations in the PrP gene. GSS is an autosomal dominant disorder that can now be classified within the spectrum of inherited prion disease.

Inherited Prion Diseases

The identification of one of the pathogenic PrP gene mutations in a case with neurodegenerative disease allows not only molecular diagnosis of an inherited prion disease but also its subclassification according to mutation (see Figure 5.2). Pathogenic mutations reported to date in the human PrP gene consist of two groups: (1) point mutations within the coding sequence, resulting in amino acid substitutions in PrP or, in one case, production of a stop codon resulting in expression of a truncated PrP and (2) insertions encoding additional integral copies of an octapeptide repeat present in a tandem array of five copies in the normal protein. A suggested notation for these diseases is *inherited prion disease (PrP mutation)*—for example, inherited prion disease (PrP 144-bp insertion) or inherited prion disease (PrP P102L).

Missense Mutations

PrP P102L PrP P102L was first reported in 1989 [22] in two families (one in the United Kingdom and the other in the United States) and has now been demonstrated in many other kindreds in the United States, United Kingdom, Germany, Italy, and Japan [22,24–27]. It has also been demonstrated in the original Austrian family reported by Gerstmann, Sträussler, and Scheinker in 1936 [28]. Progressive ataxia is the dominant clinical feature, with dementia and pyramidal features. However, marked variability both at the clinical and neuropathologic level is apparent in some families and has recently been extensively documented in the original Austrian family [125]. A family with marked amyotrophic features also has been reported [27]. Cases with severe dementia in the absence of prominent ataxia are also recognized. Histologic examination reveals PrP immunoreactive plaques in the majority of cases. Transmissibility to experimental animals has been demonstrated.

PrP P105L The proline-leucine change at codon 105 has been found in four patients from three Japanese families [126]. It has not been reported outside Japan. The patients presented with a history of spastic paraparesis and dementia. The clinical duration from onset to the development of akinetic mutism was approximately 5 years. There was no periodic synchronous discharge on EEG, but MRI scans showed atrophy of the motor cortex. Pathologic examination revealed plaques in the cerebral cortex and neuronal loss but no spongiosis. Neurofibrillary tangles were variably present among cases, and no plaques were found in the cerebellum.

PrP A117V Two nucleotide changes occur at codon 117. One is a noncoding third-base polymorphism that is found in approximately 2.5% of the population (Palmer and Collinge, unpublished data). It can be easily detected as it destroys a Pvu II restriction site in the open reading frame [127]. The other change is a coding mutation changing an alanine to valine. The mutational event generating the valine-encoding sequence seems to have occurred on a Pvu II– allele and, therefore, differs from the normal alanine encoding Pvu II+ sequence by two nucleotides. This mutation was first described in a French family [24] and subsequently in a U.S. family of German origin [128]. The U.S. family was originally described as having familial AD but was reclassified to GSS on finding PrP immunostaining amyloid plaques. The clinical features are presenile dementia associated with pyramidal signs, parkinsonism, pseudobulbar features, and cerebellar signs. Neuropathologically, PrP immunoreactive plaques are usually present. This mutation has also been identified in a large family in the United Kingdom (Collinge, et al., in preparation).

PrP Y145STOP PrP Y145STOP has been of considerable research interest because it results in the production of a truncated PrP. The mutation was detected in a Japanese patient who had a clinical diagnosis of AD. She developed memory disturbance and a slowly progressive dementia at 38 years. The duration of illness was 21 years. Histologic examination revealed typical Alzheimer pathology without spongiform change [129]. Many amyloid plaques were seen in the cortex along with diffuse neuropil threads of paired helical filaments. The plaques, however, were immunoreactive with PrP antisera. Beta-A4 immunocytochemistry was negative. Kitamoto and colleagues [129] demonstrated not only that the truncated PrP was indeed expressed in affected individuals, but that the deposited protein seemed to consist entirely of the mutant truncated protein and did not contain the wild-type protein produced by the normal allele. Such an observation is in accordance with the model of prion propagation discussed in the section on Etiology—namely that the protein-protein interaction involved preferentially involves homologous molecules. Transmission to experimental animals has not yet been reported. Of course, the clinicopathologic findings in this case emphasize the importance of PrP gene analysis in the differential diagnosis of dementias.

PrP D178N PrP D178N was originally described in two Finnish families with a CJD-like phenotype (although without typical EEG appearances) [130] and has since been demonstrated in additional CJD families in Hungary, the Netherlands, Canada, Finland, France [131,132], and the United Kingdom. The Finnish pedigree included 15 affected members in four generations. The mean age of onset was 47 years, and mean duration was 27.5 months. Brain biopsy and autopsy specimens showed spongiform change without amyloid plaques. A review of 43 patients from seven families with this mutation showed that compared to sporadic CJD, the age of onset is earlier and the duration longer [133]. As with the Finnish families, periodic sharp wave activity was absent. However, a case has been reported with onset at 57 years with a periodic EEG [134].

This mutation was also reported in two unrelated families with FFI [60,135,136]. The first cases described had a rapidly progressive disease characterized clinically by untreatable insomnia, dysautonomia, and motor signs, and neuropathologically by selective atrophy of the anterior-ventral and mediodorsal thalamic nuclei. Marked thalamic astrocytosis is present. Mild spongiform change is seen in some cases, and protease-resistant PrP demonstrated, albeit weakly, by immunoblotting. Proteinase-K treatment of extracted PrP^{Sc} from FFI cases has shown a PrP band on Western blots of a different size compared to that of PrP^{Sc} from CJD cases [137], suggesting that FFI may be caused by a distinct prion strain type.

A study by Goldfarb and colleagues [138] reported that in all the codon 178 families they studied with a CJD-like disease, the codon 178 mutation was encoded on a valine 129 allele, whereas all FFI kindreds encode the same codon 178 mutation on a methionine 129 allele. They suggested that the genotype at codon 129 determines phenotype. However, they have not demonstrated that the families they describe are unrelated; therefore, their comparison may only be based on two extended families. Insomnia is not uncommon in CJD patients, and FFI and CJD may represent extremes of a spectrum of related disease phenotypes. An inherited case with the codon 200 lysine mutation, which is normally associated with a CJD-like phenotype, has been reported with an FFI phenotype [139]. An Australian family has also been reported with the FFI genotype, but affected family members have a range of phenotypes encompassing typical CJD, FFI, and an autosomal dominant cerebellar ataxia–like illness [140]. It is of interest that the CJD-like codon 178 cases have frequently transmitted to experimental animals, whereas the FFI type did not transmit to laboratory primates [141]. Transmission of an FFI case to mice has been reported, although this case was unusual in that a single octapeptide repeat deletion was present on the same allele [142]. This individual came from an extensive kindred in which other family members with the same *PRNP* genotype had a CJD-like phenotype [143]. Two cases of FFI, however, one a U.K. case and the second an Italian case, both with the usual FFI genotype of D178N, 129M, transmitted to transgenic mice expressing human PrP [144].

PrP V180I PrP V180I was identified in two Japanese patients with subacute dementia and myoclonus [126]. The period from onset to akinetic mutism was 6–10 months. No family history was noted. EEG did not show pseudoperiodic sharp wave activity. Neuropathologic examination demonstrated spongiform change, neuronal loss, and astrocytosis. Interestingly, one of the patients with isoleucine at codon 180 also had arginine at codon 232 (see the section, PrP M232R). These were on different alleles. This disease has not been transmitted to laboratory animals [145].

PrP T183A PrP T183A was reported in a single Brazilian family with a frontotemporal dementia of mean onset at 45 years and duration of 4 years [146]. Parkinsonian features were also present in some patients. Neuropathologic examination revealed severe spongiform change and neuronal loss in deep cortical layers and putamen, but there was relatively little gliosis. PrP immunoreactivity was demonstrated in putamen and cerebellum. No transmission studies have been reported to date.

PrP F198S A variant form of GSS was described in a large Indiana kindred that has been traced back to 1792 [147]. Unlike other GSS patients with presenile onset of neurologic disability, the Indiana kindred had widespread Alzheimer-like neurofibrillary tangles composed of paired helical filaments in the cortex and subcortical nuclei, in addition to amyloid plaques. The amyloid plaques were composed of PrP and not beta-A4 [148]. Affected individuals in this kindred have a codon 198 thymine to cytosine transition resulting in a phenylalanine to serine conversion

[43]. There is an apparent codon 129 effect with this mutation in that individuals who were heterozygous at codon 129 had a later age of onset than did homozygotes. Transmission of this disease to laboratory animals has not yet been reported.

PrP E200K PrP E200K was first described in families with CJD. Affected individuals develop a rapidly progressive dementia with myoclonus and pyramidal, cerebellar, or extrapyramidal signs. Duration of illness is usually shorter than 12 months. The average age of onset for the disease is 55 years. Histologically these patients are typical of CJD; plaques are absent, but PrP^{Sc} can be demonstrated by immunoblotting. In marked contrast to other variants of inherited prion disease, the EEG usually shows the characteristic pseudoperiodic sharp wave activity seen in sporadic CJD. Interestingly, this mutation accounts for the three reported ethnogeographic clusters of CJD in which the local incidence of CJD is approximately 100-fold higher than it is elsewhere (among Libyan Jews and in regions of Slovakia and Chile) [149–153]. Now that cases can be diagnosed by PrP gene analysis, atypical forms of this condition are being detected with phenotypes other than that of classic CJD. Of interest also are reports that peripheral neuropathy can occur in this disease [154]. This mutation also shows incomplete penetrance. Elderly unaffected carriers of the mutation have been reported. Chapman and colleagues [155] have made a detailed analysis of 52 mutation-carrying patients with definite or probable CJD and 34 unaffected mutation carriers. They concluded that the cumulative penetrance reaches 50% at the age of 60 years and 80% by 80 years. There was a group of patients aged between 69 and 82 years with possible CJD, however, containing five proved and two obligate carriers of the mutation. That is to say the patients were demented but did not fulfill the clinical criteria for probable CJD. If the analysis was carried out assuming that these possible cases were actually CJD, then the penetrance reaches 100% by the age of 80 years. Individuals homozygous for the mutation have been identified and are phenotypically indistinguishable from heterozygotes, indicating that this condition is a fully dominant disorder [149]. Patients with this condition have now been reported in several other countries outside the well-recognized clusters, including the United Kingdom. At least one of the U.K. cases does not appear to be related to the ethnogeographic clusters mentioned above, suggesting a separate U.K. focus for this type of inherited prion disease [156]. Goldfarb and colleagues have found this mutation among 46 of 55 CJD-affected families studied at the National Institutes of Health (NIH) [157]. These families contain 89 affected patients and originate from seven different countries: Slovakia, Poland, Germany, Tunisia, Greece, Libya, and Chile. The codon 129 genotype does not appear to affect age at onset of this disorder. Transmission to experimental animals has been demonstrated.

PrP R208H PrP R208H has been reported in a single patient with CJD confirmed at autopsy. No details of the family history or phenotypic details are yet published [158].

PrP V210I PrP V210I has been reported only in a single case in France [159], with a rapidly progressive dementia, cerebellar signs, and myoclonus. Age of onset was 63 years. EEG showed pseudoperiodic sharp wave activity. The clinical duration was 4 months and neuropathologic examination showed spongiform change, neuronal loss, and astrocytosis. No amyloid plaques were seen. The patient's parents had died at 60 and 66 years without dementia. A sister with the mutation had died of colon cancer at 67 years. It is possible that this mutation produces a very late–onset disease or is incompletely penetrant. Transmission to experimental animals has not been reported.

PrP Q217R Reported only in a single Swedish family, individuals with PrP Q217R present with dementia followed by gait ataxia, dysphagia, and confusion [160]. As with the inherited prion disease with codon 198 serine mutation (Indiana kindred), this mutation also shows prominent neurofibrillary tangles. Transmissibility to experimental animals has not yet been demonstrated in this condition.

PrP M232R PrP M232R was first found on the opposite allele to a codon 180 mutation in a Japanese patient with prion disease [126]. It was further demonstrated in two additional Japanese patients with dementia. Both of the latter cases appeared to present as sporadic cases with no family history of neurologic disease. Both patients had progressive dementia, myoclonus, and periodic synchronous discharges in the EEG. The mean duration of illness was 3 months. Neuropathology showed spongiform change, neuronal loss, and astrocytosis. PrP immunostaining revealed diffuse gray matter staining but no plaques.

Insertional Mutations

PrP 24-bp Insertion (one extra repeat) A single octapeptide repeat insertion has been reported in a single French individual who presented at 73 years with dizziness [161]. He later developed visual agnosia, cerebellar ataxia, and intellectual impairment. Diffuse periodic activity was noted on EEG. Myoclonus and cortical blindness developed, and he progressed to akinetic mutism. Disease duration was 4 months. The patient's father had died at 70 years from an undiagnosed neurologic disorder. No neuropathologic information is available.

PrP 48-bp Insertion (two extra repeats) PrP 48-bp insertion has been reported in a single family from the United States [162]. The proband had a CJD-like phenotype both clinically and pathologically, with a typical EEG and an age at onset of 58 years. However, the proband's mother had onset of cognitive decline at 75 years with a slow progression to a severe dementia over 13 years. The maternal grandfather had a similar late onset (at 80 years) and slowly progressive cognitive decline over 15 years. The codon 129 status of these cases is not stated.

PrP 96-bp Insertion (four extra repeats) A PrP 96-bp insertional mutation encoding four octapeptide elements was first reported in an individual who died at 63 years of hepatic cirrhosis [163]. There was no history of neurologic illness, and it is unclear whether this finding indicates incomplete penetrance of this mutation. This is the only recorded case of a *PRNP* insertional mutation other than that in an affected individual with a prion disease or in an at-risk individual from an affected kindred. Two separate four–octapeptide repeat insertional mutations have been reported in affected individuals, each differing in the DNA sequence from the original four-repeat insertion, although all three of the mutations encode the same PrP. Laplanche and colleagues reported a 96-bp insertion in an 82-year-old French woman who developed progressive depression and behavioral changes [164]. She progressed over 3 months to akinetic mutism with pyramidal signs and myoclonus. EEG showed pseudoperiodic complexes. Duration of illness was 4 months. There was no known family history of neurologic illness. Another 96-bp insertional mutation was seen in a patient with classic clinical and pathologic features of CJD with the exception of the unusual finding of pronounced PrP immunoreactivity in the molecular layer of the cerebellum [165]. No family history was apparent in this case, but there was nonpaternity, and details of the biological father were unavailable.

PrP 120-bp Insertion (five extra repeats) A five additional octapeptide–repeat mutation was reported in a U.S. family with an illness characterized by progressive dementia, abnormal behavior, cerebellar signs, tremor, rigidity, hyperreflexia, and myoclonus. The age at onset was 31–45 years with a clinical duration of 5–15 years [163]. EEG showed diffuse slowing only. Histologic features were of spongiosis, neuronal loss, and gliosis. Transmission to squirrel and spider monkeys has been demonstrated.

PrP 144-bp Insertion (six extra repeats) The PrP 144-bp insertion was the first PrP mutation to be reported and was found in a small U.K. family with familial CJD [21]. The diagnosis in the family had been based on an individual who died in the 1940s with a rapidly progressive illness characteristic of CJD [166]. The reported duration of illness was 6 months. Pathologically there was gross status spongiosis and astrocytosis affecting the entire cerebral cortex, and this case is used to illustrate classic CJD histology in Greenfield's *Neuropathology* [167]. Other family members, however, had a much longer–duration GSS-like illness. Histologic features were also extremely variable. This observation led to screening of various cases of neurodegenerative disease and to the identification of a case classified on clinical grounds as familial AD [30]. More extensive screening work identified further families with the same mutation that were then demonstrated by genealogic studies to form part of an extremely large kindred [31,168]. Clinical information has been collected on approximately 50 affected individuals over seven generations. Affected individuals develop onset of a progressive dementia in the third to fourth decade associated with a varying combination of cerebellar ataxia and dysarthria, pyramidal signs, myoclonus, and occasionally extrapyramidal signs, chorea, and seizures. The dementia is often preceded by depression and aggressive behavior. A number of cases have a long-standing personality disorder characterized by aggression, irritability, antisocial and criminal activity, and hypersexuality, which may be present from early childhood, long before overt neurodegenerative disease develops. The histologic features vary from those of classic spongiform encephalopathy (with or without PrP amyloid plaques) to cases lacking any specific features of these conditions [29]. Age at onset in this condition can be predicted according to genotype at polymorphic codon 129. Because this pathogenic insertional mutation occurs on a methionine 129 PrP allele, two codon 129 genotypes for affected individuals are possible: methionine 129 homozygotes or methionine 129/valine 129 heterozygotes. Heterozygotes have an age at onset that is approximately one decade later than homozygotes [166]. Limited transmission studies to marmosets were unsuccessful. Transmission to transgenic mice expressing human PrP has been achieved (Collinge, et al., in preparation). Further families with 144-bp insertions of different nucleotide sequence have now been reported in the United Kingdom [169] and Japan [170].

PrP 168-bp Insertion (seven extra repeats) The PrP 168-bp insertion mutation has been reported in a U.S. family. The clinical features described include mood change, abnormal behavior, confusion, aphasia, cerebellar signs, involuntary movements, rigidity, dementia, and myoclonus. The age at onset was 23–35 years and the clinical duration 10 years to longer than 13 years. EEG showed diffuse slowing in two cases; a third showed slow wave burst suppression. Neuropathologic examination showed spongiform change, neuronal loss, and gliosis to varying degrees [163]. Experimental transmission to chimpanzees has been demonstrated.

PrP 192-bp Insertion (eight extra repeats) The PrP 192-bp insertion mutation has been reported in a French family with clinical features that include abnormal behavior, cerebellar signs, mutism, pyramidal signs, myoclonus, tremor, intellectual slowing, and seizures. The disease duration ranged from 3 months to 13 years. The EEG findings included diffuse slowing, slow wave burst suppression, and periodic triphasic complexes. Neuropathologic examination revealed spongiform change, neuronal loss, gliosis, and multicentric plaques in the cerebellum [163,171]. Experimental transmission to chimpanzees has been reported.

PrP 216-bp Insertion (nine extra repeats) The finding of a nine-octapeptide insertional mutation was first reported in a single case from the United Kingdom [172]. The clinical onset was approximately 54 years, with falls, axial rigidity, myoclonic jerks, and progressive dementia [173]. Although there was no clear family history of a similar illness, the mother had died at 53 years with a cerebrovascular event. The maternal grandmother died at 79 years with senile dementia. EEG was of low amplitude but did not show pseudoperiodic sharp wave activity. Neuropathologic examination showed no spongiform encephalopathy but showed marked deposition of plaques, which in the cerebellum and the basal ganglia showed immunoreactivity with PrP antisera [173]. In the hippocampus, neuritic plaques positive for both beta-A4 and *tau* were present. Some neurofibrillary tangles were also seen. In some respects, therefore, the pathology resembled AD. Experimental transmission studies have not been attempted. A second German family with a nine-octapeptide repeat insertion of different sequence has now been reported [174].

Other Polymorphic Variation in *PRNP*

PrP M129V

The role of the important coding polymorphism, PrP M129V, in determining susceptibility to acquired and sporadic prion disease and in affecting age at onset in some kindreds with inherited prion disease has been discussed in the section on Etiology.

PrP GGC-GGG^{124}

PrP GGC-GGG^{124}, a third-base change of a glycine codon from GGC to GGG, was found on the normal allele of an individual with codon 217 mutation [33]. The frequency of this polymorphism is not known, although in a screen of over 700 samples of both normal controls and patients with neurologic disease only one instance of this variation has been found, in an individual with ALS who also had a 24-bp deletion.

PrP GCA-GCG^{117}

PrP GCA-GCG^{117} is a noncoding third-base change seen in approximately 2.5% of whites (see PrP A117V, earlier).

PrP CAC-CAT^{177}

PrP CAC-CAT^{177} is a noncoding third-base change found in an 88-year-old control subject by Ripoll and colleagues [175].

PrP E219K

Originally found in a Japanese individual with schizophrenia, the PrP Glu-Lys^{219} variation has been found to be a fairly common polymorphism in the Japanese population, with an allele frequency of 6%. This variation has not yet been reported in white populations [176].

PrP 24-bp Deletion (one fewer octapeptide repeat)

Deletions in the repeat region of the PrP are now known to be polymorphisms, with a frequency of approximately 1% of alleles affected. Because of the nature of the repeat region, it is not possible to say precisely where the excision point for these 24-bp deletions lies. However, three different nucleotide sequences are recognized to be associated with the deletions. All of these deleted alleles encode the same amino acid sequence, so they are not distinguishable at the protein level [177,178].

Presymptomatic and Antenatal Testing

Because a direct gene test has become available, it has been possible to provide an unequivocal diagnosis in patients with inherited forms of the disease. This has also led to the possibility of performing presymptomatic testing of unaffected but at-risk family members, as well as antenatal testing [179]. Because of the effect of the codon 129 genotype on the age of onset of disease associated with some mutations, it is possible to determine within a family whether a carrier of a mutation will have early- or late-onset disease. Most of the mutations found so far—with the notable exception of the codon 200 mutation—appear to be fully penetrant; however, experience with many of the mutations is extremely limited. Examples of elderly unaffected gene carriers who appear to have escaped the disease are found in codon 200 families.

Genetic counseling in prion disease resembles that of Huntington's disease in many respects, and protocols established for Huntington's disease can be adapted for prion disease counseling. PrP gene analysis may have very important consequences for family members other than the individual tested, and it is preferable to discuss all the issues with the whole family before testing commences. Following the identification of a mutation, the family should be referred for genetic counseling. Testing of asymptomatic individuals should only follow adequate counseling and requires their full informed consent.

Prognosis and Treatment

All forms of prion diseases that are currently recognized are invariably fatal after a relentlessly progressive course. No currently available treatment alters the clinical course of the disease and all that can be offered at present is general supportive care for the patient and family with hospitalization in the later stages. The duration of illness in sporadic patients is very short, with a mean duration of 3–4 months. In some of the inherited cases, however, the duration can be 20 years or longer [29].

Secondary Prophylaxis after Accidental Exposure

Certain occupational groups are at risk of exposure to human prions—for instance, neurosurgeons and other operating theater staff, pathologists and morticians, and histology technicians as well as an increasing number of laboratory workers. Because of the prolonged incubation periods of prions after administration to sites other than the central nervous system (CNS), which is associated with clinically silent prion replication in the lymphoreticular tissue [180], treatments inhibiting prion replication in lymphoid organs may represent a viable strategy for rational secondary prophylaxis after accidental exposure. Although the nature of the cells responsible for prion spread from peripheral sites to the CNS is not known, adoptive bone marrow reconstitution of PrP^C-deficient mice with PrP^C-expressing hematopoietic cells restores prion accumulation in the spleen after intraperitoneal inoculation, suggesting that the crucial cells are bone-marrow derived [181]. Lymphocytes are a likely candidate because they express significant amounts of PrP^C on their surface [182]. A suggested regimen is surgical excision of inoculum along with antilymphocytic treatment using oral corticosteroids in individuals with significant accidental exposure to human prions [183].

There is hope that progress in understanding the peripheral pathogenesis will identify the precise cell types and molecules involved in prion colonization of the organism. The ultimate goal is to target the rate-limiting steps in prion spread with much more focused pharmacologic approaches, which may eventually prove useful in preventing disease even after iatrogenic and alimentary exposure.

TRANSMISSION STUDIES

Experimental transmission studies of the human prion diseases have largely involved transmission to laboratory primates, in particular chimpanzees and squirrel monkeys. The extensive experience of the NIH group, reporting over 300 successful transmissions, has been summarized [141]. Transmission studies in primates are severely limited by the expense of such studies, however, and by ethical concerns as to the use of primates in such work. Attempts by most laboratories to transmit human prions to rodents have been fairly unsuccessful, with only occasional transmissions occurring and then at very prolonged incubation periods close to the natural lifespan of the mice. Some groups have, however, reported more frequent transmissions [184]. Transgenic mice have become available that have increased susceptibility to human prions. Mice expressing a chimeric human/mouse PrP were susceptible to three CJD isolates with short incubation periods [185]. It has now become clear that transgenic mice expressing wild-type human PrP but not mouse PrP are highly susceptible to CJD, with all inoculated mice succumbing at short incubation periods, usually between 180–220 days [120,186,187]. Such mice appear to lack a species barrier to human prions and can now be used for extensive studies of the human prion diseases [187]. We have successfully transmitted more than 20 cases to mice expressing human PrP, including inherited cases that failed to transmit to primates [144,187], and larger-scale studies are in progress to establish the range of transmission characteristics of the human prion diseases and prion titers in peripheral tissues.

RISKS OF AN EPIDEMIC OF HUMAN BSE: THE BOVINE-TO-HUMAN SPECIES BARRIER

As BSE appears to have transmitted to humans, a key issue is the extent of the bovine-to-human species barrier. Clearly, this cannot be measured directly because it would require inoculation of humans with BSE. Transgenic models may offer a way to address this issue, however, at least in part. The principal determinants of the species barrier are the degree of homology between PrP molecules in the host and inoculum [39] and strain of agent; however, BSE appears to be caused by a single prion strain [49]. Transgenic mice expressing human PrP, which are competent to produce human PrP^{Sc} and "human" prions on CJD challenge, offer an opportunity to address whether it is possible for bovine prions to induce production of human PrP^{Sc}. Incubation periods of BSE were unaltered in mice expressing human PrP in addition to mouse PrP, and only mouse PrP^{Sc} appeared to be produced [187]. A potentially more revealing experiment is to challenge mice expressing only human PrP with BSE [187]. These mice are far more resistant to BSE than to CJD prions, but transmission has now occurred at more than 500 days postchallenge [120]. These mice express valine at polymorphic codon 129 of *PRNP*, and these studies are being repeated with mice transgenic for human PrP methionine 129. This is of particular importance given that all new variant CJD cases seen to date are methionine 129 homozygotes.

Even the presence of a substantial species barrier between cattle and humans, however, does not exclude extensive BSE transmission to humans given the very large numbers of people who have been exposed over a prolonged period. The extent of accumulation of risk following repeated low-dose oral exposure is unknown. The mean incubation period of BSE in humans is also unknown, making attempts to predict any epidemic exceedingly difficult at present. Genetic susceptibility is important in this regard and, in particular, *PRNP* codon 129 homozygotes would be expected to be at considerably higher risk than heterozygotes, although it is possible that heterozygotes may simply have longer incubation periods.

The production of a novel distinct molecular human PrP^{Sc} type on transmission of new variant CJD to transgenic mice expressing human PrP valine 129 [120] suggests that humans of the *PRNP* codon 129 valine homozygous genotype succumbing to BSE would have a different phenotype than new variant CJD. It remains to be seen if this new strain will present as yet another new variant or will present with a more familiar phenotype. Because route of exposure appears to be a key determinant of phenotype as well as prion strain, kuru-like features would again be expected to predominate.

EARLY DIAGNOSTIC TESTS AND THE POTENTIAL FOR THERAPEUTICS

Whereas diagnosis of sporadic CJD can usually be made with confidence on clinical and EEG criteria, and inherited forms are diagnosed definitively by *PRNP* analysis, diagnosis of new variant CJD has relied on neuropathology, either at autopsy or after brain biopsy. Interest has recently focused on the possibility of early diagnosis using tonsil biopsy to detect PrP^{Sc} by Western blot analysis [119]. This has already proved useful in the diagnosis of new variant CJD, but it is unknown how early in the disease course such a test would be positive or whether it can be used to differentiate between different forms of acquired and sporadic prion diseases. Although it is conceivable that PrP^{Sc} could be detected in blood, presumably from buffy coat preparations, the sensitivity of current detection techniques would need to be considerably improved.

The prion diseases are now perhaps the best understood of the degenerative brain diseases, and the development of rational treatments is appearing realistic. In particular, the development of drugs that selectively bind PrP^{Sc} and block prion propagation might be able to inhibit the disease process. Improved early diagnosis will be crucial.

REFERENCES

1. Gajdusek DC, Gibbs CJJ, Alpers MP. Experimental transmission of a kuru-like syndrome to chimpanzees. Nature 1966;209:794–796.
2. Gibbs CJJ, Gajdusek DC, Asher DM, et al. Creutzfeldt-Jakob disease (spongiform encephalopathy): transmission to the chimpanzee. Science 1968;161:388–389.
3. Masters CL, Gajdusek DC, Gibbs CJJ. Creutzfeldt-Jakob disease virus isolations from the Gerstmann-Sträussler syndrome with an analysis of the various forms of amyloid plaque deposition in the virus-induced spongiform encephalopathies. Brain 1981;104:559–588.
4. McGowan JP. Scrapie in sheep. Scott J Agric 1922;5:365–375.
5. Cuillé J, Chelle PL. La maladie dite tremblante du mouton est-elle inocuable? C R Acad Sci 1936; 203:1552–1554.
6. Klatzo I, Gajdusek DC, Zigas V. Pathology of kuru. Lab Invest 1959;8:799–847.
7. Hadlow WJ. Scrapie and kuru. Lancet 1959;ii:289–290.
8. Alpers MP. Epidemiology and Clinical Aspects of Kuru. In SB Prusiner, MP McKinley (eds), Prions: Novel Infectious Pathogens Causing Scrapie and Creutzfeldt-Jakob Disease. San Diego: Academic Press, 1987;451–465.
9. Spielmeyer W. Die histopathologische Forschung in der Psychiatrie. Klin Wochenschr 1922;2: 1817–1819.
10. Creutzfeldt HG. Uber eine eigenartige herdfoermige Erkrankung des Zentralnervensystems. Z Gesamte Neurol Psychiatry 1920;57:1–18.
11. Jakob A. Über eigenartige Erkrankungen des Zentralnervensystems mit bemerkenswertem anatomischen Befunde (spastische Pseudosclerose-Encephalomyelopathie mit disseminierten Degenerationsherden). Dtsch Z Nervenheilk 1921;20:132–146.
12. Jakob A. Uber eigenartige Erkrankungen des Zentralnervensystems mit bemerkenswertem anatomischem Befund. Z Gesamte Neurol Psychiatry 1921;64:147–228.
13. Jakob A. Uber eine der multiplen Sklerose klinisch nahestehende Erkrankung des Zentralnervensystems (spastische Pseudosklerose) mit bemerkenswertem anatomischen Befund. Med Klin 1921; 13:372–376.
14. Beck E, Daniel PM. Neuropathology of Transmissible Spongiform Encephalopathies. In SB Prusiner, MP McKinley (eds), Prions: Novel Infectious Pathogens Causing Scrapie and Creutzfeldt-Jakob Disease. San Diego: Academic Press, 1987;331–385.
15. Caughey B, Raymond GJ. The scrapie-associated form of PrP is made from a cell surface precursor that is both protease- and phospholipase sensitive. J Biol Chem 1991;266:18217–18223.
16. Gasset M, Baldwin MA, Fletterick RJ, Prusiner SB. Perturbation of the secondary structure of the scrapie prion protein under conditions that alter infectivity. Proc Natl Acad Sci U S A 1993;90:1–5.
17. Pan K, Baldwin MA, Nguyen J, et al. Conversion of alpha-helices into beta-sheets features in the formation of the scrapie prion proteins. Proc Natl Acad Sci U S A 1993;90:10962–10966.
18. Robakis NK, Devine Gage EA, Jenkins EC, et al. Localization of a human gene homologous to the PrP gene on the p arm of chromosome 20 and detection of PrP-related antigens in normal human brain. Biochem Biophys Res Commun 1986;140:758–765.
19. Oesch B, Westaway D, Walchli M, et al. A cellular gene encodes scrapie PrP 27-30 protein. Cell 1985;40:735–746.
20. Kretzschmar HA, Stowring LE, Westaway D, et al. Molecular cloning of a human prion protein cDNA. DNA 1986;5:315–324.
21. Owen F, Poulter M, Lofthouse R, et al. Insertion in prion protein gene in familial Creutzfeldt-Jakob disease. Lancet 1989;1:51–52.
22. Hsiao K, Baker HF, Crow TJ, et al. Linkage of a prion protein missense variant to Gerstmann-Sträussler syndrome. Nature 1989;338:342–345.
23. Doh ura K, Tateishi J, Kitamoto T, et al. Creutzfeldt-Jakob disease patients with congophilic kuru plaques have the missense variant prion protein common to Gerstmann-Sträussler syndrome. Ann Neurol 1990;27:121–126.
24. Doh ura K, Tateishi J, Sasaki H, et al. Pro-leu change at position 102 of prion protein is the most common but not the sole mutation related to Gerstmann-Sträussler syndrome. Biochem Biophys Res Commun 1989;163:974–979.
25. Brown P, Goldfarb LG, Brown WT, et al. Clinical and molecular genetic study of a large German kindred with Gerstmann-Sträussler-Scheinker syndrome. Neurology 1991;41:375–379.
26. Speer MC, Goldgaber D, Goldfarb LG, et al. Support of linkage of Gerstmann-Sträussler-Scheinker syndrome to the prion protein gene on chromosome 20p12-pter. Genomics 1991;9:366–368.

27. Kretzschmar HA, Kufer P, Riethmuller G, et al. Prion protein mutation at codon 102 in an Italian family with Gerstmann-Sträussler-Scheinker syndrome. Neurology 1992;42:809–810.
28. Kretzschmar HA, Honold G, Seitelberger F, et al. Prion protein mutation in family first reported by Gerstmann, Sträussler, and Scheinker. Lancet 1991;337:1160.
29. Collinge J, Owen F, Poulter M, et al. Prion dementia without characteristic pathology. Lancet 1990; 336:7–9.
30. Collinge J, Harding AE, Owen F, et al. Diagnosis of Gerstmann-Sträussler syndrome in familial dementia with prion protein gene analysis. Lancet 1989;2:15–17.
31. Collinge J, Brown J, Hardy J, et al. Inherited prion disease with 144 base pair gene insertion: II: clinical and pathological features. Brain 1992;115:687–710.
32. Hsiao KK, Scott M, Foster D, et al. Spontaneous neurodegeneration in transgenic mice with mutant prion protein. Science 1990;250:1587–1590.
33. Hsiao KK, Groth D, Scott M, et al. Genetic and Transgenetic Studies of Prion Proteins in Gerstmann-Sträussler-Scheinker Disease. In SB Prusiner, J Collinge, J Powell, B Anderton (eds), Prion Diseases of Humans and Animals. London: Ellis Horwood, 1992;120–128.
34. Brown P, Preece MA, Will RG. "Friendly fire" in medicine: hormones, homografts, and Creutzfeldt-Jakob disease. Lancet 1992;340:24–27.
35. Laplanche J-L, Delasnerie-Lauprêtre N, Brandel JP, et al. Molecular genetics of prion diseases in France. French Research Group on Epidemiology of Human Spongiform Encephalopathies. Neurology 1994;44:2347–2351.
36. Palmer MS, Dryden AJ, Hughes JT, Collinge J. Homozygous prion protein genotype predisposes to sporadic Creutzfeldt-Jakob disease. Nature 1991;352:340–342.
37. Salvatore M, Genuardi M, Petraroli R, et al. Polymorphisms of the prion protein gene in Italian patients with Creutzfeldt-Jakob disease. Hum Genet 1994;94:375–379.
38. Windl O, Dempster M, Estibeiro JP, et al. Genetic basis of Creutzfeldt-Jakob disease in the United Kingdom: a systematic analysis of predisposing mutations and allelic variation in the *PRNP* gene. Hum Genet 1996;98:259–264.
39. Prusiner SB, Scott M, Foster D, et al. Transgenetic studies implicate interactions between homologous PrP isoforms in scrapie prion replication. Cell 1990;63:673–686.
40. Weissmann C. Spongiform encephalopathies. The prion's progress. Nature 1991;349:569–571.
41. Collinge J, Palmer MS. CJD discrepancy. Nature 1991;353:802.
42. Baker HF, Poulter M, Crow TJ, et al. Amino acid polymorphism in human prion protein and age at death in inherited prion disease. Lancet 1991;337:1286.
43. Dlouhy SR, Hsiao K, Farlow MR, et al. Linkage of the Indiana kindred of Gerstmann-Sträussler-Scheinker disease to the prion protein gene. Nature Genetics 1992;1:64–67.
44. Collinge J, Palmer MS, Dryden AJ. Genetic predisposition to iatrogenic Creutzfeldt-Jakob disease. Lancet 1991;337:1441–1442.
45. Bueler H, Aguzzi A, Sailer A, et al. Mice devoid of PrP are resistant to scrapie. Cell 1993;73:1339–1347.
46. Bueler H, Raeber A, Sailer A, et al. High prion and PrP^{Sc} levels but delayed onset of disease in scrapie-inoculated mice heterozygous for a disrupted PrP gene. Mol Med 1995;1:19–30.
47. Brown P, Cathala F, Raubertas RF, et al. The epidemiology of Creutzfeldt-Jakob disease: conclusion of a 15-year investigation in France and review of the world literature. Neurology 1987;37:895–904.
48. Westaway D, DeArmond SJ, Cayetano-Canlas J, et al. Degeneration of skeletal muscle, peripheral nerves and the central nervous system in transgenic mice overexpressing wild-type prion proteins. Cell 1994;76:117–129.
49. Bruce M, Chree A, McConnell I, et al. Transmission of bovine spongiform encephalopathy and scrapie to mice: strain variation and the species barrier. Philos Trans R Soc Lond B Biol Sci 1994; 343:405–411.
50. Marsh RF, Kimberlin RH. Comparison of scrapie and transmissible mink encephalopathy in hamsters. II. Clinical signs, pathology, and pathogenesis. J Infect Dis 1975;131:104–110.
51. Bessen RA, Marsh RF. Biochemical and physical properties of the prion protein from two strains of the transmissible mink encephalopathy agent. J Virol 1992;66:2096–2101.
52. Bessen RA, Marsh RF. Distinct PrP properties suggest the molecular basis of strain variation in transmissible mink encephalopathy. J Virol 1994;68:7859–7868.
53. Bessen RA, Kocisko DA, Raymond GJ, et al. Non-genetic propagation of strain-specific properties of scrapie prion protein. Nature 1995;375:698–700.
54. Parchi P, Castellani R, Capellari S, et al. Molecular basis of phenotypic variability in sporadic Creutzfeldt-Jakob disease. Ann Neurol 1996;39:669–680.
55. Collinge J, Sidle KCL, Meads J, et al. Molecular analysis of prion strain variation and the aetiology of 'new variant' CJD. Nature 1996;383:685–690.

56. Somerville RA, Chong A, Mulqueen OU, et al. Biochemical typing of scrapie strains [letter]. Nature 1997;386:564.
57. Collinge J, Hill AF, Sidle KCL, Ironside J. Biochemical typing of scrapie strains [letter]. Nature 1997;386:564.
58. Wickner RB. [URE3] as an altered *URE2* protein: evidence for a prion analog in *Saccharomyces cerevisiae*. Science 1994;264:566–569.
59. Ter Avanesyan MD, Dagkesamanskaya AR, Kushnirov VV, Smirnov VN. The SUP35 omnipotent suppressor gene is involved in the maintenance of the non-Mendelian determinant [psi+] in the yeast *Saccharomyces cerevisiae*. Genetics 1994;137:671–676.
60. Medori R, Tritschler HJ, LeBlanc A, et al. Fatal familial insomnia, a prion disease with a mutation at codon 178 of the prion protein gene [see comments]. N Engl J Med 1992;326:444–449.
61. Will RG. Epidemiology of Creutzfeldt-Jakob disease. Br Med Bull 1993;49:960–970.
62. Smith PEM, Zeidler M, Ironside JW, et al. Creutzfeldt-Jakob disease in a dairy farmer. Lancet 1995;346:898.
63. Gore SM. More than happenstance: Creutzfeldt-Jakob disease in farmers and young adults. BMJ 1995;311:1416–1418.
64. Bateman D, Hilton D, Love S, et al. Sporadic Creutzfeldt-Jakob disease in an 18-year-old in the UK. Lancet 1995;346:1155–1156.
65. Britton TC, Al-Sarraj S, Shaw C, et al. Sporadic Creutzfeldt-Jakob disease in a 16-year-old in the UK. Lancet 1995;346:1155.
66. Tabrizi SJ, Scaravilli F, Howard RS, et al. Grand round. Creutzfeldt-Jakob disease in a young woman. Report of a meeting of physicians and scientists, St. Thomas' Hospital, London. Lancet 1996;347:945–948.
67. Will RG, Ironside JW, Zeidler M, et al. A new variant of Creutzfeldt-Jakob disease in the UK. Lancet 1996;347:921–925.
68. Jimi T, Wakayama Y, Shibuya S, et al. High levels of nervous system-specific proteins in cerebrospinal fluid in patients with early stage Creutzfeldt-Jakob disease. Clin Chim Acta 1992;211:37–46.
69. Otto M, Stein H, Szudra A, et al. S-100 protein concentration in the cerebrospinal fluid of patients with Creutzfeldt-Jakob disease [abstract]. J Neurol 1997;244:566–570.
70. Zerr I, Bodemer M, Räcker S, et al. Cerebrospinal fluid concentration of neuron-specific enolase in diagnosis of Creutzfeldt-Jakob disease. Lancet 1995;345:1609–1610.
71. Hsich G, Kenney K, Gibbs CJ Jr, et al. The 14-3-3 brain protein in cerebrospinal fluid as a marker for transmissible spongiform encephalopathies. N Engl J Med 1996;335:924–930.
72. Collinge J. New diagnostic tests for prion diseases. N Engl J Med 1996;335:963–965.
73. Budka H, Aguzzi A, Brown P, et al. Neuropathological diagnostic criteria for Creutzfeldt-Jakob disease (CJD) and other human spongiform encephalopathies (prion diseases). Brain Pathol 1995;5:459–466.
74. Bell JE, Gentleman SM, Ironside JW, et al. Prion protein immunocytochemistry—UK five centre consensus report. Neuropathol Appl Neurobiol 1997;23:26–35.
75. Brown P, Rodgers-Johnson P, Cathala F, et al. Creutzfeldt-Jakob disease of long duration: clinicopathological characteristics, transmissibility, and differential diagnosis. Ann Neurology 1984;16: 295–304.
76. Collinge J, Palmer MS. Molecular genetics of human prion diseases. Philos Trans R Soc Lond B Biol Sci 1994;343:371–378.
77. Gomori AJ, Partnow MJ, Horoupian DS, Hirano A. The ataxic form of Creutzfeldt-Jakob disease. Arch Neurol 1973;29:318–323.
78. Salazar AM, Masters CL, Gajdusek DC, Gibbs CJJ. Syndromes of amyotrophic lateral sclerosis and dementia: relation to transmissible Creutzfeldt-Jakob disease. Ann Neurol 1983;14:17–26.
79. Scrimgeour EM, Masters CL, Alpers MP, et al. A clinico-pathological study of a case of kuru. J Neurol Sci 1983;59:265–275.
80. Gajdusek DC, Zigas V. Untersuchungen Uber die Pathogenese von Kuru. Klin Wochenschr 1958;36: 445–459.
81. Gajdusek DC, Alpers M. Kuru in childhood: disappearance of the disease in the younger age group. J Pediatr 1966;69:886–887.
82. Klitzman RL, Alpers MP, Gajdusek DC. The natural incubation period of kuru and the episodes of transmission in three clusters of patients. Neuroepidemiology 1984;3:3–20.
83. Gajdusek DC, Zigas V. Degenerative disease of the central nervous system in New Guinea. N Engl J Med 1957;257:974–978.
84. Simpson DA, Lander H, Robson HN. Observations on kuru: II. Clinical features. Australas Ann Med 1959;8:8–15.

85. Hornabrook RW. Kuru—a subacute cerebellar degeneration. The natural history and clinical features. Brain 1968;91:53–74.
86. Alpers M, Rail L. Kuru and Creutzfeldt-Jakob disease: clinical and aetiological aspects. Proc Aust Assoc Neurol 1971;8:7–15.
87. Prusiner SB, Gajdusek DC, Alpers MP. Kuru with incubation periods exceeding two decades. Ann Neurol 1982;12:1–9.
88. Alpers M. Kuru: Age and Duration Studies [unpublished data]. Department of Medicine, University of Adelaide, 1964.
89. Cobb WA, Hornabrook RW, Sanders S. The EEG of kuru. Electroencephalogr Clin Neurophysiol 1973;34:419–427.
90. Duffy P, Wolf J, Collins G, et al. Possible person-to-person transmission of Creutzfeldt-Jakob disease [letter]. N Engl J Med 1974;290:692–693.
91. Heckmann JG, Lang CJG, Petruch F, et al. Transmission of Creutzfeldt-Jakob disease via a corneal transplant. J Neurol Neurosurg Psychiatry 1997;63:388–390.
92. Will RG, Matthews WB. Evidence for case-to-case transmission of Creutzfeldt-Jakob disease. J Neurol Neurosurg Psychiatry 1982;45:235–238.
93. Bernoulli C, Siegfried J, Baumgartner G, et al. Danger of accidental person-to-person transmission of Creutzfeldt-Jakob disease by surgery [letter]. Lancet 1977;1:478–479.
94. Thadani V, Penar PL, Partington J, et al. Creutzfeldt-Jakob disease probably acquired from a cadaveric dura mater graft. Case report. J Neurosurg 1988;69:766–769.
95. Masullo C, Pocchiari M, Macchi G, et al. Transmission of Creutzfeldt-Jakob disease by dural cadaveric graft. J Neurosurg 1989;71:954–955.
96. Marx RE, Carlson ER. Creutzfeldt-Jakob disease from allogeneic dura: a review of risks and safety. J Oral Maxillofac Surg 1991;49:272–274.
97. Willison HJ, Gale AN, McLaughlin JE. Creutzfeldt-Jacob disease following cadaveric dura mater graft. J Neurol Neurosurg Psychiatry 1991;54:940.
98. Willison HJ, Gale AN, McLaughlin JE. Creutzfeldt-Jacob disease following cadaveric dura mater graft [letter]. J Neurol Neurosurg Psychiatry 1991;54:940.
99. Pocchiari M, Masullo C, Salvatore M, et al. Creutzfeldt-Jakob disease after non-commercial dura mater graft. Lancet 1992;340:614–615.
100. Martinez-Lage JF, Poza M, Tortosa JG. Creutzfeldt-Jakob disease in patients who received a cadaveric dura mater graft—Spain, 1985–1992. MMWR Morb Mortal Wkly Rep 1993;42:560–563.
101. Esmonde T, Lueck CJ, Symon L, et al. Creutzfeldt-Jakob disease and lyophilised dura mater grafts: report of two cases. J Neurol Neurosurg Psychiatry 1993;56:999–1000.
102. Martinez Lage JF, Sola J, Poza M, Esteban JA. Pediatric Creutzfeldt-Jakob disease: probable transmission by a dural graft. Childs Nerv Syst 1993;9:239–242.
103. Lane KL, Brown P, Howell DN, et al. Creutzfeldt-Jakob disease in a pregnant woman with an implanted dura mater graft. Neurosurgery 1994;34:737–740.
104. Yamada S, Aiba T, Endo Y, et al. Creutzfeldt-Jakob disease transmitted by a cadaveric dura mater graft. Neurosurgery 1994;34:740–744.
105. Martínez-Lage JF, Poza M, Sola J, et al. Accidental transmission of Creutzfeldt-Jakob disease by dural cadaveric grafts. J Neurol Neurosurg Psychiatry 1994;57:1091–1094.
106. Clavel M, Clavel P. Creutzfeldt-Jakob disease transmitted by dura mater graft. Eur Neurol 1996;36: 239–240.
107. Antoine JC, Michel D, Bertholon P, et al. Creutzfeldt-Jakob disease after extracranial dura mater embolization for a nasopharyngeal angiofibroma. Neurology 1997;48:1451–1453.
108. Defebvre L, Destée A, Caron J, et al. Creutzfeldt-Jakob disease after an embolization of intercostal arteries with cadaveric dura mater suggesting a systemic transmission of the prion agent. Neurology 1997;48:1470–1471.
109. Yamada M, Itoh Y, Suematsu N, et al. Panencephalopathic type of Creutzfeldt-Jakob disease associated with cadaveric dura mater graft. J Neurol Neurosurg Psychiatry 1997;63:524–527.
110. Takashima S, Tateishi J, Taguchi Y, Inoue H. Creutzfeldt-Jakob disease with florid plaques after cadaveric dural graft in a Japanese woman. Lancet 1997;350:865–866.
111. Cochius JI, Burns RJ, Blumbergs PC, et al. Creutzfeldt-Jakob disease in a recipient of human pituitary-derived gonadotrophin. Aust N Z J Med 1990;20:592–593.
112. Cochius JI, Hyman N, Esiri MM. Creutzfeldt-Jakob disease in a recipient of human pituitary-derived gonadotrophin: a second case. J Neurol Neurosurg Psychiatry 1992;55:1094–1095.
113. Esmonde TFG, Will RG, Slattery JM, et al. Creutzfeldt-Jakob disease and blood transfusion. Lancet 1993;341:205–207.

114. Brown P. Can Creutzfeldt-Jakob disease be transmitted by transfusion? Curr Opin Hematol 1995;2: 472–477.
115. Chazot G, Broussolle E, Lapras CI, et al. New variant of Creutzfeldt-Jakob disease in a 26-year-old French man. Lancet 1996;347:1181.
116. Zeidler M, Johnstone EC, Bamber RWK, et al. New variant Creutzfeldt-Jakob disease: psychiatric features. Lancet 1997;350:908–910.
117. Zeidler M, Stewart GE, Barraclough CR, et al. New variant Creutzfeldt-Jakob disease: neurological features and diagnostic tests. Lancet 1997;350:903–907.
118. Collinge J, Beck J, Campbell T, et al. Prion protein gene analysis in new variant cases of Creutzfeldt-Jakob disease. Lancet 1996;348:56.
119. Hill AF, Zeidler M, Ironside J, Collinge J. Diagnosis of new variant Creutzfeldt-Jakob disease by tonsil biopsy. Lancet 1997;349:99–100.
120. Hill AF, Desbruslais M, Joiner S, et al. The same prion strain causes vCJD and BSE. Nature 1997; 389:448–450.
121. Bruce ME, Will RG, Ironside JW, et al. Transmissions to mice indicate that 'new variant' CJD is caused by the BSE agent. Nature 1997;389:498–501.
122. Gerstmann J. Über ein noch nicht beschriebenes Reflexphänomen bei einer Erkrankung des zerebellaren Systems. Wien Med Wochenschr 1928;78:906–908.
123. Gerstmann J, Sträussler E, Scheinker I. Über eine eigenartige hereditär-familiäre Erkrankung des Zentralnervensystems. Zugleich ein Beitrag zur Frage des vorzeitigen lakalen Alterns. Z Neurol 1936;154:736–762.
124. Seitelberger F. Eigenartige familiäre-hereditare Krankheit des zentralen Nervensystems in einer niederösterreichischen Sippe. Wiener Klinische Wochenschrift 1962:41/42:687–691.
125. Hainfellner JA, Brantner-Inthaler S, Cervenáková L, et al. The original Gerstmann-Sträussler-Scheinker family of Austria: divergent clinicopathological phenotypes but constant PrP genotype. Brain Pathol 1995;5:201–211.
126. Kitamoto T, Ohta M, Doh-ura K, et al. Novel missense variants of prion protein in Creutzfeldt-Jakob disease or Gerstmann-Sträussler syndrome. Biochem Biophys Res Commun 1993;191:709–714.
127. Wu Y, Brown WT, Robakis NK, et al. A PvuII RFLP detected in the human prion protein (PrP) gene. Nucleic Acids Res 1987;15:3191.
128. Hsiao KK, Cass C, Schellenberg GD, et al. A prion protein variant in a family with the telencephalic form of Gerstmann-Sträussler-Scheinker syndrome. Neurology 1991;41:681–684.
129. Kitamoto T, Iizuka R, Tateishi J. An amber mutation of prion protein in Gerstmann-Sträussler syndrome with mutant PrP plaques. Biochem Biophys Res Commun 1993;192:525–531.
130. Goldfarb LG, Haltia M, Brown P, et al. New mutation in scrapie amyloid precursor gene (at codon 178) in Finnish Creutzfeldt-Jakob kindred. Lancet 1991;337:425.
131. Nieto A, Goldfarb LG, Brown P, et al. Codon 178 mutation in ethnically diverse Creutzfeldt-Jakob disease families. Lancet 1991;337:622–623.
132. Goldfarb LG, Brown P, Haltia M, et al. Creutzfeldt-Jakob disease cosegregates with the codon 178^{Asn} *PRNP* mutation in families of European origin. Ann Neurol 1992;31:274–281.
133. Brown P, Goldfarb LG, Kovanen J, et al. Phenotypic characteristics of familial Creutzfeldt-Jakob disease associated with the codon 178^{Asn} PRNP mutation. Ann Neurol 1992;31:282–285.
134. Laplanche JL, Chatelain J, Thomas S, et al. Uncommon phenotype for a codon 178 mutation of the human PrP gene. Ann Neurol 1992;31:345.
135. Lugaresi E, Medori R, Baruzzi PM, et al. Fatal familial insomnia and dysautonomia, with selective degeneration of thalamic nuclei. N Engl J Med 1986;315:997–1003.
136. Medori R, Montagna P, Tritschler HJ, et al. Fatal familial insomnia: a second kindred with mutation of prion protein gene at codon 178. Neurology 1992;42:669–670.
137. Monari L, Chen SG, Brown P, et al. Fatal familial insomnia and familial Creutzfeldt-Jakob disease: different prion proteins determined by a DNA polymorphism. Proc Natl Acad Sci U S A 1994;91: 2839–2842.
138. Goldfarb LG, Petersen RB, Tabaton M, et al. Fatal familial insomnia and familial Creutzfeldt-Jakob disease: disease phenotype determined by a DNA polymorphism. Science 1992;258:806–808.
139. Chapman J, Arlazoroff A, Goldfarb LG, et al. Fatal insomnia in a case of familial Creutzfeldt-Jakob disease with the codon 200^{Lys} mutation. Neurology 1996;46:758–761.
140. McLean CA, Storey E, Gardner RJM, et al. The D178N (cis-129M) "fatal familial insomnia" mutation associated with diverse clinicopathologic phenotypes in an Australian kindred. Neurology 1997;49:552–558.
141. Brown P, Gibbs CJJ, Rodgers Johnson P, et al. Human spongiform encephalopathy: the National Institutes of Health series of 300 cases of experimentally transmitted disease. Ann Neurol 1994;35:513–529.

142. Tateishi J, Brown P, Kitamoto T, et al. First experimental transmission of fatal familial insomnia. Nature 1995;376:434–435.
143. Bosque PJ, Vnencak-Jones CL, Johnson MD, et al. A PrP gene codon 178 base substitution and a 24-bp interstitial deletion in familial Creutzfeldt-Jakob disease. Neurology 1992;42:1864–1870.
144. Collinge J, Palmer MS, Sidle KCL, et al. Transmission of fatal familial insomnia to laboratory animals. Lancet 1995;346:569–570.
145. Tateishi J, Kitamoto T. Inherited prion diseases and transmission to rodents. Brain Pathol 1995;5: 53–59.
146. Nitrini R, Rosemberg S, Passos-Bueno MR, et al. Familial spongiform encephalopathy associated with a novel prion protein gene mutation. Ann Neurol 1997;42:138–146.
147. Farlow MR, Yee RD, Dlouhy SR, et al. Gerstmann-Sträussler-Scheinker disease. I. extending the clinical spectrum. Neurology 1989;39:1446–1452.
148. Ghetti B, Tagliavini F, Masters CL, et al. Gerstmann-Sträussler-Scheinker disease. II. Neurofibrillary tangles and plaques with PrP-amyloid coexist in an affected family. Neurology 1989;39:1453–1461.
149. Hsiao K, Meiner Z, Kahana E, et al. Mutation of the prion protein in Libyan Jews with Creutzfeldt-Jakob disease. N Engl J Med 1991;324:1091–1097.
150. Goldfarb LG, Mitrova E, Brown P, et al. Mutation in codon 200 of scrapie amyloid protein gene in two clusters of Creutzfeldt-Jakob disease in Slovakia. Lancet 1990;336:514–515.
151. Goldfarb LG, Korczyn AD, Brown P, et al. Mutation in codon 200 of scrapie amyloid precursor gene linked to Creutzfeldt-Jakob disease in Sephardic Jews of Libyan and non-Libyan origin. Lancet 1990;336:637–638.
152. Korczyn AD, Chapman J, Goldfarb LG, et al. A mutation in the prion protein gene in Creutzfeldt-Jakob disease in Jewish patients of Libyan, Greek, and Tunisian origin. Ann N Y Acad Sci 1991;640: 171–176.
153. Brown P, Galvez S, Goldfarb LG, et al. Familial Creutzfeldt-Jakob disease in Chile is associated with the codon 200 mutation of the PRNP amyloid precursor gene on chromosome 20. J Neurol Sci 1992; 112:65–67.
154. Neufeld MY, Josiphov J, Korczyn AD. Demyelinating peripheral neuropathy in Creutzfeldt-Jakob disease. Muscle Nerve 1992;15:1234–1239.
155. Chapman J, Ben-Israel J, Goldhammer Y, Korczyn AD. The risk of developing Creutzfeldt-Jakob disease in subjects with the *PRNP* gene codon 200 point mutation. Neurology 1994;44:1683–1686.
156. Collinge J, Palmer MS, Campbell TA, et al. Inherited prion disease (PrP lysine 200) in Britain: two case reports. BMJ 1993;306:301–302.
157. Goldfarb LG, Brown P, Mitrova E, et al. Creutzfeldt-Jacob disease associated with the PRNP codon ^{200}Lys mutation: an analysis of 45 families. Eur J Epidemiol 1991;7:477–486.
158. Mastrianni JA, Iannicola C, Myers R, Prusiner SB. Identification of a new mutation of the prion protein gene at codon 208 in a patient with Creutzfeldt-Jakob disease. Neurology 1995;45(suppl 4):A201.
159. Davies PTG, Jahfar S, Ferguson IT, Windl O. Creutzfeldt-Jakob disease in individual occupationally exposed to BSE. Lancet 1993;342:680.
160. Hsiao K, Dlouhy SR, Farlow MR, et al. Mutant prion proteins in Gerstmann-Sträussler-Sheinker disease with neurofibrillary tangles. Nature Genetics 1992;1:68–71.
161. Laplanche JL, Delasnerie Laupretre N, Brandel JP, et al. Two novel insertions in the prion protein gene in patients with late-onset dementia. Hum Mol Genet 1995;4:1109–1111.
162. Goldfarb LG, Brown P, Little BW, et al. A new (two-repeat) octapeptide coding insert mutation in Creutzfeldt-Jakob disease. Neurology 1993;43:2392–2394.
163. Goldfarb LG, Brown P, McCombie WR, et al. Transmissible familial Creutzfeldt-Jakob disease associated with five, seven, and eight extra octapeptide coding repeats in the *PRNP* gene. Proc Natl Acad Sci U S A 1991;88:10926–10930.
164. Laplanche JL, Delasnerie Laupretre N, Brandel JP, et al. Two novel insertions in the prion protein gene in patients with late-onset dementia. Hum Mol Genet 1995;4:1109–1111.
165. Campbell TA, Palmer MS, Will RG, et al. A prion disease with a novel 96-base pair insertional mutation in the prion protein gene. Neurology 1996;46:761–766.
166. Meyer A, Leigh D, Bagg CE. A rare presenile dementia associated with cortical blindness (Heidenhain's syndrome). J Neurol Neurosurg Psychiatry 1954;17:129–133.
167. Adams JH, Duchen LW (eds). Greenfield's Neuropathology (5th ed). New York: Oxford, 1992.
168. Poulter M, Baker HF, Frith CD, et al. Inherited prion disease with 144 base pair gene insertion: I: genealogical and molecular studies. Brain 1992;115:675–685.
169. Nicholl D, Windl O, De Silva R, et al. Inherited Creutzfeldt-Jakob disease in a British family associated with a novel 144 base pair insertion of the prion protein gene. J Neurol Neurosurg Psychiatry 1995;58:65–69.

170. Oda T, Kitamoto T, Tateishi J, et al. Prion disease with 144 base pair insertion in a Japanese family line. Acta Neuropathol (Berl) 1995;90:80–86.
171. Guiroy DC, Marsh RF, Yanagihara R, Gajdusek DC. Immunolocalization of scrapie amyloid in non-congophilic, non-birefringent deposits in golden Syrian hamsters with experimental transmissible mink encephalopathy. Neurosci Lett 1993;155:112–115.
172. Owen F, Poulter M, Collinge J, et al. A dementing illness associated with a novel insertion in the prion protein gene. Mol Brain Res 1992;13:155–157.
173. Tagliavini F, Giaccone G, Prelli F, et al. A68 is a component of paired helical filaments of Gerstmann-Sträussler-Scheinker disease, Indiana kindred. Brain Res 1993;616:325–328.
174. Krasemann S, Zerr I, Weber T, et al. Prion disease associated with a novel nine octapeptide repeat insertion in the PRNP gene. Mol Brain Res 1995;34:173–176.
175. Ripoll L, Laplanche JL, Salzmann M, et al. A new point mutation in the prion protein gene at codon 210 in Creutzfeldt-Jakob disease. Neurology 1993;43:1934–1938.
176. Furukawa H, Kitamoto T, Tanaka Y, Tateishi J. New variant prion protein in a Japanese family with Gerstmann-Sträussler syndrome. Brain Res Mol Brain Res 1995;30:385–388.
177. Palmer MS, Mahal SP, Campbell TA, et al. Deletions in the prion protein gene are not associated with CJD. Hum Mol Gen 1993;2:541–544.
178. Laplanche JL, Chatelain J, Launay JM, et al. Deletion in prion protein gene in a Moroccan family. Nucleic Acids Res 1990;18:6745.
179. Collinge J, Poulter M, Davis MB, et al. Presymptomatic detection or exclusion of prion protein gene defects in families with inherited prion diseases. Am J Hum Genet 1991;49:1351–1354.
180. Aguzzi A. Neuro-immune connection in spread of prions in the body. Lancet 1997;349:742–743.
181. Blattler T, Brandner S, Raeber AJ, et al. PrP-expressing tissue required for transfer of scrapie infectivity from spleen to brain. Nature 1997;389:67–73.
182. Cashman NR, Loertscher R, Nalbantoglu J, et al. Cellular isoform of the scrapie agent protein participates in lymphocyte activation. Cell 1990;61:185–192.
183. Aguzzi A, Collinge J. Post-exposure prophylaxis after accidental prion inoculation. Lancet 1997;350:1519–1520.
184. Tateishi J, Koga M, Mori R. Experimental transmission of Creutzfeldt-Jakob disease. Acta Pathol Jpn 1981;31:943–951.
185. Telling GC, Scott M, Hsiao KK, et al. Transmission of Creutzfeldt-Jakob disease from humans to transgenic mice expressing chimeric human-mouse prion protein. Proc Natl Acad Sci U S A 1994;91: 9936–9940.
186. Telling GC, Scott M, Mastrianni J, et al. Prion propagation in mice expressing human and chimeric PrP transgenes implicates the interaction of cellular PrP with another protein. Cell 1995;83:79–90.
187. Collinge J, Palmer MS, Sidle KCL, et al. Unaltered susceptibility to BSE in transgenic mice expressing human prion protein. Nature 1995;378:779–783.

II
Scientific Advances in Understanding the Dementias

Introduction

John H. Growdon and Martin N. Rossor

This section contains chapters on topics in three major areas of investigation that have transformed research in dementia: molecular genetics, neuroimaging, and molecular pathology. As a result of these advances, clinicians have improved ability to diagnose Alzheimer's disease (AD) and other dementias accurately, as well as new ways to follow the course of illness and gauge response to treatment. Progress in these three broad areas will likely continue and deepen our understanding of the causes of AD and related dementias. These advances, by identifying mechanisms of neuronal death, will guide development of effective treatments to prevent, or at least retard, the course of dementia.

At the turn of the century, Emil Kraepelin challenged members of his department in Munich, Germany, to uncover the biological basis of mental illness and dementia. This was an ambitious task then, and it still occupies the attention of leading neuroscientists today. In 1906, Alois Alzheimer reported the first successful step in answering Kraepelin's challenge when he reported the histopathologic findings of neuritic plaques and neurofibrillary tangles in the brain of a 53-year-old woman with personality change and progressive dementia. From that modest beginning of a single case report, AD is recognized today as the most common cause of dementia in North America and Europe. AD is also one of the most common neurologic diseases and a major world health concern. Although familial clusters of AD have been recognized for years, it was not until 1987 that the first linkage of a chromosomal abnormality to AD was reported. In their chapter, Molecular Genetics of Alzheimer's Disease, Drs. Cruts and Van Broeckhoven review the principles of molecular genetics and describe the abnormalities on chromosomes 1, 14, and 21 that lead to autosomal dominant–inherited AD. It is remarkable that missense mutations involving single amino acids can cause AD. Although the number of families that carry these mutations is relatively small, their importance far exceeds their numbers. Discovery and characterization of these mutations open new areas for research into basic mechanisms of disease. It is also clear that further mutation(s) associated with early and familial AD unaccounted for by amyloid precursor protein and presenilin gene mutations await to be discovered.

A complementary line of research seeks to identify risk factors that do not by themselves necessarily cause AD but can modulate its appearance. For example, it is widely accepted that the incidence of AD increases with advancing age, and that apolipoprotein E (*APOE*) genotype influences the age at which AD develops. Other factors appear to protect against developing AD, including use of anti-inflammatory drugs and estrogen, consumption of red wine, and possibly cigarette smoking. Dr. Gómez-Isla and colleagues, in their chapter, Apolipoprotein E and Alzheimer's Disease, review the evidence linking the *APOE* genotype and AD. As a biomarker for AD, *APOE* is not useful in epidemiologic screening or in predicting disease in asymptomatic individuals. In an individual with suspected AD, however, determining the *APOE* genotype may add to the confidence of diagnosis. Dr. Gómez-Isla and colleagues provide clinical examples in which knowledge of the *APOE* genotype might be helpful and suggest guidelines for its use.

The chapters by Dr. Jack, Anatomic Neuroimaging in the Dementias, and by Dr. Kennedy, Functional Neuroimaging in Dementia, review the use of anatomic and physiologic neuroimaging as aids in the differential diagnosis of dementia, with emphasis on findings in AD. Adherence to the clinical criteria proposed for the diagnosis of AD, as practiced in specialized referral centers for dementia, achieves an 80–90% diagnostic accuracy rate in neuropathologically confirmed series. Across these centers, there is remarkable clinical consensus regarding the cognitive features of AD and the rate at which cognitive function fails. Memory loss is a central feature of AD, and deficits in explicit memory are generally the initial and most pervasive finding. Neuronal loss and neurofibrillary tangles in the entorhinal cortex and hippocampus are the presumed pathologic correlates of this memory loss. As pointed out by Dr. Jack, neuroimaging provides an in vivo biological correlate of these clinical features, as there is evidence of medial temporal lobe atrophy in patients with AD that exceeds that seen with normal aging. AD is a progressive dementia; even if memory loss is an isolated initial finding, it is soon joined by impairments in language function, praxis, and visuospatial capacities and accompanying personality changes. The neuropathologic correlates of progressive dementia include neuronal and synaptic loss in neocortical association areas. As described by Dr. Kennedy, positron emission tomography and single photon emission computed tomography show characteristic decreases in cerebral metabolism and perfusion in brain regions affected by AD pathology that correlate with worsening dementia.

Clues for uncovering the mechanisms of dementia must take as a starting point changes in the brain. Any theory of cell death and attempts to prevent cell death must encompass the main histopathologic signatures of AD, including neuritic plaques and neurofibrillary tangles. In his chapter, Molecular Pathology of Alzheimer's Disease: The Role of Amyloid, Dr. Selkoe presents evidence for the amyloid hypothesis of neuronal damage: Amyloid is deposited early in the course of AD, it is deposited early in the life of Down syndrome patients who develop AD histology 20–30 years later, in some experimental conditions amyloid is neurotoxic, and all genetic causes of AD have a common thread of increased amounts of the neurotoxic amyloid beta-protein (Aβ) 1–42 fragments. The theoretical amyloid cascade of neurotoxicity in AD offers multiple potential points for therapeutic intervention. Dr. Clark and colleagues, in the chapter

Molecular Pathology of Alzheimer's Disease: Neuronal Cytoskeletal Abnormalities, draw attention to changes in the neuronal cytoskeleton. Neurofilaments and microtubules are important components of the cytoskeleton and, when altered, form neurofibrillary tangles and Lewy bodies, which are the histopathologic markers of neurodegenerative diseases including Alzheimer's disease (tangles) and Parkinson's disease (Lewy bodies). The research reported by Dr. Selkoe and by Dr. Clark and colleagues is directed toward uncovering mechanisms of disease production. The research has added clinical value in generating candidate biomarkers for diagnosis. For example, in familial AD, blood levels of $A\beta_{1-42}$ are increased, whereas they are generally normal in nonfamilial sporadic AD.

In the final chapter of this section, Bioenergetics, Exitotoxicity, and Oxidative Injury in the Pathogenesis of Neurodegenerative Disease, Dr. Beal emphasizes the abnormalities in oxidative metabolism that AD shares with other neurodegenerative diseases. As specified in this line of investigation, decreased energy production renders neurons more vulnerable to environmental challenges that are not normally toxic. Further, defects in mitochondria can lead to increased production of superoxide radicals with peroxidation of lipids and proteins that eventually causes cell death. Recognizing oxidative injury as a mode of cell death has directly led to new lines of treatment. Thus, antioxidant therapies with alpha-tocopherol and selegiline have been tested in AD and found to slow some aspects of clinical decline. Although the initial results are modest, more potent and specific drugs to restore energy production and minimize the effects of superoxide radicals are likely to be discovered.

6
Molecular Genetics of Alzheimer's Disease

Marc Cruts and Christine Van Broeckhoven

Population surveys and twin and family studies have shown that Alzheimer's disease (AD) has a genetic etiology [1]. Population survey studies demonstrated that 25–40% of AD patients have a familial predisposition, with at least one other afflicted first-degree relative. Age of onset and transmission patterns of AD in different families, however, indicated a clinical heterogeneity. The distribution pattern of the age at onset is bimodal, with a cutoff age of 58 years [2]. As a result, two distinct categories of AD can be distinguished: presenile AD, or AD with early-onset age of disease (EOAD), and senile AD, or AD with late-onset age of disease (LOAD). In most studies, the cutoff age between EOAD and LOAD is arbitrarily set at 60 or 65 years. In EOAD families, the transmission pattern of AD is consistent with an autosomal dominant disorder with age-dependent penetrance [3–5]. Also, in some LOAD families the disease segregates as an autosomal dominant trait; however, the inheritance pattern in most LOAD families is less clear, suggesting that a complex set of genetic or environmental factors contribute to LOAD.

Because the underlying biochemical cause of AD is not understood and because, at least in some cases, the disease is inherited, AD has been extensively studied by the methods of positional cloning [6]. As opposed to functional cloning, in which genes and their pathologic defects are deduced from the known biochemical malfunction underlying the disease, positional cloning is a technique that attempts to localize genetic defects when the biochemistry of the disease under study is unknown. In those cases, genomic mapping techniques studying the segregation pattern of polymorphic genetic markers with known chromoso-

---

The Alzheimer's disease research work in Christine Van Broeckhoven's laboratory is funded by the Flemish Biotechnology program (COT-004), the National Fund of Scientific Research—Flanders (Belgium) (FWO), BIOMED (GENE-CT96-0015) and BIOTECH (BIO2-CT96-2056) programs of the European Community, the Alzheimer's Disease Research Program of the American Health Assistance Foundation, and by the Interuniversity Attraction Poles. Marc Cruts is a post-doctoral fellow of the FWO.

mal location are undertaken in families affected with the disease. Cosegregation of the markers with the disease is then statistically analyzed to assess the probability of linkage. The most commonly used method for studying cosegregation is the *logarithm of the odds* (LOD) score analysis, which determines the likelihood that two loci segregate together through a family as a result of their physical proximity in the human genome as opposed to chance alone. An LOD score of 3 or more (i.e., odds of cosegregation equal to or higher than 1,000 to 1) is accepted as conclusive for linkage, whereas an LOD score of less than –2 (i.e., odds of cosegregation less than 100 to 1) is accepted as conclusive evidence for two loci to segregate independent of each other. LOD scores obtained in different families can be summed, assuming that in these families the disease has a common genetic etiology.

In LOD score analyses, two different approaches are generally used. Two-point LOD score analysis calculates LOD scores between two loci at different hypothetical genetic distances, measured as a recombination fraction (θ) ranging between $\theta = 0$ (complete cosegregation) and $\theta = 0.5$ (no cosegregation). Multipoint LOD score analysis calculates LOD scores for one locus at different points in a genetic interval containing two or more fixed loci [7]. Typically, multipoint LOD score analyses yield more information on the exact genetic position of a locus than do two-point LOD score analyses; however, more detailed information on the location of the genetic markers is needed, and the computing time is considerably longer than for two-point LOD score calculations. Therefore, two-point LOD score analyses are used to localize a disease locus, after which multipoint LOD score analyses are applied to define the disease locus in further detail. When a disease locus is genetically defined, the chromosomal region showing genetic linkage is then organized in a contiguous array of overlapping clones, each containing different parts of that region. Most commonly used are yeast artificial chromosomes (YACs) that allow propagation of several hundred kilobases (kb) of human DNA in yeast. These clones are then used as a source for the isolation of unknown genes in that particular region of the human genome. The two most recently developed technologies aiming at the isolation of genes from genomic DNA fragments are direct complementary DNA (cDNA) selection [8,9] and exon amplification [10]. Once disease-related mutations have been identified, the normal and pathologic function of the disease gene(s) involved can be studied, thereby elucidating the biology of the disease.

Positional cloning was successfully used to identify gene mutations causing familial AD. To date, four genetic loci are known and their respective genes are identified. *AD1* was localized on chromosome 21q22.1 near the amyloid precursor protein gene (*APP*), and EOAD families segregating a mutation in *APP* were identified. More recently, mutations were identified in EOAD families linked to chromosome 14q24.3 (*AD3*) and chromosome 1q42.1 (*AD4*). Both loci involve novel genes that are highly homologous and are termed *presenilin-1* (*PS1*) and *presenilin-2* (*PS2*), respectively. The functions of the proteins encoded by *APP* (app) and *PS1* and *PS2* (ps1 and ps2) are currently unknown, but their pathogenic mutations all influence the processing of app into beta-amyloid (Aβ), the latter being deposited in AD brain tissue (see Chapter 10).

Unlike the three aforementioned genes, which are causative AD genes, the $\varepsilon 4$ allele of the apolipoprotein E gene (*APOE*) at chromosome 19q13.2 (*AD2*) was identified as a genetic risk factor for both EOAD and LOAD [11,12] (see Chapter 7). Other genetic risk factors have been reported; however, none of them was consistently found to be a genetic risk for AD in all AD populations.

CHROMOSOME 21—THE AMYLOID PRECURSOR PROTEIN GENE

In view of the observation that almost all middle-aged Down syndrome (DS) patients develop an AD-like brain pathology [13,14], initial genetic linkage studies mainly targeted chromosome 21, which is present in triplicate in DS patients. In DS patients, AD is presumably caused by a gene dosage effect because of overexpression of one or more otherwise normal genes on chromosome 21. In AD patients, the disease might be caused by a mutation in the same genetic region resulting in the production of an abnormal protein or the overproduction of a normal protein. Using four EOAD families in which the disease clearly segregated as an autosomal dominant trait, linkage was found to the genetic markers D21S16 and D21S1/S11 in the region 21q11.2–21q21 [15]. None of the families yielded conclusive LOD scores, but multipoint LOD scores obtained in the four AD families were conclusively positive. Two regions of D21S1/S11, one centromeric and one telomeric, each with equally strong linkage evidence were identified. At approximately the same time, *APP* was characterized and localized to the same chromosomal region as D21S1/S11 [16]. Because *APP* encodes the precursor protein from which Aβ is proteolytically generated, *APP* was a strong candidate gene for AD. Further linkage studies using genetic markers inside *APP*, however, identified recombinants in some EOAD and LOAD families, suggesting that the AD gene and *APP* were genetically separate [17,18]. Later, when the genetic maps of chromosome 21 were saturated with polymorphic markers, *APP* was localized more accurately to the region 21q21.2, telomeric of D21S1/S11 [19], whereas the AD locus showed tighter linkage to markers centromeric of D21S1/S11 (i.e., D21S13 and D21S16 in band 21q11 [20–22]). Other AD families did not show linkage to the pericentromeric region of chromosome 21, indicating that the gene defect in these families was also not located at that site [23–25]. Therefore, it was assumed that familial AD was genetically heterogeneous [26]. More extensive linkage studies involving 30 EOAD and 18 LOAD families with chromosome 21 markers excluded LOAD from chromosome 21 and demonstrated two equally possible regions of linkage in some EOAD families [26]. In addition to the locus centromeric of D21S1/S11, new evidence arose that another EOAD locus may coincide with *APP*.

In 1990, a missense mutation in *APP* was found in families with hereditary cerebral hemorrhage with amyloidosis of the Dutch type (HCHWA-D), a rare autosomal dominant disorder found in a few families in the Netherlands [27,28]. HCHWA-D is characterized by recurrent cerebral hemorrhages caused by excessive deposition of Aβ in the blood vessel walls in brain tissue [29]. The Aβ deposition in brains of HCHWA-D patients is of the same nature as that found in the brains of AD patients. In HCHWA-D patients, a missense mutation was detected in *APP* [27,30]. The *APP* gene consists of 18 exons, exons 16 and 17 of which partly encode the Aβ proteolysis fragment [31]. The HCHWA-D mutation is at codon 693 in exon 16 of *APP*, causing a glutamic acid to glutamine substitution close to the proteolytic cleavage site inside the Aβ fragment. Hence, when the mutation is present, the breakdown of Aβ is inhibited, causing its deposition in the blood vessel walls. The discovery of this mutation demonstrated that mutations in *APP* can lead to Aβ deposition and encouraged mutation analysis of *APP* in an attempt to identify mutations in EOAD families. To date, seven different AD-related *APP* mutations have been detected in 20 families with AD or a related disorder (*AD1*) [32]. All mutations are located at or near the proteolytic cleavage sites involved in the generation of Aβ, which is encoded by exons 16 and 17 of *APP* (Figure 6.1 and Table 6.1). The *APP* Val717Ile mutation was found in multiple EOAD families of different ethnicity, which underlined the causative character of the mutation. In addition, a mutation was found at codon 692 in exon 17 of *APP* in a family with a mixed phenotype, in which patients have cerebral hemorrhages or EOAD [33].

CHROMOSOMES 14 AND 1—THE PRESENILIN GENES

Of the families in which EOAD was initially linked to chromosome 21, none was found to segregate a mutation in exons 16 or 17 of *APP*. Moreover, the linkage evidence in the region centromeric of D21S1/S11 was not conclusive and could be explained by coincidental cosegregation. As a result, a genome-wide search was undertaken, using either a nonrandom approach with polymorphic genetic markers associated with candidate genes or a random approach using restriction fragment–length polymorphisms or polymorphic short tandem repeat (STR) markers evenly distributed across the whole genome. Both strategies almost simultaneously and independently led to the discovery of strong linkage evidence with markers on chromosome 14 in band 14q24.3 (*AD3*) [34–37]. The highest two-point LOD scores were obtained with STR marker D14S43. The initial linkage reports already indicated that a quantitatively important fraction of EOAD families carried a mutation at this locus. LOAD families did not appear to be linked to the *AD3* locus, although LOD scores were not conclusively negative [35,38,39]. In addition, further genetic heterogeneity was observed as some EOAD families displayed recombinants with markers from within the *AD3* locus [34]. The initial linkage studies defined an *AD3* candidate region of 22.7 cM between the flanking markers D14S53 and D14S52 [34]. Further linkage analyses using additional STR markers reduced the *AD3* candidate region to the 6.4-cM interval between D14S289 and D14S61 [40]. A physical map of this region in YACs enabled estimation of the size of the *AD3* candidate region to be between 2 and 6 megabases (Mb) [40,41]. When more STR markers became available in the *AD3* region [42], additional informative recombinants were identified, further reducing the *AD3* candidate region to a 2.2-Mb interval between D14S277 and D14S284 [43].

Because known genes residing in the *AD3* region (positional candidate genes) carried no AD-related mutations [44–47], new genes were isolated from YACs spanning the minimal *AD3* candidate region using exon amplification and direct cDNA selection techniques. This led to the identification of *PS1*, a gene of unknown function that had five missense mutations in eight EOAD families [48]. *PS1* encodes a protein of 467 residues in length that is predicted to be an integral membrane protein with six to eight transmembrane domains (TM) [49,50]. To date, 43 different *PS1* mutations have been reported in 83 families, causing AD

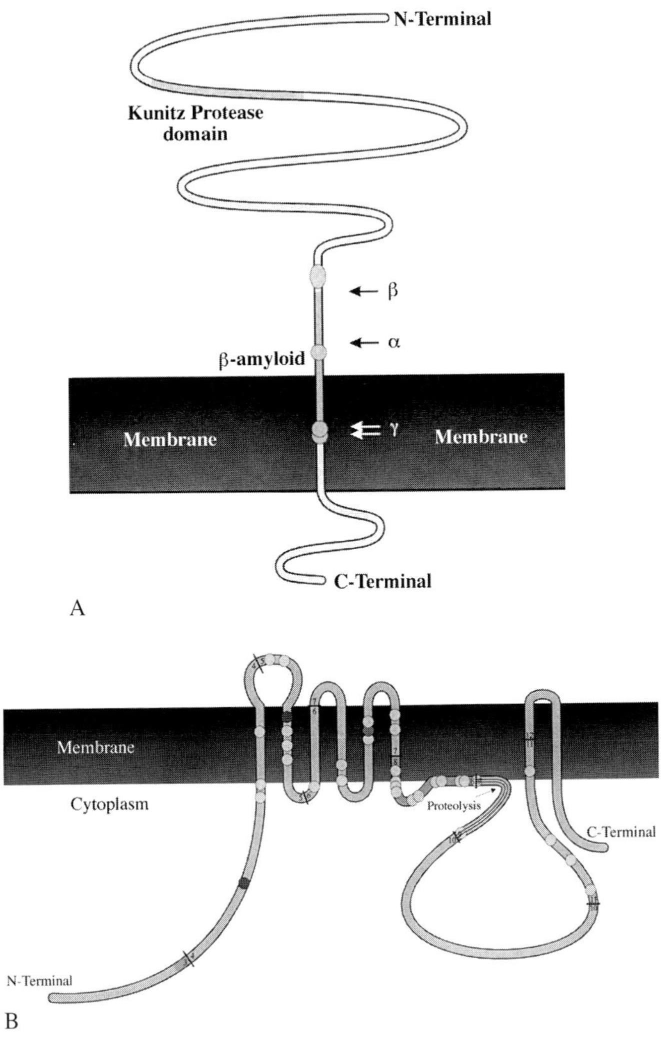

Figure 6.1 Alzheimer's disease mutations. (A) Amyloid precursor protein gene mutations. (B) Presenilin-1 (*PS1*) and presenilin-2 (*PS2*). Mutations in *PS1* are indicated by the gray circles, mutations in *PS2* are indicated by black circles.

with onset ages ranging from 35 to 64 years, with most mutations occurring in the regions encoding the second transmembrane domain (TM-II) and the sixth hydrophilic loop (HL-VI) of ps1 (Table 6.2) [51]. Remarkably, the mutations in TM-II occur every third or fourth amino acid, suggesting that they line up on the same side of an alpha helix. Disruption of such a structure might inhibit or alter the function of ps1 [52]. The large variety of mutations suggests that *PS1* has a relatively high de novo mutation frequency and raises the possibility that *PS1* mutations may also be involved in apparently nonfamilial AD cases.

Table 6.1 Amyloid precursor protein gene mutations in Alzheimer's disease*

Exon	*Mutation*	*Number of families*	*Age at onset of Alzheimer's disease (years)*
16	Lys670Asn, Met671Leu	1	55
17	Ala692Gly	1	46
	Ile716Val	1	
	Val717Ile	12	47–57
	Val717Gly	1	59
	Val717Phe	1	43

*For details, see J Hardy. Amyloid, the presenilins and Alzheimer disease. Trends Neurosci 1997;87:154–159.

Initial mutation analyses indicated that *PS1* harbored approximately 70% of disease-causing mutations in familial EOAD cases. More recent estimations, however, suggest that this initial figure was overestimated due to ascertainment bias toward *PS1*-linked families [53–55]. Indeed, mutation analyses of *PS1* in a population-based sample of presenile AD patients provided a much lower *PS1* mutation frequency of 18% in autosomal dominant AD cases [55]. In the same study, *PS1* mutation frequencies were 9% in familial EOAD and 6% in EOAD in general. The onset ages of AD in different *PS1* families are within a narrow onset age range and are directly related to the position *and* type of amino acid substitution (see Table 6.2). Because some *PS1* mutations result in a less severe disease phenotype with later onset age [51], it is possible that some mutations in *PS1* cause LOAD rather than EOAD. Indicative for this is the detection of the Ala79Val mutation causing a disease onset of 64 years of age (see Table 6.2). In addition, it is interesting to note that allelic association was reported between an intragenic polymorphism of *PS1* and LOAD [56], although not confirmed in all studies.

A distinct set of EOAD families used in molecular genetic studies is the Volga-German (VG) kindred. They are a group of nine families that descend from a single German family that emigrated first to Russia and later to the United States. Although the onset ages in these families are highly variable, it is assumed that EOAD in these families is caused by the same genetic defect inherited from a common ancestor [57]. The AD locus in the VG families did not segregate with markers confined to the *AD3* region [34]. Although a mutation in *AD3* could not be excluded in all VG families, the data strongly suggested that another genetic defect was responsible for AD. In addition, the *AD1* locus was excluded by linkage analysis, and no *APP* mutations were found [58]. Therefore, a genome-wide search was undertaken to identify the AD locus in these families. Significantly positive LOD scores were obtained with STR marker D1S479 on chromosome 1 in the region 1q31–1q42 (*AD4*). Informative recombinants defined a 14-cM candidate region between D1S225 and D1S217 [59]. At the same time, an expressed sequence tag (EST) was identified that displayed high homology with *PS1*. An EST is a short sequence, derived from an anonymous cDNA, that can be analyzed on genomic DNA using the polymerase chain reaction (PCR). EST databases enable rapid identification of gene homologues, and because they can be ampli-

Table 6.2 Presenilin-1 and presenilin-2 mutations in Alzheimer's disease[a]

Gene	*Exon*	*Mutation*	*Number of families*[b]	*Age at onset of Alzheimer's disease (years)*
Presenilin-1	4	Ala79Val	3	53–63
		Val82Leu	1	55
		Val96Phe	1	53
		3	5 (6%)	
	5	Tyr115His	1	36
		Tyr115Cys	1	42
		Gli120Lys	1	35–39
		Glu120Asp	1	
		Met139Val	4	40–49
		Met139Thr	1	49
		Met139Ile	1	
		Ile143Phe	1	55
		Ile143Thr	1	35
		Met146Leu	5	35–45
		Met146Val	4	35–37
		Met146Ile	2	40, 42
		12	23 (28%)	
	6	His163Tyr	1	47
		His163Arg	9	39–48
		2	10 (12%)	
	7	Gly209Val	1	42
		Ile213Thr	1	45
		Ala231Thr	1	51
		Ala231Val	1	63
		Met233Thr	1	35
		Leu235Pro	1	32
		Ala246Glu	2	39, 53
		Leu250Ser	1	50–55
		8	9 (11%)	
	8	Ala260Val	1	45
		Leu262Phe	1	50
		Cys263Arg	1	50
		Pro264Leu	2	50, 53
		Pro267Ser	1	35
		Arg269Gly	1	
		Arg269His	1	47
		Arg278Thr	1	37
		Glu280Ala	6	41–57
		Glu280Gly	2	47
		Ala285Val	1	55
		Leu286Val	2	46, 48
		Ser290Cys (Δ9)	2	50
		13	22 (27%)	

Table 6.2 (continued)

Gene	*Exon*	*Mutation*	*Number of families*[b]	*Age at onset of Alzheimer's disease (years)*
	9	Glu318Gly	4	35–64
		1	4 (5%)	
	11	Gly378Glu	1	35
		Gly384Ala	2	35
		Leu392Val	2	46
		Cys410Tyr	4	45–50
		4	9 (11%)	
Presenilin-2	4	Arg62His	1	62
	5	Asn141Ile	7	53
	7	Met239Val	1	50

[a]For details, see M Cruts, C Van Broeckhoven. Presenilin mutations in Alzheimer's disease. Hum Mutat 1998;11:183–190.
[b]Percentage of total number of *PS1*-mutated families appears in parentheses.

fied by PCR, the genomic location of the corresponding genes can be easily determined using chromosome mapping panels. The EST showing homology with *PS1* was localized to the region on chromosome 1 linked to AD in the VG families, making it a strong positional candidate for AD in these kindreds. The complete sequence of the cDNA represented by the EST predicted a 448 amino acids–long protein which, like ps1, resembled an integral membrane protein. Because of the high homology with *PS1*, the *AD4* gene was called *presenilin-2* (*PS2*; protein ps2). The overall homology between ps1 and ps2 is 67%, with higher homology in the transmembrane domains. The main differences between ps1 and ps2 are in their N-terminal and HL-VI domains. Together these findings led to the identification of a missense mutation in affected individuals of the VG families [60]. Two additional missense mutations in the same gene were identified in an Italian EOAD family [61] and a Dutch EOAD patient [55], indicating that mutations in this gene are not restricted to the VG kindred (see Table 6.2).

The ps proteins are expressed in all regions of the brain as well as in a variety of peripheral tissues [48]. In brain tissue, *PS1* and *PS2* transcripts are detected primarily in dendrites of neuronal cell populations [62,63]. The ps proteins are subcellularly localized in the endoplasmic reticulum and the Golgi complex. Both ps proteins occur as different isoforms due to alternative splicing events. *PS1* and *PS2* are organized in 10 coding exons, preceded by one to three 5' untranslated exons [52,64,65]. In *PS1*, alternative splicing occurs at the 3' end of exon 3 (numbering of exons is according to reference 52). The shorter splice variant lacks the amino acids Val-Arg-Ser-Gln encoded by codons 26–29 in the N-terminal of *PS1* [43,52], which constitute in part two putative phosphorylation sites. Both isoforms are present in brain tissue, fibroblasts, and lymphoblasts at a ratio of 3 to 2 for the shorter isoform [43,52]. In addition, alternative splicing of codons 257–290, corresponding to exon 8 of *PS1*, which codes for the start of HL-VI, has been reported [61]. The shorter isoform is most prominent in leukocytes [61]. Also, in *PS2*, exon

8 is alternatively spliced. In brain tissue, the longer isoform of *PS2* is predominant, although the shorter isoform can also be detected. In addition, *PS2* transcripts lacking exons 3 and 4 were identified. Because exon 3 contains the normal translation start codon, these splice variants are assumed to use an alternative start codon at position 145 in exon 5 [66]. Given that many EOAD mutations are detected in exon 8, encoding a highly conserved region, it is likely that HL-VI of ps is of particular importance for their function in the brain [67].

The normal and abnormal function of ps is currently unknown. The fact that no deletions or nonsense mutations causing EOAD have been detected so far suggests that EOAD-causing mutations in *PS1* and *PS2* result in a gain of function or dysfunction, rather than a loss of function. Furthermore, in spite of the high homology between the two ps proteins, neither one can compensate for a mutation in the other, as a mutation in one *PS* gene is sufficient to cause AD pathology.

PS are highly conserved across different species [51]. Based on homologues in other species, suggestions about possible functions of ps were put forward. One hypothesis is based on the homology of ps with *sel-12*, a component of the Notch cell–signaling pathway in *Caenorhabditis elegans* [68], which is conserved in *Drosophila* and higher species, including vertebrates [51]. *Sel-12* modulates the ability of cells to respond to *lin-12*–mediated intercellular signaling during embryonic development. Supporting evidence for a function of ps similar to that of *sel-12* is the observation that, in *C. elegans*, the defective egg-laying phenotype of mutant *sel-12* can be complemented by human *PS1* cDNA [69]. A second hypothesis is based on the function of another, weaker *ps* homologue, *spe-4* of *C. elegans*. *Spe-4* plays a role in the intracellular protein trafficking and localization of proteins during spermatogenesis. If the ps proteins were involved in a similar protein trafficking system, a disturbance in their function might result in abnormal processing of proteins, among them app [60]. In this respect it is interesting to note that in fibroblast cells, *PS1* mutations lead to an increased production of longer Aβ peptides [70]. Also, cells transfected with mutant *PS1* or *PS2* cDNA produce more of the longer Aβ [71], an increase that was also observed in brains of *PS1* transgenic mice [71,72]. Given these data, it was hypothesized that ps might affect cell sorting of app, perhaps by directing it to intracellular environments that are more conducive to the production of longer Aβ. Supporting this hypothesis is the in vitro observation of a direct protein interaction between ps2 and app [73]. Alternatively, a third hypothesis is based on the identification of a *PS* homologue in the mouse, the apoptosis-linked gene 3 (*Alg-3*) [74]. The *Alg-3* gene product (alg-3) is involved in apoptosis, functioning as an inhibitor of T-cell receptor (TCR)-induced cell death by blocking death signal transduction. Mutations in *Alg-3* can result in a decreased blocking capacity, leading to an accelerated TCR-induced cell death. By analogy, *PS* mutations could explain the observed neurodegeneration in AD brain.

CHROMOSOME 19—APOLIPOPROTEIN E GENE

In LOAD families, no mutations have been detected in either *APP* or *PS*. Moreover, regions of chromosome 21 as well as *AD3* and *AD4* were excluded by standard linkage analyses in these families. Therefore, a genome-wide search was undertaken in a set of LOAD families [75]. Genetic linkage analyses in LOAD families are complicated by a wide range of onset ages, which creates difficulty distinguishing between individuals who are at risk for the disease and those who have escaped it. This also implies that the exact pattern of inheritance is unclear in LOAD families. Therefore, the genome-wide search was performed using the affected pedigree member (APM) method, in which the segregation patterns of genetic markers are considered in affected individuals only [76]. This method is statistically less powerful than standard LOD score analyses, but it has the advantage that it does not need a definition of inheritance of the disease (i.e., nonparametric). Using the APM method, two chromosomal regions of possible linkage were identified: the pericentromeric region of chromosome 21 and the region close to the apolipoprotein CII gene at chromosome 19q13.2, to which suggestive association was reported previously [77]. Subsequent linkage analyses in LOAD families using standard LOD score calculations did not confirm linkage to chromosome 21, but they supported linkage to 19q13.2 [75]. Multipoint linkage analyses using only affected individuals mapped the disease locus between *ATP1A3* and *BCL3* (*AD2*).

In 1991, the *APOE* protein (apo E) was immunologically localized to the lesions in the brains of AD patients [78]. Two years later these findings were confirmed and *APOE* was localized to chromosome 19q13.2 near the *AD2* candidate region defined by genetic analysis [79]. Apo E is a protein involved in lipid metabolism [80]. It has three major isoforms differing in the presence of a cysteine, or arginine residue at amino acid positions 112 and 158, respectively. Apo E-ε3 ($Cys_{112}Arg_{158}$) is the most common isoform with a frequency of 75% in whites. The two other common isoforms are apo E-ε2 ($Cys_{112}Cys_{158}$) and apo E-ε4 ($Arg_{112}Arg_{158}$) with frequencies of 10% and 15% respectively.

Genetic association of *APOE* was first demonstrated with familial LOAD [75] and later also with sporadic LOAD [11]. It was observed that *APOE-ε4* heterozygotes had a threefold increased risk, and *APOE-ε4* homozygotes an eightfold increased risk of developing AD by the age of 75 years compared to *APOE-ε3* homozygotes. The finding that *APOE-ε4* is associated with a higher risk for AD was confirmed in several family and clinical case studies as well as in population-based studies (for review, see reference 81). It was also suggested that the presence of an *APOE-ε2* allele leads to a later onset age of disease and thus may offer a protective effect against AD [82]. This observation, however, has not been systematically confirmed in all studies [83].

Analysis of the *APOE* genotypes in EOAD families segregating APP mutations indicated that, except in the EOAD family segregating the APP Ala692Gly mutation, the *APOE-ε4* allele acts as a dose-dependent age of onset modifier, because its presence leads to an earlier onset age of disease. In EOAD families segregating mutations in the *PS* genes, there was no evidence for the *APOE* genotype influencing the age of onset [84–86]. This observation can be explained in two ways. Due to the early onset age of disease in *PS1* families, the genetic defect in these families could be so dramatic that the *APOE* genotype has no recognizable effect on the development of EOAD. Alternatively, it might be possible that mutations in the *PS* genes cause EOAD through a biochemical pathway in which *APOE* is not involved.

The relevance for the involvement of *APOE-ε4* in AD pathogenesis has been demonstrated. It has been shown that in cerebrospinal fluid (CSF), apo E binds with high avidity to immobilized Aβ [87], with the ε4 isoform showing much faster binding kinetics than the ε3 isoform [88]. Apo E is also capable of promoting the polymerization of Aβ into Aβ fibrils that are deposited in AD brain lesions [89]. Moreover, it was observed that the catalytic effect of the apo E-ε4 isoform was twice that of the apo E-ε3 isoform, which in turn was three times as strong as that of the apo E-ε2 isoform [89].

OTHER GENETIC FACTORS INVOLVED IN ALZHEIMER'S DISEASE

Although no missense mutations in *PS1* have been found in LOAD populations, a genetic association between LOAD and an adenine (A) to cytosine (C) polymorphism in intron 8 of *PS1* was reported [56]. In the initial study, a twofold increased risk for developing AD was associated with the *PS1* intron 8 AA genotype. This finding was replicated in some other LOAD populations [90], but not in all. In some populations, AD was associated with the CC genotype [91,92], whereas other AD populations did not show any association at all [93–97]. These findings suggest that the intron 8 polymorphism of *PS1* has no functional relevance and that the genetic association points to another variation that modulates the functionality of *PS1*. Because no mutations were detected in the coding regions of *PS1* in LOAD patients, it is possible that this variation is located in the regulatory regions or the promoter of *PS1* [51,91].

Another gene that has been associated with AD is the $alpha_1$-antichymotrypsin gene (*AACT*; protein aact) on chromosome 14q32.1. *AACT* encodes a protease inhibitor that is associated with Aβ in AD brain deposits [98]. In vitro, aact binds Aβ and is found to enhance the polymerization of Aβ into amyloid fibrils that are deposited in AD brain lesions [89]. Genetic association of AD with an adenine to thymine polymorphism in the signal peptide of *AACT* was reported, the AA genotype being significantly increased in AD patients [99]. The results of this study suggest that *AACT* acts as a modifier of the risk attributed to apo E, with the AA genotype increasing the risk associated with the *APOE-ε4* allele two to three times. AD populations were also reported, however, in which no effect of *AACT* was observed [100–104]. The polymorphism changes a threonine into an alanine in the signal peptide of *AACT*, affecting the secretion rate of the mature protein into the extracellular space, and it might have a functional significance in relation to AD. The *AACT* polymorphism, however, might also be in linkage disequilibrium with another nearby variation with biological relevance in relation to AD pathology. More profound genetic association studies need to be performed to examine the nature of the association of *AACT* with AD.

Other genes that were genetically associated with AD are the very-low-density lipoprotein receptor gene [105], the apolipoprotein J gene [106], the serotonin transporter gene [107], and HLA-DR antigens of the class II major histocompatibility complex [108,109]. However, genetic association of AD with these genes was not confirmed in other populations, and more studies are needed before final conclusions can be reached.

DIAGNOSTIC IMPLICATIONS

To date, three causative genes have been identified that when mutated lead to presenile AD: *APP*, *PS1*, and *PS2*. No mutations in these genes have been identified in LOAD patients with onset of disease after 65 years of age; however, there is some evidence that polymorphisms in *PS1* may increase an individual's risk for senile AD [56,92]. Together, the three presenile AD genes account for half of the families with autosomal dominant presenile AD, which represent approximately 10% of the whole AD population. In other words, mutations in these genes are rare genetic causes of AD in general. Current data from mutation studies indicate that mutations in *PS1* are the most frequent with 18–50% of the EOAD families [53–55], then *APP* with 5% [110], and *PS2* with less than 1% [55,111].

In general, patients with mutations in *PS1* have the earliest onset ages of AD, sometimes as early as 35 years (see Table 6.2). Considerable overlap in onset ages occurs, however, because the mean onset age in a presenile AD family segregating a mutation in one of the three causative disease genes may vary between 30 and 65 years for *PS1*, 45 and 65 years for *APP*, and 50 and 70 years for *PS2*. Therefore, the mean onset age of AD in a family cannot be used to predict which gene is more likely to be mutated. In general, however, the onset age within a family is contained within a narrow range, enabling an approximate prediction of the onset age of the disease in an asymptomatic mutation carrier. In *APP*-mutation families, some evidence suggests that the onset age is modulated by the *APOE* genotype: Mutation carriers with an *APOE-ε4* allele have onset ages approximately 5 years earlier than those with an *APOE-ε2* allele. In contrast, there is no clear evidence that the onset age in *PS*-mutation families is modulated by the *APOE* genotype [84,85,111]. Other genetic or environmental modifiers of AD expression in *PS*-mutation families cannot be excluded, however, because in *PS2*-mutation families, onset ages within the same family vary over large ranges [111]. Also, one *PS1*-mutation family was identified with a nonpenetrant *PS1* mutation carrier [112].

Screening for mutations in the three causative AD genes can be used either for predictive testing in asymptomatic at-risk individuals or as a tool in the differential diagnosis of dementia. In spite of the high risk associated with dominant mutations in *APP*, *PS1*, and *PS2*, testing for mutations in these genes in the general population is of limited value because of their low frequency. Hence, DNA testing is only useful in cases with presenile AD. Because mutations in *PS1* are most frequently observed, *PS1* should be analyzed first, before *APP* and *PS2*. Also, half of the *PS1* mutations are found in exons 5 and 8, coding in part for TM-II and HL-VI of ps1. Therefore, these regions of *PS1* should be analyzed first, either by mutation analysis of genomic DNA—for example, by single-stranded conformation polymorphism analysis—or by RT-PCR analysis of *PS1* cDNA obtained from leukocytes, lymphoblasts, or frozen tissue.

The present data indicate that other AD genes must exist to explain the genetic cause of AD in the EOAD families without mutations in *APP*, *PS1*, or *PS2*. In some AD families, the disease may be the result of the *ε4* allele of *APOE* [12], and particularly in nuclear families, its transmission may mimic an autosomal dominant inheritance pattern. However, the *APOE-ε4* allele alone is not causative to AD because the presence of an *APOE-ε4* allele is not sufficient to develop AD. Therefore, as long as the other genetic and environmental factors involved in the development of AD are unknown, *APOE* genotyping as the sole test is of no diagnostic value. Several other genetic risk factors have been suggested that, in synergy with *APOE* or not, constitute the development of AD; however, much research is still needed to elucidate their nature and contribution to AD.

REFERENCES

1. Davies P. The genetics of Alzheimer's disease: a review and a discussion of the implications. Neurobiol Aging 1986;7:459–466.
2. Farrer LA, Myers RH, Cupples LA, et al. Transmission and age-at-onset patterns in familial Alzheimer's disease: evidence for heterogeneity. Neurology 1990;40:395–403.
3. Fitch N, Becker R, Heller A. The inheritance of Alzheimer's disease: a new interpretation. Ann Neurol 1988;23:14–19.
4. Heston LL, Mastri AR, Anderson VE, White J. Dementia of the Alzheimer type. Arch Gen Psych 1981;38:1085–1090.
5. Hofman A, Schulte W, Tanja TA, et al. History of dementia and Parkinson's disease in 1st-degree relatives of patients with Alzheimer's disease. Neurology 1989;39:1589–1592.
6. Ballabio A. The rise and fall of positional cloning? Nature Genet 1994;3:277–279.
7. Lathrop GM, Lalouel JM, Julier C, Ott J. Strategies for multilocus linkage analysis in humans. Genetics 1984;81:3443–3446.
8. Lovett M, Kere J, Hinton LM. Direct selection: a method for the isolation of cDNAs encoded by large genomic regions. Proc Natl Acad Sci U S A 1991;88:9628–9632.
9. Parimoo S, Patanjali SR, Shukla H, et al. cDNA selection: efficient PCR approach for the selection of cDNAs encoded in large chromosomal DNA fragments. Proc Natl Acad Sci U S A 1991;88:9623–9627.
10. Buckler AJ, Chang DD, Graw SL, et al. Exon amplification: a strategy to isolate mammalian genes based on RNA splicing. Proc Natl Acad Sci U S A 1991;88:4005–4009.
11. Saunders AM, Strittmatter WJ, Schmechel D, et al. Association of apolipoprotein E allele ε4 with late-onset familial and sporadic Alzheimer's disease. Neurology 1993;43:1467–1472.
12. van Duijn CM, de Knijff P, Cruts M, et al. Apolipoprotein ε4 allele in a population-based study of early-onset Alzheimer's disease. Nature Genet 1994;7:74–78.
13. Wisniewski KE, Dalton AJ, Crapper-Mclachlan DR, et al. Alzheimer's disease in Down's syndrome: clinicopathologic studies. Neurology 1985;35:957–961.
14. Mann DAM. The pathological association between Down syndrome and Alzheimer disease. Mech Aging Dev 1988;43:99–136.
15. St George-Hyslop PH, Tanzi RE, Polinsky PJ, et al. The genetic defect causing familial Alzheimer's disease maps on chromosome 21. Science 1987;235:885–890.
16. Tanzi RE, Gusella JF, Watkins PC, et al. Amyloid β protein gene: cDNA, mRNA distribution, and genetic linkage near the Alzheimer locus. Science 1987;235:880–884.
17. Van Broeckhoven C, Genthe AM, Vandenberghe A, et al. Failure of familial Alzheimer's disease to segregate with the A4-amyloid gene in several European families. Nature 1987;329:153–155.
18. Tanzi RE, St George-Hyslop PH, Haines JL, et al. The genetic defect in familial Alzheimer's disease is not tightly linked to the amyloid β-protein gene. Nature 1987;329:156–157.
19. Tanzi RE, Haines JL, Watkins PC, et al. Genetic linkage map of human chromosome 21. Genomics 1988;3:129–136.
20. Van Broeckhoven C, Van Hul W, Backhovens H, et al. Genetic Linkage Analysis in Two Large Belgian Alzheimer Families with Chromosome 21 DNA Markers. In PM Sinet, Y Lamour, Y Christen (eds), Genetics and Alzheimer's Disease. Berlin: Springer-Verlag, 1988;124–129.
21. Goate AM, Owen MJ, James LA, et al. Predisposing locus for Alzheimer's disease on chromosome 21. Lancet 1989;8634:352–355.
22. Van Broeckhoven C, Backhovens H, Van Hul W, et al. Genetic Linkage Analysis in Early-Onset Familial Alzheimer's Dementia. In WE Bunney, H Hippius, G Laakmann, N Schmauss (eds), Neuropsychopharmacology. Berlin: Springer-Verlag, 1990;86–91.
23. Schellenberg GD, Bird TD, Wijsman EM, et al. Absence of linkage of chromosome 21q21 markers to familial Alzheimer's disease. Science 1988;241:1507–1510.
24. Pericak-Vance MA, Yamaoka LH, Haynes CS, et al. Genetic linkage studies in Alzheimer's disease families. Exp Neurol 1988;102:271–279.
25. Schellenberg GD, Pericak-Vance MA, Wijsman EM, et al. Linkage analysis of familial Alzheimer disease, using chromosome 21 markers. Am J Hum Genet 1991;48:563–583.

26. St George-Hyslop PH, Haines JL, Farrer LA, et al. Genetic linkage studies suggest that Alzheimer's disease is not a single homogeneous disorder. Nature 1990;347:194–197.
27. Levy E, Carman MD, Fernandez-Madrid IJ, et al. Mutation of the Alzheimer's disease amyloid gene in hereditary cerebral hemorrhage, Dutch type. Science 1990;248:1124–1126.
28. Bakker E, Van Broeckhoven C, Haan J, et al. DNA diagnosis for hereditary cerebral hemorrhage with amyloidosis (Dutch type). Am J Hum Genet 1991;49:518–521.
29. Haan J, Hardy JA, Roos RAC. Hereditary cerebral hemorrhage with amyloidosis-Dutch type: its importance for Alzheimer research. Trends Neurosci 1991;14:231–234.
30. Van Broeckhoven C, Haan J, Bakker E, et al. Amyloid β protein precursor gene and hereditary cerebral hemorrhage with amyloidosis (Dutch). Science 1990;248:1120–1122.
31. Yoshikai S, Sasaki H, Doh-ura K, et al. Genomic organization of the human amyloid beta-protein precursor gene. Gene 1990;87:257–263.
32. Hardy J. Amyloid, the presenilins and Alzheimer disease. Trends Neurosci 1997;20:154–159.
33. Hendriks L, van Duijn CM, Cras P, et al. Presenile dementia and cerebral haemorrhage linked to a mutation at condon 692 of the β-amyloid precursor protein gene. Nature Genet 1992;1:218–221.
34. Schellenberg GD, Bird TD, Wijsman EM, et al. Genetic linkage evidence for a familial Alzheimer's disease locus on chromosome 14. Science 1992;258:668–671.
35. St. George-Hyslop P, Haines J, Rogaev E, et al. Genetic evidence for a novel familial Alzheimer's disease locus on chromosome 14. Nature Genet 1992;2:330–334.
36. Van Broeckhoven C, Backhovens H, Cruts M, et al. Mapping of a gene predisposing to early-onset Alzheimer's disease to chromosome 14q24.3. Nature Genet 1992;2:335–339.
37. Mullan M, Houlden H, Windelspecht M, et al. A locus for familial early-onset Alzheimer's disease on the long arm of chromosome 14, proximal to the α_1-antichymotrypsin gene. Nature Genet 1992;2:340–342.
38. Lannfelt L, Lilius L, Appelgren H, et al. No linkage to chromosome 14 in Swedish Alzheimer's disease families. Nature Genet 1993;4:218–219.
39. Schellenberg GD, Payami H, Wijsman EM, et al. Chromosome 14 and late-onset familial Alzheimer disease (FAD). Am J Hum Genet 1993;53:619–628.
40. Cruts M, Backhovens H, Theuns J, et al. Genetic and physical characterisation of the early-onset Alzheimer's disease AD3 locus on chromosome 14q24.3. Hum Mol Genet 1995;4:1355–1364.
41. Clark RF, Cruts M, Korenblat KM, et al. A Yeast artificial chromosome contig from human chromosome 14q24 spanning the Alzheimer's disease locus AD3. Hum Mol Genet 1995;4:1347–1354.
42. Gyapay G, Morissette J, Vignal A, et al. The 1993–94 Généthon human genetic linkage map. Nature Genet 1994;7:246–249.
43. Cruts M, Backhovens H, Wang S-Y, et al. Molecular genetic analysis of familial early-onset Alzheimer's disease linked to chromosome 14q24.3. Hum Mol Genet 1995;4:2363–2372.
44. Rogaev EI, Lukiw WJ, Vaula G, et al. Analysis of the c-fos gene on chromosome 14 and the promoter of the amyloid precursor protein gene in familial Alzheimer's disease. Neurology 1993;43:2275–2279.
45. Cruts M, Backhovens H, Van Gassen G, et al. Mutation analysis of the 14q24.3 dihydrolipoyl succinyltransferase (DLST) gene in patients with early-onset Alzheimer disease. Neurosci Lett 1995;199:73–77.
46. Cruts M, Backhovens H, Martin JJ, Van Broeckhoven C. Genetic analysis of the cellular oncogene *fos* in patients with chromosome-14 encoded Alzheimer's disease. Neurosci Lett 1994;174:97–100.
47. Bonnycastle LLC, Chang-En Y, Wijsman EM, et al. The c-fos gene and early-onset familial Alzheimer's disease. Neurosci Lett 1993;160:33–36.
48. Sherrington R, Rogaev EI, Liang Y, et al. Cloning of a gene bearing missense mutations in early-onset familial Alzheimer's disease. Nature 1995;375:754–760.
49. Lehman S, Chiesa R, Harris DA. Evidence for a six-transmembrane domain structure of presenilin 1. J Biol Chem 1997;272:12047–12051.
50. Doan A, Thinakaran G, Borchelt DR, et al. Protein topology of presenilin 1. Neuron 1996;17:1023–1030.
51. Cruts M, Van Broeckhoven C. Presenilin mutations in Alzheimer's disease. Hum Mutat 1998;11:183–190.
52. Alzheimer's Disease Collaborative Group. The structure of the presenilin 1 (S182) gene and identification of six novel mutations in early onset AD families. Nature Genet 1995;11:219–222.
53. Campion D, Flaman JM, Brice A, et al. Mutations of the presenilin-1 gene in families with early-onset Alzheimer's disease. Hum Mol Genet 1995;4:2373–2377.
54. Hutton M, Busfield F, Wragg M, et al. Complete analysis of the presenilin 1 gene in families with early onset Alzheimer's disease. Neuroreport 1996;7:801–805.
55. Cruts M, van Duijn CM, Backhovens H, et al. Estimation of the genetic contribution of presenilin-1 and -2 in a population-based study of presenile Alzheimer disease. Hum Mol Genet 1998;7:43–51.
56. Wragg M, Hutton M, Talbot C, et al. Genetic association between intronic polymorphism in presenilin-1 gene and late-onset Alzheimer's disease. Lancet 1996;347:509–512.

57. Bird TD, Lampe TH, Nemens EJ, et al. Familial Alzheimer's disease in American descendants of the Volga Germans: probable genetic founder effect. Ann Neurol 1988;23:25–31.
58. Kamino K, Orr HT, Payami H, et al. Linkage and mutational analysis of familial Alzheimer disease kindreds for the APP gene region. Am J Hum Genet 1992;51:998–1014.
59. Levy-Lahad E, Wijsman EM, Nemens E, et al. A familial Alzheimer's disease locus on chromosome 1. Science 1995;269:970–973.
60. Levy-Lahad E, Wasco W, Poorkaj P, et al. Candidate gene for the chromosome 1 familial Alzheimer's disease locus. Science 1995;269:973–977.
61. Rogaev EI, Sherrington R, Rogeava EA, et al. Familial Alzheimer's disease in kindreds with missense mutations in a gene on chromosome 1 related to the Alzheimer's disease type 3 gene. Nature 1995;376:775–778.
62. Cook DG, Sung JC, Golde TE, et al. Expression and analysis of presenilin 1 in a human neuronal system: localization in cell bodies and dentrites. Proc Natl Acad Sci U S A 1996;93:9223–9228.
63. Kovacs DM, Fausett HJ, Page KJ, et al. Alzheimer-associated presenilins 1 and 2: neuronal expression in brain and localization to intracelllular membranes in mammalian cells. Nat Med 1996;2:224–229.
64. Rogaev EI, Sherrington R, Wu C, et al. Analysis of the 5' sequence, genomic structure, and alternative splicing of the presenilin-1 gene (PSEN1) associated with early onset Alzheimer's disease. Genomics 1997;40:415–424.
65. Levy-Lahad E, Poorkaj P, Wang K, et al. Genomic structure and expression of STM2, the chromosome 1 familial Alzheimer's disease gene. Genomics 1996;34:198–204.
66. Prihar G, Fuldner RA, Perez-Tur J, et al. Structure and alternative splicing of the presenilin-2 gene. Neuroreport 1996;7:1680–1684.
67. Van Broeckhoven C. Presenilins and Alzheimer disease. Nature Genet 1995;11:230–232.
68. Levitan D, Greenwald I. Facilitation of lin-12–mediated signalling by sel-12, a *Caenorhabditis elegans* S182 Alzheimer's disease gene. Nature 1995;377:351–354.
69. Levitan D, Doyle TG, Brousseau D, et al. Assessment of normal and mutant human presenilin function in *Caenorhabditis elegans*. Proc Natl Acad Sci U S A 1996;93:14940–14944.
70. Scheuner D, Eckman C, Jensen M, et al. Secreted amyloid β-protein similar to that in the senile plaques of Alzheimer's disease is increased in vivo by the presenilin 1 and 2 and APP mutations linked to familial Alzheimer's disease. Am J Med Genet 1996;67:429.
71. Borchelt DR, Thinakaran G, Eckman C, et al. Familial Alzheimer's disease-linked presenilin 1 variants elevate Abeta1-42/1-40 ratio in vitro and in vivo. Neuron 1996;17:1005–1013.
72. Duff K, Eckman C, Zehr C, et al. Increased amyloid-β42(43) in brains of mice expressing mutant presenilin 1. Nature 1996;383:710–713.
73. Weideman A, Paliga K, Durrwang U, et al. Formation of stable complexes between two Alzheimer's disease gene products: presenilin-2 and β-amyloid precursor protein. Nature Med 1997;3:328–332.
74. Vito P, Lacana E, d'Adamio L. Interfering with apoptosis: Ca-binding protein ALG-2 and Alzheimer's disease gene ALG-3. Science 1996;271:521–524.
75. Pericak-Vance MA, Bebout JL, Gaskell PC Jr, et al. Linkage studies in familial Alzheimer disease: evidence for chromosome 19 linkage. Am J Hum Genet 1991;48:1034–1050.
76. Weeks DE, Lange K. The affected-pedigree-member method of linkage analysis. Am J Hum Genet 1988;42:315–326.
77. Schellenberg GD, Deeb SS, Boehnke M, et al. Association of an apolipoprotein CII allele with familial dementia of the Alzheimer type. J Neurogenet 1987;4:97–108.
78. Namba Y, Tomonaga M, Kawasaki H, et al. Apolipoprotein E immunoreactivity in cerebral amyloid deposits and neurofibrillary tangles in Alzheimer's disease and kuru plaque amyloid in Creutzfeldt-Jakob disease. Brain Res 1991;641:163–166.
79. Wisniewski T, Frangione B. Apolipoprotein E: a pathological chaperone protein in patients with cerebral and systemic amyloid. Neurosci Lett 1992;135:235–238.
80. Mahley RW. Apolipoprotein E: cholesterol transport protein with expanding role in cell biology. Science 1988;240:622–630.
81. Hardy J. Apolipoprotein E in the genetics and epidemiology of Alzheimer's disease. Am J Med Genet (Neuropsy Genet) 1995;60:456–460.
82. Corder EH, Saunders AM, Risch NJ, et al. Protective effect of apolipoprotein E type 2 allele for late onset Alzheimer disease. Nature Genet 1994;7:180–184.
83. van Duijn CM, de Knijff P, Wehnert A, et al. The apolipoprotein E ε2 allele is associated with an increased risk of early-onset Alzheimer's disease and a reduced survival. Ann Neurol 1995;37:605–610.
84. Van Broeckhoven C, Backhovens H, Cruts M, et al. APOE genotype does not modulate age of onset in families with chromosome 14 encoded Alzheimer's disease. Neurosci Lett 1994;169:179–180.

85. Levy-Lahad E, Lahad A, Wijsman EM, et al. Apolipoprotein E genotypes and age of onset in early-onset familial Alzheimer's disease. Ann Neurol 1995;38:678–680.
86. French Alzheimer's Disease Collaborative Study Group. Apolipoprotein E genotype does not affect age at onset in patients with chromosome 14 encoded Alzheimer's disease. J Med Genet 1996;33:176.
87. Strittmatter WJ, Saunders AM, Schmechel D, et al. Apolipoprotein E: high-avidity binding to β-amyloid and increased frequency of type 4 allele in late-onset familial Alzheimer disease. Proc Natl Acad Sci U S A 1993;90:1977–1981.
88. Strittmatter WJ, Weisgraber KH, Huang D, et al. Binding of human apolipoprotein E to synthetic amyloid β peptide: isoform-specific effects and implications for late-onset Alzheimer disease. Proc Natl Acad Sci U S A 1993;90:8098–8102.
89. Ma J, Yee A, Brewer HB Jr, et al. Amyloid-associated proteins α_1-antichymotrypsin and apolipoprotein E promote assembly of Alzheimer β-protein into filaments. Nature 1994;372:92–94.
90. Matsushita S, Arai H, Muramatsu T, et al. Presenilin-1 polymorphism in Alzheimer's disease and vascular dementia. Exp Neurol 1997;146:567–569.
91. Nishiwaki Y, Kamino K, Yoshiiwa A, et al. T/G polymorphism at intron 9 of presenilin 1 gene is associated with, but not responsible for sporadic late-onset Alzheimer's disease in Japanese population. Neurosci Lett 1997;227:123–126.
92. van Duijn CM, Cruts M, Theuns J, et al. Early-onset Alzheimer's disease is associated with presenilin 1 in a population-based study. (In preparation.)
93. Perez-Tur J, Wavrant-De Vrieze F, Lambert JC, et al. Presenilin-1 polymorphism and Alzheimer's disease. Lancet 1996;347:1560–1561.
94. Cai X, Stanton J, Fallin D, et al. No association between the intronic presenilin-1 polymorphism and Alzheimer's disease in clinic and population-based samples. Am J Med Genet (Neuropsy Genet) 1997;74:202–203.
95. Sorbi S, Nacmias B, Tedde A, et al. Presenilin-1 gene intronic polymorphism in sporadic and familial Alzheimer's disease. Neurosci Lett 1997;222:132–134.
96. Tysoe C, Whittaker J, Cairns NJ, et al. Presenilin-1 intron 8 polymorphism is not associated with autopsy-confirmed late-onset Alzheimer's disease. Neurosci Lett 1997;222:68–69.
97. Scott WK, Yamaoka LH, Locke PA, et al. No association or linkage between an intronic polymorphism of presenilin-1 and sporadic or late-onset familial Alzheimer disease. Genet Epidemiol 1997;14:307–315.
98. Abraham CR, Selkoe DJ, Potter H. Immunochemical identification of the serine protease inhibitor α-1-antichymostrypsin in the brain amyloid deposits of Alzheimer's disease. Cell 1988;52:487–501.
99. Kamboh MI, Sanghera DK, Ferrell RE, DeKosky ST. APOE*4-associated Alzheimer's disease risk is modified by α_1-antichymotrypsin polymorphism. Nature Genet 1995;10:486–488.
100. Murphy GM Jr, Sullivan EV, Gallagher-Thompson D, et al. No association between the alpha 1-antichymotrypsin A allele and Alzheimer's disease. Neurology 1997;48:1313–1316.
101. Fallin D, Reading S, Schinka J, et al. No interaction between the APOE and the alpha-1-antichymotrypsin genes on risk for Alzheimer's disease. Am J Med Genet 1997;74:192–194.
102. Haines JL, Pritchard ML, Saunders AM, et al. No association between $alpha_1$-antichymotrypsin and familial Alzheimer's disease. Ann N Y Acad Sci 1996;802:35–41.
103. Muller U, Bodeker RH, Gerundt I, Kurz A. Lack of association between $alpha_1$-antichymotrypsin polymorphism, Alzheimer's disease, and allele epsilon 4 of apolipoprotein E. Neurology 1996;47:1575–1577.
104. Nacmias B, Tedde A, Latorraca S, et al. Apolipoprotein E and $alpha_1$-antichymotrypsin polymorphism in Alzheimer's disease. Ann Neurol 1996;40:678–680.
105. Okuizumi K, Onodera O, Namba Y, et al. Genetic association of the very low density lipoprotein (VLDL) receptor gene with sporadic Alzheimer's disease. Nature Genet 1995;11:207–209.
106. Tycko B, Feng L, Nguyen L, et al. Polymorphisms in the human apolipoprotein-J/clusterin gene: ethnic variation and distribution in Alzheimer's disease. Hum Genet 1996;98:430–436.
107. Li T, Holmes C, Sham PC, et al. Allelic functional variation of serotonin transporter expression is a susceptibility factor for late onset Alzheimer's disease. Neuroreport 1997;8:683–686.
108. Payami H, Schellenberg GD, Zareparsi S, et al. Evidence for association of HLA-A2 allele with onset age of Alzheimer's disease. Neurology 1997;49:512–518.
109. Curran M, Middleton D, Edwardson J, et al. HLA-DR antigens associated with major genetic risk for late-onset Alzheimer's disease. Neuroreport 1997;8:1467–1469.
110. Van Broeckhoven C. Molecular genetics of Alzheimer disease: identification of genes and gene mutations. Eur Neurol 1995;35:8–19.
111. Sherrington R, Froelich S, Sorbi S, et al. Alzheimer's disease associated with mutations in presenilin 2 is rare and variably penetrant. Hum Mol Genet 1996;5:985–988.
112. Rossor MN, Fox NC, Beck J, et al. Incomplete penetrance of familial Alzheimer's disease in a pedigree with a novel presenilin-1 gene mutation. Lancet 1996;347:1560.

7
Apolipoprotein E and Alzheimer's Disease

Teresa Gómez-Isla, G. William Rebeck, Michael C. Irizarry, Steven M. Greenberg, and Bradley T. Hyman

Alzheimer's disease (AD) represents the most common cause of dementia in the elderly. Molecular genetic studies have implicated at least four genes in the pathogenesis of the disease. Mutations in three of these, the amyloid protein precursor (APP) gene on chromosome 21, the presenilin-1 gene on chromosome 14, and the presenilin-2 gene on chromosome 1, have been identified as the causative defects that explain the majority of cases with autosomal dominant–transmitted disease that manifests before the age of 60 years [1–4] (see Chapter 6). These mutations, however, account only for a relatively small percentage of the AD population [5]. Another piece of genetic evidence concerns the probable role of one allele of the apolipoprotein E (apo E) gene (*APOE*) on chromosome 19 as a risk factor for the most common form of the disease, late-onset sporadic or familial AD [6].

Apo E is a major component of lipoproteins and has been studied for many years in the context of lipid transport and the mechanisms that lead to atherogenesis. It is well known from large population-based studies that there are several genetic variants of *APOE*. There are three common allelic variants designated *APOE-ε2*, *-ε3*, and *-ε4*. Because everyone inherits two *APOE* alleles, there are a total of six possible *APOE* genotypes: *APOE-ε2/2*, *APOE-ε2/3*, *APOE-ε3/3*, *APOE-ε2/4*, *APOE-ε3/4*, and *APOE-ε4/4*. *APOE-ε3* is the most common allele in the general population, with a frequency of approximately 80%.

Apo E2 and E4 are frequently compared against apo E3 as the standard or most common form of apo E. Apo E2, which is associated with type III hyperlipoproteinemia with increased triglyceride levels, differs from apo E3 at residue 158, where cysteine substitutes for arginine. Apo E4, which is associated with increased cholesterol levels, differs from apo E3 at residue 112, where arginine substitutes for cysteine [7] (Figure 7.1).

Given that apo E protein has a well-established function in redistributing lipids among the cells of different organs and plays a critical role in lipid metabolism, it was surprising to find that it apparently also has a role in AD. It is now well accepted that the frequency of the *ε4* allele of *APOE* is overrepresented in patients with AD. This observation was initially made in late-onset familial AD

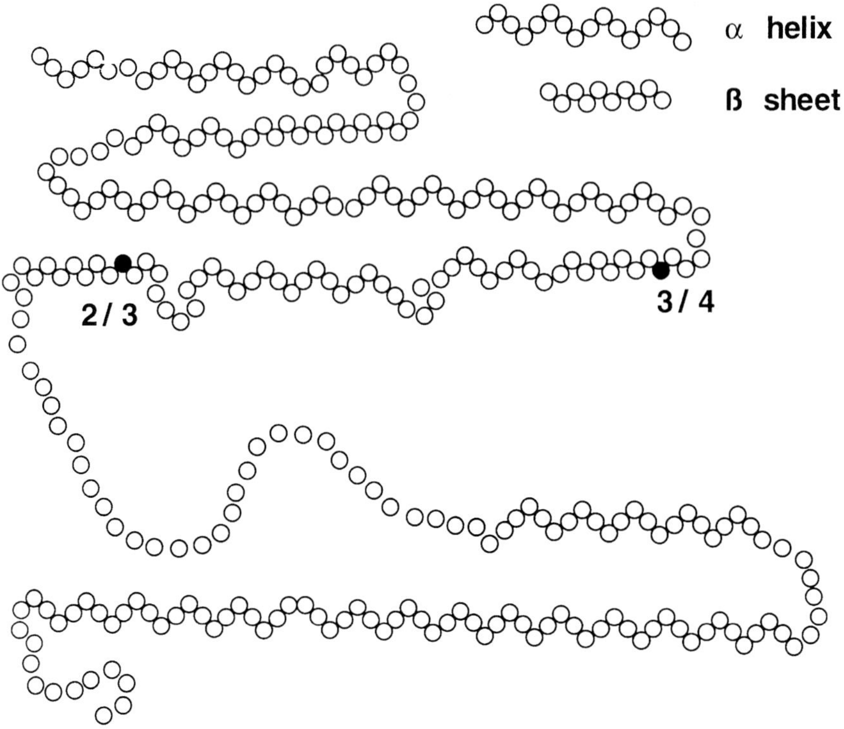

Figure 7.1 Human apolipoprotein E isoforms.

[6], but it was rapidly replicated to demonstrate that sporadic late-onset AD cases as well as young-onset cases also had approximately a threefold higher than expected likelihood of having *APOE-ε4* [8–10]. This finding suggests that inheritance of *APOE-ε4* is a risk factor for developing AD. In addition, early studies found that *APOE-ε2* is underrepresented in AD, suggesting that it is a negative or protective risk factor for AD [11,12]. These results have been replicated dozens of times in multiple populations, and even though the exact details with regard to specific risk ratios in different ethnic groups [13] and even with regard to age and gender may still need to be evaluated further, the evidence that *APOE-ε4* is a risk factor for AD is now generally accepted (Table 7.1).

The challenge we address in this chapter is to clarify how this information might help the clinician's approach to the individual patient. The goals have been to identify potential places this information could be useful:

- Are there differences in the clinical course or the pathology of the disease if a patient carries one or two copies of *APOE-ε4*?
- Does *APOE* genotype help in the differential diagnosis of a patient with dementia?
- Does *APOE* genotype help predict which individuals will develop cognitive impairment in their elder years?

Table 7.1 Apolipoprotein E genotypes and allele frequencies in controls and dementias

	Control (n = 129)	*Alzheimer's disease (n = 359)*	*Pick's disease (n = 31)*	*Progressive supranuclear palsy (n = 27)*
Apolipoprotein E genotype				
4/4	<1% (1)	16% (59)	0	0
3/4	23% (30)	42% (152)	13% (4)	15% (4)
3/3	64% (82)	33% (118)	68% (21)	74% (20)
2/4	1.5% (2)	3% (11)	0	7% (2)
2/3	11% (14)	5% (17)	16% (5)	4% (1)
2/2	0	<1% (2)	3% (1)	0
Allele frequencies				
ε4	0.13	0.39*	0.11	0.06
ε3	0.81	0.56	0.83	0.83
ε2	0.06	0.04*	0.06	0.11

*$P < .005$.

Source: Reprinted with permission from T Gómez-Isla, HL West, GW Rebeck, et al. Clinical and pathological correlates of apolipoprotein E ε4 in Alzheimer's disease. Ann Neurol 1996;39:62–70.

ARE THERE DIFFERENCES IN THE CLINICAL COURSE OR THE PATHOLOGY OF THE DISEASE IF A PATIENT HAS INHERITED *APOE-ε4* ?

Two clinical characteristics have been examined to date: age of onset and rate of progression of dementia.

APOE-ε4 and Clinical Characteristics

Age of onset of dementia appears to be an important variable with regard to the degree of *APOE*-related risk. In multiple studies, the average age of onset of individuals with AD who carry one or two copies of *APOE-ε4* is significantly lower than that of individuals with AD who do not inherit this allele. Our own clinic-based population of more than 300 AD patients showed differences in the average age of onset of several years among genotypes, with *APOE-ε4/4* individuals having an average age of onset approximately 3 years earlier than *APOE-ε3/4* individuals, which is a few years earlier than those with *APOE-ε3/3* (Table 7.2) [14]. In this population, the *APOE-ε4* allele frequency was 0.39, compared to a frequency of 0.13 in controls who were known to be cognitively intact. Although we examined a fairly small number of subjects with *APOE-ε2*, we did not detect a later age of onset for individuals who carry the *APOE-ε2* allele. Thus, on average AD patients with *APOE-ε4* have a younger age of onset, but these ages of onset are broadly overlapping among *APOE* genotypes, and the genotype–age onset relationship is not applicable to an individual patient.

It is obvious that some individuals with AD progress rapidly, whereas others have a slower clinical rate of progression. In our initial studies, we had hypoth-

Table 7.2 Apolipoprotein E genotypes and age of onset of dementia in Alzheimer's disease

Apolipoprotein E genotype	*Number of patients*	*Age of onset (mean ± SD)*
4/4	54	67.1 ± 7.6
3/4	142	72.3 ± 8.3
3/3	107	73.9 ± 11.7
2/4	11	69.4 ± 11.9
2/3	13	73.4 ± 12.9
2/2	2	69 ± 9.9

SD = standard deviation.
Source: Reprinted with permission from T Gómez-Isla, HL West, GW Rebeck, et al. Clinical and pathological correlates of apolipoprotein E ε4 in Alzheimer's disease. Ann Neurol 1996;39:62–70.

Table 7.3 Clinical characteristics of Alzheimer's patients with various apolipoprotein E genotypes

				Rate of progression	
	Number of patients	*Duration year avg (SE)*	*Follow-up year avg (SE)*	*BDS avg (SE)*	*ADL avg (SE)*
ε2/*	13	7.3 (1.2)	3.1 (0.7)	3.1 (0.7)	8.9 (1.3)
ε3/3	45	5.4 (0.4)	2.2 (0.2)	4.3 (0.6)	12.2 (1.3)
ε3/4	65	5.8 (0.4)	2.4 (0.2)	3.1 (0.4)	10.1 (1.1)
ε4/4	32	8.7 (0.9)	2.9 (0.3)	3.5 (0.5)	10.1 (1.5)

BDS = Blessed Dementia Scale rate (points per year); ADL = activities of daily living rate (points per year); avg = average; SE = standard error.
Source: Reprinted with permission from T Gómez-Isla, HL West, GW Rebeck, et al. Clinical and pathological correlates of apolipoprotein E ε4 in Alzheimer's disease. Ann Neurol 1996;39:62–70.

esized that if *APOE-ε4* was associated with an earlier age of dementia onset, it might lead as well to a more malignant clinical course with faster rates of cognitive decline. Our data and those of several other groups argue against this hypothesis [14–21], however, although a few studies reach the opposite conclusion [22,23]. In our initial study, we followed 153 probable AD patients for a mean of 31.8 months and found no differences among genotype groups in the rate of progression for a test of global cognitive ability (the information, memory, and concentration subtest of the Blessed Dementia Scale) or a measure of functional performance (the activities of daily living score) [14] (Table 7.3). A subset of these probable AD patients had been followed with an intensive battery of neuropsychometric instruments to assess explicit memory, attention, language, visuospatial function, frontal lobe function, and logical reasoning abilities. We found that the rate of decline did not consistently vary across *APOE* genotypes on these cognitive tests [16].

Several reports present different conclusions that are difficult to reconcile with our findings. Frisoni and colleagues reported that the rate of progression as judged by Mini-Mental State Examination (MMSE) scores and the Clinical Dementia Rating scale decreased significantly with increasing *ε4* gene dose

[22]. Basun and colleagues found no significant differences between *APOE-ε4* carriers and noncarriers for MMSE test scores at the first examination or after a 3-year follow-up period, despite a longer disease duration in the *APOE-ε4* carriers. They concluded that the presence of *APOE-ε4* is associated with a better prognosis in late-onset AD [23]. Overall, we believe that *APOE* genotype influences age of onset but does not affect rate of progression. Viewed in this light, the knowledge of the *APOE* genotype does not help to predict which individuals will progress faster or slower than the expected average rate of deterioration once the first clinical symptoms have appeared.

APOE-ε4 and Neuropathology

From a neuropathologic perspective, one of the initial observations was that the inheritance of the *APOE-ε4* allele is associated with an increased amount of amyloid beta-protein (Aβ) deposition in the neuropil in the form of senile plaques (SPs) [9,24]. In our prospective longitudinal study, 31 of the individuals who had been assessed at the Massachusetts Alzheimer's Disease Research Center died during the course of the study, and brain tissue was available for quantitative neuropathologic assessments. Based on image analysis and stereologic techniques on immunostained sections, we quantified the amount of Aβ deposited and the number of neurofibrillary tangles (NFTs) and neurons in each case. In addition, we were able to control for the effects of gender, age of onset, and duration of illness in these cases when comparing the degree of pathologic change among different genotypes. Our data and those from other groups reveal a clear increase in the amount of Aβ deposition in the form of SPs and also around blood vessels in association with *APOE-ε4* [9,14,24–26].

The effect of *APOE-ε4* on amyloid metabolism is not simply limited to AD: Individuals with congophilic amyloid angiopathy (but not AD) also have an increased *APOE-ε4* allele frequency [26]. Further, having an *APOE-ε4* allele is associated with the presence and earlier onset of hemorrhage in cerebral amyloid angiopathy [27]. These results are all in accord with the hypothesis that apo E binds Aβ and influences its deposition or clearance.

By contrast to Aβ deposition, in our experience, neither the rate of accumulation of NFTs nor the degree of neuronal loss appears to be influenced by *APOE* genotype when the duration of illness is taken into account [14]. Several studies share the observation that *APOE-ε4* carriers do not accumulate greater numbers of NFTs than duration- and age-matched *APOE-ε3* individuals [14,28–30]. In other studies, however, a correlation has been found between the presence of *APOE-ε4* and higher Braak and Braak staging [31,32]; this analysis does not take into account duration of illness. Duration of illness is a relevant potential confounding factor, because NFTs and neuronal loss are strongly correlated with duration of dementia. Thus, the relation between *APOE-ε4* and the rates of accumulation of NFTs in the brains of AD patients remains controversial.

Whether *APOE* genotype influences NFT formation is important, because it is a test of the hypothesis proposed by Roses and colleagues that apo E binds *tau* and that apo E3 and apo E4 might differentially affect the rates of phosphorylation of *tau* to form NFTs.

APOE and Neuroimaging

Because *APOE-ε4/4* is thought to mark a group at high risk of developing dementia, *APOE* genotype has also been investigated as a predictive factor or covariable in neuroimaging studies in dementia. The magnetic resonance imaging (MRI) volumetric data reported to date by different groups in elderly nondemented persons disagree about whether *APOE-ε4* is associated with early anatomic changes. Soininen and Reikkinen have documented minor changes in hippocampal MRI volumes in nondemented elderly individuals with an *APOE-ε4/4* genotype compared to *APOE-ε4* noncarriers [33]. Contrary to this observation, Schmidt and colleagues found no differences in the hippocampal and parahippocampal volumes of nondemented elderly *APOE-ε4* carriers, even though they tended to perform significantly worse than noncarriers in learning and memory tasks [34]. Plassman and colleagues have assessed the MRI volumes of the hippocampal formation in 10 pairs of cognitively normal twins in their early sixties. They have found no association between *APOE* status and the volume of the hippocampus or the cognitive performance in this group [35].

By contrast to the uncertainty about whether *APOE-ε4* is associated with hippocampal volume loss in nondemented individuals at high risk of developing AD, in cases of established AD, *APOE-ε4* seems to lead to more severe changes. Using MRI volumetric assessments, Lehtovirta and colleagues observed that AD patients who inherit two copies of *APOE-ε4* have more prominent and selective volume loss in the medial temporal lobe structures (hippocampus and amygdala) than do those who lack an *APOE-ε4* allele, despite similar severity of dementia [36]. A similar tendency was observed in another study, although the differences among *APOE* genotype subgroups did not reach statistical significance [37].

Along the same lines, other groups have focused on the study of relatives at risk for familial AD using positron emission tomography analysis. Small and colleagues observed that *APOE-ε4* heterozygotes with a well-documented familial history of AD had abnormally low rates of parietal lobe glucose metabolism [38]. Similarly, Reiman and colleagues have reported significantly reduced rates of glucose metabolism in asymptomatic *APOE-ε4* homozygotes, matching the regional distribution seen in AD [39].

DOES *APOE* GENOTYPE HELP IN THE DIFFERENTIAL DIAGNOSIS OF A PATIENT WITH DEMENTIA?

It has been suggested that the inheritance of *APOE-ε4* is a relatively specific risk factor for AD, and thus, the knowledge of *APOE* genotype might help in the differential diagnosis of patients with dementia. Although the number of individuals examined with other types of dementia remains fairly small, the *APOE-ε4* allele frequency does not differ in Pick's disease, progressive supranuclear palsy, Parkinson's disease, dementia with Lewy bodies without concomitant AD changes, amyotrophic lateral sclerosis, Creutzfeldt-Jakob disease, or Huntington's disease from that in the general population [14,40–45] (see Table 7.1). Some reports disagree with this conclusion, however [46,47]. Multi-infarct dementia is more controversial, in part because of difficulty in defining and identifying clinically cases with pure multi-infarct dementia without concomitant AD changes and also because of the well-established relationship between *APOE-ε4* and increased levels of cholesterol with a potential role in atherosclerosis [48,49]. In general, even though individuals with multi-infarct dementia might have a higher *APOE-ε4* allele frequency than that seen in the general population, it remains lower than that seen in AD [50,51].

How does this information impact clinical decision making? Overall, approximately half of the patients with AD probably do not have the *APOE-ε4* gene. In other words, depending on age of onset, the chance that someone with AD carries at least one copy of *APOE-ε4* is probably 50–60%, with the strongest risk seen in individuals who develop the first symptoms of dementia in the seventh decade of life [52]. Conversely, approximately one-fourth of patients with dementias other than AD have at least one copy of *APOE-ε4*. Thus, the presence of a single copy of *APOE-ε4* is not very helpful in clinical practice. On the other hand, in the case of *APOE-ε4/4*, the differences become more prominent. Fifteen percent of individuals with AD have inherited two copies of *APOE-ε4* compared with less than 2% for the general population or individuals with other types of dementia. Nonetheless, even though *APOE-ε4/4* has a higher risk and a stronger relationship to AD, the relationship does not apply to 100% of the cases. In one large population-based epidemiologic study, for example, more than half of individuals in their early eighties who are *APOE-ε4/4* remain cognitively normal on a simple mental status battery and delayed recall testing [53]. Thus, the relative benefit of the differences in *APOE* allele frequencies among different types of dementia might provide some help in the differential diagnosis of clinically atypical or difficult cases of dementia. In our hands this should be viewed with caution and treated the same way as other laboratory tests for risk factors in other medical conditions rather than as a diagnostic test itself.

For example, we consider two cases: Patient One is a 67-year-old patient who presents with a 2-year history of progressive cognitive decline, and a clinical diagnosis of probable AD is established. Should an *APOE* genotype test be requested? What would be the outcomes and interpretations of the test results?

If the *APOE* genotype is 2/2 or 2/3—genotypes somewhat less common in AD than in the general population (<1% and 5%, respectively, in the AD population)—one might reconsider the history but ultimately conclude that AD is the correct diagnosis.

If the *APOE* genotype is 3/3 (33% of the AD population), the test would not help to confirm the AD diagnosis because many AD patients are *APOE- ε3/3*; that is, they do not carry the *APOE-ε4* allele and thus only the clinical features would guide the final diagnosis.

If the *APOE* genotype is 3/4 (42% of the AD population), the diagnosis of the cause of dementia continues to rely mostly on the clinical features, because approximately 25% of individuals with non-AD pathologies have *APOE-ε4*.

If the *APOE* genotype is 4/4 (16% of the AD population), the genotype result is consistent with the clinical diagnosis but does not completely rule out other etiologies.

Patient Two is a 65-year-old patient who presents with a 3-year history of progressive dementia. During the last year, the family has noticed an accelerating cognitive deterioration and mild gait disturbances. A neuroimaging study shows generalized cortical atrophy and enlarged ventricles, slightly out of proportion to cortical atrophy. A diagnosis of normal pressure hydrocephalus (NPH) and consequent shunting is considered, although the possibility of underlying AD pathology cannot be ruled out with certainty. Repeated lumbar punctures are sometimes helpful in clarifying this situation, but in this hypothetical patient the results are equivocal. We suggest that in a case in which the differential diagnosis is unclear and a major change in management or prognosis would result from improved diagnostic accuracy, *APOE* genotyping may be useful. Thus, if this patient were *APOE-ε4/4*, the likelihood is that the symptoms are due to AD (rather than NPH), and an intracranial operation might be viewed with less enthusiasm; conversely, a genotype of *APOE-ε2/2* or *APOE-ε2/3* (less common in AD than in the general population) might sway judgment in favor of a shunt.

DOES *APOE* GENOTYPE HELP TO PREDICT WHICH INDIVIDUALS WILL DEVELOP COGNITIVE IMPAIRMENT IN THEIR ELDER YEARS?

Although *APOE-ε4* is clearly a risk factor for AD, the magnitude of that risk cannot be ascertained without knowledge from population-based studies. It is well established that a clinic-based patient with probable AD will have a high likelihood of having an *APOE-ε4* allele, but this information is based on a selected sample of individuals and may not generalize to the wider population. What is more important from a public health perspective is to know the chance that someone in the general population who is *APOE-ε4*–positive will develop cognitive impairment. How certain are we that *APOE* genotype allows an accurate prediction of dementia for asymptomatic individuals? Corder and colleagues initially estimated that in late-onset familial AD, the *APOE-ε4*–associated risk for dementia approached 100% by the age of 80 years [54]. This initial observation, however, was derived from a highly selected group of individuals with a very strong family history of AD. Therefore, it became crucial to address the risk of individuals in the general population. To date, several population-based studies have been carried out, and they have shown that the impact of *APOE* genotype on the likelihood of developing cognitive impairment in the general population is not as strong as it initially appeared [53,55–58]. In the largest study to date, we assessed the *APOE* allele frequencies in the Iowa 65+ Rural Health Study, one of the Established Populations for Epidemiological Study of the Elderly [53]. This study examined a cohort of 1,899 individuals who had been enrolled in a longitudinal 10-year population-based study. In this study, simple cognitive screening batteries (The Short Portable Mental Status Questionnaire) and a verbal memory test served as markers of individuals who developed cognitive impairment. This study confirmed that the inheritance of the *APOE-ε4* is associated with an increased risk for development of cognitive impairment, but the magnitude of this effect was fairly modest, with an odds ratio for developing impairment of 1.37 (95% confidence interval 1.01–1.85; $P = .045$). In addition, the presence of the *APOE-ε2* allele was associated with a decreased chance of developing cognitive decline, with an odds ratio of 0.53 (95% confidence interval 0.37–0.78; $P = .001$). The *APOE-ε4* and *APOE-ε2* effects were both more pronounced in women than in men. The limitations of using *APOE* genotype to identify individuals at risk for developing dementia were most clear in a subanalysis of 34 people older than 80 years who had an *APOE-ε4/4* genotype: 85% of them (n = 34, average age = 81 years) scored in the unimpaired range on a screening mental status test. Thus, the majority of individuals in this study reached old age without cognitive impairment despite inheritance of one or two *APOE-ε4* alleles. The Framingham study [58] reached a conclusion similar to ours: Approximately half of the elderly individuals in this cohort who carried two copies of *APOE-ε4* did not develop dementia.

The data derived from several population-based studies reflect a range in odds ratios associated with *APOE-ε4*, from approximately 1.4 (the Iowa study) to approximately 3.7 (the Framingham study) [53,55–58]. The differences in risk ratios among different studies might be due in part to differences in study design, population differences, and differences in age and gender distribution in those populations. Despite these differences, it is clear now that the inheritance of one or even two copies of *APOE-ε4* does not predict inevitable dementia in old age. For this reason, an *APOE* genotype test for an unimpaired individual cannot be recommended as a prognostic indicator of cognitive decline in asymptomatic individuals in the general population. This conclusion is based on scientific facts and should alone discourage *APOE* testing in the general population. There are additional considerations that reinforce this view. The concern that individuals or third parties (e.g., family, insurers, employers) might use a genetic test that is not particularly informative to make potentially unwise decisions has been raised and should be weighed even in the assessment of symptomatic individuals.

In the first patient described above, a clinical diagnosis of probable AD was made, and the *APOE* genotype was 3/4. The clinical history revealed that one of his three siblings died at 80 years with a clinical diagnosis of dementia. The patient's 40-year-old daughter wants to know what her chances are of developing AD, and she asks if she could have an *APOE* genotype performed. She was advised not to have the test due to the lack of useful information in her case, but she went to another doctor who ordered the test and she came back to clinic with the results.

The utility of this test result in an asymptomatic individual is limited by several factors:

1. The uncertain natural history of asymptomatic individuals who have inherited one or two *APOE-ε4* alleles, as highlighted by the population-based studies described above.
2. The uncertainty regarding how much of the risk associated with a positive family history of AD can be attributed to *APOE* genotype. Some estimates suggest that 50% or more of the genetic risk of late-onset AD is due to still unknown genes.

Thus, a "good" genotype—*APOE-ε3/3*, for example—might be falsely reassuring, both because many individuals who are *APOE-ε3/3* still develop AD and because the perceived genetic risk in this family might be due to a non–*APOE*-mediated mechanism.

A "bad" genotype—*APOE-ε4/4*, for example—still provides uncertainty, with approximately half of *APOE-ε4/4* individuals older than 80 years remaining cognitively unimpaired.

The complexity here relies on the fact that *APOE-ε4*, even if homozygous, remains a risk factor rather than acting as a strongly penetrant recessive gene, with which inheritance of two copies is certain to yield a phenotype.

POSSIBLE NEUROBIOLOGICAL ROLES OF *APOE* AND THEIR IMPLICATIONS IN THE PATHOGENESIS OF ALZHEIMER'S DISEASE

Apolipoprotein E and Cerebrospinal Fluid Measurements

Several observations suggest a neurobiological role for apo E. Apo E messenger RNA is abundant in the brain, where it is mostly synthesized and secreted by astrocytes [59,60]. Apo E–containing lipoproteins are present in the cerebrospinal fluid (CSF), and they appear to play a major role in lipid transport in the central nervous system (CNS) [61]. CSF levels of apo E in AD and other forms of dementia have been compared to the levels in nondemented individuals. Some studies [62–65] found that the levels of apo E in CSF from patients with AD and other forms of dementia are reduced when compared to those of nondemented controls, although they do not seem to correlate with the apo E4 isoform or the progression and severity of dementia. In other studies, and in our own data, however, no significant differences in CSF apo E level were detected between AD cases and control subjects or patients with other neurologic diseases [66,67]. The influence of *APOE* genotype has also been studied with regard to *tau* and Aβ determinations in the CSF. One or two copies of *APOE-ε4* did influence the presence of increased CSF *tau* levels in one study [68], although in other studies, *APOE* genotype has not influenced CSF levels of Aβ, soluble APP, or *tau* [69–71].

Apolipoprotein E and Amyloid

The most robust neuropathologic phenotype of the *APOE-ε4* genotype is increased Aβ deposition. There are two major hypotheses of how differences in apo E protein isoform could affect amyloid levels in the brain of AD patients: First, apo E could be involved in the clearance of Aβ; second, apo E could be involved in the deposition of Aβ. If apo E affects clearance of Aβ, apo E4 might perform this clearance function less well than apo E3, leading to an increased accumulation of Aβ. Clearance of apo E complexes could occur through several known apo E receptors. This hypothesis is composed of two components: an association of apo E with Aβ and an interaction between apo E–Aβ complexes and apo E receptors. In vitro experiments have shown that apo E isoforms on lipoproteins interact with Aβ peptide, with apo E3 displaying a more avid interaction with Aβ than apo E4 [72,73]. Other studies have also found interactions between physiologic lipoproteins and the Aβ peptide [74,75]. These apo E-lipoprotein-Aβ complexes could then be cleared by apo E receptors. We have examined the AD brain for apo E and apo E receptors by immunohistochemistry. Apo E immunostains SPs and amyloid-containing vessels [76]. One of the apo E receptors, the low-density lipoprotein receptor–related protein (LRP), is also found on plaques and amyloid-containing vessels as well as on neurons and reactive astrocytes [9]. This receptor is a multifunctional receptor that binds a variety of ligands and internalizes them for endosomal and lysosomal degradation [77,78]. Dysfunction of Aβ clearance by LRP or other apo E receptors could underlie the accumulation of Aβ seen in AD.

The second possibility is that apo E affects the deposition of Aβ. Several studies suggested that apo E promotes Aβ aggregation (with apo E4 causing greater aggregation of Aβ than does apo E3), and other studies indicated that apo E prevents Aβ aggregation (with apo E4 being less effective than apo E3). Strittmatter and colleagues [6,79] showed that purified apo E isoforms (as opposed to apo E on lipoproteins) interact with Aβ peptide in vitro and that apo E4 displayed more avid interaction and formed more stable complexes with Aβ than did apo E3. In addition, morphologic studies using electron microscopy have revealed that when apo E4 and Aβ peptide are incubated together, a dense network of very long monofibrils is formed, and the spontaneous fibrillogenesis of Aβ peptides is enhanced, whereas in the presence of apo E3, the monofibril complexes are less dense and the network simpler [80–82]. These observations favor a model in which an enhanced and more complex nature of the amyloid deposits in the presence of apo E4 in the brain might enhance the extent of amyloid deposition and plaque formation. There are also data suggesting that apo E inhibits amyloid deposition [83]. For example, Pillot and colleagues [84] found that at low concentrations, only apo E2 and apo E3 isoforms are potent inhibitors of the amyloid peptide aggregation properties in vitro, whereas the apo E4 isoform has no effect. In this study, the protective effect of apo E is suggested to be mediated by the formation of stable apo E–amyloid peptide complexes, with specific interaction between apo E2 and apo E3 (but not apo E4) and amyloid C-terminal fragments [84]. Along the same lines, Yang and colleagues have reported apo E isoform–dependent binding to Aβ with apo E2 and apo E3 (either recombinant or derived from human plasma) binding Aβ more avidly and forming more efficient apo E–Aβ complexes than the apo E4 isoform [85].

Apolipoprotein E and *Tau*

The interaction between apo E and *tau* remains controversial. *tau* is a microtubule-associated phosphoprotein that stabilizes the neuronal microtubules; when hyperphosphorylated, it loses the ability to bind with microtubules. Hyperphosphorylated *tau* is known to be one of the main components of another neuropathologic hallmark of AD, NFTs. Strittmatter and colleagues [86] initially reported that *tau* interacts with apo E3 in vitro but not with apo E4. Based on this observation, they proposed a model in which the interaction of apo E3 with *tau* could prevent its hyperphosphorylation, allowing its normal function in stabilization of microtubules. In the presence of apo E4, *tau* could become hyperphosphorylated and thus inactive, promoting the formation of NFTs. However, numerous independent observations [14,28–30] that *APOE-ε4* carriers do not accumulate a greater number of NFTs than duration- and age-matched *APOE-ε3* individuals argue against this hypothesis. The crucial link between Aβ (or other APP metabolites) and apo E4 and neuronal and synaptic alterations present in AD brains is still unknown.

Apolipoprotein E, Neurodegeneration, and Neuroprotection

Additional clues about the possible neurobiological role of apo E in the CNS come from certain analogies made several years ago on the functions that apo E plays in the peripheral nervous system. It is known that apo E plus a source of cholesterol promotes marked neurite extension in dorsal root ganglion cells in culture [87]. More than that, apo E levels dramatically increase after peripheral nerve injury [88,89]. Apo E seems to participate in the removal of lipids generated after axon degeneration as well as in their redistribution to sprouting neurites for axon regeneration [90,91]. Based on this, several groups studied the different effects of apo E isoforms on neurite extension and branching of both peripheral nervous system and cortical neurons to further understand the role of apo E in a final pathway of neuronal repair and remodeling. Using CNS-derived neuronal cell lines, Nathan and colleagues and Fagan and colleagues [92,93] observed that beta–very-low-density lipoprotein (beta-VLDL) and high-density lipoprotein (HDL) enriched with apo E3 significantly enhanced neurite outgrowth and extension, whereas apo E4 inhibited it; the apo E3 effect was mediated by interaction with the LRP receptor. Because apo E is involved in the development and regeneration of the CNS, it was proposed that apo E might also be necessary to maintain neuronal synaptic connections. In apo E–deficient (knockout) homozygous mice, Masliah and colleagues [94] documented an age-dependent 15–40% loss of synaptophysin-immunoreactive nerve terminals and microtubule-associated protein 2–immunoreactive dendrites in the hippocampus and neocortex. The dendritic alterations in these mice were present as early as 4 months of age, with extensive dendritic vacuolization and disruption of the endomembrane system and cytoskeleton. Thus, apo E may have neuroprotective as well as neuroregenerative effects.

The effect of apo E treatment on development of Aβ-induced toxicity in vitro has been evaluated using hippocampal neurons [95,96]. Puttfarcken and colleagues [96] designed an experiment to study the effects of apo E3 and apo E4 isoforms on rat hippocampal neuronal cultures treated with or without Aβ. They observed that both apo E isoforms were neurotropic and increased neurite length. Moreover, both apo E isoforms conferred significant and comparable protection, attenuating the Aβ-induced reduction in neurite length and cell viability. In addition, an antioxidant activity of apo E has been proposed [97]. Miyata and colleagues reported that apo E possesses antioxidant activity in B_{12} cell cultures with allele-specific efficacy (E2 > E3 > E4) [97]. The potential neuroprotective role of apo E has also been tested in animal models of CNS injury. Several groups have found that after transient cerebral ischemia, apo E synthesis by astrocytes and the apo E uptake by neurons are markedly and selectively increased within the hippocampal CA1 region and the neocortex [98–101]. Similarly, apo E is synthesized and secreted by astrocytes in the hippocampus after lesions of the entorhinal cortex, with a likely role in the salvage and reuse of the nonesterified cholesterol released during terminal breakdown [102]. The development of apo E knockout animals has provided further insights in elucidating the physiologic role of apo E in the CNS. Apo E–deficient mice have deficits in behavioral tests of working memory that are accompanied by specific decreases in choline acetyltransferase activity in hippocampus and neocortex [103]. These experiments highlight a possible link between the neurobiological role of apo E and one of the most noticeable biochemical deficits present in AD brains: loss of acetylcholine. In this context, preliminary data, derived from retrospective analyses of therapeutic trials with acetylcholinesterase inhibitors, hint that some medications might be more effective in individuals with certain genotypes [104,105]. Thus, tacrine apparently exerted greater benefit in AD patients with *APOE-ε3* than in those with *APOE-*

ε4 genotypes [104]. This evaluation, however, must be replicated in other trials before it can be applied to clinical practice.

SUMMARY

The observation that *APOE* genotype is related to AD is an extraordinarily important advance in our understanding of the biology of this disease. Inheritance of *APOE-ε4* is an important risk factor for AD, and *APOE-ε2* is a negative or protective risk factor. From the point of view of understanding the pathophysiology of AD, these data are of great importance, even though, to date, the exact mechanisms that link apo E4 to the neuronal and synaptic alterations that underlie the cognitive deficits in AD remain unclear. From the point of view of predicting whether or not individuals will develop cognitive decline and AD in their elder years, the data available suggest that *APOE* genotype is not particularly informative. Population-based studies have shown that the predictive value of the *APOE* genotype test for an unimpaired individual is extremely limited and it cannot be recommended as a prognostic indicator of cognitive decline in asymptomatic individuals. *APOE* genotype could be potentially more useful in the differential diagnosis of patients with dementia, particularly in the context of a difficult clinical diagnosis. Even in this case, however, the potential harm that might result from a misinterpretation of test results by patients or third parties (e.g., families, employers, insurers) should be weighed against potential benefits. Furthermore, communicating genotype information should be done in the context of appropriate counseling to the patients and their families to clarify the meaning of genetic test results. It is possible that the better understanding of the role that apo E plays in AD in the future will one day help to guide therapeutic decisions for patients with dementia; if so, the clinical utility of *APOE* genotype will obviously be enhanced. Nonetheless, current clinical data suggest that the application of *APOE* genotype to predicting fates of individuals remains an inexact science.

REFERENCES

1. Goate AM, Chartier-Harlin CM, Mullan M, et al. Segregation of a missense mutation in the amyloid protein precursor gene with familial Alzheimer's disease. Nature 1991;349:704–709.
2. Chartier-Harlin M, Crawford F, Houlden H, et al. Early-onset Alzheimer's disease caused by mutations at codon 717 of the β-amyloid precursor protein gene. Nature 1991;353:844–846.
3. Sherrington R, Rogaev EI, Rogaeva EA, et al. Cloning a gene bearing missense mutations in early-onset familial Alzheimer's disease. Nature 1995;375:754–760.
4. Levy-Lahad E, Wasco W, Poorkaj P, et al. Candidate gene for the chromosome 1 familial Alzheimer's disease locus. Science 1995;269:973–977.
5. Tanzi R, Gaston S, Bush A, et al. Genetic heterogeneity of gene defects responsible for familial Alzheimer disease [review]. Genetica 1994;91:255–263.
6. Strittmatter WJ, Saunders AM, Schmechel D, et al. Apolipoprotein E: high-avidity binding to β-amyloid and increased frequency of type 4 allele in late-onset familial Alzheimer disease. Proc Natl Acad Sci U S A 1993;90:1977–1981.
7. Mahley RW. Apolipoprotein E: cholesterol transport protein with expanding role in cell biology. Science 1988;240:622–630.

8. Saunders AM, Strittmatter WJ, Schmechel D, et al. Association of apolipoprotein E allele ε4 with late-onset familial and sporadic Alzheimer's disease. Neurology 1993;43:1467–1472.
9. Rebeck GW, Reiter JS, Strickland DK, Hyman BT. Apolipoprotein E in sporadic Alzheimer's disease: allelic variation and receptor interactions. Neuron 1993;11:575–580.
10. Poirier J, Davignon J, Bouthillier D, et al. Apolipoprotein E polymorphism and Alzheimer's disease. Lancet 1993;342:697–699.
11. Corder EH, Saunders AM, Risch NJ, et al. Apolipoprotein E type 2 allele decreases the risk of late onset Alzheimer disease. Nat Genet 1994;7:180–184.
12. West HL, Rebeck GW, Hyman BT. Frequency of the apolipoprotein E ε2 allele is diminished in sporadic Alzheimer disease. Neurosci Lett 1994;175:46–48.
13. Mayeux R, Stern Y, Ottman R, et al. The apolipoprotein ε4 allele in patients with Alzheimer's disease. Ann Neurol 1993;34:752–754.
14. Gómez-Isla T, West HL, Rebeck GW, et al. Clinical and pathological correlates of apolipoprotein E ε4 in Alzheimer's disease. Ann Neurol 1996;39:62–70.
15. Norman J, Brookes AJ, Yates C, St Clair D. Apolipoprotein E genotype and its effect on duration and severity of early and late onset Alzheimer's disease. Br J Psychiatry 1995;167:533–536.
16. Growdon JH, Locascio JJ, Corkin S, et al. Apolipoprotein E genotype does not influence rates of cognitive decline in Alzheimer's disease. Neurology 1996;47:444–448.
17. Holmes T, Levy R, McLoughlin DM, et al. Apolipoprotein E: non-cognitive symptoms and cognitive decline in late onset Alzheimer's disease. J Neurol Neurosurg Psychiatry 1996;61:580–583.
18. Li G, Silverman JM, Altstiel LD, et al. Apolipoprotein E-epsilon 4 allele and familial risk in Alzheimer's disease. Genet Epidemiol 1996;13:285–298.
19. Kurz A, Egensperger R, Haupt M, et al. Apolipoprotein E epsilon 4 allele, cognitive decline, and deterioration of everyday performance in Alzheimer's disease. Neurology 1996;47:440–443.
20. Asada T, Kariya T, Yamagata Z, et al. Apo E e4 allele and cognitive decline in patients with Alzheimer's disease. Neurology 1996;47:603.
21. Dal Forno G, Rasmusson DX, Brandt J, et al. Apolipoprotein E genotype and rate of decline in probable Alzheimer's disease. Arch Neurol 1996;53:345–350.
22. Frisoni GB, Govoni S, Geroldi C, et al. Gene dose of the ε4 allele of apolipoprotein E and disease progression in sporadic late-onset Alzheimer's disease. Ann Neurol 1995;37:596–604.
23. Basun H, Grut M, Winblad B, Lannfelt L. Apolipoprotein epsilon 4 allele and disease progression in patients with late-onset Alzheimer's disease. Neurosci Lett 1995;183:32–34.
24. Schmechel DE, Saunders AM, Strittmatter WJ, et al. Increased amyloid β-peptide deposition as a consequence of apolipoprotein E genotype in late-onset Alzheimer's disease. Proc Natl Acad Sci U S A 1993;90:9649–9653.
25. Hyman BT, West H, Rebeck GW, et al. Quantitative analysis of senile plaques in Azheimer's disease: Observation of a log-normal size distribution and molecular epidemiology of differences associated with apolipoprotein E genotype and trisomy 21 (Down syndrome). Proc Natl Acad Sci U S A 1995;92: 3586–3590.
26. Greenberg SM, Rebeck GW, Vonsattel JPG, et al. Apolipoprotein E ε4 and cerebral hemorrhage associated with amyloid angiopathy. Ann Neurol 1995;38:254–259.
27. Greenberg SM, Briggs ME, Hyman BT, et al. Apolipoprotein E epsilon 4 is associated with the presence and earlier onset of hemorrhage in cerebral amyloid angiopathy. Stroke 1996;27:1333–1337.
28. Sparks DL, Scheff SW, Liu H, et al. Increased density of senile plaques (SP), but not neurofibrillary tangles (NFT), in non-demented individuals with the apolipoprotein E4 allele: comparison to confirmed Alzheimer's disease patients. J Neurol Sci 1996;138:97–104.
29. Landen M, Thorsell A, Wallin A, Blennow K. The apolipoprotein E allele epsilon 4 does not correlate with the number of senile plaques or neurofibrillary tangles in patients with Alzheimer's disease. J Neurol Neurosurg Psychiatry 1996;61:352–356.
30. Olichney JM, Hansen LA, Galasko D, et al. The apolipoprotein E epsilon 4 allele is associated with increased neuritic plaques and cerebral amyloid angiopathy in Alzheimer's disease and Lewy body variant. Neurology 1996;47:190–196.
31. Hansen LA, Galasko D, Samuel W, et al. Apolipoprotein-E epsilon-4 is associated with increased neurofibrillary pathology in the Lewy body variant of Alzheimer's disease. Neurosci Lett 1994;182:63–65.
32. Ohm TG, Kirca M, Bohl J, et al. Apolipoprotein E polymorphism influences not only cerebral senile plaque load but also Alzheimer-type neurofibrillary tangle formation. Neuroscience 1995;66:583–587.
33. Soininen HS, Riekkinen PJJ. Apolipoprotein E, memory and Alzheimer's disease. Trends Neurosci 1996;19:224–228.
34. Schmidt H, Schmidt R, Fazekas F, et al. Apolipoprotein E ε4 allele in the normal elderly: neuropsychologic and brain MRI correlates. Clin Genet 1996;50:293–299.

35. Plassman BL, Welsh-Bohmer KA, Bigler ED, et al. Apolipoprotein E epsilon 4 allele and hippocampal volume in twins with normal cognition. Neurology 1997;48:985–989.
36. Lehtovirta M, Laakso MP, Soininen H, et al. Volumes of hippocampus, amygdala and frontal lobe in Alzheimer's patients with different apolipoprotein E genotypes. Neuroscience 1995;67:65–72.
37. Yamaguchi S, Nakagawa T, Arai H, et al. Temporal progression of hippocampal atrophy and apolipoprotein E gene in Alzheimer's disease. J Am Geriatr Soc 1996;44:216–217.
38. Small GW, Mazziotta JC, Collins MT, et al. Apolipoprotein E type 4 allele and cerebral glucose metabolism in relatives at risk for familial Alzheimer's disease. JAMA 1995;273:942–947.
39. Reiman EM, Caselli RJ, Yun LS, et al. Preclinical evidence of Alzheimer's disease in persons homozygous for the epsilon 4 allele for apolipoprotein E. N Engl J Med 1996;334:752–758.
40. Marder K, Maestre G, Cote L, et al. The apolipoprotein epsilon 4 allele in Parkinson's disease with and without dementia. Neurology 1994;44:1330–1331.
41. Mui S, Rebeck GW, McKenna-Yasek D, et al. Apolipoprotein E ε4 allele is not associated with earlier age of onset in amyotrophic lateral sclerosis. Ann Neurol 1995;38:460–463.
42. Martinoli MG, Trojanowski JQ, Schmidt ML. Association of apolipoprotein epsilon 4 allele and neuropathologic findings in patients with dementia. Acta Neuropathol (Berl) 1995;90:239–243.
43. Nakagawa Y, Kitamoto T, Furukawa H, et al. Allelic variation of apolipoprotein E in Japanese sporadic Creutzfeldt-Jakob disease patients. Neurosci Lett 1995;187:209–211.
44. Salvatore M, Seeber A, Nacmias B, et al. Apolipoprotein E in sporadic and familial Creutzfeldt-Jakob disease. Neurosci Lett 1995;199:95–98.
45. Whitehead AS, Bertrandy S, Finnan F, et al. Frequency of the apolipoprotein E epsilon 4 allele in a case-control study of early onset Parkinson's disease. J Neurol Neurosurg Psychiatry 1996;61:347–351.
46. Amouyel P, Vidal O, Launay JM, Laplanche JL. The apolipoprotein E alleles as major susceptibility factors for Creutzfeldt-Jakob disease. The French Research Group on Epidemiology of Human Spongiform Encephalopathies. Lancet 1994;344:1315–1318.
47. Helisalmi S, Linnaranta K, Lehtovirta M, et al. Apolipoprotein E polymorphism in patients with different neurodegenerative disorders. Neurosci Lett 1996;205:61–64.
48. Hofman A, Ott A, Breteler MM, et al. Atherosclerosis, apolipoprotein E, and prevalence of dementia and Alzheimer's disease in the Rotterdam Study. Lancet 1997;349:151–154.
49. Slooter AJ, Tang MX, van Duijn CM, et al. Apolipoprotein E epsilon 4 and the risk of dementia with stroke. A population-based investigation. JAMA 1997;277:818–821.
50. Kawamata J, Tanaka S, Shimohama S, et al. Apolipoprotein E polymorphism in Japanese patients with Alzheimer's disease or vascular dementia. J Neurol Neurosurg Psychiatry 1994;57:1414–1416.
51. Treves TA, Bornstein NM, Chapman J, et al. APOE-epsilon 4 in patients with Alzheimer disease and vascular dementia. Alzheimer Dis Assoc Disord 1996;10:189–191.
52. Blacker D, Haines JL, Rodes L, et al. APOE-4 and age of onset of Alzheimer's disease: the NIMH genetics initiative. Neurology 1997;48:139–147.
53. Hyman BT, Gómez-Isla T, Briggs M, et al. Apolipoprotein E and cognitive change in an elderly population. Ann Neurol 1996;40:55–66.
54. Corder EH, Saunders AM, Strittmatter WJ, et al. Gene dose of apolipoprotein E type 4 allele and the risk of Alzheimer's disease in late onset families. Science 1993;261:921–923.
55. Feskens E, Havekes L, Kalmijn S, et al. Apolipoprotein ε4 allele and cognitive decline in elderly men. BMJ 1994;309:1202–1206.
56. Kuusisto J, Koivisto K, Kervinen K, et al. Association of apolipoprotein E phenotypes with late onset Alzheimer's disease: a population based study. BMJ 1994;309:636–638.
57. Henderson A, Easteal S, Jorm A, et al. Apolipoprotein E allele 4, dementia, and cognitive decline in a population sample. Lancet 1995;346:1387–1390.
58. Myers R, Schaefer E, Wilson P, et al. Apolipoprotein E Allelle 4 Is Associated with Dementia in the Framingham Study. In K Iqbal, J Mortimer, B Winblad, H Wisniewski (eds), Research Advances in Alzheimer's Disease and Related Disorders. Chichester, England: Wiley, 1995;63–72.
59. Boyles JK, Pitas RE, Wilson E, et al. Apolipoprotein E associated with astrocytic glia of the central nervous system and with nonmyelinating glia of the peripheral nervous system. J Clin Invest 1985; 76:1501–1513.
60. Pitas RE, Boyles JK, Lee SH, et al. Astrocytes synthesize apolipoprotein E and metabolize apolipoprotein E-containing lipoproteins. Biochim Biophys Acta 1987;917:148–161.
61. Pitas RE, Boyles JK, Lee SH, et al. Lipoproteins and their receptors in the central nervous system: characterization of the lipoproteins in cerebrospinal fluid and identification of apolipoprotein B, E (LDL) receptors in the brain. J Biol Chem 1987;262:14352–14360.
62. Blennow K, Hesse C, Fredman P. Cerebrospinal fluid apolipoprotein E is reduced in Alzheimer's disease. Neuroreport 1994;5:2534–2536.

63. Lehtimaki T, Pirtilla T, Mehta PD, et al. Apolipoprotein E (apoE) polymorphism and its influence on apoE concentration in the cerebrospinal fluid in Finnish patients with Alzheimer's disease. Hum Genet 1995;95:39–42.
64. Landen M, Hesse C, Fredman P, et al. Apolipoprotein E in cerebrospinal fluid from patients with Alzheimer's disease and other forms of dementia is reduced but without any correlation to the apo E4 isoform. Dementia 1996;7:273–278.
65. Skoog I, Hesse C, Fredman P, et al. Apolipoprotein E in cerebrospinal fluid in 85-year-old subjects. Relation to dementia, apolipoprotein E polymorphism, cerebral atrophy, and white matter lesions. Arch Neurol 1997;54:267–272.
66. Lefranc D, Vermersch P, Dallongeville J, et al. Relevance of the quantification of apolipoprotein E in the cerebrospinal fluid in Alzheimer's disease. Neurosci Lett 1996;212:91–94.
67. Rosler N, Wichart I, Jellinger KA. Intra vitam lumbar cerebrospinal fluid and serum and postmortem ventricular immunoreactive apolipoprotein E in patients with Alzheimer's disease. J Neurol Neurosurg Psychiatry 1996;60:452–454.
68. Blomberg M, Jensen M, Basun H, et al. Increasing cerebrospinal fluid *tau* levels in a subgroup of Alzheimer patients with apolipoprotein E allele epsilon 4 during 14 months follow-up. Neurosci Lett 1996;214:163–166.
69. Nitsch RM, Rebeck GW, Deng M, et al. Cerebrospinal fluid levels of amyloid β-protein in Alzheimer's disease: inverse correlation with severity of dementia and effect of apoE genotype. Ann Neurol 1995;37:512–518.
70. Motter R, Vigo-Pelfrey C, Kholodenko D, et al. Reduction of beta-amyloid peptide 42 in the cerebrospinal fluid of patients with Alzheimer disease. Ann Neurol 1995;38:643–648.
71. Arai H, Terajima M, Miura M, et al. *Tau* in the cerebrospinal fluid: a potential diagnostic marker in Alzheimer's disease. Ann Neurol 1995;38:649–652.
72. LaDu MJ, Falduto MT, Manelli AM, et al. Isoform-specific binding of apolipoprotein E to β-amyloid. J Biol Chem 1994;269:23403–23406.
73. LaDu MJ, Pederson TM, Frail DE, et al. Purification of apolipoprotein E attenuates isoform-specific binding to β-amyloid. J Biol Chem 1995;270:9030–9042.
74. Biere AL, Ostaszewski B, Stimson ER, et al. Amyloid β-peptide is transported on lipoproteins and albumin in human plasma. J Biol Chem 1996;271:32916–32922.
75. Koudinov AR, Koudinova NV, Kumar A, et al. Biochemical characterization of Alzheimer's soluble amyloid beta protein in human cerebrospinal fluid: association with high density lipoproteins. Biochem Biophys Res Commun 1996;223:592–597.
76. Wisniewski T, Frangione B. Apolipoprotein E: a pathological chaperone protein in patients with cerebral and systemic amyloid. Neurosci Lett 1992;135:235–238.
77. Strickland DK, Ashcom JD, Williams S, et al. Sequence identity between the α_2-macroglobulin receptor and low density lipoprotein receptor-related protein suggests that this molecule is a multifunctional receptor. J Biol Chem 1990;265:17401–17404.
78. Herz J. The LDL-receptor–related protein—portrait of a multifunctional receptor. Curr Opin Lipidol 1993;4:107–113.
79. Strittmatter WJ, Weisgraber KH, Huang D, et al. Binding of human apolipoprotein E to βA4 peptide: isoform specific effects and implications for late onset Alzheimer disease. Proc Natl Acad Sci U S A 1993;90:8098–8102.
80. Ma J, Yee A, Brewer HB, et al. Amyloid-associated proteins α_1-antichymotrypsin and apolipoprotein E promote assembly of Alzheimer β-protein into filaments. Nature 1994;372:92–94.
81. Sanan DA, Weisgraber KH, Russell SJ, et al. Apolipoprotein E associates with beta amyloid peptide of Alzheimer's disease to form novel monofibrils. J Clin Invest 1994;94:860–869.
82. Wisniewski T, Castano EM, Golabek A, et al. Acceleration of Alzheimer's disease fibril formation by apolipoprotein E in vitro. Am J Pathol 1994;145:1030–1035.
83. Evans KC, Berger EP, Cho CG, et al. Apolipoprotein E is a kinetic but not a thermodynamic inhibitor of amyloid formation: implications for the pathogenesis and treatment of Alzheimer disease. Proc Natl Acad Sci U S A 1995;92:763–767.
84. Pillot T, Goethals M, Vanloo B, et al. Specific modulation of the fusogenic properties of the Alzheimer beta-amyloid peptide by apolipoprotein E isoforms. Eur J Biochem 1997;243:650–659.
85. Yang DS, Smith JD, Zhou Z, et al. Characterization of the binding of amyloid-beta peptide to cell culture–derived native apolipoprotein E2, E3, and E4 isoforms and to isoforms from human plasma. J Neurochem 1997;68:721–725.
86. Strittmatter WJ, Weisgraber KH, Goedert M, et al. Hypothesis: microtubule instability and paired helical filament formation in the Alzheimer disease brain are related to apolipoprotein E genotype. Exp Neurol 1994;125:163–171.

87. Handelmann GE, Boyles JK, Weisgraber KH, et al. Effects of apolipoprotein E, beta-very low density lipoproteins, and cholesterol on the extension of neurites by rabbit dorsal root ganglion neurons in vitro. J Lipid Res 1992;33:1677–1688.
88. Müller HW, Gebicke-Härter PJ, Hangen DH, Shooter EM. A specific 37,000-dalton protein that accumulates in regenerating but not in nonregenerating mammalian nerves. Science 1985;228:499–501.
89. Ignatius MJ, Gebicke-Haerter PJ, Skene JHP, et al. Expression of apolipoprotein E during nerve degeneration and regeneration. Proc Natl Acad Sci U S A 1986;83:1125–1129.
90. Ignatius MJ, Shooter EM, Pitas RE, Mahley RW. Lipoprotein uptake by neuronal growth cones in vitro. Science 1987;236:959–962.
91. Boyles JK, Zoellner CD, Anderson LJ, et al. A role for apolipoprotein E, apolipoprotein A-I, and low density lipoprotein receptors in cholesterol transport during regeneration and remyelination of the rat sciatic nerve. J Clin Invest 1989;83:1015–1031.
92. Nathan BP, Bellosta S, Sanan DA, et al. Differential effects of apolipoproteins E3 and E4 on neuronal growth in vitro. Science 1994;264:850–852.
93. Fagan AM, Bu G, Daugherty A, Holtzman DM. Apolipoprotein E-containing high density lipoprotein promotes neurite outgrowth and is a ligand for the low density lipoprotein receptor-related protein. J Biol Chem 1996;271:30121–30125.
94. Masliah E, Mallory M, Ge N, et al. Neurodegeneration in the central nervous system of apoE-deficient mice. Exp Neurol 1995;136:107–122.
95. Whitson JS, Mims MP, Strittmatter WJ, et al. Attenuation of the neurotoxic effect of amyloid peptide by apolipoprotein E. Biochem Biophys Res Commun 1994;199:163–170.
96. Puttfarcken PS, Manelli AM, Falduto MT, et al. Effect of apolipoprotein E on neurite outgrowth and beta-amyloid-induced toxicity in developing rat primary hippocampal cultures. J Neurochem 1997;68:760–769.
97. Miyata M, Smith JD. Apolipoprotein E allele–specific antioxidant activity and effects on cytotoxicity by oxidative insults and beta-amyloid peptides. Nat Genet 1996;14:55–61.
98. Kida E, Pluta R, Lossinsky AS, et al. Complete cerebral ischemia with short-term survival in rat induced by cardiac arrest. II. Extracellular and intracellular accumulation of apolipoproteins E and J in the brain. Brain Res 1995;674:341–346.
99. Hall ED, Oostveen JA, Dunn E, Carter DB. Increased amyloid protein precursor and apolipoprotein E immunoreactivity in the selectively vulnerable hippocampus following transient forebrain ischemia in gerbils. Exp Neurol 1995;135:17–27.
100. Horsburgh K, Nicoll JA. Selective alterations in the cellular distribution of apolipoprotein E immunoreactivity following transient cerebral ischemia in the rat. Neuropathol Appl Neurobiol 1996;22:342–349.
101. Ali SM, Dunn E, Oostveen JA, et al. Induction of apolipoprotein E mRNA in the hippocampus of the gerbil after transient global ischemia. Mol Brain Res 1996;38:37–44.
102. Poirier J, Baccichet A, Dea D, Gauthier S. Cholesterol synthesis and lipoprotein reuptake during synaptic remodelling in hippocampus in adult rats. Neuroscience 1993;55:81–90.
103. Gordon I, Genis I, Grauer E, et al. Biochemical and cognitive studies of apolipoprotein-E-deficient mice. Mol Chem Neuropathol 1996;28:97–103.
104. Poirier J, Delisle MC, Quirion R, et al. Apolipoprotein E4 allele as a predictor of cholinergic deficits and treatment outcome in Alzheimer disease. Proc Natl Acad Sci U S A 1995;92:12269–12264.
105. Farlow MR, Lahiri DK, Poirier J, et al. Apolipoprotein E genotype and gender influence response to tacrine therapy. Ann NY Acad Sci 1996;802:101–110.

8 Anatomic Neuroimaging in the Dementias

Clifford R. Jack, Jr.

Many pathologic conditions are associated with dementia. This chapter is limited, however, to a discussion of dementia in the elderly. Many of the conditions discussed are neurodegenerative disorders. The discussion focuses on those neurodegenerative disorders for which dementia is a cardinal feature of the clinical presentation. The chapter emphasizes magnetic resonance imaging (MRI) over computed tomography (CT). MRI is now a widely available technology. Due to superior soft tissue contrast, multiplanar imaging capability, and freedom from bone-hardening artifacts, virtually every anatomic feature of the brain that is relevant to aging and dementia is depicted with greater precision and greater sensitivity with MRI than with CT.

IMAGE EVALUATION—QUANTITATION

Cross-sectional imaging studies, both MRI and CT, contain two primary types of information, morphologic information about the size and shape of an anatomic structure and intensity information. Cross-sectional images may be evaluated either qualitatively or quantitatively. For most clinical applications, images are evaluated qualitatively, whereas for many research applications some form of image quantitation is used. The most common morphologic alteration associated with dementing neurodegenerative disorders is atrophy, and atrophy has been quantified in different ways. Images may be ranked visually by assigning a degree of atrophy on the basis of visual impression. The most sophisticated schemes for qualitative ranking of images use a set of exemplar scans that illustrate the prescribed ranking scheme—for example, minimum, mild, moderate, and severe atrophy [1,2]. A panel of trained expert reviewers ranks the images of each study participant against those in the exemplar set. Measures of inter- and intra-rater reproducibility are established for the expert reviewers. A second approach to quantitation of brain morphology involves performing anatomically based measurements, which can be linear, planimetric, or volumetric. Because of the complex three-dimensional anatomic nature of the brain, volume measurements are more accurate descriptors of the clinical and pathologic process of interest than either linear or planimetric measurements. Linear measurements have an advantage, however, in terms of speed and simplicity.

Volume measurements of a brain structure from a set of cross-sectional images may be accomplished in two ways. With image-based stereologic techniques, a computerized or hard-copy grid is superimposed on the images, and the number of grid points that fall within the anatomic structure of interest is counted [3,4], and structure volume is estimated by Cavalieri's principle [5]. Alternatively, structure volume can be measured using the volume of interest approach, which requires that the boundaries be defined in all three dimensions and then segmented from adjacent tissues. Once that is accomplished, the number of voxels (or volume imaging elements) inside the volume of interest that has been defined by the segmentation procedure is counted, and the structure's volume is calculated by multiplying voxel number by voxel dimensions. Segmentation of an image may be accomplished manually, automatically, or with hybrid semi-automated approaches. The optimal approach depends on the intrinsic contrast properties of the imaging sequence used, the degree to which the anatomic structure of interest has contrast properties that differ significantly from adjacent tissue, and the desired precision of the measurement. For example, if the measurement of the volume of the ventricular system is the objective, then an automated or nearly automated approach is feasible due to the high intrinsic contrast on MRI or CT between the signal intensity of cerebrospinal fluid (CSF) and that of adjacent brain. Two commonly used semi-automated approaches to measure global and hemispheric brain or CSF volume are threshold-based techniques and feature-space techniques [6–8]. If, on the other hand, volume measurements of individual brain structures or brain regions are desired, then manual tracing of some or all of the structure boundaries is usually used (Figure 8.1). For example, the hippocampus is a structure of interest in the study of aging and dementia. Although much of the border between the hippocampus and adjacent structures is high contrast—CSF in the choroidal fissure and temporal horn and white matter in the underlying parahippocampal gyrus—some is low contrast. For this reason, nearly all investigators who have performed volumetric measurements of the hippocampus have manually outlined the borders of the hippocampus on serial planimetric images to segment the hippocampus from adjacent tissues.

Brain atrophy is a negative phenomenon. Measurements of atrophy do not lend themselves to traditional positive counting criteria (e.g., counting the number of senile plaques or neurofibrillary tangles per high-power field). To quantify atrophy, the volume of a given brain structure in any patient must be measured and compared to what it "should be" in the absence of disease. To accomplish this, measurements in any individual patient must be compared to those in an appropriate control group [9–11]. Moreover, because the numeric values that result from any image-based volume measurement are highly dependent on technique, normative technique-specific volumetric values in control individuals should be generated for each laboratory.

A volume measure of any given brain structure will contain several important sources of variability [12]. For the sake of discussion, assume that the structure of interest is the hippocampus, and volume measurements of this structure are being

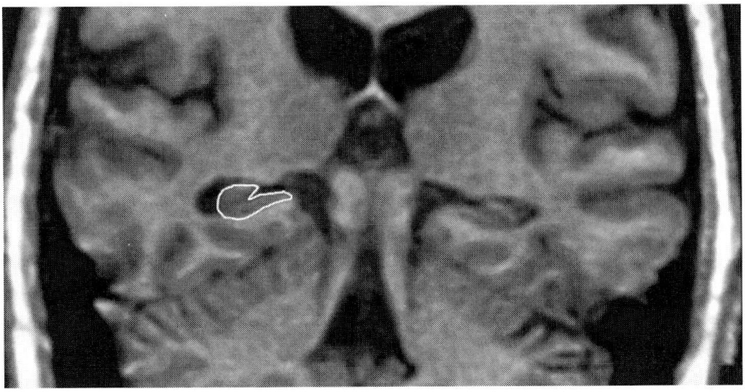

Figure 8.1 Hippocampal boundary tracing. Portions of the hippocampal boundary do not lend themselves to automated image segmentation routines. Therefore, the boundary of the hippocampus is typically traced (illustrated on the patient's right) on successive planimetric images to segment the hippocampus from neighboring structures.

performed in a study of Alzheimer's disease (AD). The hippocampal volume measurement in any AD patient will contain variability that is due to (1) the disease process itself; (2) measurement error; (3) intersubject variability in hippocampal size due to age, gender, and head size; and (4) normal intersubject baseline differences in hippocampal size. The quantity that is desired from the measurement is variation in volume due to the disease process. To eliminate or minimize the variance in volume measurements due to measurement error, scrupulous attention must be paid to the technical quality of the images at the time they are acquired, rigorous anatomically based borders of the hippocampus must be established, and reliability of the measurements must be documented through measurements of test-retest reproducibility [10]. A common approach used to accommodate variability in hippocampal volume due to intersubject differences in head size is to normalize each hippocampal volume measurement by that individual's total intracranial volume. This can be accomplished either by forming the ratio of the hippocampus to the total intracranial volume or by adjusting the raw hippocampal volume by the individual's total intracranial volume using a covariance approach [9,13]. Hippocampal volume will also vary as a function of gender and age. An approach we have taken is to estimate normal percentiles for hippocampal volume based on a large number of elderly control individuals [14]. The effects of gender and age are identified through regression analysis. The hippocampal volume measurement of any AD patient can then be assigned a z score relative to controls that have been appropriately adjusted for that particular patient's age, gender, and head size.

The second major MRI and CT finding that may be quantified is parenchymal signal change. Like atrophy, signal change has been quantified by viewer ranking as well as by direct quantitative measurement. A topic of interest in aging and dementia has been the significance of the severity of leukoariosis. The most common approach used has been ranking individual scans by expert reviewers on an ordinal severity scale—for example, minimum, mild, moderate, or severe leukoariosis. Formal measurements of tissue intensity have been tried as well, although less frequently. CT measures of intensity in Hounsfield units are directly related to the tissue x-ray attenuation coefficient. MRI measures of tissue intensity are more complicated and are influenced by multiple MRI parameters, the most important being tissue T1 and T2 relaxation times. These intrinsic properties of any tissue are exponential functions that are ideally measured by the acquisition of multiple images with varying echo times or repetition times. Several groups, including our own, have explored the feasibility of formal tissue T2 relaxation measurements in AD without much success [15,16].

NORMAL AGING

A distinction is often made between usual aging and successful aging [17]. With advancing age, the prevalence of a number of vascular risk factors increases, such as hypertension, atherosclerotic disease, and diabetes mellitus. Declines in a number of other physiologic indices as well as cognitive performance are also observed. *Usual aging* is defined as the absence of overt neurologic symptoms and includes individuals with the aforementioned comorbid conditions. In contrast, *successful aging* refers to aging that is not accompanied by any noticeable decline in physiologic or cognitive measures when compared to younger individuals. Most imaging studies of aging have included subjects who fall into the category of usual aging. Nearly all such imaging studies find an increase in the prevalence of three imaging findings with advancing age: (1) cerebral atrophy, accompanied by passive enlargement of cerebral CSF spaces, (2) areas of altered signal in the white matter and the central nuclei (increased signal on T2-weighted MRI, decreased signal on T1-weighted MRI, and hypointensity on CT), and (3) progressive decrease in the MRI signal intensity of the extrapyramidal nuclei [17]. Given the makeup of the subjects included in most imaging studies of aging, however, it is unclear whether the aforementioned imaging changes represent an inevitable consequence of aging or the result of conditions, such as hypertension, that promote global neuroanatomic degeneration and also increase in prevalence with age, thus imposing an increasing burden of cerebral degenerative changes on the population with increasing age. In support of the latter notion, DeCarli and colleagues [18] studied a group of successfully aging elderly individuals and found no evidence of age-related atrophy of the temporal lobe.

Atrophy

Numerous studies have been performed with CT and MRI documenting the relationship between cerebral atrophy and usual aging. Measurements have included qualitative ranking of cerebral atrophy by experts; linear measurements such as the bicaudate ratio; planimetric measurements of brain and CSF spaces; and volume measurements of cerebral CSF spaces, whole brain, gray matter, and white matter [19]. One point that has been controversial is the rate of cerebral atrophy in usual aging. Most studies report a linear decline in brain volume with advancing age, beginning sometime in middle to old age. The "knee" of the volume versus age curve has been variably located in the fifth, sixth, or seventh decade [20–26]. The rate of age-related brain atrophy was noted to be different in men than in women [20,22,27]. Whereas most studies have assessed global and hemispheric atrophy with advancing age, studies during the 1990s indicate that different portions of the brain may be more susceptible to age-related atrophy than are others [18,20,21,24–29].

Normal Focal Brain Hyperintensities

A widely recognized phenomenon is the increase in prevalence of focal and confluent areas of increased signal intensity on T2-weighted MRI in the white matter and central nuclei of individuals with increasing age, which is discussed in the section on Leukoariosis and Usual Aging. Elevated signal intensity in several areas of the brain, however, is a normal finding even in young individuals. The parietal-pontine tracts in the posterior portion of the internal capsule normally have less intense myelin staining than do adjacent white matter tracks. These areas, therefore, may appear as bilaterally symmetric focal bright areas as a normal variant [30].

Hyperintense foci exist in many normal younger and middle-aged individuals anterior and lateral to the frontal horns [31]. The myelin content generally is decreased in this area accounting in part for the increased signal. In addition, the ependymal lining may be focally discontinuous in this area, with adjacent gliosis, a benign variant termed *ependymitis granularis*.

Dilated perivascular spaces are commonly seen in the anterior-inferior portion of the putamen and along the course of penetrating hemispheric medullary arterioles. Although dilated perivascular spaces can normally be seen in younger individuals, the prevalence and size increase with advancing age, presumably due to increased tortuosity of penetrating medullary arterioles with advancing age. Distinction between dilated perivascular spaces and lacunar infarction is a common problem. The following guidelines are useful: Lacunar infarctions are not isointense to CSF on all imaging sequences unless they have undergone cystic change, larger than 5 mm in diameter, usually asymmetric, and located in the upper two-thirds of the putamen. Conversely, dilated perivascular spaces are isointense to CSF on all pulse sequences, bilaterally symmetric, less than 5 mm in diameter, and typically located in the inferior one-third of the putamen [32–34].

Leukoariosis and Usual Aging

Leukoariosis is a popular term used to describe a radiographic abnormality seen frequently in the hemispheric white matter and central nuclei of elderly individuals [35]. The pathologic findings are discussed in the section on Vascular Dementia. The prevalence of leukoariosis varies among different studies, but in the Cardiovascular Health Study it was 87% in all subjects and 83% in subjects without a clinical history of prior stroke [28]. Leukoariosis increases in prevalence with age and the presence of vascular disease risk factors. The published literature on the subject of leukoariosis and impaired cognition in usual aging can be divided into three relevant categories.

1. *The association between leukoariosis and impaired cognition.* Some publications do [36–45] and some do not [46–52] support the idea that among normally functioning elderly people, those with the greater volumetric burden of leukoariosis tend to perform more poorly on cognitive tasks. Worth noting, however, is that the Cardiovascular Health Study, which is by far the largest such study published, found a relationship between cognitive impairment and volumetric burden of leukoariosis [42].

2. *The association between hypertension and cognition.* Several large epidemiologic studies have conclusively documented a link between hypertension and cognitive dysfunction in otherwise healthy elderly people [53–58]. Hypertension in midlife has been linked with cognitive dysfunction in those same individuals decades later [59].

3. *The association between hypertension and leukoariosis.* Virtually all studies have found a positive association between leukoariosis and hypertension [28,44,60–69]. These strong epidemiologic links support the notion that hypertension is fundamental to the pathogenesis of leukoariosis and that leukoariosis is a marker of chronic or episodic hypoperfusion in the distribution of the penetrating arterioles. It is found frequently enough in elderly persons, however, that a legitimate argument may be raised that it is a feature of usual aging.

Iron Deposition

The third distinct change in the brain associated with aging is progressive decrease in signal intensity of the extrapyramidal nuclei, which is most pronounced on T2-weighted imaging sequences [17]. This is believed to be due to deposition of storage iron in the brain, although the precise site of iron storage and the form of stored iron has been controversial [70–72]. During the first decade of life, the signal intensity of the extrapyramidal nuclei is equal to that of cortical gray matter. In most usual aging subjects thereafter, there is a progressive decrease in signal intensity of the globus pallidus, red nucleus, pars reticula of the substantia nigra, caudate, and putamen [73,74] (Figure 8.2). The signal intensity of the thalamus normally remains unchanged throughout life. Low-intensity changes in the cortical ribbon, particularly in the motor cortex, presumably due to iron deposition, have also been correlated with usual aging as well as certain neurodegenerative disorders such as amyotrophic lateral sclerosis (ALS) [75].

ALZHEIMER'S DISEASE

The pathologic hallmarks of AD are senile plaques, neurofibrillary tangles, cell death of selectively vulnerable neuronal populations, and decreased density of synapses and dendritic spines [76–87]. On a macroscopic level, the primary abnormality associated with AD is cerebral atrophy, which is more advanced than that in age-matched controls. It is this feature of the pathology of AD that anatomic neuroimaging techniques seek to capture. Which of the preceding histologic abnormalities represents the "primary event" of AD is a highly contested topic. Nonetheless, it has been firmly established that neurofibrillary change does not

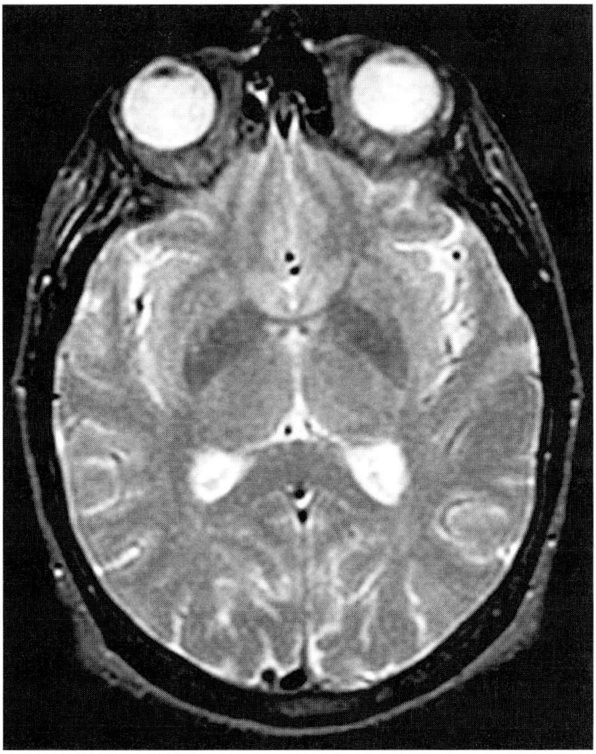

Figure 8.2 Iron deposition in usual aging. Decreased signal intensity in the putamen and other central nuclei on T2-weighted magnetic resonance images is a feature of usual aging, as illustrated in a cognitively normal 68-year-old woman.

progress globally at a constant rate. Rather, neurofibrillary changes begin locally in a laminar and cell-specific fashion in the entorhinal cortex, then spread to the hippocampus and related medial temporal lobe limbic areas, and ultimately to higher-order association cortices, sparing primary sensory and sensorimotor areas [76,78,80,81,88–90]. National Institutes of Health neuropathologic criteria for diagnosing AD include the Braak [78–80] criteria for staging neurofibrillary change, which are based on the concept of stereotypic progression of the disease from the medial temporal lobe to other areas of the brain. The concept of AD, or at least early AD, as a medial temporal lobe limbic disorder is strengthened by the observations that the earliest functional deficit found in patients who progress to AD is one of declarative memory, and the regions of the brain that are most closely linked with declarative memory function are the medial temporal lobe limbic areas [77,91–99].

Imaging Cerebral Atrophy in Alzheimer's Disease

Quantitation of cerebral atrophy by cross-sectional imaging has been used extensively in the study of AD. A variety of measurements have been used in an

Table 8.1 Methods for quantifying cerebral atrophy in Alzheimer's disease

Measures of global and hemispheric atrophy	
	Qualitative assessment and ranking of ventricular size and brain atrophy
	Linear measures of the width of the frontal horns, third ventricle, foramen of Monro, and cortical sulci
	Area measures of the lateral ventricles, frontal horns, and third ventricle interhemispheric fissure
	Volumetric measures of the ventricles and subarachnoid space
Measures of medial temporal atrophy	
	Qualitative assessment and ranking of the temporal horn, choroidal-hippocampal fissure, and suprasellar cistern
	Linear measurements of the interuncal distance and width of the medial temporal lobe
	Area measurements of the choroidal-hippocampal fissure complex, and the hippocampal formation itself
	Volume measurements of the hippocampus, amygdala, parahippocampal gyrus, and temporal horn

attempt to separate patients with clinically probable AD from age-matched controls. The various measures for the diagnosis of AD that are outlined in Table 8.1 can be divided into those that are designed to assess global and hemispheric atrophy [7,100–108] and those that are designed primarily to assess medial temporal lobe atrophy [11,14,106,109–137]. Likewise, the anatomic features that have been measured can be divided into measurements of CSF spaces as indirect markers of cerebral atrophy and measurements of brain parenchyma itself as direct markers of cerebral atrophy.

All approaches have been successful to some degree. The usefulness of anatomic measures for the diagnosis of AD in individual patients is limited, however, because although mean values of AD patients and controls were significantly different, overlap between the two groups was present in most studies. More emphasis has been placed on MRI-based volumetric medial temporal lobe measurements, particularly of the hippocampi [11,14,125–135]. This trend was driven by (1) recognition that the most sensitive imaging markers were likely to be found in the areas of the brain in which the disease initially manifested itself [76,78,80,81,88–90], and (2) the widespread introduction of MRI technology, which made high-quality images of the medial temporal lobe regions feasible (Figure 8.3).

Early Diagnosis of Alzheimer's Disease

In each person who develops AD, the transition from normal cognition to clearly recognizable AD occurs gradually over a number of years, without an abrupt transition point. It is widely presumed that the pathologic substrate of the cognitive decline that characterizes AD follows a similar slowly progressive course. Progressive accumulation of the degenerative pathologic markers of AD is ongoing for years before manifestation of any obvious clinical symptoms. At the time that a clinical diagnosis of AD can be made with a relatively high degree of certainty, extensive and presumably irreversible degenerative pathologic changes have already occurred. No definitive therapeutic interventions that retard, arrest, or

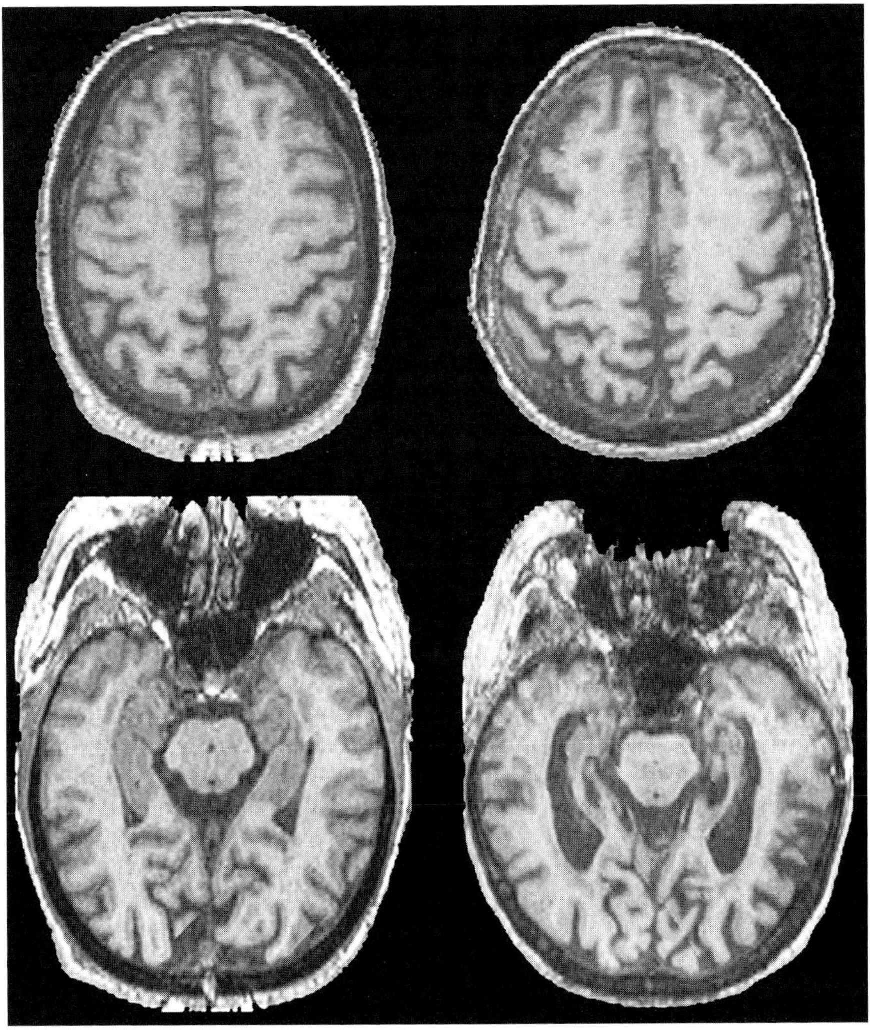

A

Figure 8.3 Medial temporal lobe atrophy in Alzheimer's disease. (A) Axial T1-weighted images through the supraventricular portion of the brain (*top row*) and through the temporal lobes (*bottom row*) in an elderly control (*left*) and a probable AD patient (*right*). Both the control and AD patient demonstrate some degree of generalized global/ hemispheric cerebral atrophy on the cephalad anatomic sections (*top row*); however, the degree of atrophy in the hippocampus and medial temporal lobe is significantly more severe in the patient with AD (*right*) when compared to the control subject (*left*).

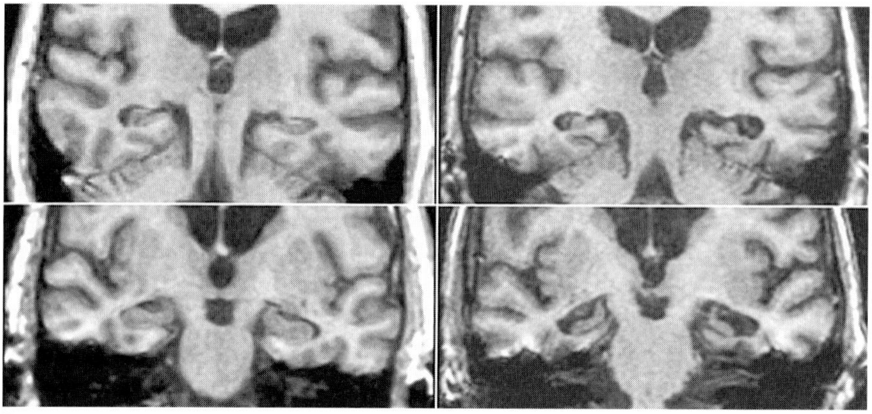

B

Figure 8.3 (continued) (B) Coronal T1-weighted images of a control subject (*left*) and an AD patient (*right*) through the body of the hippocampus (*top row*) and the head of the hippocampus (*bottom row*). Note the striking atrophy of the hippocampus in the AD patient compared to that of the control.

reverse the disease process of AD have been identified. If and when effective therapies are developed, however, the appropriate point at which to intervene must be before the development of extensive, irreversible pathologic damage. The challenge that exists in the diagnosis of AD, therefore, is to develop an approach that will enable the diagnosis to be made before the development of the fully manifest clinical syndrome. Several investigators have pursued MRI-based volume measurements of the hippocampus as a means of early diagnosis of AD and have shown that the hippocampi of patients in the earliest or mildest stages of AD, as well as patients with an age-associated memory impairment, have significant hippocampal atrophy with respect to age-matched control subjects [14,125,135,138].

In a study of probable AD patients at our institution, 94 AD patients were ranked with respect to disease severity by the clinical dementia rating (CDR) score [14]. Thirty-six of these had very mild disease (CDR = 0.5), 43 had mild disease (CDR = 1), and 15 had moderate disease (CDR = 2). Thirty-five of the 36 AD patients (97%) with CDR = 0.5 had hippocampal volumes that fell below the mean value of age- and gender-matched controls, indicating that MRI-based volume measurements of the hippocampus are sensitive markers of the pathology of AD in its earliest and mildest clinically evident form. In this same study, a direct correlation was seen between CDR score and mean hippocampal volume among the 94 AD patients. The mean hippocampal volume for AD patients by severity of disease were as follows: CDR = 0.5, fourth percentile relative to age- and gender-matched controls; CDR = 1, second percentile; and CDR = 2, first percentile. These findings indicate a direct correlation between in vivo hippocampal volume measurements and clinically relevant measures of disease severity.

Little information is present in the literature on the topic of the prediction of AD by anatomic imaging in individuals who were asymptomatic or "presymptomatic" at the time a baseline imaging study was performed. DeLeon and colleagues [112] reported that cross-sectional viewer ratings of medial temporal lobe atrophy were able to predict which subjects would develop AD versus which would remain stable. Fox and colleagues [139,140] found that serial hippocampal volume measurements completely separated cognitively stable controls from patients known to have a familial autosomal dominant mutation for AD at the point when the patients began to experience cognitive decline (presumably the earliest manifestation of the disease itself). In a study of the "oldest old," Kaye and colleagues [141], on the other hand, found no difference in the rate of hippocampal volume loss over time between cognitively stable subjects and patients who later became demented, but did find a greater rate of temporal lobe atrophy in patients who became demented.

Longitudinal Imaging Studies

The number of true longitudinal (serial measurements) studies reported in the literature is relatively small. Several CT studies of ventricular volume have shown that the rate at which the ventricular system increases in size over time in AD patients exceeds that in elderly controls [116,142–145]. Few studies using serial measurements of medial temporal lobe structures have been reported to date. Smith and Jobst [146] found that serial CT-based linear measurements of medial temporal lobe thickness completely separated controls from patients with AD. Our own data on serial MRI measurements indicate that although the mean annualized rates of hippocampal atrophy and temporal horn enlargement are significantly different between controls and AD patients, there is substantial overlap between the two groups [147].

Parenchymal Signal Intensity Alterations in Alzheimer's Disease

Gliosis is a feature of the pathology of AD; therefore, one might expect T2 measurements in areas of the brain most severely affected (the medial temporal lobe) to differ between AD patients and controls. Increased T2 signal intensity in the hippocampus has been reported in AD patients [148,149]. Kirsch and colleagues [150], using a two-point fit, measured the T2 relaxation time in the hippocampus of probable AD patients and reported that the values exceeded those of nondemented, age-matched elderly individuals. They concluded that measurements of hippocampal T2 relaxation times were clinically useful as a marker of both the presence and severity of AD. On the other hand, Laasko and colleagues [16] measured the T2 relaxation times of the hippocampus and found considerable overlap among the study groups and reported that T2 relaxometry was not a useful method for diagnosing early AD. To resolve the conflicting results from these studies, we measured the T2 relaxation times in the hippocampi in 123 subjects: 62 AD patients and 61 elderly nondemented controls [15]. We found complete overlap in the distribution of T2 relaxation values between the two clinical groups, with no difference in the mean hippocampal T2 relaxation values between controls and AD patients. We concluded that hippocampal T2 relaxation measurements are not useful in distinguishing between controls and AD patients.

Although a few publications have indicated that a correlation exists between leukoariosis and AD, the majority of the literature supports the notion that there is no correlation between the two, and therefore leukoariosis is not a direct manifestation of the pathology of AD [149,151–165].

FRONTOTEMPORAL LOBE DEGENERATION

Nearly all published attempts at formal quantification of cerebral atrophy in the neurodegenerative dementias have centered on the diagnosis of AD. The published literature on neuroimaging of the remaining neurodegenerative dementia syndromes typically consists of phenomenologic descriptions of observed imaging findings in small groups of patients. Frontotemporal dementias are considerably less common primary neurodegenerative dementing illnesses than AD (see Chapters 1 and 2). The pathologic findings of microvacuolation, gliosis in the cortex and white matter, myelin loss, swollen neurons with or without intracytoplasmic inclusions (Pick bodies), and neuron loss are localized rather than diffusely distributed throughout the brain [166,167]. The neuroimaging findings mirror the gross pathologic description of the disorder and occur whether or not Pick bodies are present histologically. Significant focal atrophy affects the frontal and anterior temporal lobes [106,168–173]. The atrophy is usually bilaterally symmetric but may be asymmetric in cases of Pick's disease (PcD) (Figure 8.4). When a hemispheric predominance is identified, the atrophy is typically more pronounced on the left. The affected gyri become paper thin, and at pathology, the involved areas of the brain resemble the kernel of a dried walnut. This characteristic has led to the radiologic description of *knife-blade atrophy*. Severe atrophy is sharply localized to the frontal and anterior temporal lobes, whereas the occipital lobes, perirolandic region, the posterior two-thirds of the superior temporal gyrus, and usually the parietal lobes are spared. The extrapyramidal nuclei, especially the caudate nucleus, insular cortex, and the anterior corpus callosum are affected as well. MRI may show a hyperintense signal in the cortex and underlying white matter of the affected areas. These MRI findings in an appropriate clinical setting may support the diagnosis of a frontotemporal-like dementia.

Asymmetric cortical degenerative syndromes are characterized by progressive focal neurologic deficits that result from a relatively circumscribed degenerative process. The specific clinical symptoms expressed are tightly coupled to the functional area(s) of the brain that is involved by the focal degenerative process. A number of specific clinical syndromes associated with focal cortical degeneration have been described, including progressive aphasia with and without dementia, progressive apraxia with and without dementia, and progressive prosopagnosia [174–176]. Frontotemporal lobe dementia described earlier in this section is the most well-recognized member of this family of focal cortical degenerative syndromes. The neuropathologic substrates differ among patients and include increased neuronal lipofuscin, gliosis, spongiform atrophy, and nonspecific pathology as well as pathologic changes suggestive of PcD and AD. The clinical syndrome itself is determined by the neuroanatomic location(s) of the degenerative process rather than specific histopathologic features (see Chapter 17). The term *asymmetric cerebral degenerative syndrome* has been proposed to

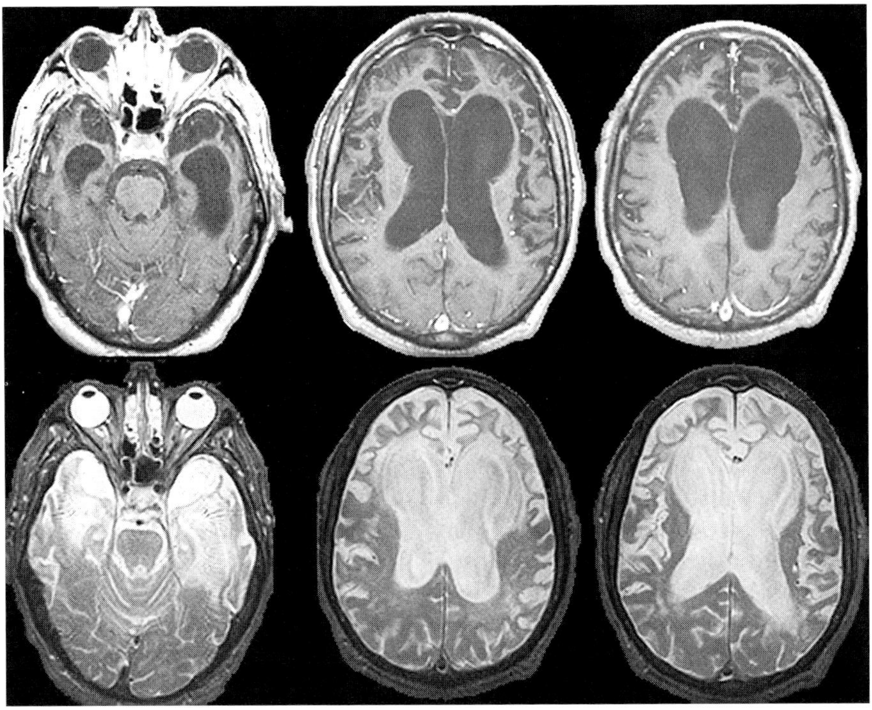

Figure 8.4 Axial T2-weighted magnetic resonance images of a 55-year-old man with pathologically confirmed Pick's disease. Severe atrophy is restricted to the anterior temporal and frontal lobes, with sparing of the posterior portions of both hemispheres. T1-weighted images are on the top row with T2-weighted images at matching anatomic sections on the bottom row. From left to right, the three columns display different axial anatomic sections of the brain, moving from inferior to superior.

describe this family of disorders because although patients may present with a clinical syndrome that is dominated by focal features, affected patients often display cognitive and pathologic evidence of more widespread but milder cortical degeneration [175,176]. Cross-sectional imaging studies can be a useful aid in the diagnosis when an area of focal cortical atrophy is identified that matches the clinical deficits observed (Figure 8.5).

LEWY BODY AND PARKINSONIAN DEMENTIA SYNDROMES

Dementia is a common feature of advanced Parkinson's disease (PD) (see Chapter 4). Relating specific imaging findings to the clinical dementia in PD is tenuous, however. It has become increasingly clear that the pathology of AD (neurofibrillary tangles and senile plaques) and the pathology of Lewy body dementia commonly coexist (see Chapter 3). A spectrum, therefore, exists, with pure AD

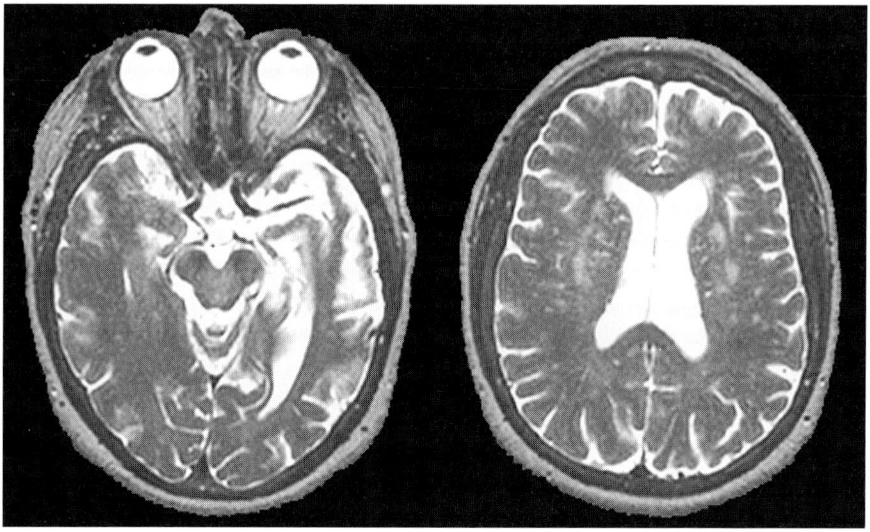

Figure 8.5 Asymmetric cortical degeneration. This 69-year-old woman presented with an aphasic dementia. Axial T2-weighted images through the temporal lobes (*left*) and through the ventricular system (*right*) demonstrate selective atrophy of the left temporal lobe with sparing of the remainder of the brain. This pattern corresponded to the patient's focal clinical presentation.

dementia at one end, pure Lewy body dementia at the other, and mixed cases between [177]. Although preferential atrophy of medial temporal lobe structures has been identified as a characteristic feature of AD, specifically early AD, the only imaging finding that has been identified as a feature of parkinsonian dementia is nonspecific generalized cerebral atrophy. To identify specific imaging criteria that characterize each of the three aforementioned neurodegenerative syndromes (pure AD, mixed Lewy body–AD, pure Lewy body dementia) rigorous radiologic-pathologic studies will have to be carried out in which premortem imaging studies are correlated with clinical features and postmortem pathologic features.

The cardinal pathologic features of PD are found in the substantia nigra, locus ceruleus, and dorsal motor nucleus of the vagus. These pigmented nuclei show a depletion of pigmented cells, gliosis, and Lewy bodies. An imaging finding that is putatively characteristic of PD is narrowing of the pars compacta [70,178–184]. Decreased T2 signal intensity in the pars compacta has been reported as well [185]. Unilateral narrowing of the pars compacta has been correlated with a hemi-parkinsonian clinical presentation [186,187]. The pars compacta is visualized as the nonpigmented band of tissue with normal cortical signal intensity that is interposed between the red nucleus and pars reticularis of the substantia nigra. Both the pars reticularis of the substantia nigra and the red nucleus have large amounts of storage iron and, therefore, decreased signal intensity on T2-weighted MRI. Substantial overlap, however, exists in the width of the pars compacta between patients with PD and normal controls. Excessive iron deposition in the putamen has been advanced as an imaging finding of striatonigral degeneration, Shy-Drager syndrome, and progressive supranuclear palsy [188–192]. Beyond non-

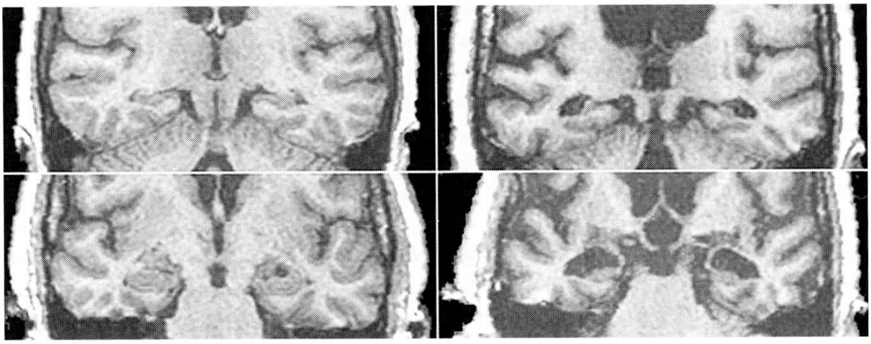

Figure 8.6 Parkinsonian–Alzheimer's disease–amyotrophic lateral sclerosis complex of Guam. Coronal T1-weighted images demonstrate severe hippocampal atrophy in a 54-year-old woman with this mixed neurodegenerative syndrome (*right*). On the left, a 55-year-old female control subject from the same population demonstrates no appreciable hippocampal atrophy.

specific generalized cerebral atrophy, anatomic imaging findings have not been correlated specifically with parkinsonian dementias [187]. The aforementioned basal ganglionic and midbrain findings have been primarily correlated with the clinical movement disorder symptoms of PD. Whether these imaging findings have any diagnostic significance with respect to the differentiation of Lewy body dementias from AD is unknown. With respect to the imaging diagnosis of AD versus the Lewy body variant of AD versus pure Lewy body dementia, it is tantalizing to hypothesize that medial temporal lobe atrophy is a specific finding of AD pathology. If this were the case, then imaging measures of medial atrophy may ultimately be useful in clarifying the clinical diagnoses along the spectrum from pure AD to Lewy body dementia. Patients with the parkinsonian–AD–ALS complex of Guam who are demented do demonstrate the classic hippocampal–medial temporal lobe atrophy seen with AD (Figure 8.6), indicating that this imaging finding may indeed be a marker of the AD pathology in these mixed degenerative disorder syndromes.

HUNTINGTON'S DISEASE

Huntington's disease is an inherited neurodegenerative movement disorder with dementia as a prominent feature of the clinical syndrome. Atrophy of the caudate and putamen late in the course of the disease are clearly recognizable on cross-sectional imaging studies (Figure 8.7). Both increased and decreased signal intensity in the striatum have been described in Huntington's disease [193]. Increased signal is likely a reflection of reactive gliosis plus the loss of small myelinated fibers [34]. Accumulation of iron in the striatum would be the reasonable explanation for the hypointense signal on T2-weighted images that may be observed as well. Volumetric studies as well as measures of the bicaudate width in Huntington's disease have documented a significant decline in volume

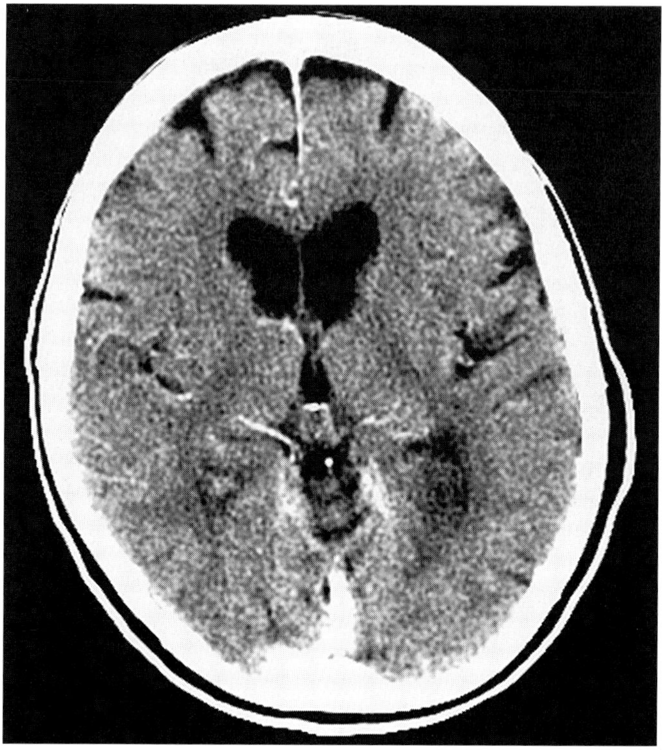

Figure 8.7 Computed tomographic section of a 67-year-old woman with Huntington's disease demonstrates significant bilaterally symmetric atrophy of the caudate nuclei and no apparent atrophy of the neocortex.

of the caudate, putamen, and to a less severe degree, the thalamus, medial temporal lobe, and neocortex [194,195]. Volume loss in the neocortex, medial temporal lobe, and caudate have been correlated with the cognitive deficit [195–200]. Serial measurements demonstrate measurable volume loss in the basal ganglia over time that parallel the declining clinical course [201,202].

VASCULAR DEMENTIA

Cerebrovascular disease is regarded by some to be the second most common cause of dementia in the elderly (see Chapter 15). From a pathologic and mechanistic standpoint, two general forms of cerebrovascular disease are recognized as causes of dementia: multi-infarct dementia (MID) and subcortical vascular dementia. The cerebrovascular arterial tree can be divided into two general categories: conducting arterial supply and penetrating arterial supply. An infarction in the distribution of one of the large conducting arteries on the surface of the

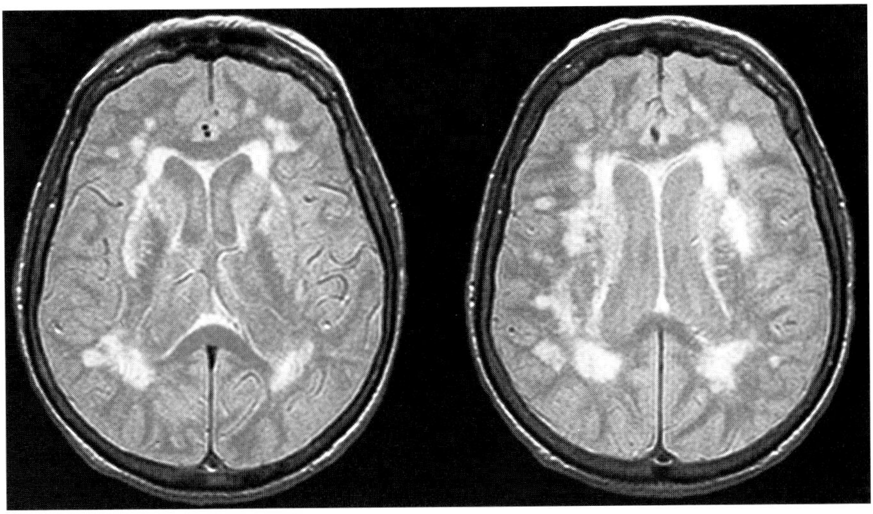

Figure 8.8 Vascular dementia. Axial spin density magnetic resonance images that demonstrate ischemic white matter disease in an 85-year-old woman with a clinical diagnosis of vascular dementia that was called Binswanger's disease at autopsy.

brain involves the gray matter ribbon and underlying white matter. Infarction or impaired blood flow in the distribution of the penetrating arterioles involves the hemispheric white matter or the central gray matter nuclei [203,204].

Multi-Infarct Dementia

Cortical infarction is due to thromboembolic occlusive disease involving the conducting arterial vessels of the brain. Mechanisms of arterial occlusion are either embolic (typically from a cardiac, ascending aorta, or cervical carotid arterial source) or local thrombotic occlusion. Dementia typically may result from the cumulative effect of several episodes of thromboembolic cortical infarction, and MID is attributed to this mechanism when a volumetric burden of infarction exceeding 60–80 ml of cortical tissue is reached [205–208].

Subcortical Ischemia

The second form of vascular disease associated with dementia, subcortical infarction/ischemia, is more controversial [209–214]. The vascular distribution of subcortical ischemic change can be divided into two recognized forms [35,215] (Figure 8.8). An occlusion in the distribution of the short penetrating arterioles that arise from the circle of Willis produces lacunar infarction. Ischemic change in the distribution of the long penetrating medullary arteries affects the hemispheric white matter. The blood flow to the deep gray nuclei is similar to that of the deep hemispheric white matter in that both are subserved by penetrating end arterioles with little collateral circulation. For this reason, white matter ischemic disease and lacunar infarctions tend to occur in the same patients and are often ascribed to similar etiologic mechanisms. A number of clinical terms have been applied to this process, particularly deep white matter ischemic change—*senile dementia of the Binswanger type*, *subcortical arterial sclerotic encephalopathy*, and *Binswanger's disease*. Numerous radiographic terms have been coined to describe the varying levels of severity of white matter ischemic disease, the most popular perhaps is *leukoariosis* [28,46,62,179,216–220]. Pathologically, at the mild end of the spectrum, one finds periventricular myelin pallor, astrocytosis, and partial loss of periventricular myelin in oligodendroglia [31,221–238]. In the most mild cases, these changes are limited to the periventricular zones. In more advanced cases, however, the changes extend away from the ventricular surface throughout the centrum semiovale. Changes in the centrum semiovale are generally felt to result from chronic or episodic subacute ischemia. The magnitude of the ischemic change can range from myelin loss to frank cavitary necrosis. The process is characterized by sparing of the cortex and subarcuate fibers. Leukoariosis is associated with tortuosity, fibrohyalinoid thickening, and sclerosis of the long penetrating medullary arterioles [204,239].

A number of risk factors has been associated with leukoariosis, most prominently age and hypertension [28,44,60–69,240–242]. Other associated risk factors are cigarette smoking, postural hypotension, and nocturnal hypotension. The proposed link between leukoariosis and hypertension is progressive sclerosis of long penetrating medullary arterioles, which is said to occur in response to chronic hypertension. This predisposes the vascular territory subserved by the long medullary arterioles to chronic hypoperfusion or renders them vulnerable during periods of systemic hypoperfusion. It also accounts for the association between leukoariosis and episodic hypotension.

CREUTZFELDT-JAKOB DISEASE

Creutzfeldt-Jakob disease (CJD) is transmitted by a "slow virus," or prion (see Chapter 5). Dementia is a prominent feature of the clinical presentation. Pathologically, neuron loss, gliosis, and spongiform change are seen. The initial MR change, which is quite characteristic, is bilaterally symmetric, increased T2 signal in the caudate, putamen, and sometimes the thalamus [243–247] (Figure 8.9). Elevated T2 signal in the cortical ribbon has been described as well [248]. As the disease progresses, the striatum and neocortex become visibly atrophic [249].

NORMAL PRESSURE HYDROCEPHALUS

Normal pressure hydrocephalus (NPH) is a controversial entity that is mentioned in this chapter because cross-sectional MRI findings have been described that putatively are not only characteristic of this disorder but also may predict response to ventricular shunting procedures [250–252]. The use of MRI in predicting

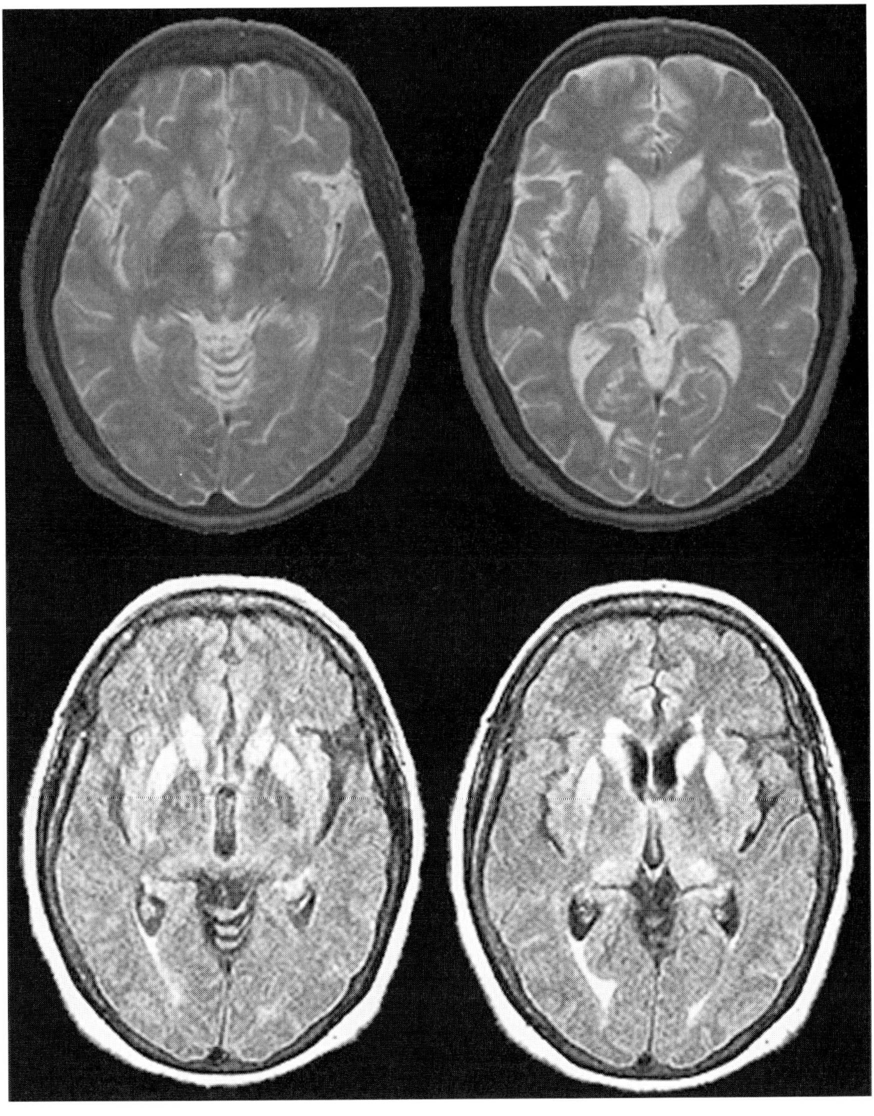

Figure 8.9 A 63-year-old woman with autopsy-proved Creutzfeldt-Jakob disease. T2-weighted images (*top row*) and fast-fluid attenuated inversion recovery images (*bottom row*) demonstrate the characteristic increased signal intensity restricted to the caudate, putamen, and in this case, the thalami in a bilaterally symmetric fashion.

response to shunting, however, is not universally embraced [253]. Two competing theories exist to explain the etiology of this syndrome: impaired extraventricular CSF resorption due to prior subarachnoid hemorrhage or meningitis, and decreased white matter tensile strength due to deep white matter infarction/ischemic change

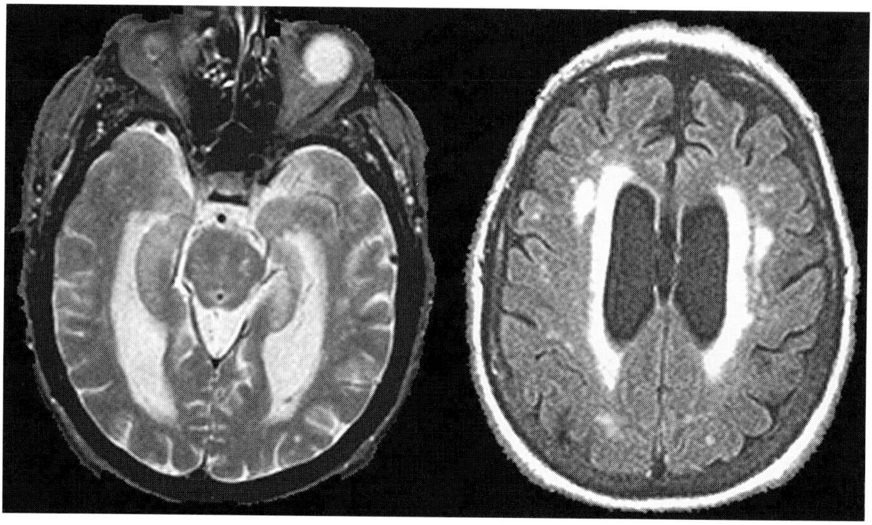

Figure 8.10 Normal pressure hydrocephalus. This 67-year-old man presented with the classic clinical triad of gait apraxia, dementia, and incontinence. Clinical symptoms improved after a ventricular shunting procedure. Aqueductal cerebrospinal fluid velocity was calculated with cinephase-contrast magnetic resonance imaging and was significantly elevated with respect to values obtained in normal elderly controls. Note also ventricular enlargement and the prominent periventricular halo.

[254,255]. Three primary MRI findings have been described in NPH: (1) enlargement of the ventricular system out of proportion to the subarachnoid space, (2) a prominent periventricular halo, and (3) a prominent CSF flow void in the cerebral aqueduct [256] (Figure 8.10). The prominent periventricular halo has been ascribed to centrifugal flow of CSF from the ventricular system radially into the periventricular white matter. The prominent flow void in the cerebral aqueduct has been attributed to excessively rapid pulsatile CSF flow [250,257]. The putative result of loss of brain elasticity in this condition produces excessively forceful transmission of the arterial pressure pulse during cardiac systole to the incompressible CSF in the ventricular system. This forceful pressure wave is transmitted from the CSF in the lateral ventricles through the third ventricle to the CSF in the aqueduct, resulting in pulsatile flow in the aqueduct that is more prominent than normal. This in turn results in a loss of coherent signal in aqueductal CSF, which is more prominent than normal. MRI markers of this hyperdynamic aqueductal CSF flow have been prominent signal loss, excessive anteroposterior extent of the aqueductal CSF signal void, and excessive aqueductal flow velocity using formal velocity measurements with cine phase contrast methods. At some sites, measurements of aqueductal CSF velocity that exceed normal limits are used to indicate which patients suspected of having NPH will respond favorably to shunting [258]. Another measure derived from CSF velocity mapping that has been used to predict response to shunting is the CSF stroke volume, which is a measure of the volume of CSF flow through the aqueduct over the cardiac cycle [252].

RECOMMENDATIONS FOR CROSS-SECTIONAL IMAGING

The traditional role of cross-sectional imaging in dementia has been to identify treatable causes of dementia, such as hydrocephalus, brain tumor, and subdural hematoma. The reported yield of cross-sectional studies in identifying surgically treatable causes of dementia in newly diagnosed cases varies considerably among different publications [259]. Although cost containment concerns have been raised as an argument against imaging, many clinicians would agree with the advisability of performing a cross-sectional imaging study as part of the routine workup for dementia [260–262]. Most clinicians would agree that a cross-sectional imaging study is also indicated in patients who carry a diagnosis of a dementing illness if the clinical course becomes atypical or if the patient experiences a precipitous decline in cognition or sudden onset of neurologic symptoms.

No universally accepted guidelines exist with regard to the selection of MRI versus CT as the cross-sectional imaging modality of choice. In the past, substantially lower cost and greater availability favored CT. With declining reimbursement for MRI and proliferation of MRI scanning units, however, the gap in cost and availability between MRI and CT is narrowing, thus eroding the impetus to recommend CT as the cross-sectional imaging modality of choice for screening patients with dementia. While the search for additional positive imaging diagnostic criteria which are specific for different dementing illnesses continues, at least four of the imaging findings discussed in this chapter seem to be both sensitive and specific enough to serve as useful ancillary diagnostic criteria in the appropriate clinical settings: (1) atrophy of the medial temporal lobes—for the diagnosis of AD; (2) focal cortical atrophy—for the diagnosis of frontotemporal dementias including PcD and other asymmetric cortical degenerative syndromes; (3) cortical and subcortical infarction/ischemic changes—for the diagnosis of vascular dementia or clinically silent stroke(s); and (4) elevated T2 signal in the striatum bilaterally—for the diagnosis of CJD. All of these imaging findings are depicted with greater sensitivity with MRI than with CT [263,264].

There are situations in which CT is preferable in the imaging of patients with dementia. In the event of sudden new neurologic symptoms or sudden decline in consciousness, CT is preferable to MRI for the visualization of acute subarachnoid hemorrhage. Patients with cardiac pacemakers, intraocular and intracranial foreign bodies, or other medical contraindications to MRI should be imaged by CT, as should patients who are severely claustrophobic. A single CT slice can be acquired in less than 1 second, whereas the minimal amount of time required to acquire the data for reconstruction of an MRI study is on the order of minutes. Therefore, patients who are too demented to remain still should probably be imaged by CT as well.

REFERENCES

1. Bryan RN, Manolio TA, Schertz LD, et al. A method for using MR to evaluate the effects of cardiovascular disease on the brain: the Cardiovascular Health Study. AJNR Am J Neuroradiol 1994;15: 1625–1633.
2. Davis PC, Gearing M, Gray L, et al. The CERAD experience, part VIII: neuroimaging-neuropathology correlates of temporal lobe changes in Alzheimer's disease. Neurology 1995;45:178–179.

3. Escalona PR, McDonald WM, Doraiswamy PM, et al. In vivo sterological assessment of human cerebellar volume: effects of gender and age. AJNR Am J Neuroradiol 1991;12:927–929.
4. Gunderson HJG, Jensen EG. The efficiency of systematic sampling in sterology and its prediction. J Microsc 1987;147:229–263.
5. Cavalieri B. Geometra degli indivisibili. Unione Tipograficao Editrice 1966.
6. Jernigan TL, Zatz L, Naeser MA. Semiautomated methods for quantiating CSF volume on cranial computed tomography. Radiology 1979;132:463–466.
7. Tanna NK, Kohn MI, Horwich DN, et al. Analysis of brain and cerebrospinal fluid volumes with MR imaging: impact on PET data correction for atrophy. Part II. Aging and Alzheimer dementia. Radiology 1991;178:123–130.
8. Blatter DD, Bigler ED, Gale SD, et al. Quantitative volumetric analysis of brain MR: normative database spanning 5 decades of life. AJNR Am J Neuroradiol 1995;16:241–251.
9. Jack CR Jr, Twomey CK, Zinsmeister AR, et al. Anterior temporal lobes and hippocampal formations: normative volumetric measurements for MR images in young adults. Radiology 1989;172:549–554.
10. Jack CR Jr, Bentley M, Twomey CK, Zinsmeister AR. MR-based volume measurements of the hippocampal formation and anterior temporal lobe: validation studies. Radiology 1990;176:205–209.
11. Jack CR Jr, Petersen RC, O'Brien PC, et al. MR-based hippocampal volumetry in the diagnosis of Alzheimer's disease. Neurology 1992;42:183–188.
12. Jack CR Jr. MRI-based hippocampal volume measurements in epilepsy. Epilepsia 1994;35(suppl 6):S21–S29.
13. Free SL, Bergin PS, Fish DR, et al. Methods for normalization of hippocampal volumes measured with MR. AJNR Am J Neuroradiol 1995;16:637–643.
14. Jack CR Jr, Petersen RC, Xu YC, et al. Medial temporal atrophy on MRI in normal aging and very mild Alzheimer's disease. Neurology 1997;49:786–794.
15. Campeau NG, Petersen RC, Felmlee JP, et al. Hippocampal magnetic resonance transverse relaxation times in patients with Alzheimer disease. Radiology 1997;205:197–201.
16. Laakso MP, Partanen K, Soininen H, et al. MR T2 relaxometry in Alzheimer's disease and age-associated memory impairment. Neurobiol Aging 1996;17:1–5.
17. Drayer BP. Imaging of the aging brain. Part I. Normal findings. Radiology 1988;166:785–796.
18. DeCarli C, Murphy DGM, Gillette JA, et al. Lack of age-related differences in temporal lobe volume of very healthy adults. AJNR Am J Neuroradiol 1994;15:689–696.
19. DeCarli C, Kaye JA, Horwitz B, Rapoport SI. Critical analysis of the use of computer-assisted transverse axial tomography to study human brain in aging and dementia of the Alzheimer type. Neurology 1990;40:872–883.
20. Kaye JA, DeCarli C, Luxenberg JS, Rapoport SI. The significance of age-related enlargement of the cerebral ventricles in healthy men and women measured by quantitative computed x-ray tomography. J Am Geriatr Soc 1992;40:225–231.
21. Jernigan TL, Archibald SL, Berhow MT, et al. Cerebral structure on MRI, part I: Localization of age-related changes. Biol Psychiatry 1991;29:55–67.
22. Laffey PA, Peyster RG, Nathan R, et al. Computed tomography and aging: results in a normal elderly population. Neuroradiology 1984;26:273–278.
23. Zatz LM, Jernigan TL, Ahumada AJ. Changes on computed cranial tomography with aging. Intracranial fluid volume. AJNR Am J Neuroradiol 1982;3:1–11.
24. Coffey CE, Wilkinson WE, Parashos IA, et al. Quantitative cerebral anatomy of the aging human brain: a cross-sectional study using magnetic resonance imaging. Neurology 1992;42:527–536.
25. Murphy DGM, DeCarli C, Schapiro MB, et al. Age-related differences in volumes of subcortical nuclei, brain matter, and cerebrospinal fluid in healthy men as measured with magnetic resonance imaging. Arch Neurol 1992;49:839–845.
26. Pfefferbaum A, Mathalon DH, Sullivan EV, et al. A quantitative magnetic resonance imaging study of changes in brain morphology from infancy to late adulthood. Arch Neurol 1994;51:874–887.
27. Gur RC, Mozley PD, Resnick SM, et al. Gender differences in age effect on brain atrophy measured by magnetic resonance imaging. Proc Natl Acad Sci 1991;88:2845–2849.
28. Manolio TA, Kronmal RA, Burke GL, et al. Magnetic resonance abnormalities and cardiovascular disease in older adults. The Cardiovascular Health Study. Stroke 1994;25:318–327.
29. Sullivan EV, Marsh L, Mathalon DH, et al. Age-related decline in MRI volumes of temporal lobe gray matter but not hippocampus. Neurobiol Aging 1995;16:591–606.
30. Mirowitz S, Sartor K, Gado M, Torack R. Focal signal-intensity variations in the posterior internal capsule: normal MR findings and distinction from pathologic findings. Radiology 1989;172:535–539.
31. Sze G, DeArmond SJ, Brant-Zawadzki M, et al. Foci of MRI signal (pseudo lesions) anterior to the frontal horns: histologic correlations of a normal finding. AJNR Am J Neuroradiol 1986;7:381–387.

32. Heier L, Bauer CJ, Schwartz L. Large Virchow-Robin spaces: MR-clinical correlation. AJNR Am J Neuroradiol 1989;10:929–936.
33. Jungreis CA, Kanal E, Hirsch WL, et al. Normal perivascular spaces mimicking lacunar infarction: MR imaging. Radiology 1988;169:101–104.
34. Lexa FJ, Trojanowski JQ, Braffman BH, Atlas SW. The Aging Brain and Neurodegenerative Diseases. In SW Atlas (ed), Magnetic Resonance Imaging of the Brain and Spine. Philadelphia: Lippincott–Raven Publishers, 1996:803–870.
35. Hachinski VC, Potter P, Merskey H. Leuko-araiosis: an ancient term for a new problem. Can J Neurol Sci 1986;13:533–534.
36. Almkvist O, Wahlund LO, Andersson-Lundman G, et al. White-matter hyperintensity and neuropsychological functions in dementia and healthy aging. Arch Neurol 1992;49:626–632.
37. Austron MG, Thompson RF, Hendrie HC, et al. Foci of increased T2 signal intensity in MR images of healthy elderly subjects. A follow-up study. J Am Geriatr Soc 1990;38:1133–1138.
38. Boone KB, Miller BL, Lesser IM, et al. Neuropsychological correlates of white-matter lesions in healthy elderly subjects. A threshold effect. Arch Neurol 1992;49:549–554.
39. Breteler MMB, van Amerongen NM, van Swieten JC, et al. Cognitive correlates of ventricular enlargement and cerebral white matter lesions on magnetic resonance imaging. The Rotterdam Study. Stroke 1994;25:1109–1115.
40. Breteler MMB, van Swieten JC, Bots ML, et al. Cerebral white matter lesions, vascular risk factors, and cognitive function in a population-based study: the Rotterdam Study. Neurology 1994;44:1246–1252.
41. Junque C, Pujol J, Vendrell P. Leuko-araiosis on magnetic resonance imaging and speed of mental processing. Arch Neurol 1990;47:151–156.
42. Longstreth WT, Manolio TA, Arnold A, et al. Clinical correlates of white matter findings on cranial magnetic resonance imaging of 3301 elderly people. The Cardiovascular Health Study. Stroke 1996; 27:1274–1282.
43. Steingart A, Hachinski VC, Lau C. Cognitive and neurologic findings in subjects with diffuse white matter lucencies on computed tomographic scan (leukoaraiosis). Arch Neurol 1987;44:32–35.
44. van Swieten JC, Geyskes GG, Derix MMA, et al. Hypertension in the elderly is associated with white matter lesions and cognitive decline. Ann Neurol 1991;30:825–830.
45. Wahlund LO, Andersson-Lundman G, Julin P, et al. Quantitative estimation of brain white matter abnormalities in elderly subjects using magnetic resonance imaging. Magn Reson Imaging 1992;10:859–865.
46. Hendrie HC, Farlow MR, Austrom MG, et al. Foci of increased T2 signal intensity on brain MR scans of healthy elderly subjects. AJNR Am J Neuroradiol 1989;10:703–707.
47. Kozachuk WE, DeCarli C, Schapiro MB. White matter hyperintensities in dementia of Alzheimer's type and in healthy subjects without cerebrovascular risk factors. Arch Neurol 1990;47:1306–1310.
48. Lopez OL, Becker JT, Jungreis CA, et al. Computed tomography but not magnetic resonance imaging identified periventricular white matter lesions predict symptomatic cerebrovascular disease in probable Alzheimer's disease. Arch Neurol 1995;52:659–664.
49. Rao SM, Mittenberg W, Bernardin L, et al. Neuropsychological test findings in subjects with leukoaraiosis. Arch Neurol 1989;46:40–44.
50. Schmidt R, Fazekas F, Offenbacher H, et al. Neuropsychologic correlates of MRI white matter hyperintensities: a study of 150 normal volunteers. Neurology 1993;43:2490–2494.
51. Schmidt R, Fazekas F, Offenbacher H, et al. Magnetic resonance imaging white matter lesions and cognitive impairment in hypertensive individuals. Arch Neurol 1991;48:417–420.
52. Tupler LA, Coffey CE, Logue PE, et al. Neuropsychological importance of subcortical white matter hyperintensity. Arch Neurol 1992;49:1248–1252.
53. Elias MF, Schultz NR Jr, Robbins MA, Elias PK. A longitudinal study of neuropsychological performance by hypertensives and normotensives: a third measurement point. J Gerontol 1989;44: P25–P28.
54. Elias MF, Wolf PA, D'Agostino RB, et al. Untreated blood pressure level is inversely related to cognitive functioning: the Framingham Study. Am J Epidemiol 1993;138:353–364.
55. Sands LP, Meredith W. Blood pressure and intellectual functioning in late midlife. J Gerontol B Psychol Sci Soc Sci 1992;47:P81–P84.
56. Starr JM, Whalley LJ, Inch S. Blood pressure and cognitive function in healthy old people. J Am Geriatr Soc 1993;41:753–756.
57. Wallace RB, Lemke JH, Morris MC, et al. Relationship of free-recall memory to hypertension in the elderly. The Iowa 65+ Rural Health Study. J Chron Dis 1985;38:475–481.
58. Wilkie F, Eisdorfer C. Intelligence and blood pressure in the aged. Science 1971;172:959–962.
59. Launer LJ, Masaki K, Petrovitch H, et al. The association between midlife blood pressure levels and late-life cognitive function. JAMA 1995;274:1846–1851.

60. Awad IA, Spetzler RF, Hodak JA, et al. Incidental subcortical lesions identified on magnetic resonance imaging in the elderly. I. Correlation with age and cerebrovascular risk factors. Stroke 1986; 17:1084–1089.
61. Fukuda H, Kitani M. Cigarette smoking is correlated with the periventricular hyperintensity grade on brain magnetic resonance imaging. Stroke 1996;27:645–649.
62. Kertesz A, Black SE, Tokar G, et al. Periventricular and subcortical hyperintensities on magnetic resonance imaging. Arch Neurol 1988;45:404–408.
63. Kobayashi S, Okada K, Yamashita K. Incidence of silent lacunar lesion in normal adults and its relation to cerebral blood flow and risk factors. Stroke 1991;22:1379–1383.
64. Liao D, Cooper L, Cai J, et al. Presence and severity of cerebral white matter lesions and hypertension, its treatment, and its control. The ARIC study. Stroke 1996;27:2262–2270.
65. Watanabe N, Imai Y, Nagai K, et al. Nocturnal blood pressure and silent cerebrovascular lesions in elderly Japanese. Stroke 1996;27:1319–1327.
66. Blennow K, Wallin A, Uhlemann C, et al. White-matter lesions on CT in Alzheimer patients: relation to clinical symptomatology and vascular factors. Acta Neurol Scand 1991;83:187–193.
67. DeCarli C, Murphy DGM, Tranh M, et al. The effect of white matter hyperintensity volume on brain structure, cognitive performance, and cerebral metabolism of glucose in 51 healthy adults. Neurology 1995;45:2077–2084.
68. Inzitari D, Diaz F, Fox A, et al. Vascular risk factors and leukoariosis. Arch Neurol 1987;44:42–47.
69. Salerno JA, Murphy DGM, Horwitz B, et al. Brain atrophy in hypertension. A volumetric magnetic resonance imaging study. Hypertension 1992;20:340–348.
70. Rutledge JN, Hilal SK, Silver AJ, et al. Study of movement disorders and brain iron by MR. AJR Am J Roentgenol 1987;149:365–379.
71. Rutledge JN, Schallert T, Hall S. Magnetic resonance imaging in parkinsonisms. Adv Neurol 1993; 60:529–534.
72. Chen JC, Hardy PA, Clauberg M, et al. T2 values in the human brain: comparison with quantitative assays of iron and ferritin. Radiology 1989;173:521–526.
73. Milton WJ, Atlas SW, Lexa FJ, et al. Deep gray matter hypointensity patterns with aging in healthy adults: MR imaging at 1.5T. Radiology 1991;181:715–719.
74. Aoki S, Okada Y, Nishimura K, et al. Normal deposition of brain iron in childhood and adolescence: MR imaging at 1.5T. Radiology 1989;172:381–385.
75. Imon Y, Yamaguchi S, Yamamura Y, et al. Low intensity areas observed on T2-weighted magnetic resonance imaging of the cerebral cortex in various neurological diseases. J Neurol Sci 1995; 134(suppl):27–32.
76. Arnold SE, Hyman BT, Flory J, et al. The topographical and neuroanatomical distribution of neurofibrillary tangles and neuritic plaques in the cerebral cortex of patients with Alzheimer's disease. Cerebral Cortex 1991;1:103–116.
77. Brun A, Englund E. Regional pattern of degeneration in Alzheimer's disease: neuronal loss and histopathological grading. Histopathology 1981;5:549–564.
78. Braak H, Braak E, Bohl J. Staging of Alzheimer-related cortical destruction. Eur Neurol 1993; 33:403–408.
79. Braak H, Braak E. Morphological criteria for the recognition of Alzheimer's disease and the distribution pattern of cortical changes related to this disorder. Neurobiol Aging 1994;15:355–356.
80. Braak H, Braak E. Neuropathological staging of Alzheimer-related changes. Acta Neuropathol (Berl) 1991;82:239–259.
81. Hyman BT, Gomez-Isla T. Alzheimer's disease is a laminar, regional, and neural system specific disease, not a global brain disease. Neurobiol Aging 1994;15:353–354.
82. Mann DMA. Pathological correlates of dementia in Alzheimer's disease. Neurobiol Aging 1994;15: 357–360.
83. Price JL, Davis PB, Morris JC, White DL. The distribution of tangles, plaques, and related immunohistochemical markers in healthy aging and Alzheimer's disease. Neurobiol Aging 1991;12:295–312.
84. Swaab DF, Hofman MA, Lucassen PJ, et al. Neuronal atrophy, not cell death, is the main hallmark of Alzheimer's disease. Neurobiol Aging 1994;15:369–371.
85. Terry RD, Masliah E, Salmon DP, et al. Physical basis of cognitive alterations in Alzheimer's disease: synapse loss is the major correlate of cognitive impairment. Ann Neurol 1991;30: 572–580.
86. Terry RD, Peck A, DeTeresa R, et al. Some morphometric aspects of the brain in senile dementia of the Alzheimer type. Ann Neurol 1981;10:184–192.
87. Tomlinson BE, Blessed G, Roth M. Observations on the brains of demented old people. J Neurol Sci 1970;11:205–242.

88. Hyman BT, Van Hoesen GW, Damasio AR, Barnes CL. Alzheimer's disease: cell-specific pathology isolates the hippocampal formation. Science 1984;225:1168–1170.
89. Hyman BT, Van Hoesen GW, Kromer LJ, Damasio AR. Perforant pathway changes and the memory impairment of Alzheimer's disease. Ann Neurol 1986;20:472–481.
90. Arriagada PV, Growdow JH, Hedley-Whyte ET, Hyman BT. Neurofibrillary tangles but no senile plaques parallel duration and severity of Alzheimer's disease. Neurology 1992;42:631–639.
91. Ball MJ, Hachinski V, Fox A, et al. A new definition of Alzheimer's disease: a hippocampal dementia. Lancet 1985;1:14–16.
92. Shefer VF. Hippocampal pathology as a possible factor in the pathogenesis of senile dementia. Neurosci Behav Physiol 1977;8:236–239.
93. Brun A, Gustafson L. Distribution of cerebral degeneration in Alzheimer's disease. Arch Psychiatr Nervenkr 1976;223:15–33.
94. Brun A. Regional rather than global pathology decides symptoms in senile dementia of Alzheimer's type. Neurobiol Aging 1994;15:367–368.
95. Herzog AG, Kemper TL. Amygdaloid changes in aging and dementia. Arch Neurol 1980;37:625–629.
96. Hooper MW, Vogel FS. The limbic system in Alzheimer's disease: a neuropathologic investigation. Am J Pathol 1976;85:1–19.
97. Reyes PF, Golden GT, Fagel PL, et al. The prepiriform cortex in dementia of the Alzheimer type. Arch Neurol 1987;44:644–645.
98. Scott SA, DeKosky ST, Scheff SW. Volumetric atrophy of the amygdala in Alzheimer's disease. Quantitative serial reconstruction. Neurology 1991;41:351–356.
99. Wilcock GK, Esiri MM. Plaques, tangles, and dementia: a quantitative study. J Neurol Sci 1982;56: 343–356.
100. Tanabe JL, Amend D, Schuff N, et al. Tissue segmentation of the brain in Alzheimer's disease. AJNR Am J Neuroradiol 1997;18:115–123.
101. Albert M, Naeser MA, Levine HL, Garvery AJ. Ventricular size in patients with presenile dementia of the Alzheimer's type. Arch Neurol 1984;41:1258–1263.
102. Bigler ED, Hubler DW, Cullum CM, Turkheimer E. Intellectual and memory impairment in dementia computerized axial tomography volume correlations. J Nerv Ment Dis 1985;173:347–352.
103. Brinkman SD, Sarwar M, Levin HS, Morris HH. Quantitative indexes of computed tomography in dementia and normal aging. Radiology 1981;138:89–92.
104. Creasey H, Schwartz M, Frederickson H, et al. Quantitative computed tomography in dementia of the Alzheimer type. Neurology 1986;36:1563–1568.
105. Gado M, Hughs CP, Danziger W, et al. Volumetric measurements of the cerebrospinal fluid spaces in demented subjects and controls. Radiology 1982;144:535–538.
106. LeMay M. CT changes in dementing diseases: a review. AJR Am J Roentgenol 1986;147:963–975.
107. Huckman MS, Fox J, Topel J. The validity of criteria for the evaluation of cerebral atrophy by computed tomography. Radiology 1975;116:85–92.
108. Rusinek H, de Leon MJ, George AE, et al. Alzheimer's disease measuring loss of cerebral gray matter with MR imaging. Radiology 1991;178:109–114.
109. George AE, de Leon MJ, Stylopoulos LA, et al. CT diagnostic features of Alzheimer's disease: importance of the choroidal/hippocampal fissure complex. AJNR Am J Neuroradiol 1990;11:101–107.
110. Kido DK, Caine ED, LeMay M, et al. Temporal lobe atrophy in patients with Alzheimer's disease: a CT study. AJNR Am J Neuroradiol 1989;10:551–555.
111. Sandor T, Albert M, Stafford J, Harpley S. Use of computerized CT analysis to discriminate between Alzheimer patients and normal control subjects. AJNR Am J Neuroradiol 1988;9:1181–1187.
112. de Leon MJ, Golomb J, George AE, et al. The radiologic prediction of Alzheimer disease: the atrophic hippocampal formation. AJNR Am J Neuroradiol 1993;14:897–906.
113. de Leon MJ, Golomb J, Convit A, et al. Measurement of medial temporal lobe atrophy in diagnosis of Alzheimer's disease. Lancet 1993;341:125–126.
114. de Leon MJ, Convit A, George AE, et al. In vivo structural studies of the hippocampus in normal aging and in incipient Alzheimer's disease. Ann N Y Acad Sci 1996;777:1–13.
115. de Leon MJ, George AE, Golomb J, et al. Frequency of hippocampal formation atrophy in normal aging and Alzheimer's disease. Neurobiol Aging 1997;18:1–11.
116. de Leon MJ, George AE, Stylopoulos LA, et al. Early marker for Alzheimer's disease: the atrophic hippocampus. Lancet 1989;2:672–673.
117. Early B, Escalona PR, Boyko OB, et al. Interuncal distance measurements in healthy volunteers and in patients with Alzheimer disease. AJNR Am J Neuroradiol 1993;14:907–910.
118. Erkinjuntti T, Lee DH, Gao F, et al. Temporal lobe atrophy on magnetic resonance imaging in the diagnosis of early Alzheimer's disease. Arch Neurol 1993;50:305–310.

119. Frisoni GB, Bianchetti A, Geroldi C, Trabucchi M. Measures of medial temporal lobe atrophy in Alzheimer's disease. J Neurol Neurosurg Psychiatry 1994;57:1438–1439.
120. Frisoni GB, Beltramello A, Weiss C, et al. Linear measures of atrophy in mild Alzheimer's disease. AJNR Am J Neuroradiol 1996;17:913–923.
121. Howieson J, Kaye JA, Holm L, Howieson D. Interuncal distance: marker of aging and Alzheimer disease. AJNR Am J Neuroradiol 1993;14:647–650.
122. Jobst KA, Smith AD, Szatmari M, et al. Detection in life of confirmed Alzheimer's disease using a simple measurement of medial temporal lobe atrophy by computed tomography. Lancet 1992;340: 1179–1183.
123. Scheltens P, Leys D, Barkhof F, et al. Atrophy of medial temporal lobes on MRI in "probable" Alzheimer's disease and normal aging: diagnostic value and neuropsychological correlates. J Neurol Neurosurg Psychiatry 1992;55:967–972.
124. Seab JB, Jagust WJ, Wong STS, et al. Quantitative NMR measurements of hippocampal atrophy in Alzheimer's disease. Magn Reson Med 1988;8:200–208.
125. Convit A, de Leon MJ, Golomb J, et al. Hippocampal atrophy in early Alzheimer's disease: anatomic specificity and validation. Psychiatr Q 1993;64:371–387.
126. Cuenod CA, Denys A, Michot JL, et al. Amygdala atrophy in Alzheimer's disease. An in vivo magnetic resonance imaging study. Arch Neurol 1993;50:941–945.
127. Kesslak JP, Nalcioglu O, Cotman CW. Quantification of magnetic resonance scans for hippocampal and parahippocampal atrophy in Alzheimer's disease. Neurology 1991;41:51–54.
128. Killiany RJ, Moss MB, Albert MS, et al. Temporal lobe regions on magnetic resonance imaging identify patients with early Alzheimer's disease. Arch Neurol 1993;50:949–954.
129. Laakso MP, Soininen H, Partanen K, et al. Volumes of hippocampus, amygdala and frontal lobes in the MRI-based diagnosis of early Alzheimer's disease: correlation with memory functions. J Neural Transm Park Dis Dement Sect 1995;9:73–86.
130. Laakso MP, Partanen K, Riekkinen P, et al. Hippocampal volumes in Alzheimer's disease, Parkinson's disease with and without dementia, and in vascular dementia: an MRI study. Neurology 1996; 46:678–681.
131. Lehericy S, Baulac M, Chiras J, et al. Amygdalohippocampal MR volume measurements in the early stages of Alzheimer disease. AJNR Am J Neuroradiol 1994;15:927–937.
132. Lehtovirta M, Laakso MP, Soininen H, et al. Volumes of hippocampus, amygdala and frontal lobe in Alzheimer's patients with different apolipoprotein E genotypes. Neuroscience 1995;67:65–72.
133. Lehtovirta M, Soininen H, Laakso MP, et al. SPECT and MRI analysis in Alzheimer's disease: relation to apolipoprotein E epsilon 4 allele. J Neurol Neurosurg Psychiatry 1996;60:644–649.
134. Pearlson G, Harris GJ, Powers RE, et al. Quantitative changes in mesial temporal volume, regional cerebral blood flow, and cognition in Alzheimer's disease. Arch Gen Psychiatry 1992;49:402–408.
135. Soininen HS, Partanen K, Pitkanen A, et al. Volumetric MRI analysis of the amygdala and the hippocampus in subjects with age-associated memory impairment: correlation to visual and verbal memory. Neurology 1994;44:1660–1668.
136. Jobst KA, Hindley NJ, King E, Smith AD. The diagnosis of Alzheimer's disease: a question of image? J Clin Psychiatry 1994;55:22–31.
137. Maunoury C, Michot JL, Caillet H, et al. Specificity of temporal amygdala atrophy in Alzheimer's disease: quantitative assessment with magnetic resonance imaging. Dementia 1996;7:10–14.
138. Convit A, de Leon MH, Tarshish C, et al. Hippocampal volume losses in minimally impaired elderly. Lancet 1995;345:266.
139. Fox MC, Warrington EK, Freeborough PA, et al. Presymptomatic hippocampal atrophy in Alzheimer's disease. A longitudinal MRI study. Brain 1996;119:2001–2007.
140. Fox NC, Warrington EK, Stevens JM, et al. Atrophy of the hippocampal formation in early familial Alzheimer's disease. A longitudinal MRI study of at-risk members of a family with an amyloid precursor protein 717Val-Gly mutation. Ann N Y Acad Sci 1996;777:226–232.
141. Kaye JA, Swihart T, Howieson D, Dame A. Volume loss of the hippocampus and temporal lobe in healthy elderly persons destined to develop dementia. Neurology 1997;48:1297–1304.
142. Gado M, Hughes CP, Danzinger W, Chi D. Aging, dementia, and brain atrophy: a longitudinal computed tomographic study. AJNR Am J Neuroradiol 1983;4:699–702.
143. DeCarli C, Haxby JV, Gillette JA, et al. Longitudinal changes in lateral ventricular volume in patients with dementia of the Alzheimer type. Neurology 1993;42:2029–2036.
144. Luxenberg JS, Haxby JV, Creasey H, et al. Rate of ventricular enlargement in dementia of the Alzheimer type correlates with rate of neuropsychological deterioration. Neurology 1987;37:1135–1140.
145. Wippold FJ, Gado MH, Morris JC, et al. Senile dementia and healthy aging: a longitudinal CT study. Radiology 1992;179:215–219.

146. Smith AD, Jobst KA. Use of structural imaging to study the progression of Alzheimer's disease. Br Med Bull 1996;52:575–586.
147. Jack CR Jr, Petersen RC, Xu YC, et al. Hippocampal and temporal horn MRI volumetrics in normal aging and Alzheimer's disease: a longitudinal study. (In press.)
148. Bondareff W, Raval J, Woo B, et al. Magnetic resonance imaging and the severity of dementia in older adults. Arch Gen Psychiatry 1990;47:47–51.
149. Fazekas F, Chawluk JB, Alavi A, et al. MR signal abnormalities at 1.5T in Alzheimer's dementia and normal aging. AJR Am J Roentgenol 1987;149:351–356.
150. Kirsch SJ, Roland WJ, Butcher LL, Beatty J. Prolongation of magnetic resonance T2 time in hippocampus of human patients marks the presence and severity of Alzheimer's disease (letter). Neuroscience 1992;134:187–190.
151. Brilliant M, Hughes L, Anderson D, et al. Rarefield white matter in patients with Alzheimer disease. Alzheimer Dis Assoc Disord 1995;9:39–46.
152. DeCarli C, Grady CL, Clark CM, et al. Comparison of positron emission tomography, cognition, and brain volume in Alzheimer's disease with and without severe abnormalities of white matter. J Neurol Neurosurg Psychiatry 1996;60:158–167.
153. Erkinjuntti T, Gao F, Lee DH, et al. Lack of difference in brain hyperintensities between patients with early Alzheimer's disease and control subjects. Arch Neurol 1994;51:260–268.
154. Fazekas F, Kapeller P, Schmidt R, et al. The relation of cerebral resonance signal hyperintensities to Alzheimer's disease. J Neurol Sci 1996;142:121–125.
155. George AE, deLeon MJ, Kalnin A. Leukoencephalopathy in normal and pathologic aging. 2. MRI of brain lucencies. AJNR Am J Neuroradiol 1986;7:567–570.
156. Harrell LE, Duvall E, Folks DG, et al. The relationship of high-intensity signals on magnetic resonance images to cognitive and psychiatric state in Alzheimer's disease. Arch Neurol 1991;48:1136–1140.
157. Kumar A, Yousem D, Souder E, et al. High-intensity signals in Alzheimer's disease without cerebrovascular risk factors: a magnetic resonance imaging evaluation. Am J Psychiatry 1992;149:348–250.
158. Leys D, Soetaert G, Petit H, et al. Periventricular and white matter magnetic resonance imaging hyperintensities do not differ between Alzheimer's disease and normal aging. Arch Neurol 1990;47:524–527.
159. Marder K, Richards M, Bello J, et al. Clinical correlates of Alzheimer's disease with and without silent radiographic abnormalities. Arch Neurol 1995;52:146–151.
160. McDonald WM, Krishnan KRR, Doraiswamy PM, et al. Magnetic resonance findings in patients with early-onset Alzheimer's disease. Biol Psychiatry 1991;29:799–810.
161. Mirsen TR, Lee DH, Wong CJ, et al. Clinical correlates of white-matter changes on magnetic resonance imaging scans of the brain. Arch Neurol 1991;48:1015–1021.
162. Rezek DL, Morris JC, Fulling KH, Gado MH. Periventricular white matter lucencies in senile dementia of the Alzheimer type and in normal aging. Neurology 1987;37:1365–1368.
163. Scheltens P, Barkhof F, Leys D, et al. Histopathologic correlates of white matter changes on MRI in Alzheimer's disease and normal aging. Neurology 1995;45:883–888.
164. Scheltens P, Barkhof F, Valk J, et al. White matter lesions on magnetic resonance imaging in clinically diagnosed Alzheimer's disease. Brain 1992;115:735–748.
165. Waldemar G, Christiansen P, Larsson HW, et al. White matter magnetic resonance hyperintensities in dementia of the Alzheimer type: morphological and regional cerebral blood flow correlates. J Neurol Neruosurg Psychiatry 1994;57:1458–1465.
166. Brun A. Neuropathological brain mapping. Dement Geriatr Cogn Disord 1997;8:123–127.
167. Neary D, Snowden J. Fronto-temporal dementia: nosology, neuropsychology, and neuropathology. Brain Cogn 1996;31:176–187.
168. Cummings JL, Duchen LW. Kluver-Bucy syndrome in Pick's disease: clinical and pathologic correlations. Neurology 1981;31:1415–1422.
169. Groen JJ, Hekster REM. Computed tomography in Pick's disease: findings in a family affected in three consecutive generations. J Comput Assist Tomogr 1982;6:907–911.
170. Gustafson L. Clinical picture of frontal lobe degeneration of non-Alzheimer type. Dementia 1993; 41:143–148.
171. Julin P, Wahlund LO, Basun H. Clinical diagnosis of frontal lobe dementia and Alzheimer's disease: relation to cerebral perfusion, brain atrophy, and electroencephalography. Dementia 1995;6:142–147.
172. Kitagaki H, Mori E, Hirono N, et al. Alteration of white matter MR signal intensity in frontotemporal dementia. AJNR Am J Neuroradiol 1997;18:367–378.
173. Weschler AF, Verity MA, Rosenschein S, et al. Pick's disease. A clinical, computed tomographic, and histologic study with Golgi impregnation observations. Arch Neurol 1982;39:287–290.
174. Hodges JR, Patterson K, Oxbury S, Funnell E. Semantic dementia. Progressive fluent aphasia with temporal lobe atrophy. Brain 1992;115:1783–1806.

175. Caselli RJ, Jack CRJ. Asymmetric cortical degeneration syndromes. A proposed clinical classification. Arch Neuol 1992;49:770–780.
176. Caselli RJ, Jack CRJ, Petersen RC, et al. Asymmetric cortical degenerative syndromes. Clinical and radiologic correlations. Neurology 1992;42:1462–1468.
177. Perry RH, Irving D, Blessed G, et al. Senile dementia of Lewy body type. A clinically and neuropathologically distinct form of Lewy body dementia in the elderly. J Neurol Sci 1990;95:119–139.
178. Braffman BH, Grossman RI, Goldberg HI, et al. MR imaging of Parkinson disease with spin-echo and gradient-echo sequences. AJNR Am J Neuroradiol 1988;9:1093–1099.
179. Drayer BP. Imaging of the aging brain. Part II. Pathologic conditions. Radiology 1988;166:797–806.
180. Drayer BP. Magnetic resonance imaging and extrapyramidal movement disorders. Eur Neurol 1989; 29:9–12.
181. Pujol J, Junque C, Vendrell P, et al. Reduction of the substantia nigra width and motor decline in aging and Parkinson's disease. Arch Neurol 1992;49:1119–1122.
182. Duguid JR, De La Paz R, DeGroot J. Magnetic resonance imaging of the midbrain in Parkinson's disease. Ann Neurol 1986;20:744–747.
183. Lisanby SH, McDonald WM, Massey EW, et al. Diminished subcortical nuclei volumes in Parkinson's disease by MR imaging. J Neural Transm Suppl 1993;40:13–21.
184. Huber SJ, Chakeres DW, Paulson GW, Khanna R. Magnetic resonance imaging in Parkinson's disease. Arch Neurol 1990;47:735–737.
185. Ryvlin P, Broussolle E, Piollet H, et al. Magnetic resonance imaging evidence of decreased putamenal iron content in idiopathic Parkinson's disease. Arch Neurol 1995;52:583–588.
186. Kume A, Shiratori M, Takahashi A, et al. Hemi-parkinsonism in multiple system atrophy: a PET and MRI study. J Neurol Sci 1992;110:37–45.
187. Huber SJ, Shuttleworth EC, Christy JA, et al. Magnetic resonance imaging in dementia of Parkinson's disease. J Neurol Neurosurg Psychiatry 1989;52:1221–1227.
188. Brown RT, Polinsky RJ, Di Chiro G, et al. MRI in autonomic failure. J Neurol Neurosurg Psychiatry 1987;50:913–914.
189. Stern MB, Braffman BH, Skolnick BE, et al. Magnetic resonance imaging in Parkinson's disease and parkinsonian syndromes. Neurology 1989;39:1524–1526.
190. Savoiardo M, Girotti F, Strada L, Ciceri E. Magnetic resonance imaging in progressive supranuclear palsy and other parkinsonian disorders. J Neural Transm Suppl 1994;42:93–110.
191. Drayer BP, Olanow W, Burger P, et al. Parkinson plus syndrome: diagnosis using field MR imaging of brain iron. Radiology 1986;159:493–498.
192. Ye FQ, Allen PS, Martin WR. Basal ganglia iron content in Parkinson's disease measured with magnetic resonance. Mov Disord 1996;11:243–249.
193. Oliva D, Carella F, Savoiardo M, et al. Clinical and magnetic resonance features of the classic and akinetic-rigid variants of Huntington's disease. Arch Neurol 1993;50:17–19.
194. Harris GJ, Pearlson GD, Peyser CE, et al. Putamen volume reduction on magnetic resonance imaging exceeds caudate changes in mild Huntington's disease. Ann Neuol 1992;31:69–75.
195. Jernigan TL, Salmon DP, Butters N, et al. Cerebral structure on MRI. Part II. Specific changes in Alzheimer's and Huntington's disease. Biol Psychiatry 1991;29:68–81.
196. Bamford KA, Caine ED, Kido DK, et al. Clinical-pathologic correlation in Huntington's disease: a neuropsychological and computed tomography study. Neurology 1989;39:796–801.
197. Bamford KA, Caine ED, Kido DK, et al. A prospective evaluation of cognitive decline in early Huntington's disease: functional and radiographic correlates. Neurology 1995;45:1867–1873.
198. Harris GJ, Aylward EH, Peyser CE, et al. Single photon emission computed tomographic blood flow and magnetic resonance volume imaging of basal ganglia in Huntington's disease. Arch Neurol 1996; 53:316–324.
199. Starkstein SE, Brandt J, Bylsma F, et al. Neuropsychological correlates of brain atrophy in Huntington's disease: a magnetic resonance imaging study. Neuroradiology 1992;34:487–489.
200. Grafton ST, Mazziotta JC, Pahl JJ, et al. Serial changes of cerebral glucose metabolism and caudate size in persons at risk for Huntington's disease. Arch Neurol 1992;49:1161–1167.
201. Aylward EH, Li Q, Stine OC, et al. Longitudinal change in basal ganglia volume in patients with Huntington's disease. Neurology 1997;48:394–399.
202. Aylward EH, Codori AM, Barta PE, et al. Basal ganglia volume and proximity to onset in presymptomatic Huntington disease. Arch Neurol 1996;53:1293–1296.
203. Ostrow PT, Miller LL. Pathology of Small Artery Disease. In LR Caplan, PM Pullicino, M Hommel (eds), Advances in Neurology. New York: Raven Press, 1993;93–123.
204. Furuta A, Ishii N, Nishihara Y, Horie A. Medullary arteries in aging and dementia. Stroke 1991;22: 442–446.

205. Caplan LR, Schoene WC. Clinical features of subcortical arteriosclerotic encephalopathy (Binswanger disease). Neurology 1978;28:1206–1215.
206. Fields WS. Multi-infarct dementia. Neurologic Clinics 1986;4:405–413.
207. Roman GC, Tatemichi TK, Erkinjuntti T, et al. Vascular dementia: diagnostic criteria for research studies. Report of the NINDS-AIREN international workshop. Neurology 1993;43:250–260.
208. Scheinberg P. Dementia due to vascular disease—a multifactorial disorder. Stroke 1988;19:1291–1299.
209. Hachinski VC, Lassen NA, Marshall J. Multi-infarct dementia: a cause of mental deterioration in the elderly. Lancet 1974;2:207–210.
210. Fukuda H, Kobayashi S, Okada K, Tsunematusu T. Frontal white matter lesions and dementia in lacunar infarction. Stroke 1990;21:1143–1149.
211. Liu CK, Miller BL, Cummings JL, et al. A quantitative MRI study of vascular dementia. Neurology 1992;42:138–143.
212. Loeb C, Gandolfo C, Bino G. Intellectual impairment and cerebral lesions in multiple cerebral infarcts. Stroke 1988;19:560–565.
213. Loeb C, Gandolofo C, Croce R. Dementia associated with lacunar infarction. Stroke 1992;23:1225–1229.
214. Roman GC. Senile dementia of the Binswanger type: a vascular form of dementia in the elderly. JAMA 1987;258:1782–1788.
215. Hachinski VC, Potter P, Merskey H. Leuko-araiosis. Arch Neurol 1987;44:21–23.
216. Bradley WG, Waluch V, Brant-Zawadzki M, et al. Patchy, periventricular white matter lesions in the elderly: a common observation during NMR imaging. Noninvasive Medical Imaging 1984;1:35–41.
217. Brant-Zawadzki M, Fein G, Van Dyke C, et al. MR imaging of the aging brain: patchy white-matter lesions and dementia. AJNR Am J Neuroradiol 1985;6:675–682.
218. Mineura K, Sasajima H, Kikuchi K, et al. White matter hyperintensity in neurologically asymptomatic subjects. Acta Neurol Scand 1995;92:151–156.
219. Ylikoski A, Erkinjuntti T, Raininko R, et al. White matter hyperintensities on MRI in the neurologically nondiseased elderly. Analysis of cohorts of consecutive subjects aged 55 to 85 years living at home. Stroke 1995;26:1171–1177.
220. Zimmerman RD, Fleming CA, Lee BCP, et al. Periventricular hyperintensity as seen by magnetic resonance: prevalence and significance. AJNR Am J Neuroradiol 1986;7:13–30.
221. Awad IA, Johnson PC, Spetzler RF, Hodak JA. Incidental subcortical lesions identified on magnetic resonance imaging in the elderly. II. Postmortem pathological correlations. Stroke 1986;17:1090–1097.
222. Braffman BH, Zimmerman RA, Trojanowski JQ, et al. Brain MR: pathologic correlation with gross and histopathology. 2. Hyperintense white matter foci in the elderly. AJNR Am J Neuroradiol 1988;9:629–636.
223. Brun A, Englund E. A white matter disorder in dementia of the Alzheimer type: a pathoanatomical study. Ann Neurol 1986;19:253–262.
224. Chimowitz MI, Estes ML, Fulan AJ, et al. Further observations on the pathology of subcortical lesions identified on magnetic resonance imaging. Arch Neurol 1992;49:747–752.
225. Englund E, Brun A, Alling C. White matter changes in dementia of Alzheimer's type. Brain 1988; 11:1425–1439.
226. Fazekas F, Kleinert R, Offenbacher H, et al. The morphologic correlate of incidental punctate white matter hyperintensities on MR images. AJNR Am J Neuroradiol 1991;12:915–921.
227. Fazekas F, Kleinert R, Offenbacher H, et al. Pathologic correlates of incidental MRI white matter signal hyperintensities. Neurology 1993;43:1683–1689.
228. George AE, deLeon MJ, Gentes CI, et al. Leukoencephalopathy in normal and pathologic aging: 1. CT of brain lucencies. AJNR Am J Neuroradiol 1986;7:561–566.
229. Grafton ST, Sumi SM, Stimac GK, et al. Comparison of postmortem magnetic resonance imaging and neuropathologic findings in the cerebral white matter. Arch Neurol 1991;48:293–298.
230. Gupta SR, Naheedy MH, Young JC, et al. Periventricular white matter changes and dementia. Arch Neurol 1988;45:637–641.
231. Kirkpatrick JB, Hayman LA. White-matter lesions in MR imaging of clinically healthy brains of elderly subjects: possible pathologic basis. Radiology 1987;162:509–511.
232. London E, deLeon MJ, George AE, et al. Periventricular lucencies in the CT scans of aged and demented patients. Biol Psychiatry 1986;21:960–962.
233. Leifer D, Buonanno FS, Richardson EP. Clinicopathologic correlations of cranial magnetic resonance imaging of periventricular white matter. Neurology 1990;40:911–918.
234. Lotz PR, Ballinger WE, Quisling RG. Subcortical arteriosclerotic encephalopathy: CT spectrum and pathologic correlation. AJNR Am J Neuroradiol 1986;7:817–822.
235. Marshall VG, Bradley WG Jr, Marshall CE, et al. Deep white matter infarction: correlation of MR imaging and histopathologic findings. Radiology 1988;167:517–522.

236. Moody DM, Brown WR, Challa VR, Anderson RL. Periventricular venous collagenosis: association with leukoariosis. Radiology 1995;194:469–476.
237. Munoz DG, Hastak SM, Harper B, et al. Pathologic correlates of increased signals of the centrum ovale on magnetic resonance imaging. Arch Neurol 1993;50:492–497.
238. van Swieten JC, van den Hout JHW, van Ketel BA, et al. Periventricular lesions in the white matter on magnetic resonance imaging in the elderly. Brain 1991;114:761–774.
239. Reed D, Jacobs DR, Hayashi T, et al. A comparison of lesions in small intracerebral arteries among Japanese men in Hawaii and Japan. Stroke 1994;25:60–65.
240. Gerard G, Weisberg LA. MRI periventricular lesions in adults. Neurology 1986;36:998–1001.
241. Lechner H, Schmidt R, Bertha G, et al. Nuclear magnetic resonance image white matter lesions and risk factors for stroke in normal individuals. Stroke 1988;19:263–265.
242. Yetkin FZ, Fischer ME, Papke RA, Haughton VM. Focal hyperintensities in cerebral white matter on MR images of asymptomatic volunteers: correlation with social and medical histories. AJR Am J Roentgenol 1993;161:855–858.
243. Barboriak DP, Provenzale JM, Boyko OB. MR diagnosis of Creutzfeldt-Jakob disease: significance of high signal intensity of the basal ganglia. AJR Am J Roentgenol 1994;162:137–140.
244. Finkenstaedt M, Szudra A, Zerr I, et al. MR imaging of Creutzfeldt-Jakob disease. Radiology 1996; 199:793–798.
245. Pearl GS, Anderson RE. Creutzfeldt-Jakob disease: high caudate signal on magnetic resonance imaging. South Med J 1989;82:1177–1180.
246. Rother J, Schwartz A, Harle M, et al. Magnetic resonance imaging follow-up in Creutzfeldt-Jakob disease. J Neurol 1992;239:404–406.
247. Milton WJ, Atlas SW, Lavi E, Mollman JE. Magnetic resonance imaging of Creutzfeldt-Jacob disease [see comments]. Ann Neurol 1991;29:438–440.
248. Falcone S, Quencer RM, Bowen B, et al. Creutzfeldt-Jakob disease: focal symmetrical cortical involvement demonstrated by MR imaging. AJNR Am J Neuroradiol 1992;13:403–406.
249. Uchino A, Yoshinaga M, Shiokawa O, et al. Serial MR imaging in Creutzfeldt-Jakob disease. Neuroradiology 1991;33:364–367.
250. Bradley WGJ, Kortman KE, Burgoyne B. Flowing cerebrospinal fluid in normal and hydrocephalic states: appearance on MR images. Radiology 1986;159:611–616.
251. Bradley WG, Whittemore AR, Watanabe AS, et al. Association of deep white matter infarction with chronic communicating hydrocephalus: implications regarding the possible origin of normal-pressure hydrocephalus. AJNR Am J Neuroradiol 1991;12:31–39.
252. Bradley WG Jr, Scalzo D, Queralt J, et al. Normal-pressure hydrocephalus: evaluation with cerebrospinal fluid flow measurements at MR imaging. Radiology 1996;198:523–529.
253. Krauss JK, Regel JP, Vach W, et al. Flow void of cerebrospinal fluid in idiopathic normal pressure hydrocephalus of the elderly: can it predict outcome after shunting? Neurosurgery 1997;40:67–74.
254. Adams RD, Fisher CM, Hakim S, et al. Symptomatic occult hydrocephalus with "normal" cerebrospinal-fluid pressure: a treatable syndrome. N Engl J Med 1965;273:117–126.
255. Huckman MS. Normal pressure: evaluation of diagnostic and prognostic tests. AJNR Am J Neuroradiol 1981;2:385–395.
256. Jack CR Jr, Mokri B, Laws ER Jr, et al. MR findings in normal-pressure hydrocephalus: significance and comparison with other forms of dementia. J Comput Assist Tomogr 1987;11:923–931.
257. Sherman JL, Citrin CH, Gangarosa RE, et al. The MR appearance of CSF flow in patients with ventriculomegaly. AJNR Am J Neuroradiol 1986;7:1025–1031.
258. Mascalchi M, Arnetoli G, Inzitari D, et al. Cine-MR imaging of aqueductal CSF flow in normal pressure hydrocephalus syndrome before and after CSF shunt. Acta Radiol 1993;34:586–592.
259. Larson EB. Alzheimer's disease in the community. JAMA 1989;262:2591–2592.
260. de Leon MJ, Convit A, DeSanti S, et al. The hippocampus in aging and Alzheimer's disease. Neuroimaging Clin North Am 1995;5:1–17.
261. Davis PC, Mirra SS, Alazraki N. The brain in older persons with and without dementia: findings on MR, PET, and SPECT images. AJR Am J Roentgenol 1994;162:1267–1278.
262. Katzman R. Should a major imaging procedure (CT or MRI) be required in the workup of dementia? An affirmative view. J Fam Pract 1990;31:401–405.
263. Johnson KA, Davis KR, Buonanno FS, et al. Comparison of magnetic resonance and roentgen ray computed tomography in dementia. Arch Neurol 1987;44:1075–1080.
264. Brown JJ, Hesselink JR, Rothrock JF. MR and CT of lacunar infarcts. AJNR Am J Neuroradiol 1988;9:477–482.

9
Functional Neuroimaging in Dementia

Angus M. Kennedy

Since the 1980s, advances have been made in neuroimaging technology that provide clinicians with an expanding armamentarium for imaging the shape, size, and function of the human brain. These developments, particularly the advent of computerized tomography (CT) and magnetic resonance imaging (MRI), have had enormous impact on neurologic practice. Scans that assess brain morphology are central to the differential diagnosis of dementia (see Chapter 8). In many instances of dementia, however, brain anatomy appears normal even though clinical examinations indicate that the brain is not functioning normally. In these situations, functional imaging (FI) has the potential to complement morphologic brain imaging and provide a biological measure of the behavioral abnormalities observed in dementia. This chapter provides a comprehensive account of FI in dementia and includes (1) a critical review of the different functional techniques and methodologies that have been used to investigate cognitive impairment, (2) a summary of the key scientific findings from studies that describe metabolic or perfusion deficits in patients with different types of dementia, (3) current views about the pathophysiologic basis of the metabolic patterns, and (4) practical guidelines for the use of FI in investigation of cognitive impairment.

NUCLEAR MEDICINE TECHNIQUES

FI measures neural activity indirectly using surrogate markers to calculate resting brain glucose metabolism or cerebral blood flow (CBF). The two nuclear medicine methods used are positron emission tomography (PET) and single photon emission computed tomography (SPECT). Two different techniques have been developed to measure glucose metabolism or CBF with PET. The ^{18}F fluorodeoxyglucose (FDG) technique estimates cerebral glucose metabolism after intravenous injection of an artificial radiolabeled form of glucose, which is only partly metabolized by brain cells [1,2]. PET brain images depend on detecting the gamma rays produced by annihilation of a positron and an electron from the decaying ^{18}F isotope. The PET camera records the location and extent of such events, which are subsequently used to form a radioactive decays distribution map after computer analysis. The $^{15}O_2$ oxygen method simultaneously measures cerebral oxygen metabolism and CBF following inhalation of ^{15}O-labeled oxygen incorporated into $C^{15}O$, $^{15}O_2$, and $C^{15}O_2$ [3]. Complex kinetic models allow both methods to quantify absolute values for metabolism and CBF from the reconstructed images and a measured plasma input function. Regional radioactivity can be estimated from the scan by manual placement of regions of interest (ROI). Subsequently, the number of radioactive counts from each ROI can be used to quantify metabolism or CBF. Improved imaging processing enables absolute quantification of entire image sets.

The methods used for PET scan interpretation have varied considerably between laboratories; styles of depicting data are equally diverse. Visual assessment of color-coded images is favored by some, although others believe this technique to be insufficiently sensitive for diagnostic purposes [4]. Most investigators agree that some attempt to control for the wide variations in global cerebral metabolism found between individual subjects should be made. The best theoretical solution is to adjust the raw data by calculating a ratio between the regional cerebral metabolic rate for glucose (rCMRGlu) and the global cerebral metabolic rate for glucose (gCMRGlu) for the whole brain. This procedure provides an index of metabolism at a given location of the brain and facilitates comparison between subjects. In practice, regional data from patients with dementia have been normalized to a cerebellar internal reference standard [5–7] because the cerebellum is assumed to be unaffected by the majority of degenerative diseases [5]. Although this assumption is usually correct, some types of dementia, such as prion disease, may affect the cerebellum [8]. Other reference points, therefore, have been used, including the occipital [9,10] and sensorimotor cortex [11,12]. Some laboratories calculate an asymmetry ratio, which determines the variation in regional metabolism between the left and right side of the brain [6,9,13–20]. Alternatively, more complex metabolic ratios have been proposed that compare the mean rCMRGlu at predefined locations affected by Alzheimer's disease (AD) pathology with the mean rCMRGlu from areas thought to be relatively unaffected by the disease [17]. This composite formula has been subsequently used to compare individual patients scanned with different PET cameras [21] and with different ages at onset [22]. One disadvantage of the analysis using ratios is that it fails to make complete use of the data set. Consequently, automated means of analysis that enable statistical comparison of the entire scan on a pixel-by-pixel basis have been suggested [23–25]. These techniques make fewer a priori assumptions about the nature and extent of metabolic deficits and are useful for comparing different groups of patients or for analyzing individual subjects versus normal control data. The analyses take advantage of the linear relationship between regional radioactivity and the absolute values for the metabolic rate for glucose metabolism or CBF. Each scan is stereotactically realigned so that the brains are identically oriented to all the others included in the analysis group. Corrections are then made for variations in global flow between individuals before pixel-by-pixel statistical analyses are performed. Correction for multiple statistical test comparisons are frequently required in this sort of analysis, and various statistical procedures can be used to determine the significance threshold. Several approaches have been proposed for dementia studies, including a *z* score surface projection method [23], a regression-type statistical analysis method, [26] and the statistical parametric mapping (SPM) method, which is commonly used for scans obtained during cognitive activation analysis [25,27]. There has been concern that brain images from individuals with dementia may be less easily manipulated during these analyses; in practice, however, the results are similar to those using more labor-intensive methods.

SPECT provides estimates of cerebral perfusion; unlike PET, it does not measure glucose metabolism. SPECT uses lipophilic tracers of CBF such as technetium Tc 99m hexamethyl propyleneamine oxamine (HMPAO) or *N*-isopropyl-*p*-iodoamphetamine, which cross the blood-brain barrier where they are metabolized to less-lipid-soluble products. The distribution of these breakdown products is thought to reflect CBF at the time of injection. Some of the methods used to analyze PET data have been used for SPECT scan analysis and include visual assessments of images by blinded observers [28–35], manual placement of ROIs with normalization of CBF to reference values, semiautomated ROI placement, and combinations of all three. Because the SPECT images are not absolutely quantifiable, there is controversy about which location should be used for normalization of ROI data. Some authors believe the cerebellum should be used [36–44], but others prefer the occipital cortex [45–49], basal ganglia [50], or hemispheric values of flow [51]. The different reference points may account for some of the discrepancies found between studies [44,52]. Artificial neural network classifiers have been proposed as a means of discriminating perfusion patterns found in elderly controls and those of patients with dementia. Two studies now suggest that this type of scan analysis shows considerable promise because they outperformed other techniques and correctly classified between 88% and 94% of subjects [53,54].

Advantages and Disadvantages of Positron Emission Tomography and Single Photon Emission Computed Tomography

PET is primarily a research tool, although it is available as a clinical service in a number of centers. Its widespread clinical application is unlikely, mainly because a cyclotron is required to produce the radioactive isotopes, such as oxygen 15 and fluorine 18, on which the techniques are based. Its advantage has been to provide sensitive quantitative measures of brain function, and its future as a method for assessing physiologic parameters such as receptor binding should not be dismissed. In contrast to PET, the radioactive tracers used in SPECT are relatively inexpensive and easy to prepare and administer. Because SPECT uses a standard gamma ray detection camera, SPECT brain scans can be performed in nearly all nuclear medicine departments. Modern PET cameras have resolutions approaching 6-mm full-width-half-maximum (FWHM) with a uniform field of view, which may have theoretical advantages when it comes to determining the earliest metabolic consequences of dementia. Even with the best camera, the PET technique can only just resolve the 3-cm × 1-cm human hippocampus. Modern SPECT gamma cameras have image resolutions approaching that of PET; however, some differences in resolution are attributed to the nonuniform field sensitivity of

SPECT, which may hinder its ability to quantify some parts of the brain, particularly central brain structures such as the hippocampus.

Overall, the technical limitations of SPECT have to be compared with the expense and restricted availability of PET. It remains to be determined whether the nonbiological, nonuniform tracers used in SPECT, which also has generally poorer resolution, will limit its ability to distinguish the CBF changes associated with early Alzheimer's disease (AD). Although some advocates are confident about the potential ability of SPECT to do this [55], others do not share such optimism [56]. To address these issues, several authors have directly compared PET and SPECT in the same group of patients with dementia and concluded that the metabolic patterns of deficits are most accurately evaluated with PET [50,57]. One study suggested that glucose metabolism may be more sensitive than CBF for detecting deficits in mildly affected individuals [58]. Although an early study that compared CT, MRI, and PET found that FI was more sensitive than structural techniques, there have been no subsequent large-scale studies that compare volumetric hippocampal MRI, neuropsychological assessment, and PET and SPECT imaging [59]. This deficiency has been partly due to the logistic difficulties associated with performing a multimodal study of this nature in patients with AD. Furthermore, the data from longitudinal studies in subjects at risk of familial AD suggest that PET, MRI, and neuropsychological methods can all detect presymptomatic deficits in those who go on to become demented [25,60,61]. It remains to be seen, however, whether these findings can be extrapolated to the wider AD population. SPECT seems less sensitive than PET in detecting early disease: In two separate studies, approximately one-third of patients with mild probable AD had a normal perfusion pattern [49,62].

Positron Emission Tomography and Alzheimer's Disease

There are many studies in the world literature that describe resting cerebral metabolism and CBF measured by PET in patients with AD (Table 9.1). Frackowiak and colleagues [63] were the first to show a global reduction in CBF and oxygen metabolism using PET $^{15}O_2$ in 20 patients with degenerative dementia. The deficits were not uniform and appeared greatest in the temporal and parietal cortices, with additional frontal hypometabolism in those who were more severely demented. These abnormalities were in contrast to other regions of the brain, such as the cerebellum, motor cortex, occipital cortex, and the basal ganglia, in which the values for CBF and metabolism remained within normal limits. In addition, the study showed that blood flow and metabolism remained physiologically coupled in both degenerative and vascular dementia, thereby disproving any suggestion that chronic ischemia might contribute to the pathophysiology of these conditions.

The majority of PET studies have used ^{18}F FDG to measure cerebral glucose metabolism. As with ^{15}O, most investigators report a temporoparietal (TP) pattern of hypometabolism in patients with AD [64–67]. Although initial studies were performed before the advent of the National Institute of Neurological Communication Disorders and Stroke–Alzheimer's Disease and Related Disorders Association (NINCDS-ADRDA) criteria for AD, subsequent experiments have confirmed that this pattern is consistently observed in probable AD patients selected using these criteria. Table 9.1 summarizes nearly 60 PET AD studies accumulated between 1980 and 1996 performed on more than 1,000 patients with probable AD. The following conclusions can be drawn. The majority of the studies show significant reductions in global cerebral glucose metabolism or CBF, with maximal regional decreases in the parietal and temporal association cortices [6,13,17,21,67–73]. The extent of the decreases when compared with age-matched controls ranges between 30% and 70%. The TP deficits have usually been bilateral [6,12,13,16,17,21–23,63,68–70,72,74–76], although unilateral TP hypometabolism has been noted by some authors in a small percentage of subjects [13,16,21,72,77,78] (Figure 9.1). Hypometabolism in frontal association cortices is usually less severe [6,17,21,22,63,67,71,72,75,79,80] and is most apparent in patients with advanced disease [22,63,69,71,72,80]. The sensorimotor, visual cortices, basal ganglia, and cerebellum usually have metabolic values that are not significantly different from those found in controls [17,63,67].

TEMPOROPARIETAL METABOLIC DEFICIT

Although a TP deficit is a frequent observation in probable AD, this pattern is not pathognomonic of AD because occasionally it is described in other neurologic conditions, including multi-infarct dementia (MID) [76,81], Parkinson's disease (PD) without dementia [82], PD with dementia [76,83], diffuse Lewy body disease (LBD) [84], and Creutzfeldt-Jakob disease (CJD) [76,83,85]. It would be important to know the specificity and sensitivity of the TP pattern for AD, but there have been numerous obstacles to deriving this information. First, insufficient numbers of AD patients with a TP deficit have undergone postmortem examination. The data in Table 9.1 show that 73 patients with autopsy-confirmed AD had the TP pattern, which represented less than 1% of all patients studied [6,14,63,71,72,76,78,86–89]. Also, the NINCDS-ADRDA criteria are not completely reliable and sometimes fail to exclude non-AD causes of dementia, which complicates interpretation of studies that use the criteria as the sole method for selecting AD cases [90]. Other limitations include the diagnostic power of PET, the quality of image analysis, the variety of non-AD dementia control subjects, and the types of classification methods that were used. Few have calculated the positive predictive value attributable to PET imaging or estimated the additional diagnostic benefit that the scan provides.

Visual analysis of PET data is widely used but may not be sufficiently sensitive. For example, Powers and colleagues [4] tested the value of bilateral TP deficits as a marker of AD in a blinded analysis of low-resolution CBF images. Little useful diagnostic information was obtained because the pattern was associated with a sensitivity of 0.38 (five of 13 AD cases were correctly identified) and a specificity of 0.88 (the deficit was seen in only three of 26 controls). Others report similar data: Duara and colleagues [81] found that a parietal to occipital lobe ratio achieved an acceptable degree of sensitivity (91% for detecting abnormality in AD patients) but only a 54% specificity. This ratio also failed to distinguish MID patients, included in the study as dementia controls, from AD patients. This group also reported better results with a neural network

Table 9.1 Summary of all positron emission tomography studies involving Alzheimer's disease patients between 1980 and 1997

Year	*Author*	*Reference*	*Alzheimer's disease patients (n)*	*Severity of dementia*[a]	*Controls (n)*	*Other dementia types*[b]
1980	Ferris et al.	64	7	ns	3	—
1981	Frackowiak et al.	63	13	B	14	9 MID
1982	Farkas et al.	65	11	ns	6	—
1983	Benson et al.	67	8	M se	8	3 MID
1983	de Leon et al.	246	23	R (3–6)	21	—
1983	Foster et al.	13	13	M	10	—
1983	Friedland et al.	68	10	M	6	—
1984	Chase et al.	79	17	M	5	—
1984	Foster et al.	69	20	NPB	8	—
1984	Friedland et al.	66	2	M (91–111)	7	—
1985	Cutler et al.	71	7	F (16)	25	—
1985	Cutler et al.	89	1	B (1.5)	12	—
1985	Friedland et al.	98	—	M	—	—
1985	Haxby et al.	74	10	F (20.7)	26	—
1985	Jagust et al.	97	7	M (93)	17	3 NPH
1985	Koss et al.	18	18	M mi,mo	7	—
1985	Kuhl et al.	70	6	M mo,se	6	6 MID; DEP
1986	Durara et al.	72	21	B (3–18)	29	—
1986	Foster et al.	111	17	NPB	6	—
1986	Grady et al.	19	16	F	0	—
1986	Haxby et al.	12	22	F (12–29)	29	—
1986	McGeer et al.	100	1	ns	10	—
1986	McGeer et al.	6	14	NPB	11	—
1986	Polinsky et al.	73	2	B (10)	4	—
1987	Chalwuck et al.	110	24	F	17	—
1987	Grady et al.	11	34	F (17)	28	—
1988	Haxby et al.	80	32	F (0–30)	29	—
1988	Jagust et al.	15	6	M	7	—
1989	Adams et al.	117	1	R (6)	0	—
1989	Durara et al.	81	87	F (20.2)	36	12 MID
1989	Small et al.	116	24	F (19)	0	—
1989	Fazekas et al.	59	30	F (29–4)	25	—
1989	Foster et al.	78	10	ns	9	—
1989	Lowenstein et al.	77	31	F (19)	45	11 MID
1990	Haxby et al.	14	33	F (30–0)	29	—
1990	Herholtz et al.	17	19	F (14.5)	19	—
1990	McGeer et al.	16	57	NPB	20	—
1991	Guze et al.	95	—	F	—	DEP
1991	Kumar et al.	9	47	Range	30	—
1991	Nyback et al.	75	13	R	9	—
1992	Mielke et al	22	38	F (16)	20	—
1992	DeCarli et al.	86	6	ns	0	—
1992	Kippenhan et al.	91	80	F (15)	?	—
1992	Powers et al.	4	13	CDR	11	13 PD
1993	Goto et al.	83	14	ns	5	3 PSP; 9 P; 2 CJD; 5 PD

Analysis method[c]	*Maximum deficit (%)*	*Parietal*	*Temporal*	*Frontal*	*Occipital*	*Autopsy confirmation (n)*
		Rank order				
Ab: ROI	37	—	2	1	—	0
Ab: ROI	29	1	2	3	—	4
Ab: ROI	45		No pattern			0
Ab: ROI	49	1	1	2	—	0
Ab: ROI	23		No pattern			0
Ab: ROI	19	1	2	3	—	0
R: LR	ns	2	1	—	—	0
Ab: ROI	42	1	2	—	—	0
Ab: ROI	49	1	2	3	—	0
Ab: ROI	ns	2	1	—	—	0
Ab: ROI	20–55	1	2	3	—	1
Ab: ROI	40	1	2	—	—	1
Ab: ROI	ns	1	2	—	—	0
R: LR	14	1	2	3	—	0
Ab: ROI	40	2	1	3	—	0
R: LR	ns	ns	ns	ns	ns	0
R: global	54	1	—	3	2	0
Ab: ROI; R: LR	15–50	1	—	—	—	3
Ab: ROI	ns	ns	ns	ns	ns	0
R: LR	ns	ns	ns	ns	ns	0
R: motor	ns	1	—	—	—	0
Absol	60	2	1	3	—	1
R: cereb; R: LR	35	3	1	2	4	2
R: global	36	1	2	—	—	FAD
R: global	ns	ns	ns	ns	ns	0
R: motor; R: LR	ns	ns	ns	ns	ns	0
R: motor	16	1	—	2	—	0
—	ns	1	2	3	—	0
Ab: ROI	ns	2	1	3	—	1
Ab: ROI; R: occ	ns	1	1	—	—	0
R: global	30	1	2	3	—	0
V	—	2	3	1	—	0
—	—	2	1	—	—	10
R: LR	ns	2	—	1	—	0
R: LR	ns	2	1	3	—	10
R: H	—	—	—	—	—	0
Ab: ROI; R: LR	12	2	1	3	—	8
hippo, ?dlpf	30	—	—	—	—	0
R: occ; R: LR	34	1	2	3	—	6
Ab: ROI; R: LR	60	1	2	—	—	—
R: H	30	—	—	—	—	—
Ab: ROI	ns	ns	ns	ns	ns	6
Multiple	ns	—	—	—	—	0
V	ns	1	2	—	—	4
V	ns	1	2	3	—	0

Table 9.1 (continued)

Year	*Author*	*Reference*	*Alzheimer's disease patients (n)*	*Severity of dementia*[a]	*Controls (n)*	*Other dementia types*[b]
1993	Herholtz et al.	21	37	F	34	—
1993	Jagust et al.	105	22	F (21)	8	—
1993	Kennedy et al.	247	—	F (16)	—	—
1994	Ichimiya et al.	20	61	F (18)	—	—
1994	Mesna et al.	50	21	F (19)	10	—
1994	Salmon et al.	76	65	ns	—	28 MID; 1 PSP; 5 P; 3 CJD; 13 PD
1995	Ishii et al.	7	16	F (17.7)	14	—
1995	Kennedy et al.	25	3	—	—	—
1995	Kennedy et al.	119	18	—	—	—
1995	Minoshima et al.	23	37	CDR	22	5 MID
1995	Penniello et al.	112	11	F (10–26)	0	—
1996	DeCarli et al.	88	28	F (12)	14	—
1996	Mielke et al.	87	4	ns	ns	—
1996	Salmon et al.	10	10	F (15.8)	10	—

ns = not stated; FAD = familial Alzheimer's disease.

[a]Capital letters indicate the type of test; lowercase letters give a broad indication of the severity of dementia (e.g., mild, moderate, severe). Numeric values shown in parentheses indicate the mean score or range on the appropriate scale. (B = Blessed Dementia Scale; M = Mattis dementia rating; R = Reisberg dementia scale; NPB = neuropsychological battery; F = Folstein Mini-Mental State Examination; Range = range of different severity; CDR = Clinical Dementia Rating scale; mi = mild; mo = moderate; se = severe.)

[b]This column lists the types and numbers of other dementias studied. (MID = multi-infarct dementia; NPH = normal pressure hydrocephalus; DEP = depression; PD = Parkinson's disease with dementia; PSP = progressive supranuclear palsy; P = Pick's disease; CJD = Creutzfeldt-Jakob disease.)

[c]Ab: ROI = absolute quantification using an ROI method; R: LR = ratio method: left right asymmetry; R: global = ratio method: global metabolism used as denominator; R: motor = ratio method: motor cortex used as denominator; Absol = absolute; R: cereb = ratio method: cerebellar cortex used as denominator; R: occ = ratio method: occipital; V = visual analysis; R: II = composite ratio, hippo = hippocampal; dlpf = dorsolateral prefrontal cortex; PCA = principal component analysis; R: occ bg = ratio method: occipital: basal ganglia; PBPA = pixel-by-pixel analysis; R: temp = ratio method: temporal.

Analysis method[c]	*Maximum deficit (%)*	*Parietal*	*Temporal*	*Frontal*	*Occipital*	*Autopsy confirmation (n)*
		Rank order				
V; R: H	ns	ns	ns	ns	ns	—
Absol; ratio regions	35	—	1	—	—	0
—	ns	1	2	3	—	C21
R: cereb; PCA	ns	ns	ns	ns	ns	—
R: occ bg	25	2	1	—	—	—
V	ns	ns	ns	ns	ns	5
Ab: ROI; R: cereb	—	2	1	3	—	No
Ab: ROI; PBPA	ns	1	2	3	—	C14
PBPA	—	1	2	3	—	FAD
PBPA	20	1	2	3	—	0
R: temp	ns	ns	ns	ns	ns	0
Ab: ROI	—	1	2	3	—	10
R: global	—	2	1	3	—	4
R: occ	28	2	1	3	—	No

classifier, which performed at a specificity of 80% and a sensitivity of 80–85% [91]. Indeed, these findings were better than discriminant function analysis, which has also been used for scan classification [26]. Herholz and colleagues [17] reported results using a composite metabolic ratio (see the section on Nuclear Medicine Techniques, above), which was used to test diagnostic power in 56 probable AD patients and achieved a sensitivity of 92% and a specificity of 80% for predicting the disease. Further impressive results with the composite ratio have been reported, although non-AD dementia controls were not included in the subsequent study [21]. The specificity and sensitivity of metabolic patterns in AD will remain a subject of controversy until large, randomly chosen samples can be studied and followed to a definitive pathologic diagnosis. The suggestion at present is that visual analyses involving the TP pattern are insufficiently sensitive, in that fewer abnormalities are detected than with other methods.

Another way to gauge the clinical utility of PET in dementia derives from studies that report the different metabolic profiles obtained in consecutive referrals to a dementia clinic. Salmon and colleagues [76] studied 65 cases with probable or definite AD from a total of 129 patients with dementia. Abnormal scans were found in 97% of patients, with 83% of AD patients having a bilateral or unilateral TP deficit. Frontal deficits were more likely to be found in non-AD subjects, and the unilateral TP deficit was found in less than one-fourth of all AD patients. Other studies of this type have corroborated these findings [83]. In retrospect, it was optimistic to view the TP pattern in isolation as a specific marker for AD, especially because considerable clinical overlap is already known to exist

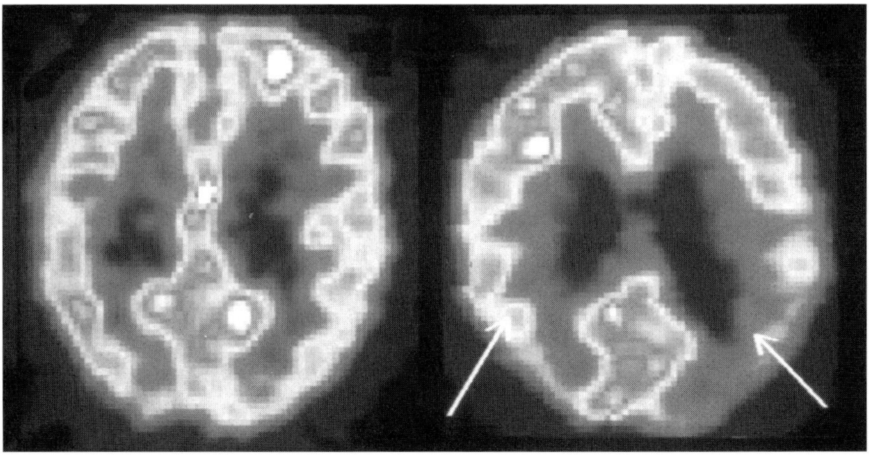

Figure 9.1 Fluorodeoxyglucose positron emission tomography. Normal control (*left*) and typical temporoparietal hypometabolism (*right*) in probable Alzheimer's disease.

between the different causes of dementia. Based on our current knowledge, it is reasonable to conclude that the TP deficit is frequently found in AD and is significantly distinct from some patterns found in other pathologic entities, particularly those that manifest themselves as frontal lobe syndromes. Importantly, isolated frontal hypometabolism has not been convincingly described as an early metabolic feature of definite AD. Two accounts of unusual "apparent" frontal AD are reported, although insufficient details are provided [76,92]. The TP pattern has greatest utility in distinguishing AD patients from those with probable Pick's disease (PcD) [93,94] or frontal lobe dementia (FLD) [76,83] and other conditions, including depression [95,96] and normal pressure hydrocephalus [76,97], which have different patterns of dysmetabolism. For these reasons, the TP pattern when present can be used to add weight to a clinical diagnosis of probable AD.

What Causes the Metabolic Deficit?

The precise pathophysiologic mechanism(s) for the TP deficits is unclear, and many theories have been proposed. The prevailing hypothesis is that the metabolic deficits in some way reflect neuronal dysfunction because they parallel the distribution of AD histopathology, showing predilection for the association neocortices [98,99]. McGeer and colleagues [100] followed a single patient to autopsy and showed a qualitative relationship between the severity of the metabolic deficit and the extent of neuronal loss as well as the severity of gliosis. They concluded that the deficits were likely to be due to depressed metabolism in less actively functioning neurons and not due to partial volume effects. DeCarli and colleagues [86] reported five of six subjects who showed a clear relationship between the antemortem pattern of regional metabolism and the density of neurofibrillary tangles (NFTs) found at postmortem. No correlations were found between neuritic plaque or neuronal density, however, and they concluded that the metabolic pattern reflected neuronal dysfunction due to tangle accumulation, although the precise relationship was probably more complicated. Such reports are limited by the supposition that little or no alteration occurs in either variable in the intervening period between final scan and death. These observations are similar to other quantitative pathologic studies in AD that show correlations between tangle density and clinical markers of disease severity [101]. In the only study in which these conditions were met, no correlations were detected between regional metabolism and tangle density. Mega and colleagues [102] described an AD patient who had an FDG scan shortly before death. The digitized brain specifically stained for NFTs was subsequently coregistered with the PET data. No correlations between the scan and NFTs were apparent, but a correlation between FDG metabolism and the concentration of amyloid beta-protein (Aβ) was later reported [103].

An alternative view holds that the TP deficit may occur as a result of lesions at distant locations, which may be influential in determining the initial location of metabolic patterns. In this instance, the earliest metabolic changes in AD may not be in the brain region that shows the earliest or most severe pathologic changes, such as the entorhinal cortex and hippocampus [101,104]. Jagust and colleagues [105,106] addressed this point and studied the medial temporal cortex of 22 mildly affected AD patients using a single slice PET camera with high resolution (2.6 mm FWHM). The results suggested that the early maximal deficits were to be found in the temporal neocortex and not the medial temporal cortex or hippocampus. They concluded that maximal initial reductions in rCMRGlu can occur remote from the cortex that is maximally affected by early AD pathology. The studies of individuals at risk for familial AD also show that maximal early deficits occur remote from medial temporal structures [25]. These conclusions arc consistent with functional disconnection of neurons projecting to and from the entorhinal cortex and hippocampus. Meguro and colleagues [107] have tested this theory in experiments that show that bilateral focal rhinal lesions cause long-standing alterations in the pattern of rCMRGlu abnormality in association cortices. A further PET autopsy series also suggests that tangle formation may disrupt projection neurons, which may in turn be responsible for cortical dysfunction [87]. MRI and PET studies also support this view, and Yamaguchi and colleagues [108] report a correlation between hippocampal atrophy and ipsilateral cortical metabolism in the temporal lobe.

Other slightly different hypotheses have been put forward. Salmon and colleagues [10] compared the extent of cortical tissue loss as measured with ^{11}C methionine with the pattern of glucose metabolism. The regional tissue loss was insufficient to explain cortical glucose metabolism decreases, which they concluded reflected reduced synaptic connectivity. It is also possible that partial volume effects may contribute to the TP pattern. This problem is largely a consequence of the poor spatial resolution of PET, which cannot differentiate between enlarged ventricles and relatively shrunken brain. Attempts to correct for these effects have been made that diminish the calculated reductions in cerebral metabolism [109,110], but it is important to note that deficits sometimes occur in the absence of any atrophy whatsoever [98]. The majority opinion suggests that dysmetabolism reflects neuronal loss, although the other mechanisms described above may contribute.

Correlations between Neuropsychological Markers and Metabolic Patterns in Alzheimer's Disease

In many studies, regional hypometabolism has been correlated with clinical measures of disease severity [6,7,10,14,20,22,63,64,69,79,80,87,88,105]; however, a significant association has not always been found [13,21,77]. Some investigators have correlated regional metabolic deficits with various behavioral measures, including tests of language [12,13,63,74,75,79,80], visuospatial function [12,13,18,74,75,79,111], praxis [63,111], and spelling [112]. Foster and colleagues [111] reported that AD patients who showed a predominance of apraxia as judged by a composite test of praxis in response to verbal commands and visual demonstration showed more profound right parietal hypometabolism, whereas those with predominant language impairment had greater left hemisphere hypometabolism [13]. Haxby and colleagues [74] investigated the relationship between regional asymmetry and neuropsychological function by calculating a single ratio that expressed the difference between regional metabolism at identical locations on the left and right side of the brain: (right – left)/(right + left/2) × 100. Whereas the mean value for this ratio in AD did not differ overall from that found in controls, the variance was significantly greater [74]. This finding has subsequently been confirmed in many similar studies [9,12, 14–20,75]. In most cases the variance in metabolic asymmetry has been found to correlate with the behavioral data. For instance, those who have greater language deficits have more pronounced left frontotemporal asymmetry, and those who have impairment in visuospatial function show right parietal asymmetry. The ratio has been used in an important series of longitudinal studies that show that the pattern of metabolic asymmetry becomes more apparent over time and can be used to predict subsequent cognitive decline [12,14,19,74]. Although most investigators have not reported overall asymmetries in metabolism, Lowenstein and colleagues [113] did note predominant left hemisphere hypometabolism in 33 AD subjects that was unrelated to severity or duration of dementia. This striking observation supports a priori speculations that the left hemisphere is more vulnerable in AD than the right [114,115].

POSITRON EMISSION TOMOGRAPHY AND SUBTYPES OF ALZHEIMER'S DISEASE

Many investigators have hoped that PET would identify clinical subtypes of AD, each with distinctive metabolic patterns. This idea relies heavily on the assumption that etiologic subtypes of AD have distinct pathophysiologic mechanisms that selectively affect different populations of vulnerable neurons and ultimately cause distinct patterns of symptoms. PET investigators had hoped that the metabolic variability reported in large cross-sectional studies of AD subjects could be related to etiologic subgroups. On balance, however, the current results fail to show reliable metabolic patterns in different etiologic subtypes of AD. Initial attempts at subtype analysis used age of onset to classify AD patients into early-onset and late-onset cases. In retrospect, it was probably optimistic to expect that this classification would neatly subdivide patients into two etiologic subgroups. Koss and colleagues [18] described right hemisphere asymmetry in seven of 11 presenile onset patients, which was not apparent in an older cohort that conversely had a greater degree of frontal asymmetry. The results were confounded by the fact that the older patients also had a greater severity of dementia. Grady and colleagues [11] studied early- and late-onset groups of AD patients with no difference in baseline neuropsychological profiles or in the rate of cognitive decline and found greater parietal metabolic deficits in the younger onset cases. These observations have been confirmed by subsequent studies [22,116]. Mielke and colleagues [22] found more focal metabolic deficits in presenile patients than in senile AD and attributed this observation to a partial reduction in the contrast between association cortex and other brain regions. This effect may partly reflect diffuse reductions in glucose metabolism associated with normal aging. Subsequently, principal component analyses have been used and show a more prominent right temporoparietal deficit associated with presenile-onset individuals [11,18,20,22,116].

Subtypes of AD based on molecular genetic classification may be a more meaningful way to subdivide patients than is age of onset. In general, cases of familial AD have a metabolic pattern similar to the sporadic form of the disease [73,89,117]. Similarly, age-matched cohorts both with and without a family history do not differ in their pattern of cerebral metabolism [118]. Genetic advances have identified at least three genetic loci associated with familial AD, which are often characterized by consistent pedigree-specific ages of onset (see Chapter 6). A TP and frontal deficit is common to both amyloid precursor protein mutation [119] and presenilin-1 mutation–type AD [24]. Kennedy and colleagues [25] studied asymptomatic individuals at risk of autosomal dominant familial AD to determine whether PET scans could detect preclinical metabolic deficits. They studied gCMRGlu in 24 at-risk individuals and compared these data to normal controls and to clinically affected individuals. The at-risk group showed a significant decrease in gCMRGlu compared to the controls, which was less extensive than that seen in those affected by the disease. An SPM regional analysis of the at-risk data revealed TP and dorsolateral prefrontal deficits, which were also seen in one individual who became symptomatic during the course of the study. This distribution has also been noted in other studies that report those at risk for or affected by early familial AD [25,73,120]. In a related vein, the *ε4* allele of the apolipoprotein E gene (*APOE*) confers increased risk of developing AD (see Chapter 7) and may be detected by PET scans status. Thus, Small and colleagues [121] reported that 12 age-matched cognitively normal subjects with an *APOE-ε4* allele had lower parietal metabolism and greater hemispheric asymmetry than 19 subjects without an *ε4* allele. Reiman and colleagues [122] subsequently confirmed this finding in 11 cognitively normal *ε4* homozygotes who had significant reductions in glucose metabolism in TP, cingulate, and prefrontal cortices compared to 22 control subjects who did not carry an *ε4* allele. One SPECT study that examined the relationship between *APOE* in AD and the pattern of cerebral perfusion suggested that those with an *ε4* allele had more prominent temporal perfusion deficits [123]. Corder and colleagues [124], however, studied 46 dementia clinic patients, including 31 probable AD patients and 12 individuals with mild memory disorders. No specific pattern of metabolism identified individuals with and without an *APOE-ε4* allele, which calls the *ε4* at-risk PET studies into question. Although the at-risk studies confirm earlier work suggesting that metabolic dysfunction precedes the onset of clinical symptoms, the current data argue against different metabolic subtypes in AD.

Cognitive Activation Studies in Alzheimer's Disease

Measuring changes in CBF detected by ^{15}O PET and its application to mapping brain regions involved in different cognitive functions in normal volunteers has gained wide acceptance. Despite the power of the technique, surprisingly few studies have been reported in AD. The scarcity of studies probably reflects the practical difficulties associated with asking cognitively impaired patients to perform intricate behavioral tasks during a PET scan. Some neuropsychological functions, for instance, explicit memory, are preferentially affected in early AD, and for this reason there has been considerable interest to perform studies in amnesic AD patients (for review in normal controls see reference 125). Interpretation of activation data in AD patients, however, is more complicated. What exactly does a different pattern of CBF activation mean in a cognitively impaired patient as compared to a normally performing control subject? It may suggest that additional neuronal circuits are recruited to process the task by an alternative strategy, but on the other hand, such activations may be nonspecific CBF increases arising from the patient's inability to perform the task. Kessler and colleagues [126,127] used a visual recognition task and showed a greater increase in global metabolism in normal controls as compared to the AD subjects. This result was difficult to interpret because the task presentation was adjusted to each subjects' performance. Miller and colleagues [128] used a verbal task and reported a relative shift in glucose metabolism to the right hemisphere in AD patients as opposed to the left hemisphere in normal controls. Grady and colleagues [129] performed a face-matching task and reported that the AD cohort showed a similar pattern of CBF activation associated with sensory and perceptual processing, although additional frontal activation in the AD group was attributed to increased attentional demands. Becker and colleagues used a memory task and suggested a reallocation of brain resources in AD subjects [130], although a subsequent paper used principal component analysis to examine the same data set and showed similar patterns of activation for both groups [131]. Activation studies are probably unlikely to be immediately useful for the clinical evaluation of patients with dementia. The present controversies about the exact CBF correlates of explicit memory in normal control subjects makes it quite unlikely that a simple, highly specific diagnostic activation paradigm can be designed to aid clinical evaluation.

SINGLE PHOTON EMISSION COMPUTED TOMOGRAPHY AND ALZHEIMER'S DISEASE

Early studies by Gemmell and colleagues [132] involving small numbers of subjects suggested that the characteristic TP deficit identified by PET could also be seen with SPECT tracers. Since that original report, 43 different studies including information from more than 950 AD patients scanned with different CBF tracers at a range of scanner resolutions have been published (Table 9.2). Most patients were selected using the NINCDS-ADRDA guidelines, although the context in which the criteria have been applied has varied because different ways of recruiting patients have been used, including referrals to dementia clinics [45,49,62,133] and nuclear medicine departments [134]. The majority of studies have measured dementia severity using the Mini-Mental State Examination (MMSE) [40,43,45,49,62,135,136], Blessed Dementia Scale (BDS) [37], or other scales [30,38,137]. Most patients have been moderately to severely affected [43,45,46,48,138], and only recently have mildly affected subjects with an MMSE greater than 20 out of 30 been evaluated [49,55,123,139]. A variety of other patient groups have been assessed to determine the spectrum of perfusion deficits found in other dementing conditions. These include those with PD [43,135,140], MID [28–30,33,34,40,51,138,140,141], progressive supranuclear palsy (PSP) [34,43,133], and FLD [33,58,133].

Single Photon Emission Computed Tomography and the Temporoparietal Pattern

As with the PET literature, a preponderance of SPECT studies have confirmed the bilateral TP deficit either in isolation [28–32,34,36,39,41,50,51,62,133–137, 142,143] or together with less severe frontal deficits (Figure 9.2). A variable proportion of AD patients have asymmetric or even unilateral TP deficit [28,30,32, 36,38,40,41,50], which indicates that the bilateral TP deficit is unlikely to be a completely reliable diagnostic marker for AD. As in the PET studies, the extent of frontal blood flow deficits in AD has been debated, and although the majority find these in association with the TP pattern [28,31,34,38,40,41,43,46, 50,133,134,137,143–145], some find them in isolation [41,50,133,134]. Many have noted additional frontal deficits in individuals who are severely demented [31,34,40,136,142,144], although not all series report this [43]. The SPECT literature is just as confused as the PET field about the alleged "pure frontal" perfusion pattern in probable AD. Most consider this unusual because it has been rarely documented, and the majority of these patients may not have AD. Despite the large number of reported studies, very few postmortem follow-up studies have been published to clarify these issues. An exception is the study of Bonte and colleagues [146], who compared the clinical, imaging, and histopathologic diagnosis in 18 dementia patients at postmortem examination. The TP pattern correctly identified 11 of the 13 cases with definite AD, whereas a ratio method performed perfectly. Of interest, one patient with diffuse LBD showed the TP pattern; a frontal pattern was noted both in a patient with clinical PcD who had a "multisystem disorder" at autopsy and an individual with adult polyglucosan body disease. This study included a patient with frontal perfusion deficits and pathologically possible AD, even though the hippocampus was said to be uninvolved. Obviously, this patient does not fulfill usual pathologic criteria for AD. In a similar postmortem series, Read and colleagues [147] found the bilateral TP pattern in 11 patients with definite AD; two AD patients also had cortical Lewy bodies, and one had diffuse LBD also. Seven patients with frontal perfusion deficits were found to have either PcD or other types of frontotemporal dementia (FTD). A mottled appearance was observed in two individuals with CJD. Other studies have reported the TP deficit in individuals with pathologically

Table 9.2 Summary of all single photon emission computed tomography studies involving Alzheimer's disease patients between 1980 and 1997

Year	*Author*	*Reference*	*AD patients (n)*	*Severity of dementia*[a]	*Controls (n)*
1984	Gemmell et al.	131	—	ns	ns
1986	Cohenet al.	29	6	ns	6
1986	Sharp et al.	136	14	ns	ns
1987	Celcis et al.	151	6	ns	20
1987	Gemmell et al.	30	17	ns	3
1987	Jagust et al.	51	9	F (15)	5
1987	Johnson et al.	36	15	R	9
1987	Neary et al.	132	23	ns	8
1987	Smith et al.	137	17	ns	9
1988	Johnson et al.	37	37	B	9
1988	Perani et al.	38	16	Crichon	16
1989	Burns et al.	39	20	CAMCOG	6
1989	Hellman et al.	31	10	R (45)	7
1989	Hunter et al.	248	12	F (15)	12
1989	Jagust et al.	45	26	F (10–18)	—
1989	Montaldi et al.	46	26	F (9)	10
1989	Gemmell et al.	28	35	ns	17
1990	Battistin et al.	40	19	F (9)	11
1990	Frelich et al.	143	15	R	0
1990	Gemmell et al.	140	10	—	—
1990	Kuwabara et al.	139	21	ns	75
1990	Kuwabara et al.	58	9	—	—
1990	Spampinato et al.	134	19	F (9)	13
1991	Habert et al.	43	19	F (10)	0
1991	Hurwitz et al.	249	7	F (10)	10
1991	Launes et al.	33	36	ns	—
1991	O'Brien et al.	141	35	F (17)	35
1992	Holman et al.	133	52	ns	—
1992	Liu et al.	32	37	F	19
1992	Pearlson et al.	148	26	F (18)	16
1992	Syed et al.	142	—	M (18)	
1993	Bonte et al.	145	13	ns	ns
1993	Curran et al.	47	20	M (16)	30
1993	Eberling et al.	48	50	F (12–26)	8
1994	Claus et al.	135	48	F (19)	60
1994	Messa et al.	50	21	—	10
1994	Mielke et al.	57	20	F (20)	13
1994	Waldemar et al.	41	25	M (14)	25
1994	Waldemar et al.	35	45	F (13)	13
1995	Ohnishi et al.	149	13	ns	ns
1995	Read et al.	146	16	F (16)	—
1995	Villa et al.	34	23	F (15–21)	ns
1995	Van Gool et al.	62	68	F (16)	18
1996	Greene et al.	49	33	F (23)	30
1996	Lehtovira et al.	123	58	F (21)	34

ns = not stated; FAD = familial Alzheimer's disease.
[a]The letters indicate the type of test. Numeric values shown in parentheses indicate the mean score or range on the appropriate scale. (F = Folstein Mini-Mental State Examination; R = Reisberg dementia scale; B = Blessed Dementia Scale; Crichon = Crichon Dementia Rating Scale; CAMCOG = Cambridge Cognition Dementia Rating Scale; M = Mattis dementia rating)
[b]This column lists the types and numbers of other dementias studied. (MID = multi-infarct dementia; PSP = progressive supranuclear palsy; PD = Parkinson's disease with dementia; P = Pick's disease;

Other dementia types[b]	*Analysis method*[c]	*Parietal*	*Temporal*	*Frontal*	*Occipital*	*Autopsy confirmation (n)*
		Rank order				
—	V	2	1	—	—	—
3 MID	V	—	1	—	2	0
—	—	2	1	—	3	0
—	R: LR	—	—	—	—	0
10 MID	V	—	—	—	—	0
2 MID	R: global	2	1	—	—	0
—	R: cereb	1	—	—	—	1
9 MID 9 PSP	V	—	—	—	—	4
10 MID	V	2	1	—	3	—
—	R: cereb	1	—	—	—	0
—	R: cereb	—	2	1	—	0
—	R: cereb	2	1	—	—	0
—	V; R: cereb	1	—	—	—	0
—	R: occ	2	1	—	—	0
—	R: occ; R: LR	2	1	—	—	3
—	R: occ	—	1	—	—	1
15 MID 22 PD	V	2	1	3	—	—
15 MID	R: cereb; R: LR	1	2	—	—	0
—	R: cereb	2	1	—	—	0
8 MID	Multiple	3	1	1	—	0
17 MID 5 PD	R: motor	1	—	—	—	0
5 MID 3 P	R: motor	—	—	—	—	0
30 PD	R: cereb	1	2	3	—	0
5 P; 5 PSP; 15 PD	R: cereb	1	2	—	—	0
—	R: cereb	1	2	—	—	1
33 MID 5 P	V	—	—	—	—	0
—	R: cereb	—	—	—	—	0
—	V	2	1	—	—	0
—	V	—	—	—	—	0
—	—	—	—	—	—	0
—	V	—	—	—	—	0
3 FTD; 1 LBD; 1 PD	V	—	—	—	—	18
—	R: occ	—	—	—	—	0
—	R: occ Regn anal	ns	ns	ns	ns	0
—	R: cereb	ns	ns	ns	ns	0
—	R: occ bg	1	2	—	—	0
—	R: cereb H	—	—	—	—	0
—	R: cereb		No pattern			1
—	V	2	1	—	—	2
6 MID; 4 MND; 3 TGA	R: cereb	—	1	—	—	0
7 FTD; 2 CJD; 2 LBD	V	1	2	3	—	27
12 MID 7 PSP	V	—	—	—	—	0
—	R: cereb	—	—	—	—	0
—	R: occ		No pattern			0
—	R: cereb	—	—	—	—	0

FTD = frontotemporal dementia; LBD = Lewy body disease; MND = motor neuron disease; TGA = transient global amnesia; CJD = Creutzfeldt-Jakob disease.)

[c] V = visual analysis; R: LR = ratio method: left right asymmetry; R: global = ratio method: global metabolism used as denominator; R: cereb = ratio method: cerebellar cortex used as denominator; R: occ = ratio method: occipital; R: motor = ratio method: motor cortex used as denominator; R: occ Regn anal = ratio method: occipital regional analysis; R: occ bg = ratio method: occipital: basal ganglia; R: cereb H = ratio method: cerebral hemisphere used as denominator.

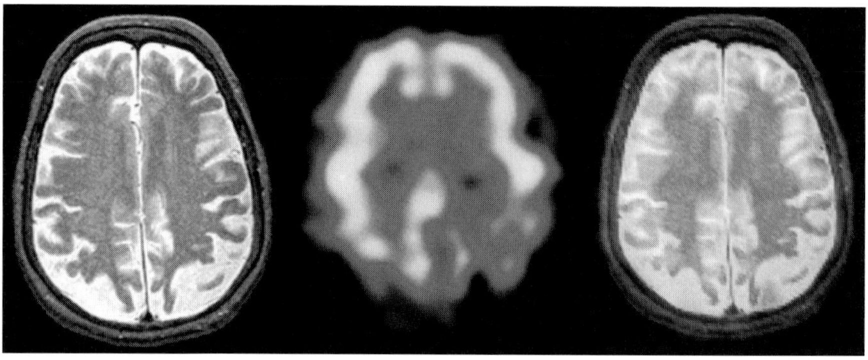

Figure 9.2 Single photon emission computed tomography (SPECT) cerebral blood flow using technetium Tc 99m hexamethyl propylenamine oxime in a 73-year-old woman with probable Alzheimer's disease (*center*). A transaxial T2-weighted magnetic resonance imaging (MRI) scan (*left*) shows global widening of the cerebral sulci. The center image illustrates the typical posterior parietal perfusion deficit from the SPECT scan, left side worse than right. Posterior cingulate hypoperfusion is also seen. The image on the right shows the SPECT and MRI scans coregistered together. (Courtesy of Dr. Keith Johnson, Department of Neurology, Brigham and Women's Hospital, Boston.)

confirmed MID [140], mitochondrial encephalopathy with stroke-like episodes [148], hypoglycemia [140], and carbon monoxide poisoning [140].

Specificity and Sensitivity of the Temporoparietal Single Photon Emission Computed Tomography Pattern

Some believe that the sensitivity and specificity of the SPECT TP pattern may be inferior to that found in PET, although few studies directly compare the two modalities with similar resolution cameras using patients with early disease [50,57,58]. Comparing the value of SPECT to that of neuropsychological assessment in the diagnosis of AD, Villa and colleagues [34] noted that they showed similar degrees of sensitivity (91%), but a SPECT hippocampal CBF deficit was considerably less specific (71% versus 81%) than cognitive testing. Another study also reported more favorable performance for neuropsychological evaluation, and SPECT was believed to be of limited use in staging AD [62]. In both these and a further study by Green and colleagues [49], approximately one-third of the AD patients had normal perfusion patterns, which subsequently limited the sensitivity of the TP pattern for diagnosis, even though a respectable specificity was noted (89%). The superior performance of neuropsychological measures over SPECT might reflect a selection bias on account of the NINCDS-ADRDA criteria, selecting patients based partly on neuropsychological performance. If the TP pattern is present, SPECT can aid in the diagnosis of AD, because there is an 82% probability for AD compared to a 19% probability of AD if it is absent [134]. Claus and colleagues [136] assessed 48 AD subjects with 60 population controls and showed that when the specificity was set at 90%, sensitivity figures varied between 42% for mild and 79% for severe AD. They concluded that the diagnostic gain was likely to be greatest for those patients in whom there was most diagnostic doubt. Johnson and colleagues [36] also found that sensitivity was lower for mild than for severe AD. Pearlson and colleagues [149] have claimed 100% discrimination using a combination of SPECT and MRI hippocampal volume measurement to differentiate 24 moderately affected AD patients and 16 control subjects. When the TP pattern is absent or there is a heterogeneous pattern of deficit, diagnostic classification based on SPECT alone is unreliable [41]. To resolve these issues, it will be important to establish whether SPECT has sufficient sensitivity to detect the TP deficit early in the course of the disease.

The precise anatomic locations of the maximal and earliest SPECT CBF deficits are also disputed. Although they are nearly always reported to involve posterior structures, maximal hypoperfusion is variably in either the parietal [31,36,37,40,135,137,140,147] or temporal cortices [28,30,39,45,46,51, 138,144]. Although these are association areas known to be affected by AD pathology, it is not entirely certain that the CBF reductions necessarily reflect those structures associated with greatest pathologic damage. This problem could be a consequence of the poor resolution of SPECT, which has particular difficulty resolving the medial temporal lobe and hippocampus. More recent studies with higher-resolution cameras have claimed that significant hippocampal blood flow deficits can be observed [41]. Ohnishi and colleagues [150] concluded that hippocampal flow was a more sensitive marker of dementia than parietal flow in 13 AD patients. This finding was nonspecific because it was also found in six MID patients included in the study. Data from Villa and colleagues [34] support the view that decreased CBF in hippocampal regions reflect dementia in general without regard to specific diseases. These investigators found that hippocampal hypoperfusion occurred in all types of dementia, including AD.

Although SPECT detects more abnormalities in AD patients than in normal control subjects, its value in the differential diagnosis of dementia remains controversial. Neary and colleagues [133] evaluated three well-characterized clinical groups including 23 probable AD patients, nine patients with FLD, and nine patients with PSP. The FLD patients were differentiated from the AD patients on account of their distinct clinical profile combined with the presence of isolated frontal oligemia found in all but one individual. Frontal oligemia was noted in all the PSP patients, but only three individuals with AD. This important study emphasized the value of determining patterns of cerebral perfusion in dementia syndromes and documented the distinction between AD (TP pattern) and FLD (frontal pattern). Other investigators have verified these findings [43]. Launes and colleagues [33], however, scanned 36 patients with AD, 33 with MID, and five with FLD and were unable to differentiate FLD from AD, although abnormalities were found in 87% of those with mild and 100% of those with severe dementia.

Single Photon Emission Computed Tomography and Neuropsychological Correlations

Many investigators have correlated the pattern of perfusion deficit with measures of dementia severity, such as the MMSE [31,35,40,51,143,144] or BDS

[37]. An association between the regional blood flow pattern and more specific cognitive tests, such as explicit memory [49,151], visuospatial function, and frontal lobe function are reported [48]. Some studies have correlated CBF with scores from structured neuropsychological batteries [39,46,142,143,145]. Burns and colleagues [39] showed a correlation between CBF and scores on tests of memory, praxis, and language. These results have been confirmed by others, although no correlation with the memory test were found [46]. For completeness, it should be noted that associations such as these are not universally described [41,43,49,133,135].

Attempts to correlate CBF with age at onset have also been variable. Some results are difficult to interpret because the data are confounded by increased dementia severity in the presenile group who had prominent left frontal deficits [45]. On the other hand, positive correlations between age at onset and left parietal deficit and negative associations with right medial temporal activity have been documented [39]. Some studies, however, fail to correlate age at onset and CBF at all [142]. The literature suggesting that AD may have a focal onset has been supported by a study that showed that six probable AD patients with circumscribed neuropsychological impairments had focal cerebral perfusion deficits [152].

IMAGING OF NEUROTRANSMITTER SYSTEMS

Many postmortem studies report reduced presynaptic and postsynaptic cholinergic activity in individuals with AD. In view of these observations, there have been preliminary attempts to use specific PET and SPECT radioligands to quantify the distribution of cholinergic receptors in vivo. Data interpretation from these studies has been complicated because apparent reductions in receptor binding may be secondary to tissue loss or alterations in receptor regulation and not merely due to the loss of receptors themselves. One study showed a small age-related loss of muscarinic cholinergic receptors in controls and more dramatic losses in those with AD and PD with dementia. A dissociation between the pattern of muscarinic receptor loss and FDG metabolism was noted, indicating that the receptor deficits were not secondary to the loss of neurons in this instance [153,154]. Nicotinic receptor function has also been investigated in AD and used to assess the long-term effects of drug treatment [155,156]. One study has reported preliminary data with an acetylcholine analog with high specificity for acetylcholinesterase, which also showed maximal reductions in the TP cortex. It is unclear, however, what proportion of the reduction was due to generalized loss of neurons [157]. Other neurotransmitters, such as 5-hydroxytryptamine, have also been evaluated [158]. The rationale for receptor binding studies such as these needs to be critically assessed, because it seems unlikely that a single neurotransmitter deficit will explain the cognitive decline in AD. Tyrrell and colleagues [159] adopted a different strategy and speculated that AD patients with extrapyramidal signs have presynaptic dopaminergic deficits similar to those found in PD. Subsequent PET data showed normal ^{18}F dihydroxyphenylalanine uptake, which indicated that the extrapyramidal symptoms in their AD group were unlikely to be due to this mechanism [160]. Other investigators have tried to develop ligands specific for

Aβ. Although this seems an attractive idea, the current results do not suggest that this is a realistic possibility at present [161]. Other studies that attempt to map the degree of microgliosis have been similarly unrewarding [162].

FUNCTIONAL IMAGING IN VASCULAR DEMENTIA

The FI literature concerning vascular dementia (VaD) is somewhat bewildering because it is impossible to identify clearly a pattern of altered perfusion specific to this diagnosis. The lack of conformity is probably a consequence of the variable criteria used to select VaD patients and the different arterial territories that may lead to cognitive impairment (see Chapter 15). Although terms such as *MID* have been proposed [163], it is now understood that VaD is heterogeneous and includes many conditions, such as subcortical arteriosclerotic encephalopathy or Binswanger's disease (BD); cortical vascular dementia, often associated with atrial fibrillation, vasculitis, or hemorrhage; as well as rarer entities such as cerebral autosomal dominant arteriopathy with subcortical infarcts and leukoencephalopathy (CADASIL) and amyloid angiopathy. MRI is exceptionally good at identifying both the site and the extent of infarction, and for this reason, FI should only be interpreted in light of the corresponding MRI scan appearance (see Chapter 8). FI has been used to investigate the pathophysiology of white matter hyperintensities or leukoariaosis found on T2-weighted MRI in individuals with dementia [164]. Periventricular white matter lesions (WMLs) are seen in diverse groups, including those with vascular risk factors such as stroke or hypertension [165–167], asymptomatic normal aging [168–170], dementia [171,172], and probable AD [167,173–175]. Although ischemia is a likely cause for these lesions, PET has been used to determine whether there is a mismatch between CBF and metabolism, indicating chronic underlying ischemia as a causal mechanism.

Initial PET studies were based on earlier CBF studies that had suggested that cortical perfusion was abnormal in MID [176]. Patients diagnosed according to the Hachinski criteria were evaluated in an attempt to compare their pattern of regional metabolism or CBF with individuals with AD [163]. Some described similar perfusion patterns to those with AD [63], whereas others showed variable deficits with asymmetric, random, and even focal deficits affecting both cortical and subcortical regions [67,70]. The protean appearances presumably reflected the different vascular territories that had been involved. It was also suggested that parietal metabolism was significantly lower in AD patients as compared to those with MID. One report that supported this theory noted that although both types of patients had significant hypometabolism in occipital, TP, and frontal association cortices, the AD patients had additional deficits in the superior parietal and primary visual cortices. Additionally, the VaD patients commonly had lesions in basal ganglia, thalamus, and cerebellum; a metabolic ratio was significantly lower in the AD group because the cerebellum and thalamus were used as the denominator in this calculation [57]. A follow-up study replicated these findings and showed that the severity of dementia related to the volume of metabolically impaired tissue [177]. The variability of the MID pattern was emphasized by Sultzer and colleagues [178], who studied 11 elderly vascular patients and showed a correlation between the severity of subcortical damage, judged by their MRI, and the degree of cortical hypometabolism. These data support the idea that cortical hypometabolism in VaD often results from subcortical damage and subsequent disconnection. Overall, the VaD patients had variable regional deficits that were dependent on the precise location of the subcortical lesion. A consistent frontal deficit was associated with basal ganglia and thalamic infarcts. Other studies have also shown the effect of thalamic infarction on the pattern of cortical metabolism [179].

The distinction between AD and MID is no more clearly resolved with SPECT than with PET. Several reports stress that parietal deficits are more prominent in AD [40,150,180], but this observation is not universal [181]. Other investigators suggest that focal deficits without the TP pattern of hypoperfusion support the diagnosis of MID [30,33,137]. These broad conclusions stem more from expectations than from postmortem confirmed data. In two rare reports, two demented patients who had focal parietal deficits on SPECT scans showed evidence of mixed AD and vascular lesions at autopsy [147,150]. These case reports indicate that an FI approach for differentiating VaD from AD cannot be recommended because focal lesions also occur in degenerative causes of dementia.

PATHOGENESIS OF LEUKOARIOSIS

Other FI studies have concentrated on trying to determine the pathophysiologic basis of leukoariosis. Kawamura and colleagues [182] quantified the degree of leukoariosis and correlated it with SPECT CBF in 35 cases with MID. CBF was reduced for all cerebral regions apart from the parietal white matter when compared with normal control subjects. Regression analysis showed that the frontal leukoariosis best correlated with reduced perfusion in the putamen and thalamus and was used to support the hypothesis that hypoperfusion in the deep penetrating arterioles contributed to the pathogenesis of WMLs. A subsequent study examined AD patients in addition to individuals with MID. Correlations with frontal leukoariosis were confined to the MID cohort alone, which the authors cryptically suggested implicated alternative pathogenic mechanisms for white matter changes associated with AD [183]. AD patients with and without leukoariosis have been studied. Smaller metabolic deficits are found in those individuals with the most severe WMLs, which is also attributed to additional pathogenic mechanisms (presumably ischemia) [88].

FUNCTIONAL IMAGING IN BINSWANGER'S DISEASE

A number of authors have focused on BD because it is a pathologically well-defined form of vascular dementia. Initial studies reported frontal perfusion deficits in BD [51], which have subsequently been confirmed in larger series [184]. Shyu and colleagues [185] studied BD patients who were divided into two groups according to severity of dementia. Those who were mildly affected had white matter changes and perfusion deficits restricted to the frontal lobes, whereas severely afflicted BD patients had generalized white matter changes and CBF deficits. Other investigators have demonstrated ischemia early in the course of BD but not when the disease is more severe, because the oxygen extraction fraction is normal in this instance [186,187]. Other PET studies also support the hypothesis that progressive ischemia occurs during the development of BD [188]. It has also been suggested that the cerebrovascular response to hypercapnia can be used to distinguish BD from AD [189]. More recently, a specific form of vascular dementia named *CADASIL* has been described [190,191]. FI studies in one affected individual showed a diffuse reduction in cortical metabolism due to basal ganglia infarction. An asymptomatic individual with white matter changes without infarction had a 40% reduction in CBF, although oxygen metabolism was normal on account of the increased oxygen extraction fraction. These provisional data confirm that underlying chronic oligemia occurs in CADASIL [192].

FUNCTIONAL IMAGING IN PATIENTS WITH BOTH DEMENTIA AND MOVEMENT DISORDERS

A variety of FI abnormalities have been observed in nondemented patients with PD, including decreased global CBF but not oxygen metabolism [193], increased striatal but not cortical metabolism [194], and focal reductions in parietal metabolism [195]. PD patients who show signs of dementia appear to have regional deficits similar to those found in AD [196]. In the largest series, Peppard and colleagues [197] studied 14 demented PD patients and compared them with individuals who were cognitively normal. The nondemented patients had reductions in global metabolism, whereas the demented PD patients had TP deficits resembling those found in AD. This observation has been confirmed in numerous other studies, but there is little postmortem confirmation of the underlying histopathology [76,83,135,198]. In the single study reported to date, the brain of a demented PD patient without senile plaques and NFTs had the TP pattern [82]. The situation has now been complicated by the recognition of cortical LBD as a cause of dementia in PD patients [199]. The metabolic profiles of three subjects with autopsy confirmed diffuse LBD, as well as three with combined AD and LBD have been reported [84]. The deficits were identical to AD, apart from conspicuous occipital hypometabolism, which has been described in AD patients with prominent visuospatial symptoms [84]. No particular relationship between the distribution of Lewy bodies and cerebral metabolism was noted.

Cognitive impairment may occur in parkinsonian syndromes such as PSP and cortical basal degeneration (CBD). In PSP, the cognitive impairment and behavioral abnormality stem from frontal lobe dysfunction. Both SPECT and PET detect bifrontal CBF and metabolic deficits in PSP patients that correlate with the degree of intellectual deterioration [200–202]. CBD is an asymmetric akinetic rigid syndrome with apraxia, myoclonus, and sometimes dementia that shows markedly asymmetric patterns of cortical dysmetabolism [203,204]. It has been suggested that the PSP and CBD patterns are sufficiently distinct to aid in diagnosis. Metabolism contralateral to the affected limb in the CBD cohort was lower in inferior parietal, lateral temporal, and sensory motor cortex than in PSP [205]. Patients with Huntington's disease have decreased glucose metabolism in

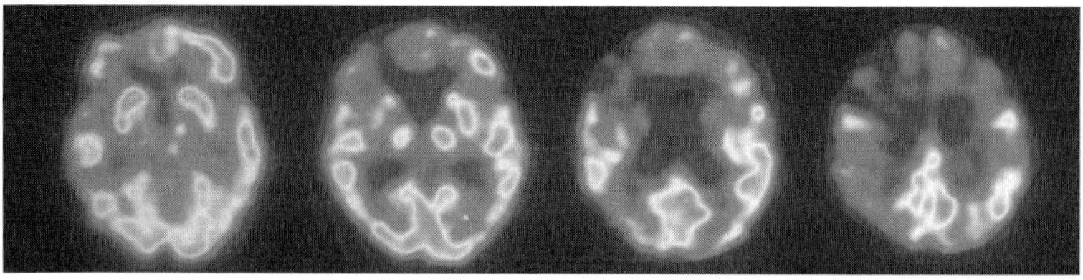

Figure 9.3 Positron emission tomographic scan shows frontal hypometabolism in a patient with frontal lobe dementia.

the caudate nuclei in advance of clinical symptoms, which can help to identify individuals at risk for this disease [206,207].

FUNCTIONAL IMAGING IN FRONTOTEMPORAL DEMENTIA

A variety of pathologic entities can cause FTD [51] including PcD, dementia lacking specific pathologic features, motor neuron disease, and progressive subcortical gliosis [208] (see Chapters 1, 2, and 17). An FI scan can usefully be requested for the investigation of FTD, because a frontotemporal pattern of deficit may distinguish these individuals from those with the TP pattern found in AD (Figure 9.3). No particular frontal pattern appears to identify any specific pathologic type of FTD. Thus, single patients who show frontal temporal hypometabolism have been found to have histopathologically verified PcD [93,94,209], and similar deficits are associated with individuals with FLD and amyotrophic lateral sclerosis (ALS) [210–212]. Some suggest that classic motor neuron disease, FTD, and motor neuron disease with frontal dementia are part of a continuum because frontal perfusion deficits and neuropsychological impairments can be identified in each subgroup [211]. In some instances, frontal CBF deficits can be detected in advance of focal atrophy found on MRI. Calculating the ratio between CBF in the parietal and frontal cortices has been proposed as a sensitive way to distinguish FTD from AD patients [213]. CBF correlates of disinhibited behavior show orbitofrontal, anterior temporal, and basal ganglia deficits that distinguish mildly demented disinhibited FTD patients from AD patients who also had this symptom complex [214]. Graff-Radford and colleagues [215] examined eight FTD and 43 probable AD patients diagnosed according to clinical criteria and found that an anterior to posterior ratio of less than 0.89 correctly identified the FTD group. Julin and colleagues [216] have also reported similar findings including more severe frontal deficits in eight FTD patients as compared to 28 AD patients studied simultaneously. Pasquier and colleagues [217] failed to correlate verbal fluency performance and the pattern of perfusion deficit in patients with FTD and AD. Kew and colleagues reported non-ALS patients without dementia who had impaired resting CBF in the anterior cingulate gyrus. In addition, the same patients had an attenuated CBF response during motor activation [218,219], which was proposed as evidence for cortical adaptation following loss of motor neurons.

FUNCTIONAL NEUROIMAGING IN PRION DISEASE

There have been relatively few FI studies in prion disease. The most common abnormality is diffuse metabolic deficits affecting all regions of the brain [220]. A wide variety of focal deficits have also been described, including TP deficits similar to those found in AD [76,85], a TP and frontal pattern, and foci of hypometabolism and hypermetabolism throughout the brain [76]. One patient with familial prion disease had the AD pattern of TP deficit as well as additional cerebellar hypometabolism [8]. A recent abstract drew attention to thalamic hypometabolism in an individual with a new variant of CJD [221] that was similar to that found in another prion disease—familial fatal insomnia [222].

FUNCTIONAL NEUROIMAGING IN FOCAL COGNITIVE DEFICITS

Functional neuroimaging has value for studying brain behavior relationships as well as in diagnosis. For this reason, it has been especially valuable in studying patients with isolated cognitive deficits such as primary progressive aphasia, which may either herald dementia or remain as a relatively isolated cognitive disorder [223]. Patients with progressive aphasia [224,225], progressive apraxia [111], posterior cortical atrophy [226], progressive orofacial apraxia with reduced speech output [227], and prosopagnosia [228] have been described and show correlations between the well-circumscribed neuropsychological impairments and the focal metabolic deficits. Often these focal metabolic lesions have been identified in advance of structural abnormalities. A recent review of this literature highlights the underlying pathologic diversity of focal cognitive deficits, which include PcD [229], AD, CJD, and CBD [230].

MAGNETIC RESONANCE TECHNIQUES FOR FUNCTIONAL IMAGING

Alternative methods for measuring CBF with MRI are being developed in which dynamic cerebral blood volume images contain information comparable to PET. Gonzalez and colleagues [231] conducted a study to determine the correspondence between perfusion abnormalities in patients with dementia detected by functional magnetic resonance imaging (fMRI) and PET. They found significant correlations between PET and fMRI with an overall concordance of 78% (Figure 9.4). This technique required echoplanar imaging and gadolinium contrast injection. Sandson and colleagues [232] reported similar results and detected TP perfusion deficits in seven out of 11 patients with probable AD. There has also been speculation that fMRI cognitive activation studies may one day prove to be clinically useful in the assessment of patients with cognitive impairment [233]. Although the development of integrated tests of cognitive function, which assess neuropsychological function and CBF simultaneously, are attractive, there are many practical and methodologic issues to be overcome before such

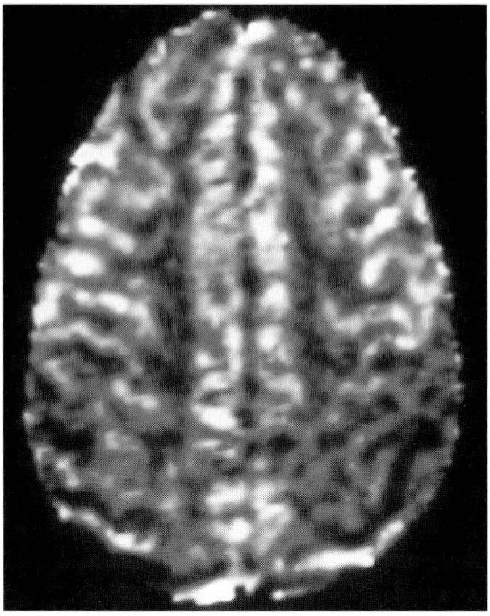

Figure 9.4 Functional magnetic resonance imaging scan shows typical temporoparietal hypometabolism in probable Alzheimer's disease. (Courtesy of Dr. Gilberto Gonzalez, Department of Radiology, Massachusetts General Hospital, Boston.)

tests can be seriously considered. Despite these concerns, Corkin and colleagues [234] reported provisional results in AD patients who were tested with a picture encoding/recognition task. The same cognitive task activated the hippocampus, fusiform, and lingual gyri in an earlier fMRI study of explicit memory in young normal control subjects [235]. Figure 9.5 shows a representative fMRI activation map from a patient with AD who was able to perform the task successfully. A similar distribution of activations to normal controls is observed.

Magnetic resonance spectroscopy (MRS) is a research technique for measuring indices of brain chemistry in a living subject. To date, MRS has had little clinical application, but the technique may assume greater importance in the future. There are two molecules of MRS interest: protons (^{1}H) and phosphorus (^{31}P). ^{1}H MRS produces a spectrum that includes *myo*-inositol, *N*-acetyl aspartate (NAA), choline, and creatinine (Cr). These compounds provide indices of neuronal loss, membrane phospholipids, and cell energy metabolism. The NAA signal is specific for neurons because the amino acid is absent in tissues of glial origin; it is, therefore, an indirect measure of neuronal number. MRS studies in AD have quantified regional neuronal loss by comparing the NAA peak relative to the Cr peak, which is presumed to be unaltered by AD pathology. The most prominent reductions in the NAA-Cr ratio have been found in the frontal, parietal, and occipital association cortices [236–238]. In AD patients with mild to moderate dementia, Shonk and colleagues [239] found increased *myo*-inositol and decreased NAA signals. It has been proposed that MRS can quantify the degree of neuronal loss in the frontal lobes and be used to distinguish FTD from AD [240]. MRS signal from choline-containing compounds reflects phospholipid metabolism and total choline stores. Choline

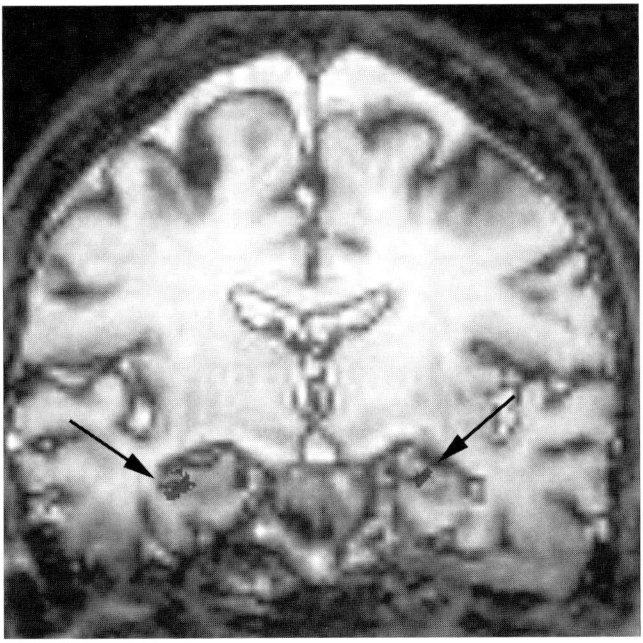

Figure 9.5 Functional magnetic resonance imaging scan shows hippocampal activations in an Alzheimer's disease subject. (Courtesy of Professor Suzanne Corkin, Department of Brain and Cognitive Sciences, Massachusetts Institute of Technology, Boston.)

signal in the white matter of AD patients appears to be variably decreased [241], normal, or even increased [236,238]. The variability presumably reflects the alterations that occur in phospholipid and membrane metabolism during the different stages of dementia. ^{31}P MRS is theoretically the most direct way to examine alterations in phospholipid metabolism and to measure energy sources such as phosphocreatine and adenosine triphosphate (ATP). ^{31}P MRS detected minor changes in phospholipid metabolites in AD patients compared to control subjects. Pettigrew and associates [242] reported that high-energy phosphates were decreased in the frontal lobes of AD patients, whereas Bottomley and colleagues [243] and Gonzalez and colleagues [244] detected normal ATP peaks in AD patients. One study evaluated whole-brain phosphorous metabolism with MRS and PET and suggested that PET metabolic deficits are due to synaptic loss as opposed to abnormalities in high-energy phosphate production [245].

FUNCTIONAL IMAGING AND DEMENTIA: CLINICAL IMPLICATIONS

FI should be considered as an adjunct to other investigations in several specific clinical situations. There is no evidence to support its use in routine assessment of individuals with cognitive impairment and little practical utility in requesting it in those with advanced neurodegenerative dementia. The situations in which FI can be appropriately considered and may yield helpful information are the following:

1. Patients with symptoms of cognitive impairment without a clear diagnosis. The issue in this situation is to clarify rapidly the exact diagnosis in an individual who often has a normal neurologic examination, normal MRI brain scan, and a borderline mental status examination or equivocal neuropsychological test score. Options include repeating the neuropsychological testing at a delayed interval (usually 6 months to 1 year) or arranging some form of FI. A classic pattern of TP deficit would add weight to a diagnosis of AD. A normal scan, however, does not completely exclude the possibility of a degenerative etiology, but may shift the focus to nonstructural causes of cognitive impairment, such as depressive pseudodementia. A proportion of individuals may show progressive cognitive decline, and it is important therefore that some form of longitudinal assessment is undertaken.
2. Patients in whom it is necessary to confirm the clinical suspicion of AD. In certain situations, the presence of the PT deficit may be used to corroborate the clinical diagnosis. This is especially useful in mildly affected individuals in which FI deficits can be used to indicate both to the patient and the patient's family the likely ultimate diagnosis and suggest some of the potential consequences.
3. Patients with early frontal lobe symptoms. These individuals usually have behavioral abnormalities, show few neurologic signs, lack prominent memory loss, and perform satisfactorily on other neuropsychological tests. An isolated frontal perfusion deficit in this instance may correctly distinguish FTD from primary psychiatric illness or AD.
4. Individuals with focal neuropsychological deficits such as progressive aphasia. Focal FI in regions predicted by the clinical signs are valuable biological markers of disease, especially in circumstances in which the MRI scan is normal.

Situations in which FI is inappropriate include (1) routine assessment of dementia patients and (2) investigation of asymptomatic individuals worried about the risk of developing dementia. Although several studies have suggested preclinical metabolic deficits in asymptomatic individuals at risk for familial AD, these have been aptly confined to specific research studies [25]. It is likely that sensitive biochemical markers, molecular genetic assays, neuropsychological tests, quantitative MRI, and FI will be developed for detecting individuals at risk for dementia. The ethical implications of all investigations that assess dementia risk or presymptomatic deficits should be carefully monitored.

REFERENCES

1. Phelps ME, Huang SC, Hoffman EJ, et al. Tomographic measurement of local cerebral glucose metabolic rate in humans with (F-18)2-fluoro-2-deoxy-D-glucose: validation of method. Ann Neurol 1979;6: 371–388.
2. Sokoloff L, Reivich M, Kennedy C. The (^{14}C) deoxyglucose method for the measurement of local cerebral glucose utilization; theory, procedure and normal values in the conscious and anaesthetized albino rat. J Appl Physiol 1977;28:897–916.

3. Frackowiak RSJ, Lenzi GL, Jones T, Heather JD. Quantitative measurements of regional cerebral blood flow and oxygen metabolism in man using ^{15}O and positron emission tomography; theory, procedure and normal values. J Comput Assist Tomogr 1980;4:727–736.
4. Powers WJ, Perlmutter JS, Videen TO, et al. Blinded clinical evaluation of positron emission tomography for diagnosis of probable Alzheimer's disease. Neurology 1992;42:765–771.
5. Kushner M, Tobin M, Alavi A, et al. Cerebellar glucose consumption in normal and pathologic states using fluorine-FDG and PET. J Nucl Med 1987;28:1667–1670.
6. McGeer PL, Kamo H, Harrop R, et al. Positron emission tomography in patients with clinically diagnosed Alzheimer's disease. J Can Med Assoc 1986;134:597–607.
7. Ishii K, Kitagaki H, Kono M, Mori E. Decreased medial temporal oxygen metabolism in Alzheimer's disease shown by PET. J Nucl Med 1996;37:1159–1165.
8. Kennedy AM, Tyrrell PJ, Collinge J, Rossor MN. Positron emission tomography (PET) demonstrates cerebellar hypometabolism in a case of inherited prion disease [abstract]. J Neurol Neurosurg Psychiatry 1992;55(suppl):422.
9. Kumar A, Schapiro M, Grady C, et al. High resolution PET studies in Alzheimer's disease. Neurolpsychopharmacology 1991;4:35–46.
10. Salmon E, Gregoire MC, Delfiore G, et al. Combined study of cerebral glucose metabolism and [^{11}C] methionine accumulation in probable Alzheimer's disease using positron emission tomography. J Cereb Blood Flow Metab 1996;16:399–408.
11. Grady CL, Haxby JV, Horwitz B, et al. Neuropsychological and cerebral metabolic function in early vs late onset dementia of the Alzheimer type. Neuropsychologia 1987;25:807–816.
12. Haxby JV, Grady C, Durara R, et al. Neocortical metabolic deficit precede nonmemory cognitive defects in early Alzheimer's-type dementia. Arch Neurol 1986;43:882–885.
13. Foster NL, Chase TN, Fedio P, et al. Alzheimer's disease: focal cortical changes shown by positron emission tomography. Neurology 1983;33:961–965.
14. Haxby J, Grady C, Koss E, et al. Longitudinal study of cerebral metabolic asymmetries and associated neuropsychological patterns in early dementia of the Alzheimer type. Arch Neurol 1990;47:753–760.
15. Jagust W, Friedland RP, Budiner T, et al. Longitudinal studies of regional cerebral metabolism in Alzheimer's disease. Neurology 1988;38:909–912.
16. McGeer EG, Peppard RP, McGeer PL, et al. ^{18}Fluorodeoxyglucose positron emission tomography studies in presumed Alzheimer cases, including 13 serial scans. Can J Neurol Sci 1990;17:1–11.
17. Herholz K, Adams R, Kessler R, et al. Criteria for the diagnosis of Alzheimer's disease with positron emission tomography. Dementia 1990;1:156–164.
18. Koss E, Friedland RP, Ober BA, Jagust WJ. Differences in lateral hemispheric asymmetries of glucose utilization between early- and late-onset Alzheimer-type dementia. Am J Psychiatry 1985;142:5:638–640.
19. Grady CL, Haxby JV, Schlageter NL, et al. Stability of metabolic and neuropsychological asymmetries in dementia of the Alzheimer type. Neurology 1986;36:1390–1392.
20. Ichimiya A, Herholz K, Mielke R, et al. Difference of regional cerebral metabolic pattern between presenile and senile dementia of the Alzheimer type: a factor analytic study. J Neurol Sci 1994;123:11–17.
21. Herholz K, Perani D, Salmon E, et al. Comparability of FDG PET studies in probable Alzheimer's disease. J Nucl Med 1993;34:1460–1466.
22. Mielke R, Herholz K, Grond M, et al. Differences of regional cerebral blood glucose metabolism between presenile and senile dementia of the Alzheimer type. Neurobiol Aging 1992;13:93–98.
23. Minoshima S, Frey KA, Koeppe RA, et al. A diagnostic approach in Alzheimer's disease using three-dimensional stereotactic surface projections of fluorine-18-FDG PET. J Nucl Med 1995;36:1238–1248.
24. Kennedy AM, Newman SK, Frackowiak RS, et al. Chromosome 14 linked familial Alzheimer's disease. A clinico-pathological study of a single pedigree. Brain 1995;118:185–205.
25. Kennedy AM, Frackowiak RS, Newman SK, et al. Deficits in cerebral glucose metabolism demonstrated by positron emission tomography in individuals at risk of familial Alzheimer's disease. Neurosci Lett 1995;186:17–20.
26. Azari N, Pettigrew K, Schapiro M, et al. Early detection of Alzheimer's disease: a statistical approach using positron emission tomographic data. J Cereb Blood Flow Metab 1993;13:438–447.
27. Friston K, Frith C, Liddle P, Frackowiak RSJ. Comparing functional (PET) images; the assessment of significant change. J Cereb Blood Flow Metab 1991;11:690–699.
28. Gemmell HG, Sharp PF, Smith FW, et al. Cerebral blood flow measured by SPECT as a diagnostic tool in the study of dementia. Psychiatry Res 1989;29:327–329.
29. Cohen MB, Graham LS, Lake R, et al. Diagnosis of Alzheimer's disease and multiple infarct dementia by tomographic imaging of iodine-123 IMP. J Nucl Med 1986;27:769–774.
30. Gemmell HG, Sharp PF, Besson JA, et al. Differential diagnosis in dementia using the cerebral blood flow agent ^{99m}Tc HM-PAO: a SPECT study. J Comput Assist Tomogr 1987;11:398–402.

31. Hellman RS, Tikofsky RS, Collier BD, et al. Alzheimer disease: quantitative analysis of I-123-iodoamphetamine SPECT brain imaging. Radiology 1989;172:183–188.
32. Liu HC, Liu RS, Lin KN, et al. Single photon emission computed tomography using 99Tcm-HMPAO in Alzheimer's disease. Nucl Med Commun 1992;13:535–541.
33. Launes J, Sulkava R, Erkinjuntti T, et al. 99Tcm-HMPAO SPECT in suspected dementia. Nucl Med Commun 1991;12:757–765.
34. Villa G, Cappa A, Tavolozza M, et al. Neuropsychological tests and [^{99m}Tc]-HM PAO SPECT in the diagnosis of Alzheimer's dementia. J Neurology 1995;242:359–366.
35. Waldemar G, Walovitch RC, Andersen AR, et al. ^{99m}Tc-bicisate (neurolite) SPECT brain imaging and cognitive impairment in dementia of the Alzheimer type: a blinded read of image sets from a multicenter SPECT trial. J Cereb Blood Flow Metab 1994;14:S99–S105.
36. Johnson KA, Mueller ST, Walshe TM, et al. Cerebral perfusion imaging in Alzheimer's disease. Use of single photon emission computed tomography and iofetamine hydrochloride I 123. Arch Neurol 1987;44:165–168.
37. Johnson KA, Holman BL, Mueller SP, et al. Single photon emission computed tomography in Alzheimer's disease. Abnormal iofetamine I 123 uptake reflects dementia severity [see comments]. Arch Neurol 1988;45:392–396.
38. Perani D, Di Piero V, Vallar G, et al. Technetium-99m HM-PAO-SPECT study of regional cerebral perfusion in early Alzheimer's disease. J Nucl Med 1988;29:1507–1514.
39. Burns A, Philpot M, Costa D, et al. The investigation of Alzheimer's disease with single photon emission tomography. J Neurol Neurosurg Psychiatry 1989;52:248–253.
40. Battistin L, Pizzolato G, Dam M, et al. Regional cerebral blood flow study with ^{99m}Tc-hexamethylpropyleneamine oxime single photon emission computed tomography in Alzheimer's and multi-infarct dementia. Eur Neurol 1990;30:296–301.
41. Waldemar G, Bruhn P, Kristensen M, et al. Heterogeneity of neocortical cerebral blood flow deficits in dementia of the Alzheimer type: a [^{99m}Tc]-*d,l*-HMPAO SPECT study. J Neurol Neurosurg Psychiatry 1994;57:285–295.
42. O'Brien M. Cerebral blood flow in dementia. Neurology 1986;36:1542–1540.
43. Habert MO, Spampinato U, Mas JL, et al. A comparative technetium 99m hexamethylpropylene amine oxime SPET study in different types of dementia. Eur J Nucl Med 1991;18:3–11.
44. Talbot PR, Lloyd JJ, Snowden JS, et al. Choice of reference region in the quantification of single-photon emission tomography in primary degenerative dementia. Eur J Nucl Med 1994;21:503–508.
45. Jagust W, Reed B, Seab P, Budinger T. Alzheimer's disease. Age at onset and single photon emission computed tomographic patterns of regional cerebral blood flow. Arch Neurol 1990;47:628–633.
46. Montaldi D, Brooks D, McColl J, et al. Measurements of regional cerebral blood flow and cognitive performance in Alzheimer's disease. J Neurol Neurosurg Psychiatry 1990;53:33–38.
47. Curran SM, Murray CM, Van Beck M, et al. A single photon emission computerised tomography study of regional brain function in elderly patients with major depression and with Alzheimer-type dementia. Br J Psychiatry 1993;163:155–165.
48. Eberling JL, Reed BR, Baker MG, Jagust WJ. Cognitive correlates of regional cerebral blood flow in Alzheimer's disease. Arch Neurol 1993;50:761–766.
49. Greene JD, Miles K, Hodges JR. Neuropsychology of memory and SPECT in the diagnosis and staging of dementia of Alzheimer type. J Neurology 1996;243:175–190.
50. Messa C, Perani D, Lucignani G, et al. High-resolution technetium-99m-HMPAO SPECT in patients with probable Alzheimer's disease: comparison with fluorine-18-FDG PET. J Nucl Med 1994;35:210–216.
51. Jagust WJ, Budinger TF, Reed BR. The diagnosis of dementia with single photon emission computed tomography. Arch Neurol 1987;44:258–262.
52. Syed GM, Eagger S, Toone BK, et al. Quantification of regional cerebral blood flow (rCBF) using 99Tcm-HMPAO and SPECT: choice of the reference region. Nucl Med Commun 1992;13:811–816.
53. Page MP, Howard RJ, O'Brien JT, et al. Use of neural networks in brain SPECT to diagnose Alzheimer's disease. J Nucl Med 1996;37:195–200.
54. deFigueiredo RJ, Shankle WR, Maccato A, et al. Neural-network-based classification of cognitively normal, demented Alzheimer disease and vascular dementia from single photon emission with computed tomography image data from brain. Proc Natl Acad Sci U S A 1995;92:5530–5534.
55. Johnson KA, Jones KJ, Becker A, et al. Preclinical diagnosis with SPECT [abstract]. Neurology 1997;48:A207.
56. Kerwin R. Functional neuroimaging in Alzheimer's disease: how far should we go? [editorial]. Eur J Nucl Med 1994;21:1041–1043.

57. Mielke R, Pietrzyk U, Jacobs A, et al. HMPAO SPET and FDG PET in Alzheimer's disease and vascular dementia: comparison of perfusion and metabolic pattern [see comments]. Eur J Nucl Med 1994; 21:1052–1060.
58. Kuwabara Y, Ichiya Y, Otsuka M, et al. Comparison of I-123 IMP and Tc-99m HMPAO SPECT studies with PET in dementia. Ann Nucl Med 1990;4:75–82.
59. Fazekas F, Alavi A, Chawluk J, et al. Comparison of CT, MRI and PET in Alzheimer's disease and normal aging. J Nucl Med 1989;30:1607–1615.
60. Fox NC, Warrington EK, Freeborough PA, et al. Presymptomatic hippocampal atrophy in Alzheimer's disease. A longitudinal MRI study. Brain 1996;119:2001–2007.
61. Newman S, Warrington E, Kennedy A, Rossor M. Initial cognitive changes in an individual with familial Alzheimer's disease [abstract]. J Neurol Neurosurg Psychiatry 1994;57:967–972.
62. Van Gool WA, Walstra GJ, Teunisse S, et al. Diagnosing Alzheimer's disease in elderly, mildly demented patients: the impact of routine single photon emission computed tomography. J Neurology 1995;242:401–405.
63. Frackowiak RSJ, Pozzilli C, Legg NJ, et al. Regional cerebral oxygen supply and utilization in dementia. A clinical and physiological study with oxygen 15 and positron emission tomography. Brain 1981;104:753–778.
64. Ferris S, de Leon M, Wolf AP. Positron emission tomography in the study of aging and senile dementia. Neurobiol Aging 1980;1:127–131.
65. Farkas T, Ferris SH, Wolf AP, et al. 18F-2-deoxy-2-fluoro-D-glucose as a tracer in the positron emission tomographic study of senile dementia. Am J Psychiatry 1982;139:352–353.
66. Friedland RP, Budinger TF, Brant-Zawadzki M, Jagust WJ. The diagnosis of Alzheimer-type dementia. A preliminary comparison of positron emission tomography and proton magnetic resonance. JAMA 1984;252:2750–2752.
67. Benson DF, Kuhl DE, Hawkins RA, et al. The fluorodeoxy-glucose (^{18}F) scan in Alzheimer's disease and multi-infarct dementia. Arch Neurol 1983;40:711–714.
68. Friedland R, Budinger T, Ganz E, et al. Regional cerebral metabolic alterations in dementia of the Alzheimer type: positron emission tomography with 18-F-fluorodeoxyglucose. J Comput Assist Tomogr 1983;7:590–598.
69. Foster NL, Chase TN, Mansi L, et al. Cortical abnormalities in Alzheimer's disease. Ann Neurol 1984;16:649–654.
70. Kuhl DE, Metter EJ, Reige WH. Patterns of Cerebral Utilization in Depression, Multi-Infarct Dementia, and Alzheimer's Disease. In L Sokoloff (ed), Brain Imaging and Brain Function. New York: Raven Press, 1985;211–226.
71. Cutler N, Haxby JV, Duara R, et al. Clinical history, brain metabolism, and neuropsycholgical function in Alzheimer's disease. Ann Neurol 1985;18:298–309.
72. Duara R, Grady CL, Haxby JV, et al. Positron emission tomography in Alzheimer's disease. Neurology 1986;36:879–887.
73. Polinsky RJ, Noble H, Chiro G, et al. Dominantly inherited Alzheimer's disease: cerebral glucose metabolism. J Neurol Neurosurg Psychiatry 1987;50:725–757.
74. Haxby JV, Duara R, Grady CL, Cutler NR. Relations between neuropsychological and cerebral metabolic asymmetries in early Alzheimer's disease. J Cereb Blood Flow Metab 1985;5:193–200.
75. Nyback H, Nyman H, Blomqvist G, et al. Brain metabolism in Alzheimer's dementia; studies of 11 C deoxyglucose accumulation, CSF monoamine metabolites and neuropsychological test performance in patients and healthy subjects. J Neurol Neurosurg Psychiatry 1990;54:672–678.
76. Salmon E, Sadzot B, Maquet P, et al. Differential diagnosis of Alzheimer's disease with PET. J Nucl Med 1994;35:391–398.
77. Loewenstein DA, Barker W, Chang JY, et al. Predominant left hemisphere metabolic dysfunction in dementia. Arch Neurol 1989;46:146–152.
78. Foster N, Mann U, Mohr E, et al. Focal cerebral glucose hypometabolism in definite Alzheimer disease. Ann Neurol 1989;26:132–133.
79. Chase TN, Foster N, Fedio P, et al. Regional cortical dysfunction in Alzheimer's disease as determined by positron emission tomography. Ann Neurol 1984;15:S170–S174.
80. Haxby JV, Grady C, Koss E, et al. Heterogeneous anterior-posterior metabolic patterns in dementia of the Alzheimer type. Neurology 1988;38:1853–1863.
81. Duara R, Barker W, Lowenstein D, et al. Sensitivity and specificity of positron emission tomography and magnetic resonance imaging studies in Alzheimer's disease and mulit-infarct dementia. Eur Neurol 1989;29(suppl 3):9–15.

82. Schapiro M, Grady C, Ball M, et al. Reductions in parieto-temporal cerebral glucose metabolism are not specific for Alzheimer's disease [abstract]. Neurology 1990;40(suppl 1):152.
83. Goto I, Taniwaki T, Hosokawa S, et al. Positron emission tomographic (PET) studies in dementia. J Neurol Sci 1993;114:1–6.
84. Albin RL, Minoshima S, D'Amato CJ, et al. Fluoro-deoxyglucose positron emission tomography in diffuse Lewy body disease. Neurology 1996;47:462–466.
85. Friedland RP, Pruisner SB, Jagust WJ, et al. Bitemporal hypometabolism in Creutzfeldt-Jakob disease measured by positron emission tomography with [^{18}F] fluorodeoxyglucose. J Comput Assist Tomogr 1984;8:978–981.
86. DeCarli C, Atack J, Ball M, et al. Post-mortem regional neurofibrillary tangle densities but not senile plaque densities are related to regional cerebral metabolic rates for glucose during life in Alzheimer's disease patients. Neurodegeneration 1992;1:113–121.
87. Mielke R, Schroder R, Fink GR, et al. Regional cerebral glucose metabolism and postmortem pathology in Alzheimer's disease. Acta Neuropathol (Berl) 1996;91:174–179.
88. DeCarli C, Grady CL, Clark CM, et al. Comparison of positron emission tomography, cognition, and brain volume in Alzheimer's disease with and without severe abnormalities of white matter. J Neurol Neurosurg Psychiatry 1996;60:158–167.
89. Cutler N, Haxby J, Duara R, et al. Brain metabolism as measured with positron emission tomography: serial assessment in a patient with familial Alzheimer's disease. Neurology 1985;35:1556–1561.
90. Tierney M, Fisher R, Lewis A. The NINCDS-ADRDA work group criteria for the clinical diagnosis of probable Alzheimer's disease; a clinopathological study of 57 cases. Neurology 1988;38:359–364.
91. Kippenhan JS, Barker WW, Pascal S, et al. Evaluation of a neural-network classifier for PET scans of normal and Alzheimer's disease subjects. J Nucl Med 1992;33:1459–1467.
92. Braak H, Braak E. Neuropathological stageing of Alzheimer-related changes. Acta Neuropathol (Berl) 1991;82:239–259.
93. Kamo H, McGeer PL, Harrop R, et al. Positron emission tomography and histopathology in Pick's disease. Neurology 1987;37:439–445.
94. Salmon E, Franck G. Positron emission tomographic study in Alzheimer's disease and Pick's disease. Arch Gerontol Geriatr 1989;8(suppl):241–247.
95. Guze BH, Baxter LR Jr, Schwartz JM, et al. Changes in glucose metabolism in dementia of the Alzheimer type compared with depression: a preliminary report. Psychiatry Res 1991;40:195–202.
96. Bench CJ, Friston KJ, Brown RG, et al. Regional cerebral blood flow in depression measured by positron emission tomography: the relationship with clinical dimensions. Psychol Med 1993;23:579–590.
97. Jagust WJ, Friedland RP, Budinger TF. Positron emission tomography with [^{18}F]fluorodeoxyglucose differentiates normal pressure hydrocephalus from Alzheimer-type dementia. J Neurol Neurosurg Psychiatry 1985;48:1091–1096.
98. Friedland RP, Brun A, Budinger TF. Pathological and positron emission tomographic correlates in Alzheimer's disease. Lancet 1985;26:228.
99. Brun A, Englund E. Regional pattern of degeneration in Alzheimer's disease: neuronal loss and histopathological grading. Histopathology 1981;5:549–564.
100. McGeer PL, Kamo H, Harrop R, et al. Comparison of PET, MRI, and CT with pathology in a proven case of Alzheimer's disease. Neurology 1986;36:1569–1574.
101. Gomez-Isla T, Price JL, McKeel DW Jr, et al. Profound loss of layer II entorhinal cortex neurons occurs in very mild Alzheimer's disease. J Neurosci 1996;16:4491–4500.
102. Mega MS, Chen SS, Thompson PM, et al. Mapping histology to metabolism: coregistration of sustained whole brain sections to premortem PET in Alzheimer's disease. Neuroimage 1997;5:147–153.
103. Mega M, Chu T, Thompson P, et al. Amyloid beta protein density and cortical metabolism on FDG PET and Alzheimer's disease [abstract]. Neuroimage 1997;5(suppl 2):S346.
104. Hyman BT, Van Horsen GW, Damasio AR, Barnes CL. Alzheimer's disease: cell-specific pathology isolates the hippocampal formation. Science 1984;225:1168–1170.
105. Jagust WJ, Eberling JL, Richardson BC, et al. The cortical topography of temporal lobe hypometabolism in early Alzheimer's disease. Brain Research 1993;629:189–198.
106. Jagust WJ. Functional imaging patterns in Alzheimer's disease. Relationships to neurobiology. Ann N Y Acad Sci 1996;777:30–36.
107. Meguro K, Chavoix C, Blaizot X, et al. Effects of bilateral neurotoxic lesion of the rhinal cortex on cerebral glucose utilization (CMRglu) in baboons: a PET study [abstract]. Soc Neurosci 1995;21:1723.
108. Yamaguchi S, Meguro K, Itoh M, et al. Decreased cortical glucose metabolism correlates with hippocampal atrophy in Alzheimer's disease as shown by MRI and PET. J Neurol Neurosurg Psychiatry 1997;62:596–600.

109. Videen T, Perlmutter J, Mintun, Raichle M. Regional correction of positron emission tomography data for the effects of cerebral atrophy. J Cereb Blood Flow Metab 1988;8:662–670.
110. Chawluk J, Alavi A, Dann R, et al. Positron emission tomography in aging and dementia: effect of cerebral atrophy. J Nucl Med 1987;28:431–437.
111. Foster N, Chase T, Patronas N, et al. Cerebral mapping of apraxia in Alzheimer's disease by positron emission tomography. Ann Neurol 1986;19:139–143.
112. Penniello MJ, Lambert J, Eustache F, et al. A PET study of the functional neuroanatomy of writing impairment in Alzheimer's disease. The role of the left supramarginal and left angular gyri. Brain 1995;118:697–706.
113. Lowenstein D, Barker W, Chang J, et al. Predominant left hemisphere metabolic dysfunction in dementia. Arch Neurol 1989;46:146–152.
114. Rossor MN, Garrett NJ, Johnson AJ, et al. A postmortem study of the cholinergic and GABA system in senile dementia. Brain 1982;105:313–330.
115. Seltzer B, Sherwin I. A comparison of clinical features in early and late onset primary degenerative dementia. Arch Neurol 1983;40:143–146.
116. Small B, Kuhl D, Reige W, et al. Cerebral glucose metabolic patterns in Alzheimer's disease. Effect of gender and age at dementia onset. Arch Gen Psychiatry 1989;46:527–532.
117. Adams R, Kessler C, Herholz K, et al. Positron emission tomography for differential diagnosis of dementia: a case of familial dementia [abstract]. J Neural Transm Park Dis Dement Sect 1989;1:36–30.
118. Guze B, Hoffman J, Mazziotta J, et al. Positron emission tomography and familial Alzheimer's disease: a pilot study. J Am Geriatr Soc 1992;40:120–123.
119. Kennedy AM, Rossor MN, Frackowiak RS. Positron emission tomography in familial Alzheimer's disease. Alzheimer Dis Assoc Disord 1995;9:17–20.
120. Pietrini P, Azari N, Grady C, et al. Pattern of cerebral metabolic interaction in a subject with isolated amnesia at risk for Alzheimer's disease: a longitudinal evaluation. Dementia 1993;4:94–101.
121. Small GW, Mazziotta JC, Collins MT, et al. Apolipoprotein E type 4 allele and cerebral glucose metabolism in relatives at risk for familial Alzheimer disease. JAMA 1995;273:942–947.
122. Reiman EM, Caselli RJ, Yun LS, et al. Preclinical evidence of Alzheimer's disease in persons homozygous for the epsilon 4 allele for apolipoprotein E [see comments]. N Engl J Med 1996;334:752–758.
123. Lehtovirta M, Soininen H, Laakso MP, et al. SPECT and MRI analysis in Alzheimer's disease: relation to apolipoprotein E epsilon 4 allele. J Neurol Neurosurg Psychiatry 1996;60:644–649.
124. Corder EH, Jelic V, Basun, H, et al. No difference in cerebral glucose metabolism in patients with Alzheimer's disease and differing apolipoprotein E genotypes. Arch Neurol 1997;54:273–277.
125. Fletcher PC, Frith CD, Rugg MD. The functional neuroanatomy of episodic memory. Trends Neurosci 1997;20:213–218.
126. Kessler J, Herholz K, Ground M, Heis WD. Impaired metabolic activation in Alzheimer's disease: a PET study during continous visual recognition. Neuropsychologia 1991;29:229–243.
127. Kessler J, Ghaemi M, Mielke R, et al. Visual versus auditory memory stimulation in patients with probable Alzheimer's disease. A PET study with 18 FDG. Ann N Y Acad Sci 1996;777:233–238.
128. Miller JD, de Leon MJ, Ferris SH, et al. Abnormal temporal lobe response in Alzheimer's disease during cognitive processing as measured by ^{11}C-2-deoxy-D-glucose and PET. J Cereb Blood Flow Metab 1987;7:248–251.
129. Grady CL, Haxby JV, Horwitz B. Activation of cerebral blood flow during a visuospatial task in patients with Alzheimer type dementia. Neurobiol Aging 1993;14:35–44.
130. Becker JT, Mintun MA, Aleva K, et al. Compensatory reallocation of brain resources supporting verbal episodic memory in Alzheimer's disease. Neurology 1996;46:692–700.
131. Herbster AN, Nichols T, Wiseman M, et al. Functional connectivity in auditory verbal short term memory in Alzheimer's disease. Neuroimage 1996;4:67–77.
132. Gemmell HG, Sharp PF, Evans NT, et al. Single photon emission tomography with 123-isopropylamphetamine in Alzheimer's disease and multi-infarct dementia. Lancet 1984;2:1348.
133. Neary D, Snowden J, Shields R, et al. Single photon emission tomography using 99m Tc HM-PAO in the investigation of dementia. J Neurol Neurosurg Psychiatry 1987;50:1101–1109.
134. Holman BL, Johnson KA, Gerada B, et al. The scintigraphic appearance of Alzheimer's disease: a prospective study using technetium-99m-HMPAO SPECT [see comments; published erratum appears in J Nucl Med 1992;33:484]. J Nucl Med 1992;33:181–185.
135. Spampinaton U, Habert M, Mas J, et al. (99m Tc) HM-PAO SPECT and cognitive impairment in Parkinson's disease: a comparison with dementia of the Alzheimer type. J Neurol Neurosurg Psychiatry 1991;54:787–792.

136. Claus JJ, van Harskamp F, Breteler MM, et al. The diagnostic value of SPECT with Tc 99m HMPAO in Alzheimer's disease: a population-based study. Neurology 1994;44:454–461.
137. Sharp P, Gemmell H, Cherryman G, et al. Application of iodine-123-labeled isopropylamphetamine imaging to the study of dementia. J Nucl Med 1986;27:761–768.
138. Smith FW, Gemmell HG, Sharp PF. The use of 99Tcm-HM-PAO for the diagnosis of dementia. Nucl Med Commun 1987;8:525–533.
139. Luxenberg JS, May C, Haxby JV, et al. Cerebral metabolism, anatomy and cognition in monozygotic twins discordant for dementia of the Alzheimer type. J Neurol Neurosurg Psychiatry 1987;50:333–340.
140. Kuwabara Y, Ichiya Y, Otsuka M, et al. Differential diagnosis of bilateral parietal abnormalities in I-123 IMP SPECT imaging. Clin Nucl Med 1990;15:893–899.
141. Gemmell HG, Evans NT, Besson JA, et al. Regional cerebral blood flow imaging: a quantitative comparison of technetium-99-HMPAO SPECT with $C^{15}O_2$ PET. J Nucl Med 1990;31:1595–1600.
142. O'Brien JT, Eagger S, Syed GM, et al. A study of regional cerebral blood flow and cognitive performance in Alzheimer's disease. J Neurol Neurosurg Psychiatry 1992;55:1182–1187.
143. Syed GM, Eagger S, O'Brien J, et al. Patterns of regional cerebral blood flow in Alzheimer's disease. Nucl Med Commun 1992;13:656–663.
144. Frlich L, Eilles C, Ihl R, et al. Stage-dependent reductions of regional cerebral blood flow measured by HMPAO-SPECT in dementia of Alzheimer type. Psychiatry Res 1989;29:347–350.
145. Eagger S, Syed GM, Burns A, et al. Morphologic (CT) and functional (rCBF-SPECT) correlates in Alzheimer's disease. Nucl Med Commun 1992;13:644–647.
146. Bonte FJ, Tintner R, Weiner MF, et al. Brain blood flow in the dementias: SPECT with histopathologic correlation. Radiology 1993;186:361–365.
147. Read SL, Miller BL, Mena I, et al. SPECT in dementia: clinical and pathological correlation. J Am Geriatr Soc 1995;43:1243–1247.
148. Grunwald F, Zierz S, Broich K, et al. HMPAO-SPECT imaging resembling Alzheimer-type dementia in mitochondrial encephalomyopathy with lactic acidosis and stroke-like episodes (MELAS). J Nucl Med 1990;31:1740–1742.
149. Pearlson GD, Harris GJ, Powers RE, et al. Quantitative changes in mesial temporal volume, regional cerebral blood flow, and cognition in Alzheimer's disease. Arch Gen Psychiat 1992;49:402–408.
150. Ohnishi T, Hoshi H, Nagamachi S, et al. High-resolution SPECT to assess hippocampal perfusion in neuropsychiatric diseases. J Nucl Med 1995;36:1163–1169.
151. Besson JA, Crawford JR, Parker DM, et al. Neuroimaging, cognitive, and pathological changes in dementia of the Alzheimer type (DAT). Psychiatry Res 1989;29:447–448.
152. Celsis P, Agniel A, Rascol A, Marc-Vergnes J. Focal cerebral hypoperfusion and selective cognitive deficit in dementia of the Alzheimer type. J Neurol Neurosurg Psychiatry 1987;50:1602–1612.
153. Weinberger DR, Gibson R, Coppola R, et al. The distribution of cerebral muscarinic acetylcholine receptors in vivo in patients with dementia. A controlled study with ^{123}IQNB and single photon emission computed tomography [see comments]. Arch Neurol 1991;48:169–176.
154. Kuhl DE, Minoshima S, Fessler JA, et al. In vivo mapping of cholinergic terminals in normal aging Alzheimer's disease and Parkinson's disease. Ann Neurol 1996;40:399–410.
155. Nordberg A, Hartvig P, Lilja A, et al. Decreased uptake and binding of C-nicotine in brain of Alzheimer patients as visualized by positron emission tomography. J Neural Transm 1992;2:215–224.
156. Nordberg A, Lundqvist H, Hartvig P, et al. Kinetic analysis of regional (S)(-)^{11}C-nicotine binding in normal and Alzheimer brains—in vivo assessment using positron emission tomography. Alzheimer Dis Assoc Disord 1995;9:21–27.
157. Iyo M, Namba H, Fukushi K, et al. Measurement of acetylcholinesterase by positron emission tomography in the brains of healthy controls and patients with Alzheimer's disease. Lancet 1997;349:1805–1809.
158. Blin J, Baron JC, Dubois B, et al. Loss of brain 5-HT_2 receptors in Alzheimer's disease. In vivo assessment with positron emission tomography and [^{18}F] setoperone. Brain 1993;116:497–510.
159. Tyrrell PJ, Sawle GV, Ibanez V, et al. Clinical and positron emission tomographic studies in the "extrapyramidal syndrome" of dementia of the Alzheimer type. Arch Neurol 1990;47:1318–1323.
160. Itoh M, Meguro K, Fujiwara T, et al. Assessment of dopamine metabolism in brain of patients with dementia by means of ^{18}F-fluorodopa and PET. Ann Nucl Med 1994;8:245–251.
161. Majocha R, Reno J, Friedland R, et al. Development of monoclonal antibody specific for beta/A4 amyloid in Alzheimer's disease brain for application to in vivo imaging of amyloid angiopathy. J Nucl Med 1992;33:2184–2189.
162. Groom GN, Junck L, Foster NL, et al. PET of peripheral benzodiazepine binding sites in the microgliosis of Alzheimer's disease. J Nucl Med 1995;36:2207–2210.
163. Hachinski V, Lassen N, Marshall J. Multi-infarct dementia. A cause of mental deterioration in the elderly. Lancet 1974;2:207–209.

164. Hachinski V, Potter P, Merskey H. Leuko-araiosis. Arch Neurol 1987;44:21–23.
165. Inzitari D, Diaz F, Fox A, et al. Vascular risk factors and leuko-araiosis. Arch Neurol 1987;44:42–47.
166. van Swieten JC, Geyskes GG, Derix MMA, et al. Hypertension in the elderly is associated with white matter lesions and cognitive decline. Ann Neurol 1991;30:825–830.
167. Kozachuk WE, DeCarli C, Schapiro MB, et al. White matter hyperintensities in dementia of Alzheimer's type and in healthy subjects without cerebrovascular risk factors. Arch Neurol 1990;47:1306–1310.
168. Coffman JA, Torello W, Bornstein RA, et al. Leukoaraiosis in asymptomatic adult offspring of individuals with Alzheimer's disease. Biol Psychiatry 1992;27:1244–1248.
169. Brant-Zawadzki M, Fein G, Van Dyke C, et al. MR imaging of the aging brain: patchy white-matter lesions and dementia. AJNR Am J Neuroradiol 1985;6:675–681.
170. Kobari M, Meyer JS, Ichijo M. Leuko-araiosis, cerebral atrophy, and cerebral perfusion in normal aging. Arch Neurol 1990;47:161–165.
171. Gerard G, Weisberg LA. MRI periventricular lesions in adults. Neurology 1986;36:998–1001.
172. Sarpel G, Chaudry F, Hindo W. Magnetic resonance imaging of periventricular hyperintensity in a Veterans Administration hospital population. Arch Neurol 1987;44:725–731.
173. Steingart A, Hachinski V, Lau C, et al. Cognitive and neurologic findings in demented patients with diffuse white matter lucencies on computed tomographic scan (leuko-araiosis). Arch Neurol 1987;44:36–39.
174. Blenlow K, Wallin A, Uhlemann C, Gottfries CG. White-matter lesions on CT in Alzheimer patients: relation to clinical symptomatology and vascular factors. Acta Neurol Scand 1991;83:187–193.
175. Fukuda H, Kobayashi S, Okada K, Tsunematsu T. Frontal white matter lesions and dementia in lacunar infarction. Stroke 1990;21:1143–1149.
176. Hachinski V, Hiff L, Zilhk E, et al. Cerebral blood flow in dementia. Arch Neurol 1975;32:632–637.
177. Mielke RM, Herholz K, Grond M, et al. Severity of vascular dementia is related to volume of metabolically impaired tissue. Arch Neurol 1992;49:909–913.
178. Sultzer DL, Mahler ME, Cummings JL, et al. Cortical abnormalities associated with subcortical lesions in vascular dementia. Clinical and positron emission tomographic findings. Arch Neurol 1995;52: 773–780.
179. Baron JC, D'Antona R, Pantano P, et al. Effects of thalamic stroke on energy metabolism of the cerebral cortex. A positron tomography study in man. Brain 1986;109:1243–1259.
180. Deutsch G, Tweedy JR. Cerebral blood flow in severity-matched Alzheimer and multi-infarct patients. Neurology 1987;37:431–438.
181. Starkstein SE, Sabe L, Vazquez S, et al. Neuropsychological, psychiatric, and cerebral blood flow findings in vascular dementia and Alzheimer's disease. Stroke 1996;27:408–414.
182. Kawamura J, Meyer JS, Terayama Y, Weathers S. Leukoaraiosis correlates with cerebral hypoperfusion in vascular dementia. Stroke 1991;22:609–614.
183. Kawamura J, Meyer JS, Ichijo M, et al. Correlations of leuko-araiosis with cerebral atrophy and perfusion in elderly normal subjects and demented patients. J Neurol Neurosurg Psychiatry 1993;56:182–187.
184. Sacquegna T, de Carolis P, Daidone R, Dondi M. Single-photon emission tomography with technetium Tc 99m hexamethylpropylene amine oxime in Binswanger's disease [letter]. Arch Neurol 1988; 45:603–604.
185. Shyu WC, Lin JC, Shen CC, et al. Vascular dementia of Binswanger's type: clinical, neuroradiological and ^{99m}Tc-HMPAO SPET study. Eur J Nucl Med 1996;23:1338–1344.
186. Yao H, Sadoshima S, Kuwabara Y, et al. Cerebral blood flow and oxygen metabolism in patients with vascular dementia of the Binswanger type. Stroke 1990;21:1694–1699.
187. Yao H, Sadoshima S, Ibayashi S, et al. Leukoaraiosis and dementia in hypertensive patients. Stroke 1992;23:1673–1677.
188. Meguro K, Hatazawa J, Yamaguchi T, et al. Cerebral circulation and oxygen metabolism associated with subclinical periventricular hyperintensity as shown by magnetic resonance imaging. Ann Neurol 1990;28:378–383.
189. Kuwabara Y, Ichiya Y, Otsuka M, et al. Cerebrovascular responsiveness to hypercapnia in Alzheimer's dementia and vascular dementia of the Binswanger type [see comments]. Stroke 1992; 23:594–598.
190. Joutel A, Corpechot C, Ducros A, et al. Notch3 mutations in CADASIL, a hereditary adult-onset condition causing stroke and dementia [see comments]. Nature 1996;383:707–710.
191. Chabriat H, Vahedi K, Iba-Zizen MT, et al. Clinical spectrum of CADASIL: a study of 7 families. Cerebral autosomal dominant arteriopathy with subcortical infarcts and leukoencephalopathy [see comments]. Lancet 1995;346:934–939.
192. Chabriat H, Bousser MG, Pappata S. Cerebral autosomal dominant arteriopathy with subcortical infarcts and leukoencephalopathy: a positron emission tomography study in two affected family members [letter]. Stroke 1995;26:1729–1730.

193. Wolfson LI, Leenders KL, Brown LL, Jones T. Alterations of regional cerebral blood flow and oxygen metabolism in Parkinson's disease. Neurology 1985;35:1399–1405.
194. Rougemont D, Baron JC, Collard P, et al. Local cerebral glucose utilisation in treated and untreated patients with Parkinson's disease. J Neurol Neurosurg Psychiatry 1984;47:824–830.
195. Lenzi GL, Jones T, Reid JL, Moss S. Regional impairment of cerebral oxidative metabolism in Parkinson's disease. J Neurol Neurosurg Psychiatry 1979;42:59–62.
196. Kuhl DE, Metter EJ, Riege WH. Patterns of local cerebral glucose utilization determined in Parkinson's disease by the [^{18}F] fluorodeoxyglucose method. Ann Neurol 1984;15:419–424.
197. Peppard RF, Martin WR, Carr GD, et al. Cerebral glucose metabolism in Parkinson's disease with and without dementia. Arch Neurol 1992;49:1262–1268.
198. Liu RS, Lin KN, Wang SJ, et al. Cognition and 99Tcm-HMPAO SPECT in Parkinson's disease. Nucl Med Commun 1992;13:744–748.
199. McKeith LG, Galasko D, Kosaka K, et al. Consensus guidelines for the clinical and pathologic diagnosis of dementia with Lewy bodies (DLB): report of the Consortium on DLB International Workshop. Neurology 1996;47:1113–1124.
200. D'Antona R, Baron JC, Samson Y, et al. Subcortical dementia. Frontal cortex hypometabolism detected by positron tomography in patients with progressive supranuclear palsy. Brain 1985;108:785–799.
201. Neary D, Snowden JS, Shields RA, et al. Single photon emission tomography using ^{99m}Tc-HM-PAO in the investigation of dementia. J Neurol Neurosurg Psychiatry 1987;50:1101–1109.
202. Blin J, Baron JC, Dubois B, et al. Positron emission tomography study in progressive supranuclear palsy. Brain hypometabolic pattern and clinicometabolic correlations. Arch Neurol 1990;47:747–752.
203. Sawle GV, Brooks D, Marsden CD, Frackowiak RJS. Corticobasal degeneration; a unique pattern of regional cortical oxygen metabolism and striatal fluoro DOPA uptake demonstrated by positron emission tomography. Brain 1991;114:541–556.
204. Eidelberg D, Dhawan V, Moeller J, et al. The metabolic landscape of cortico basal ganglionic degeneration; regional asymmetries studied with positron emission tomography. J Neurol Neurosurg Psychiatry 1991;54:856–862.
205. Nagahama Y, Fukuyama H, Turjanski N, et al. Cerebral glucose metabolism in cortical basal degeneration: comparison with progressive supranuclear palsy and normal controls. Mov Disord 1997;12: 691–696.
206. Kuhl D, Phelps M, Markham C, et al. Cerebral glucose metabolism and atrophy in Huntington's disease determined by 18 FDG and computed tomographic scan. Ann Neurol 1982;12:425–434.
207. Mazziotta JC, Phelps M, Pahl J, et al. Reduced cerebral glucose metabolism in asymptomatic subjects at risk for Huntington's disease. New Engl J Med 1987;316:357–362.
208. Lantos P. Overview of Neuropathology. In MN Rossor (ed), Unusual Dementias (13th ed). London: Balliere Tindall, 1992;485–516.
209. Friedland RP, Koss E, Lerner A, et al. Functional imaging, the frontal lobes, and dementia. Dementia 1993;4:192–203.
210. Ludolph AC, Langen KJ, Regard M, et al. Frontal lobe function in amyotrophic lateral sclerosis: a neuropsychologic and positron emission tomography study. Acta Neurol Scand 1992;85:81–89.
211. Talbot PR, Goulding PJ, Lloyd JJ, et al. Inter-relation between "classic" motor neuron disease and frontotemporal dementia: neuropsychological and single photon emission computed tomography study. J Neurol Neurosurg Psychiatry 1995;58:541–547.
212. Sam M, Gutmann L, Schochet S, Doshi H. Pick's disease: a case clinically resembling amyotrophic lateral sclerosis. Neurology 1991;41:1831–1833.
213. Miller BL, Cummings JL, Villanueva-Meyer J, et al. Frontal lobe degeneration: clinical, neuropsychological, and SPECT characteristics [see comments]. Neurology 1991;41:1374–1382.
214. Starkstein SE, Migliorelli R, Teson A, et al. Specificity of changes in cerebral blood flow in patients with frontal lobe dementia. J Neurol Neurosurg Psychiatry 1994;57:790–796.
215. Graff-Radford NR, Russell JW, Rezai K. Frontal degenerative dementia and neuroimaging [discussion]. Adv Neurol 1995;66:37–47.
216. Julin P, Wahlund LO, Basun H, et al. Clinical diagnosis of frontal lobe dementia and Alzheimer's disease: relation to cerebral perfusion, brain atrophy and electroencephalography. Dementia 1995;6:142–147.
217. Pasquier F, Lebert F, Grymonprez L, et al. Verbal fluency in dementia of frontal lobe type and dementia of Alzheimer type. J Neurol Neurosurg Psychiatry 1995;58:81–84.
218. Kew JJ, Goldstein LH, Leigh PN, et al. The relationship between abnormalities of cognitive function and cerebral activation in amyotrophic lateral sclerosis. A neuropsychological and positron emission tomography study. Brain 1993;116:1399–1423.
219. Kew JJ, Leigh PN, Playford ED, et al. Cortical function in amyotrophic lateral sclerosis. A positron emission tomography study. Brain 1993;116:655–680.

220. Matochick J, Molchan S, Zametkin A, Warden D. Regional cortical glucose metabolism in autopsy confirmed Creutzfeldt-Jackob disease. Acta Neurol Scand 1995;91:153–157.
221. Reed LJ, O'Docherty MO, Scaravilli F, Kopelman MD. Identification of the thalamic hypometabolism in new variant Creutzfeld-Jakob disease using 18 FDG PET and statistical parametric mapping. Correlation with neuropathological findings [abstract]. Neuroimage 1997;5:S347.
222. Perani G, Cortelli P, Lucignani G, et al. FDG PET in familial fatal insomnia. The functional affects of thalamic lesions. Neurology 1993;43:2565–2569.
223. Mesulam MM. Slowly progressive aphasia without generalized dementia. Ann Neurol 1982;11:592–598.
224. Chawluk JB, Mesulam MM, Hurtig H, et al. Slowly progressive aphasia without generalized dementia: studies with positron emission tomography. Ann Neurol 1986;19:68–74.
225. Tyrrell PJ, Warrington EK, Frackowiak RSJ, Rossor MN. Heterogeneity in progressive aphasia due to focal cortical atrophy. A clinical and PET study. Brain 1990;113:1321–1336.
226. Kennedy AM, Tyrrell P, Warrington EK, et al. Progressive posterior cortical atrophy studied with positron emission tomography. J Cereb Blood Flow Metab 1991;11(suppl 2):S174.
227. Tyrrell PJ, Kartounis LD, Frackowiak RSJ, et al. Progressive loss of speech output and orofacial dyspraxia associated with frontal lobe hypometabolism. Ann Neurol 1991;54:351–357.
228. Tyrrell PJ, Warrington EK, Frackowiak RSJ, Rossor MN. Progressive degeneration of the right temporal lobe studied with positron emission tomography. J Neurol Neurosurg Psychiatry 1990;53:1046–1050.
229. Graff-Radford NR, Damasio AR, Hyman BT, et al. Progressive aphasia in a patient with Pick's disease: a neuropsychological, radiologic, and anatomic study. Neurology 1990;40:620–626.
230. Turner RS, Kenyon LC, Trojanowski JQ, et al. Clinical, neuroimaging, and pathologic features of progressive nonfluent aphasia. Ann Neurol 1996;39:166–173.
231. Gonzalez RG, Fischman AJ, Guimaraes AR, et al. Functional MR in the evaluation of dementia: correlation of abnormal dynamic cerebral blood volume measurements with changes in cerebral metabolism on positron emission tomography with fluorodeoxyglucose F 18. AJNR Am J Neuroradiol 1995;16:1763–1770.
232. Sandson TA, O'Connor M, Sperling RA, et al. Noninvasive perfusion MRI in Alzheimer's disease: a preliminary report. Neurology 1996;47:1339–1342.
233. Prichard JW, Cummings JL. The insistent call from functional MRI. Neurology 1997;48:797–800.
234. Corkin S, Amaral DG, Gonzalez RG. H. M.'s medial temporal lesion: findings from magnetic resonance imaging. J Neurosci 1997;10:3964–3979.
235. Stern CE, Corkin S, Gonzalez RG, et al. The hippocampal formation participates in novel picture encoding: evidence from functional magnetic resonance imaging. Proc Natl Acad Sci U S A 1996;93: 8660–8665.
236. MacKay S, Meyerhoff DJ, Constans JM, et al. Regional gray and white matter metabolite differences in subjects with AD, with subcortical ischemic vascular dementia, and elderly controls with ^{1}H magnetic resonance spectroscopic imaging. Arch Neurol 1996;53:167–174.
237. MacKay S, Ezekiel F, Di Sclafani V, et al. Alzheimer disease and subcortical ischemic vascular dementia: evaluation by combining MR imaging segmentation and H-1 MR spectroscopic imaging. Radiology 1996;198:537–545.
238. Meyerhoff DJ, MacKay S, Constans JM, et al. Axonal injury and membrane alterations in Alzheimer's disease suggested by in vivo proton magnetic resonance spectroscopic imaging. Ann Neurol 1994;36:40–47.
239. Shonk TK, Moats RA, Gifford P, et al. Probable Alzheimer disease: diagnosis with proton MR spectroscopy [see comments]. Radiology 1995;195:65–72.
240. Ernst T, Chang L, Melchor R, Mehringer CM. Frontotemporal dementia and early Alzheimer's disease: differentiation with frontal lobe H1 MR spectroscopy. Radiology 1997;203:829–836.
241. Tedeschi G, Bertolino A, Lundbom N, et al. Cortical and subcortical chemical pathology in Alzheimer's disease as assessed by multislice proton magnetic resonance spectroscopic imaging. Neurology 1996;47:696–704.
242. Pettigrew JW, Kopp SJ, Minshew NJ, et al. ^{31}P Nuclear magnetic resonance studies on phosphoglyceride metabolism in developing and degenerating brain: preliminary observations. J Neuropathol Exp Neurol 1987;46:419–430.
243. Bottomley PA, Cousins JP, Pendrey DL, et al. Alzheimer dementia: quantification of energy metabolism and mobile phosphoesters with P-31 NMR spectroscopy. Radiology 1992;183:695–699.
244. Gonzalez RG, Guimaraes AR, Moore GJ, et al. Quantitative in vivo ^{31}P magnetic resonance spectroscopy of Alzheimer disease. Alzheimer Dis Assoc Disord 1996;10:46–52.
245. Murphy DG, Bottomley PA, Salerno JA, et al. An in vivo study of phosphorus and glucose metabolism in Alzheimer's disease using magnetic resonance spectroscopy and PET. Arch Gen Psychiat 1993;50:341–349.

10

Molecular Pathology of Alzheimer's Disease: The Role of Amyloid

Dennis J. Selkoe

Few subjects in the study of Alzheimer's disease (AD) have generated more interest and, at times, more controversy than that of beta-amyloid (Aβ). In his original paper, Alzheimer himself wrote prophetically: "Scattered through the entire cortex, especially in the upper layers, one found miliary foci that were caused by the deposition of a peculiar substance in the cerebral cortex." Evidence emerging from many laboratories since 1984 indicates that this "peculiar substance" is a protein fragment, approximately 40–42 amino acids long, referred to as *amyloid beta-protein*. It arises from cleavage by unknown proteases of a much larger precursor polypeptide, the beta-amyloid precursor protein (APP), encoded by a gene on human chromosome 21 (*APP*).

Whether the innumerable foci of neuritic and glial alteration that constitute the senile plaques of the disease are *caused* by Aβ deposition, as Alzheimer seemed to imply, and whether this deposition is the key pathogenetic trigger that initiates the long and complex cascade of AD remain matters of some debate. Nevertheless, rapidly accumulating evidence from many laboratories worldwide suggests that the answer to both questions may turn out to be yes. The strongest support has come from the elucidation of the genotype-to-phenotype relationships for each of the four genes implicated to date in familial forms of AD. In each case, mutations or polymorphisms in genes that cause the premature development of AD have been shown to increase the cellular production or cerebral deposition of Aβ. In view of this finding and its attendant therapeutic implications, it is important for neurologists and other specialists caring for demented patients to become familiar with APP metabolism, its links to the genetics of the disease, and its potential role in the diagnosis and treatment of AD. These topics are considered in detail here.

EXPRESSION, METABOLISM, AND FUNCTION OF AMYLOID PRECURSOR PROTEIN

Knowledge of the specific proteins comprising the neurofibrillary tangles and senile plaques found in AD and of the mutant gene products causing familial forms of the disease has led to substantial progress in deciphering the mechanisms that underlie the development of the AD phenotype. Advances in this area have in turn provided important new information about protein structure and function of interest to biologists in general. Nowhere is this interrelationship more true than in the case of APP, the study of which has drawn interest from many scientists outside of the disciplines of neurology and neuropathology. The identification and cloning of APP [1–4] resulted directly from the original isolation by Glenner and Wong [5] of its Aβ fragment in the meningovascular amyloid of AD and Down syndrome (DS) and the subsequent confirmation of this protein as the subunit of amyloid filaments in senile plaque cores [6–8]. APP actually comprises a heterogeneous group of polypeptides that undergo alternative exon splicing (the longest spliced transcript encoding 770 amino acids) and extensive post-translational processing, including the addition of sugar, phosphate, and sulfate groups to the protein. Whereas the 770–amino acid form and the slightly shorter 751-residue alternatively spliced version are the most common isoforms expressed in non-neural cells throughout the body, neurons express both these and a shorter 695-residue form. The difference between the 751/770 forms and the 695 form resides in the presence in the former of a 56-amino acid exon that encodes a region homologous to the Kunitz family of serine protease inhibitors (Figure 10.1). The presence of this so-called Kunitz protease inhibitor (KPI) motif suggests one of the functions of the longer APP isoforms—namely, their ability to inhibit certain serine proteases. That this actually occurs has been shown by in vitro studies in which trypsin, chymotrypsin, and some other serine proteases undergo inhibition [9,10]. Indeed, the 751/770 forms of APP present in platelets have been shown to serve as an inhibitor of factor XIa in the coagulation cascade [11]. Although the shorter 695 form of APP is expressed almost exclusively in neurons, these cells also express the KPI-containing 751 and 770 isoforms. Therefore, a special role for APP_{695} in the pathogenesis of AD has never been confirmed. The almost ubiquitous expression of $APP_{751/770}$ in cells and tissues throughout the body (with particularly high expression in kidney and muscle) raises the question of why substantial Aβ deposition occurs only in the brain, although very small deposits of nonfibrillar (diffuse) Aβ have been seen in some non-neural tissues, including skin, spleen, and intestine [12]. The reasons for this anatomic discrepancy could include both the relatively higher rate of Aβ production by neurons and potential differences in the fate of Aβ following its release from neural versus non-neural cells—for example, an adverse balance between degradation and aggregation of the peptide in the brain.

The APP sequence has been highly conserved during evolution in mammals (e.g., all 695 residues of APP_{695} are identical in monkey and human [13]), and close homologs have been found in the fruit fly, *Drosophila* [14], and the round worm, *Caenorhabditis elegans* [15]. This conservation implies that the polypeptide is functionally important. Nevertheless, the use of recombinant DNA methods ("genetic engineering") to delete both copies of *App* from mice results in neither mortality nor severe morbidity; only cerebral gliosis and some change in

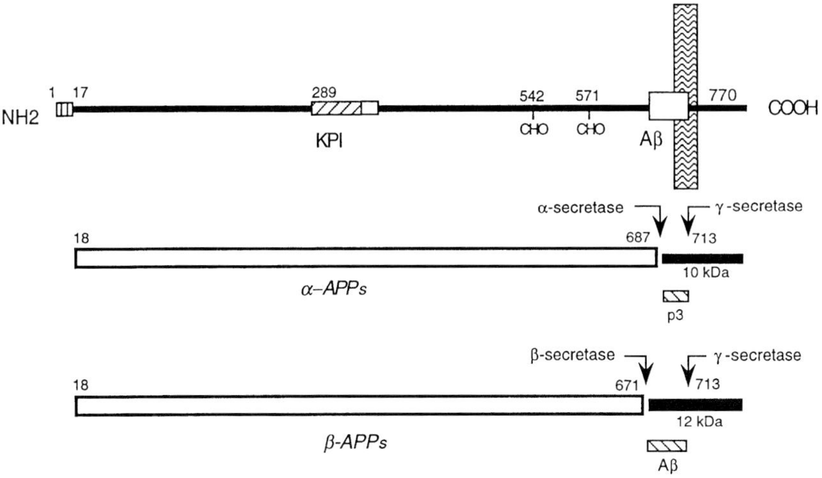

Figure 10.1 Schematic diagrams of the beta-amyloid (AB) precursor protein (APP) and its principal metabolic derivatives. The upper diagram depicts the largest of the known APP alternate transcripts, comprising 770 amino acids. Regions of interest are indicated at their correct relative positions. A 17-residue signal peptide occurs at the amino terminus (*box with vertical lines*). Two alternatively spliced exons of 56 and 19 amino acids are inserted at residue 289; the first contains a serine protease inhibitor domain of the Kunitz type (KPI). Two sites of N-glycosylation (CHO) are found at residues 542 and 571. A single membrane-spanning domain at amino acids 700–723 is indicated by the vertical hatched bar. The Aβ fragment (*white box*) includes 28 residues just outside the membrane plus the first 12–14 residues of the transmembrane domain. In the middle diagram, the arrow indicates the site (after residue 687) of a constitutive proteolytic cleavage made by an unknown protease(s), designated *alpha-secretase*, that enables secretion of the large, soluble ectodomain of APP (α-APP_S) into the medium and retention of the 83-residue carboxy-terminal fragment (approximately 10 kd) in the membrane. The 10-kd fragment can undergo cleavage by an unknown protease(s) called *gamma-secretase* at residue 711 or residue 713 to release the p3 peptides. The bottom diagram depicts the alternative proteolytic cleavage after residue 671 by an unknown enzyme(s) called *beta-secretase* that results in the secretion of a truncated APP_s (β-APP_S) molecule and the retention of a 99-residue (approximately 12-kd) carboxy-terminal fragment. The 12-kd fragment can also undergo cleavage by gamma-secretase to release the Aβ peptides.

locomotor behavior over time have been described initially in these animals [16]. This lack of a vital consequence may be explained by the fact that mammals have other genes homologous to *APP*, the amyloid precursor–like protein genes (*APLP*s) [17,18].

As regards in vitro studies of APP function, the physiologic consequences of the secretion of alpha-APP_s (see Figure 10.1) and Aβ have not been clearly defined. In particular, a specific receptor for alpha-APP_s is not known, although this major secreted derivative is capable of stimulating a mitogen-activated protein kinase–mediated, $p21^{ras}$-dependent signal transduction cascade in cultured cells [19]. As stated above, the KPI-like amino acid motif of exon 7 of *APP* can serve as a serine protease inhibitor. Other functions of alpha-APP_s or cell surface holo-APP that have been postulated on the basis of cell culture experiments include roles as a trophic [20] or neuroprotective [21] molecule and as a mediator of cell-cell [22] and cell-substrate [23,24] interactions. The true functions of APP in vivo, however, have not yet been determined.

The intracellular trafficking and processing of APP have been extensively studied since the late 1980s. After its synthesis on ribosomes, APP is cotranslationally translocated into the endoplasmic reticulum (ER) via its signal peptide and then "matures" through the central secretory pathway. In the Golgi apparatus, the protein undergoes N- and O-linked glycosylation [25] as well as phosphorylation of its ectodomain [26,27]. APP is a single transmembrane protein; that is, it has one approximately 23-residue hydrophobic stretch (located near its end [carboxy terminus]) that serves to anchor APP in the phospholipid bilayer of internal (e.g., Golgi, endosome) and external (plasmalemma) membranes (see Figure 10.1). The addition of sugars to a protein-like APP within the Golgi apparatus is not unexpected, but it is unusual that APP is phosphorylated selectively in its ectodomain in this secretory compartment [27]. The functional reason for the addition of phosphates here rather than in the cytoplasmic domain, a far more common locus for this protein modification, is unclear.

During and after its maturation in the central secretory pathway (i.e., the ER, Golgi, and trans-Golgi network) by the addition of sugar, phosphate, and sulfate groups, APP can undergo specific endoproteolytic cleavages, particularly by a scission between residues 16 and 17 of the Aβ region, which is located just a few amino acids before the beginning of the single transmembrane sequence (see Figure 10.1). This principal secretory cleavage—first described in APP molecules that had trafficked to the cell surface, but now known to occur also in APP molecules in the secretory pathway before reaching the surface—is referred to as the *alpha-secretory cleavage*, and the as-yet-unknown enzyme(s) that creates the cleavage is designated *alpha-secretase*. The enzyme's action creates (1) a large, soluble fragment (virtually the entire ectodomain) that is released into the lumina of vesicles and from the cell surface (alpha-APP_s) and (2) a membrane-retained carboxy terminal fragment (CTF) of 83 amino acids that is sometimes referred to as the *10-kd CTF* [25,28,29]. The creation and release of alpha-APP_s is presumably important for APP function, because it is the secreted derivative that may confer the properties of APP observed so far in in vitro studies (e.g., its inhibition of serine proteases, including factor XIa). Alpha-secretase most likely is itself a membrane-anchored protease capable of cleaving a variety of other cell-surface transmembrane proteins, but the responsible enzyme has not been specifically defined and cloned.

The cleavage of APP molecules by alpha-secretase(s) appears to be a highly regulated event in both neural and non-neural cells. For example, activation of certain phosphate-adding enzymes (kinases), such as protein kinase C, by stimulating various cell-surface receptors (e.g., muscarinic receptors) linked to this kinase results in a substantial increase in the secretion of alpha-APP_s [30,31]. Electrical depolarization of neurons has also been shown to enhance alpha-APP_s release [32]. These and similar data indicate that the cleavage of APP and release of its ectodomain is physiologically important and thus well regulated by a variety of first and second messenger systems in cells. Nevertheless, the significance of this regulation for the mechanism of Aβ buildup in AD remains unclear. Only a minority of total cellular APP undergoes alpha-secretory cleavage, so that an increase in this scission would still leave many APP molecules that could be subjected to the alternative cleavages (made by proteases designated beta- and gamma-secretases) that lead to Aβ formation.

Even before the alpha-secretory pathway was described, it was assumed that the formation and release of Aβ into the extracellular space, where it constituted the subunit of amyloid plaques, must represent a strictly pathologic event. This assumption was based not only on the occurrence of Aβ deposits under pathologic circumstances—namely, in AD, DS, and with great age—but also because one of the proteolytic cleavages generating Aβ, the gamma-secretase cut, would need to occur within the membranes of cells. This requirement suggested that some pre-existing injury to cell membranes would be necessary before the gamma-secretase could access this region and clip it to release Aβ. In 1992, however, three groups unexpectedly showed that this concept was wrong. Aβ was found to be constitutively secreted by normal, healthy cells in culture and could actually be detected as a circulating peptide in both the plasma and cerebrospinal fluid (CSF) of normal humans and lower mammals [33–35]. The discovery of normal Aβ production carries implications for the proteolytic processing of transmembrane proteins in general and for the role of Aβ production in AD in particular (reviewed in reference 36). In our laboratory, we observed that not only Aβ but also a smaller fragment thereof, which we called *p3*, were constitutively released by APP-expressing cells during normal metabolism [33,37]. These and many subsequent studies have clearly shown that the amino terminus of p3 is generated when alpha-secretase cleaves APP between residues 16 and 17 of the Aβ region, and the carboxy terminus of p3 is subsequently generated when the resultant of 10-kd CTF is cleaved by gamma-secretase (see Figure 10.1). In an entirely analogous fashion, other APP holoproteins can instead be cleaved by beta-secretase just before aspartic $acid_1$ (asp_1) of the Aβ region to create this amino terminus, followed by cleavage of the resultant approximately 12-kd (or "C99") CTF by the same gamma-secretase to create Aβ (see Figure 10.1). Although precise quantitation is not available, it appears that an even smaller proportion of total cellular APP molecules undergoes beta-secretase processing than undergoes alpha-secretase cleavage. Not all of the resultant 12- and 10-kd CTFs are processed to Aβ and p3 respectively; other so-called nonspecific proteolytic pathways can degrade these CTFs to very small peptides and individual amino acids, perhaps principally in lysosomes [38,39].

To summarize the proteolytic pathways just reviewed, Aβ is created when APP is cleaved sequentially by beta- and gamma-secretase, whereas p3 is created when APP is cleaved sequentially by alpha- and gamma-secretase. To make matters considerably more complicated, we now know that both beta- and gamma-secretases do not cleave only at a single amino acid position. Aβ peptides found in culture medium, in human spinal fluid and, notably, in the amyloid deposits of AD brains show both N- and C-terminal heterogeneity. At the N-terminus, Aβ peptides may begin at residues $pyroglutamate_3$, $arginine_5$, or $glutamate_{11}$, in addition to the principal N-terminus of asp_1. There is evidence that certain of these N-terminally truncated Aβ species, particularly those beginning with a pyroglutamate at residue 3, are detectable relatively early in the course of progressive cerebral Aβ deposition in AD and DS [40]. These N-terminal species are generally assumed to arise from modification of the Aβ N-terminus after an initial beta-secretase clip at asp_1, but they could also arise in part from direct endoproteolytic cleavages at those respective residues. Their significance for the pathogenesis of plaque formation remains unclear. In contrast, the importance of C-terminal heterogeneity is more apparent. Immunocytochemical studies using antibodies that selectively recognize either the valine$_{40}$ or the alanine$_{42}$ C-termini have clearly shown that the first Aβ form deposited in DS and AD brain tissue ends at residue 42. In other words, the so-called diffuse plaques of Aβ that neuropathologists have come to recognize as the earliest form of Aβ deposit to be detectable in DS and AD brains are virtually exclusively composed of Aβ peptides ending at residue 42 [41–43]. Indeed, in studies of the temporal progression of plaque formation in DS brains of increasing age, it was shown that $Aβ_{42}$ peptides could form numerous diffuse plaques as early as age 12 years, whereas $Aβ_{40}$ reactivity in the plaques was first observed almost two decades later near age 30 years [43]. This immunocytochemical evidence of initial $Aβ_{42}$ deposition in AD and DS patients appears to fit well with a number of in vitro studies showing that the $Aβ_{42}$ peptide, with its two extra hydrophobic residues (isoleucine and alanine) aggregates into amyloid fibrils far more avidly and rapidly than does the $Aβ_{40}$ peptide [44,45]. It may seem surprising that just two amino acids can make such a difference in the apparent pathogenicity of a peptide, but then of course single amino acid mutations in many proteins are known to precipitate devastating and fatal diseases.

Both in cell culture and in normal human CSF and plasma, $Aβ_{40}$ peptides are far more abundant than $Aβ_{42}$ peptides, comprising roughly 90% of total secreted Aβ. This disparity in basal concentrations of the two peptides underscores the strong aggregation properties of $Aβ_{42}$, which despite its minor levels, accumulates first and foremost in the form of myriad diffuse plaques in AD and DS brains. As a result, there is great interest in understanding the basic mechanism of the putatively intramembranous cleavage of APP by gamma-secretases and determining whether there are distinct proteases cleaving after residues 40 and 42. The two cleavages can be differentially blocked by certain protease inhibitors, suggesting that two distinct proteases or at least two distinct proteolytic activities of one enzyme exist [46,47]. Given the apparently seminal role of $Aβ_{42}$ formation and deposition in AD, it would be desirable to identify protease inhibitors that selectively block only $Aβ_{42}$ production and leave all other aspects of APP metabolism unchanged.

Because the beta- and gamma-secretases have not yet been identified and cloned, it is difficult to determine precisely where they are located in the cell. An approximate localization can be established, however, by defining where their respective cleavage products are detectable—namely, the free C-terminus of the truncated form of APP_s (beta-APP_s) created by the beta-secretase cleavage event and the free C-termini of $Aβ_{40}$ and $Aβ_{42}$ created by the respective gamma-secretase cleavages. It has become clear that a sizable portion (probably the majority) of $Aβ_{40}$ peptides is generated in recycling endosomes after internalization of APP molecules from the cell surface [48,49]. Several lines of evidence support early endosomes as a principal site of $Aβ_{40}$ generation (Table 10.1). That surface APP indeed undergoes endocytosis and rapid recycling to the surface has been established directly in both non-neural [50] and neural [51] cells. The strongest evidence that Aβ is directly generated from surface APP molecules comes from experiments in which APP at the surface of living cells is labeled and then allowed to internalize at 37°C; this leads to the release within 15–30 minutes of labeled Aβ that could only have arisen from the surface-labeled molecules

Table 10.1 Data supporting early endosomes as the principal site of beta-amyloid generation

Deleting beta-amyloid (Aβ) precursor protein (βAPP) cytoplasmic domain (containing a gly-tyr-glu-asn-pro-thr-tyr signal) lowers Aβ production
Mild alkalinization lowers Aβ production
Altering vesicular H^+ transport lowers Aβ production
Late endosome/lysosome fractions do not contain Aβ
Endocytosis of surface-labeled βAPP molecules leads directly to release of labeled Aβ
Kinetics of labeled Aβ release are slightly slower than those of APP_s and consistent with those of recycling endosomes
Depleting cellular K^+ inhibits clathrin-mediated endocytosis and lowers Aβ production

[48]. C-terminal–specific $A\beta_{40}$ and $A\beta_{42}$ antibodies, however, have not yet been used in this experiment to determine the relative amounts of these two species generated in the endosomal system; it is assumed that it is mostly $A\beta_{40}$. As regards the loci for $A\beta_{42}$ formation, the use of sensitive sandwich enzyme-linked immunosorbent assays (ELISA) combined with manipulations that block the forward transport of APP through the secretory pathway suggest that $A\beta_{42}$ is generated in considerable part during early secretory processing of APP—namely, in the ER [52]. We have directly measured both Aβ species in subcellular fractions and found that $A\beta_{42}$ is by far the most abundant form in ER fractions, whereas both $A\beta_{42}$ and $A\beta_{40}$ are detectable in Golgi fractions [53]. The conclusion that Aβ can be generated during the secretory processing of APP is also supported by biochemical and immunocytochemical experiments detecting beta-APP_s in post-Golgi secretory vesicles [54]. One reason for establishing precisely the intracellular milieu in which different Aβ species are generated is to design highly specific inhibitors that operate under certain subcellular conditions.

A special feature of the endocytosis of APP in neurons is that some APP molecules are inserted at the surface of axon terminals, where they can be internalized and then traffic in a retrograde manner up axons to the cell body [55]; some of this APP can subsequently be further transported to the somatodendritic surface [56]. This means that APP can undergo full transcytosis from the axonal to the somatodendritic compartment. APP is the first example of an endogenous neuronal protein shown to undergo full transcytosis, but the functional significance of this trafficking is unclear. It should be noted that APP is not significantly present in synaptic vesicles per se [57] but rather occurs in other vesicles at axon terminals that are capable of undergoing retrograde transport.

Additional in vitro and in vivo studies of both APP trafficking and APP function are underway. Nevertheless, there is currently no convincing evidence that the normal functions of APP are perturbed in some way in AD. Rather, the involvement of the protein in the disease seems to arise through enhanced generation, decreased clearance, or increased aggregation of its Aβ fragment. It appears that only after excessive cerebral accumulation of Aβ fragments and the subsequent occurrence of many cellular and molecular changes do symptoms of dementia appear. One line of support for this conclusion is that all of the missense mutations in APP that have been found to cause AD are located at or near the alpha-, beta-, or gamma-secretase sites. These mutations thus act by altering APP proteolysis. If AD involved altered APP function in general, one would expect mutations to be distributed more randomly in other physiologically important regions of the molecule.

THE FATE OF BETA-AMYLOID PROTEIN AFTER ITS PRODUCTION: METABOLISM, DEPOSITION, AND CYTOTOXIC EFFECTS

In contrast to the substantial information just reviewed about APP trafficking and proteolytic processing, the fate of Aβ once it is generated in different subcellular compartments is still poorly understood. In most cell types, Aβ is quantitatively released from cells into the extracellular fluid, with much smaller amounts of total Aβ remaining intracellularly. Nonetheless, some Aβ, particularly $A\beta_{42}$, has been detected inside cells, including neural cell lines [52,53,58]. The presence of Aβ in human extracellular fluids, including plasma, CSF, and urine, and the accumulation of extracellular Aβ in the form of innumerable diffuse and compacted plaques in aged and AD brain tissue suggest that much of the activity and metabolic fate of Aβ occurs in the extracellular space.

Although there has been much interest in the mechanisms of Aβ generation, the manner in which the peptide is degraded and cleared from tissue has been much less studied. One possibility is that Aβ is taken back up by cells after its secretion and then degraded intracellularly, presumably in the endosomal/lysosomal system. Some evidence for the uptake of synthetic Aβ peptides incubated with cultured cells has been reported [59]. If this is a principal mechanism for Aβ removal from tissue, the peptide must be rapidly degraded once internalized because little or no intracellular Aβ has been detected in neurons or other brain cells by light or electron microscopic immunocytochemistry. An alternate manner of clearance would be by proteolytic degradation in the extracellular space. A few studies have described protease activities that are capable of degrading $A\beta_{40}$ and $A\beta_{42}$ peptides in vitro. One protease that is receiving increasing attention and has been studied in several laboratories is the insulin-degrading enzyme (IDE) [60,61]. This well-known metalloprotease is capable of degrading insulin, glucagon, and other small peptides in a variety of tissues and is present in normal brain tissue. Isolation of Aβ binding proteins from rodent brain extracts has revealed that IDE is one such protein [60]. Recent screening for Aβ-degrading proteases released into the media of a variety of cultured cell lines has shown that the principal Aβ degrading activity in several cell types, including microglia, is a metalloprotease very similar to, if not indistinguishable from, IDE [62]. Further information confirming that IDE constitutively degrades Aβ in neural and non-neural tissues and establishing what role it might play in AD is likely to emerge. Beyond this protease, there is currently little specific information about other candidate enzymes that degrade Aβ under normal or pathologic circumstances.

Competing with the cellular reuptake or extracellular degradation of Aβ is the peptide's tendency to polymerize into extracellular aggregates that are far more stable than the monomer and can apparently exert cytotoxic activities. Because of growing evidence that Aβ in its aggregated but not in its monomeric form is neurotoxic, the mechanisms of its aggregation have come under increasing scrutiny. Both $A\beta_{40}$ and $A\beta_{42}$ have a tendency to self-assemble into oligomers and polymers based on their hydrophobic properties. The Aβ_{42} species, however, with its two extra hydrophobic residues, has a particularly strong tendency to aggregate rapidly into insoluble oligomeric and polymeric material [45]. In general, the association of Aβ monomers into polymers appears kinetically unfavorable unless there is a preformed "seed" or initial oligomeric species present to accelerate the reaction. The nature and mechanism of formation of such seeds remain unclear. It may be that other proteins (so-called pathologic chaperones) can bind Aβ monomers or dimers and serve as a nidus for subsequent accrual of further monomers or oligomers and their progressive aggregation. In addition, nonprotein substances, for example metal ions or fragments of phospholipid membranes, could also serve as a stimulant of initial Aβ aggregation. In short, a number of inducers of Aβ aggregation may exist in the extracellular space of the brain. The recent observations that Aβ_{42} occurs as a stable species intracellularly (reviewed in the previous section) raise the possibility that it may dimerize or oligomerize intracellularly and that these early oligomers are released as seeds for extracellular Aβ aggregation.

The first morphologic form in which Aβ is detectable in AD, DS, or normal-aged brain tissue is the material comprising diffuse plaques. The Aβ in these early plaque-like deposits is particulate and insoluble in aqueous buffer [63,64]. Nonetheless, it is not filamentous in the diffuse plaques according to electron microscopic descriptions [65]; these plaques are largely devoid of the typical approximately 8-nm amyloid fibrils that comprise the cores of neuritic plaques. The recent detection in vitro of so-called Aβ protofilaments that are approximately half the size of amyloid fibrils (approximately 4 nm) and appear to be a metastable intermediate in the assembly of synthetic Aβ has raised the question of whether similar filaments occur in diffuse plaques in vivo [66]. The apparent dearth of typical Aβ fibrils in diffuse plaques and the fact that diffuse plaques always precede the appearance of fibrillar, compacted plaques in DS and normal brain aging suggest that Aβ exists in intermediate aggregated forms that undergo conversion to filaments before or while they become associated with surrounding cytotoxicity. If this is so, it may be possible to design small molecules that bind to these intermediates and prevent their association into larger fibrils. On the other hand, it may be preferable to prevent the initial oligomerization of the Aβ monomer in the first place.

Biochemists studying the accrual of Aβ in AD brain tissue are increasingly separating the phenomena of Aβ aggregation and Aβ deposition. It is likely that soluble Aβ monomers accumulate to supranormal concentrations before any aggregation occurs. Soluble oligomers of Aβ have been detected in normal and AD brain tissue [67]. Moreover, studies of Aβ deposition in transgenic mice overexpressing mutant human *APP* [68–70] suggest that Aβ accumulates to high levels in soluble and then insoluble forms before the appearance of diffuse plaques. It may be that after soluble monomers achieve a critical concentration, oligomers begin to form, presumably with the help of other molecules, such as protein "chaperones" that promote aggregation but do not necessarily become part of the aggregates. One example of aggregation-mediating molecules may be heparan sulfate proteoglycans (HSPGs), which are present in diffuse as well as compacted plaques [71,72]. Once initial Aβ oligomers or polymers are formed, they could be deposited onto a permissive substrate such as HSPG-containing basement membranes (e.g., in capillaries) or onto the plasma membranes of neurons or other brain cells. The further accrual of Aβ monomers onto pre-existing deposits has been studied using cryostat sections of AD brain [73], and the data suggest that Aβ deposition has kinetics that are distinct from those of Aβ aggregation [74]. Whether Aβ is deposited in the form of monomers or as already formed oligomers or larger aggregates in vivo remains unclear.

One curious feature of Aβ deposition in the human brain is that most plaques are roughly spherical in form, suggesting some organizing factor such as a local point source of Aβ (either within a cell or by being secreted from a cell) or an extracellular nidus of aggregated Aβ that serves as the template for further accrual of monomeric Aβ present at substantial levels in the local interstitial fluid. In the case of the vascular Aβ deposits that occur both in AD and in sporadic and familial forms of cerebral amyloid angiopathy, the vascular basement membrane, including proteoglycans, has been considered to be a potential nidus for progressive Aβ deposition. In this locus, Aβ has been recognized solely in filamentous form, without a clearly nonfilamentous form analogous to that in diffuse plaques [75]. It has even been hypothesized that amyloid plaques form initially around a nidus of Aβ deposited onto a capillary basement membrane, and light and electron microscopic evidence has suggested that many amyloid plaques are intimately associated with capillary basement membranes [76]. It is also known that spherical deposits of filamentous Aβ with surrounding dystrophic neurites can form around amyloid-laden microvessels that occur in AD cortex. Nevertheless, the lack of obvious juxtaposition of many diffuse and compacted Aβ deposits to capillaries in AD, DS, and transgenic mouse brains has so far precluded widespread acceptance of the theory that vascular basement membranes represent the organizing principle for cerebral Aβ deposition.

A number of other proteins that are normally synthesized and secreted by neurons, astrocytes, microglia, or other brain cells have been documented in association with Aβ in amyloid plaques. Most of those identified have clearly been shown to be present in fibrillar (usually neuritic) plaques, but some have also been found to varying degrees in diffuse plaques. Some consistently detectable Aβ-associated proteins include HSPG [71,72], $alpha_1$-antichymotrypsin [77], serum amyloid P component [78], various complement components [79,80], and apolipoprotein E (apo E) [43,81,82]. These are but a few of the polypeptides normally produced by brain cells that apparently become associated with developing Aβ deposits. The exact sequence of accrual of these polypeptides and their possible roles in inducing surrounding glial and neuritic cytopathology remain to be determined. In the case of apo E, for example, it is clear from studies of DS that $A\beta_{42}$ is the first protein to be detectable in diffuse plaques (which can appear as early as age 12 years in these individuals) and that many of these are initially unreactive for apo E but later steadily accrue apo E. Indeed, in DS, the appearance of apo E–positive plaques occurs virtually as a linear function of age, with a correlation coefficient of approximately 0.90 [43]. Here, we are talking about all isoforms of apo E in patients with varying genotypes for apo E; there is no current evidence as to whether a particular isoform of apo E (e.g., apo E-ε4) accrues onto Aβ deposits before another isoform. It is important to emphasize that some of the various plaque-associated proteins that accumulate in brain regions in which fibrillar, neuritic plaques form (e.g., hippocampus, neocortex) do so much less in areas such as cerebellum and striatum in which very few such mature plaques develop. In summary, the addition to plaques of various Aβ-associated proteins and perhaps also some nonproteinaceous constituents (e.g., gangliosides) is a complex, heterogeneous process, the temporal sequence of which is not yet well understood.

With regard to the biological activities of Aβ itself, the normal functions of the monomeric Aβ secreted by neural and non-neural cells at low nanomolar concentration are not known. There has been some evidence that Aβ in either a soluble or particulate form at low concentrations may have neurotrophic functions or may support neuron attachment and neurite outgrowth [83–85]. Whether these in vitro activities actually have physiologic significance in vivo is difficult to say, however. We know that mice in which *App* is knocked out have minimally abnormal phenotypes and develop and reproduce normally [16]. Because the *App* gene homologues (*APLP*s) that continue to be expressed in these knockout mice lack the Aβ region, one can conclude that deletion of *App*, with its unique Aβ sequence, has no critical consequences for mice. On the other hand, rodents in general do not convert much of their APP molecules to Aβ compared to humans, and it could be that constitutive Aβ production has a salutary function only in higher mammals that are also prone to excessive Aβ accumulation with age.

Most of the information about the biological activities of Aβ rests on the observed neurotoxicity of aggregated but not monomeric Aβ [86,87]. In general, knowledge of cytotoxic events have derived from short-term in vitro studies in which cultured neurons, astrocytes, or microglia are exposed to relatively high concentrations (10–50 μM) of aggregated synthetic Aβ of a single length, usually $A\beta_{1-40}$. A wide range of cytotoxic mechanisms for the effects of these synthetic Aβ aggregates has been reported. These include altered calcium homeostasis [88], free radical generation [89], various forms of peroxidative injury [90], and the potentiation by Aβ of other, more subtle cytotoxic events. Clearly, the various mechanisms hypothesized on the basis of in vitro neurotoxicity studies are not mutually exclusive. Aβ could exert direct neurotoxicity, could potentiate minor neurotoxic events that occur during normal cerebral metabolism in aged humans, or could act initially by proinflammatory mechanisms (i.e., stimulating local microglia and astrocytes to release cytokines and acute phase proteins). Whether the aggregated forms of Aβ that induce cytotoxicity act via specific receptors or generally perturb the function of the neuronal plasma membrane remains to be established. At least two types of cell surface receptors capable of binding and being activated by Aβ have been described: the scavenger receptor [91,92] and the receptor for advanced glycation end products [93]. These receptors, however, have not yet been confirmed to bind the oligomeric or polymeric forms of Aβ that are apparently capable of inducing neurotoxicity in vitro and in vivo. A classic ligand-receptor interaction that has saturable and competable kinetics has not yet been clearly demonstrated for Aβ aggregates. An alternative to a specific receptor-mediated mechanism would be a nonspecific contact of the aggregates with the plasma membrane, thereby altering the local microenvironment for numerous surface proteins rather than acting via one or two specific receptors. Such a mechanism has generally been assumed for systemic amyloidoses, although precisely how non-neural amyloid fibrils injure local cells is also not established. The early appearance of diffuse Aβ deposits in transgenic mouse models before noticeable microglial, astrocytic, and neuritic alterations suggests that it is compacted, largely fibrillar Aβ that is associated with a subsequent cellular response, but some participation by high levels of soluble monomers or oligomers is not yet excluded. A finer dissection of the temporal progression of Aβ-related cellular changes in the transgenic mice may provide better clues to the mechanisms of Aβ toxicity.

GENOTYPE-TO-PHENOTYPE CONVERSIONS IN FAMILIAL ALZHEIMER'S DISEASE: INVOLVEMENT OF BETA-AMYLOID PROTEIN

At the same time that studies of APP processing and Aβ biochemistry were proceeding, molecular geneticists combined forces with physicians to search for loci in the human genome that might contain defective genes underlying autosomal dominant cases of AD (familial AD [FAD]). Geneticists needed a compelling clue as to where in the human genome to begin their search for a faulty gene. This clue came with the recognition that patients with trisomy 21 invariably developed a neuropathologic phenotype indistinguishable from that of AD and that *APP* was located on chromosome 21. First, a linkage of some cases of FAD to markers on the long arm of chromosome 21 was suggested by analysis in a few families [94], and then, four years later, a mutation in the coding region of *APP* was identified in two families as the first specific molecular cause of AD [95]. Extensive further studies have revealed only six missense mutations in *APP* occurring in a very small number of autosomal dominant cases of the disease. The rarity of this initially defined genetic form of AD does not detract from its mechanistic importance for understanding AD pathogenesis in general, however, because all of the *APP* missense mutations cluster within or immediately flanking the Aβ region of *APP*. Indeed, the mutations are found at or near the alpha-secretase, beta-secretase, or gamma-secretase cleavage sites for APP proteolysis.

All of the known *APP* missense mutations linked to FAD have now been modeled in cultured cells or in transgenic mice, and some of them have also been analyzed directly in the plasma and CSF of mutation-bearing patients. In each case, the *APP* mutations have been shown to increase the secretion of Aβ into the extracellular fluid, particularly that of the $A\beta_{42}$ form (reviewed in reference 96). There is now virtually universal agreement among investigators that the rare *APP*-linked form of familial AD operates via an amyloid-promoting mechanism (Table 10.2). An important corollary of this conclusion is that the neuropathologic and clinical phenotypes of the *APP*-caused cases are highly similar to or indistinguishable from those of the other, more common genetic and sporadic forms of the disease.

Another gene to be implicated by genetic studies turned out to be a major risk factor for the late-onset form of AD. Biochemical studies searching for CSF proteins capable of binding to Aβ identified apo E as one such protein [97]. Subsequent genetic analyses showed that the naturally occurring ε4 polymorphism of the apo E gene (*APOE*) was substantially overrepresented in AD subjects compared to age-matched controls, and thus appeared to represent a major risk factor for the development of the disease (see Chapter 7). It has since been confirmed that inheritance of one or two *APOE-ε4* alleles significantly increases the likelihood of developing late-onset AD and decreases its age of onset [98]. Conversely, inheritance of the infrequent *APOE-ε2* allele appears to confer a

Table 10.2 Genetic factors predisposing to Alzheimer's disease and their relationship to the beta-amyloid phenotype

Chromosome	*Gene defect*	*Age of onset*	*Beta-amyloid ($A\beta$) phenotype*
21	Beta-amyloid precursor protein mutations	50s	Increases in production of total Aβ peptides or of $A\beta_{42}$ peptides
19	Apolipoprotein E-*ε4* allele polymorphism	60s and older	Increases in density of Aβ plaques and vascular deposits
14	Presenilin-1 mutations	40s and 50s	Increases in production of $A\beta_{42}$ peptides
1	Presenilin-2 mutations	50s	Increases in production of $A\beta_{42}$ peptides

Note: Additional chromosomal loci exist but are not yet specifically identified.

decreased risk of developing the disorder compared to that seen in humans harboring the common *ε3* allele [99].

The molecular mechanism by which the apo E-ε4 protein (which lacks cysteines and therefore cannot undergo intramolecular or intermolecular disulfide cross-linking) increases the likelihood of AD, whereas apo E-ε3 and apo E-ε2 proteins (which contain cysteines) do not remain unclear. A major clue to the mechanism, however, has come from the observation, now confirmed in numerous laboratories, that AD subjects with two *ε4* alleles have a significantly higher number and density of Aβ deposits in their brains than subjects with no *ε4* alleles, whereas subjects with one *ε4* allele generally fall in between [100–104]. In vitro biochemical studies have suggested that apo E-ε4 protein may be less effective in retarding the self-aggregation of Aβ into amyloid fibrils than is apo E-ε2 or apo E-ε3 [105]. Alternative hypotheses for the effect of apo E-ε4 in AD have been proposed. These include (1) the evidence that apo E-ε4 does not support neurite outgrowth in vitro and is less salutary for normal neuronal structure and function than is apo E-ε3 [106], and (2) that apo E-ε4 may permit *tau* to become dissociated from microtubules and participate in enhanced paired helical filament formation [107]. The latter hypothesis, however, is inconsistent with the observation that amyloid plaque density, not neurofibrillary tangle density, correlates with *APOE-ε4* gene dosage in AD patients [100,101].

In 1995, linkage analysis and positional cloning led to the identification of a gene on chromosome 14 that turned out to be responsible for a sizable fraction of early-onset FAD cases [108] (see Chapter 6). This novel gene, currently called *presenilin-1* (*PS1*), encodes a protein that appears to have six to eight transmembrane domains and thus resembles certain kinds of cell-surface receptors, channel proteins, or structural proteins of internal membrane vesicles. Shortly after *PS1* was cloned, a highly homologous second gene, termed *presenilin-2* (*PS2*), was identified as the cause of early-onset familial AD in at least two families, one of which was the renowned Volga-German pedigree that contains many members with presenile AD [109,110]. Both presenilin gene products are highly homologous to a *C. elegans* protein called *sel-12* that appears to function in the recognition of certain cells by other cells during development [111].

Based again on the observation that cells normally secrete Aβ, various *PS1* and *PS2* gene mutations, more than 45 of which have been identified, have been studied in transfected cells and, in some cases, in the plasma and skin fibroblast media of mutation-bearing patients. These analyses demonstrate a selective and statistically significant increase in the cellular production of the highly amyloidogenic $A\beta_{42}$ peptides [112–115]. Moreover, direct analysis of the brain tissue from several patients bearing a particular *PS1* missense mutation shows that there are many more $A\beta_{42}$-immunoreactive amyloid plaques in the brains of these subjects than in sporadic AD subjects with comparable overall neuropathologic severity [116]. The elevation of $A\beta_{42}$ has also been confirmed in the brains of transgenic mice harboring *PS1* mutations [113,114,117]. Because $A\beta_{42}$ has been shown to be the initially deposited species in DS and conventional AD [41–43], it is highly likely that the *PS1* and *PS2* mutant genes confer the AD phenotype by selectively enhancing $A\beta_{42}$ production throughout life. Precisely how they do this is under study, but recent data indicate that APP and presenilin proteins can form stable complexes that can be found in the ER and Golgi, and that mutant presenilins elevate $A\beta_{42}$ production in these compartments [118].

AMYLOID-RELATED MARKERS AS ANTIGENS IN THE DIAGNOSIS OF ALZHEIMER'S DISEASE

It has been widely assumed that few, if any, markers in biological fluids are useful in confirming a specific clinical diagnosis of AD. This assumption, however, is now changing with the advent of highly sensitive assays that can detect very small quantities of the proteins implicated in AD pathogenesis, such as Aβ and *tau*. Both of these molecules are now measurable in normal human CSF, and both the $A\beta_{42}$ and $A\beta_{40}$ peptides can be quantitated. Initial attempts to find diagnostically useful alterations of APP metabolites led to reports of possible decreases in alpha-APP_s or total Aβ levels. Further studies, however, have not clearly confirmed a diagnostic useful change in these analytes in most AD cases. On the other hand, a significant lowering of $A\beta_{42}$ concentrations in the CSF of AD compared to non-AD subjects has been reported [119], and additional studies from other laboratories have confirmed this finding [120]. Approximately one-half to two-thirds of subjects with clinically typical AD show a significant lowering of $A\beta_{42}$ levels. The reason soluble $A\beta_{42}$ falls in the CSF in AD is not entirely clear, but it is assumed to be due to the progressive aggregation and insolubilization of the peptide in the form of plaques and microvascular deposits. Thus, the total *soluble* pool of $A\beta_{42}$ in brain extracellular fluid is apparently reduced during progressive $A\beta_{42}$ aggregation and deposition, and this change is reflected in lower CSF levels. Correlation of CSF $A\beta_{42}$ levels with the extent of cerebral Aβ deposition seen postmortem, however, has not yet been accomplished.

Studies suggest that correlating low $A\beta_{42}$ levels with high *tau* levels in a CSF sample is more useful for supporting a presumptive clinical diagnosis of AD than measurement of either analyte alone [119,120]. A significant elevation of *tau* protein by itself has been reported in more than a dozen studies of AD patient CSF (see Chapter 11). Presumably, the rise reflects the release of excess *tau* protein from neurons undergoing neurofibrillary degeneration and its subsequent clearance into the CSF. Further clinical experience with combined $A\beta_{42}$/*tau* assay in the CSF will determine whether its sensitivity for supporting a diagnosis of AD can exceed the current range of 50–65% and whether its relatively high specificity (currently in the range of 85–90%) can be sustained or increased.

Another diagnostic assay that holds promise for the future is that of plasma Aβ levels. The very limited data published to date come from the laboratory of Younkin and colleagues [112] and suggest that a subset of "sporadic" AD patients, perhaps in the range of 15–20%, have elevated plasma $A\beta_{42}$ levels. These data need confirmation and extension in other studies before they can be interpreted. In the case of subjects bearing presenilin or *APP* mutations, elevated $A\beta_{42}$ in plasma has been documented during the symptomatic phase of the illness and even presymptomatically [112]. Although the elevations are presumably caused by the increased production of $A\beta_{42}$ by cells throughout the body in these familial forms of AD, it has generally been assumed that there is no increase in Aβ production per se in the large majority of conventional AD cases. This assumption could be incorrect; there may yet be other genetic defects discovered in late-onset patients that lead to altered APP metabolism in a way that enhances Aβ production, and this could be reflected in elevated plasma levels. Furthermore, genetically based alterations of Aβ clearance mechanisms, which are poorly understood, could also lead to intermittent or chronic elevation of $A\beta_{42}$ in plasma. It is generally assumed at present, however, that most cases of AD involve local accumulation of Aβ in brain tissue, without this being reflected in the peripheral circulation. Thus, the determination of plasma Aβ (both $A\beta_{42}$ and $A\beta_{40}$) may only prove to be helpful diagnostically in a subset of AD cases. Even so, this could still be meaningful, as there are other biological markers of disease states that are only altered in a subset of patients afflicted with the disease.

Detection of minor Aβ deposition in non-neural tissues such as skin has been observed by several investigators [12,121,122], but such deposits have also been seen in a percentage of normal aged subjects. Therefore, at least the current methods for detecting non-neural Aβ deposits do not show high diagnostic specificity, and further work will be needed to determine whether certain forms of non-neural deposits or certain tissue locations correlate in a specific way with the occurrence of excessive cerebral Aβ deposition and symptomatic AD.

PROGRESS IN UNDERSTANDING AMYLOID PRECURSOR PROTEIN AND BETA-AMYLOID METABOLISM IN FAMILIAL ALZHEIMER'S DISEASE POINTS TO A COMMON PATHOGENETIC MECHANISM FOR ALZHEIMER'S DISEASE

To summarize, four genes that are unequivocally associated with the development of AD have been identified to date, and linkage analyses of other families make it clear that additional genes may be responsible. Three of the known genes, *APP* on chromosome 21, *PS1* on chromosome 14, and *PS2* on chromosome 1, can be said to be causative of AD in the respective families in which mutations in these genes occur. In each of these three cases, there is now compelling evidence that the mechanism involves altered APP catabolism to generate increased amounts of Aβ peptides, particularly the highly amyloid-prone 42 residue form (see Table 10.2). In the case of *APOE* on chromosome 19, its *ε4* allele is a major genetic risk factor for the development of AD, perhaps contributing to the development of the disorder in some 30–40% of all AD patients. *APOE-ε4* is not causative, per se, because some patients with one or two *APOE-ε4* alleles show no signs of the clinical disease even late in life, and conversely, half or more of all AD patients do not bear an *ε4* allele.

The discussion thus far has emphasized the possible role of APP metabolism and the gradual accumulation of insoluble Aβ deposits in the pathogenesis of the disease. However, many other biochemical and structural abnormalities have also been observed in the brains of AD patients. Although at this moment it is impossible to arrange the heterogeneous molecular and cellular changes found at the end of the disease into a precise temporal sequence of progression, the outlines of a pathogenetic cascade are emerging. Insights into the temporal course of the disorder in its preclinical phase derive primarily from three sources: (1) the study of the accrual of AD-type brain changes in patients with trisomy 21 who have died of other causes at various ages from early childhood to late adulthood; (2) similar analyses of the development of AD-type lesions during the normal aging process in humans and other primates; and (3) studies of small animal models of AD, in particular transgenic mice that overexpress mutant forms of APP that cause early-onset AD in humans [68,69].

Analyses of DS brains have provided perhaps the most relevant information about how AD may progress. Numerous investigators have reported that the earliest AD-like morphologic change found in very young (e.g., 12- to 15-year-old) DS brains is the accrual of amorphous, largely nonfibrillar forms of Aβ deposits, the diffuse plaques. Some or many such deposits are found in limbic and association cortices (and often in striatum, cerebellum, and elsewhere) in trisomic individuals dying after age 12 years or so [43,123,124]. Importantly, many such diffuse plaques are also found in the brains of late middle-aged (≥60 years) or older people with normal cognition who have died of other causes. Diffuse plaques are also abundantly present in typical AD brains at the end of the patients' lives.

Light and electron microscopic studies of diffuse plaques in AD and in DS demonstrate very little or no structural alteration of axons, dendrites, astrocytes, and microglia within and immediately surrounding these amorphous Aβ deposits. This lack of cytopathology appears to correlate with a relative dearth of fibrillar amyloid in the diffuse deposits. As the brains of DS patients of increasing age are examined, fibrillar plaques with surrounding neuritic and glial dystrophy are detected increasingly after approximately age 30 years [43,124]. At approximately the same time, neurofibrillary tangles also begin to appear. Although such temporal correlation is imprecise in the relatively limited number of DS patients reported to date, a consensus has emerged that diffuse Aβ plaques clearly precede the other AD-type changes that occur in DS. The early accumulation of diffuse plaques is assumed to be caused by the elevated *APP* gene dosage and the consequent increase in APP expression and Aβ levels documented in these patients [125].

APP transgenic mice experience high brain expression of APP from birth and are thus analogous in some respects to patients with DS. However, the mice reported to date have the additional influence of an FAD-linked missense mutation flanking the Aβ region of *APP* [68,69]. Although such animals have high neuronal expression of the *APP* transgene as well as high levels of soluble Aβ within their brains from birth, they develop diffuse and compacted Aβ plaques resembling those of AD beginning at approximately 5–8 months (mice normally live approximately 2–3 years). During the next several months, the transgenic mice show increasing numbers of Aβ deposits, many of which are now Congo red–positive (suggesting that they contain fibrillar amyloid), and electron microscopy clearly reveals filamentous amyloid cores [126]. Moreover, after Aβ plaques develop, the mice show morphologically and immunocytochemically abnormal neurites intimately associated with the amyloid plaques [68,69,126]. Cytoskeletal proteins such as the microtubule-associated protein 2, the neurofilament protein, and even the *tau* protein can show abnormal immunoreactivity in these dystrophic neurites and in some nearby neuronal cell bodies [68,69,126, 127], although human-type neurofibrillary tangle formation has not been reported to date. A brisk reactive astrocytosis occurs within and around the Aβ plaques, and activated microglial cells occur near the centers of many of the plaques [126,127]. Confocal microscopy of the mouse plaques and immunostaining for synaptic proteins indicate that degeneration and loss of synapses is occurring, particularly in the vicinity of the plaques [68,126]. To what extent the progressive amyloidotic, neuritic, astrocytic, and microglial pathology observed in the transgenic mice leads to reproducible behavioral impairment is not yet clear [68,69], but the degree of neuropathologic abnormality makes this occurrence of behavioral impairment likely.

Although the rather rapid acquisition of AD-like lesions in the transgenic mice resulting from high expression of *APP* from birth cannot be considered an ideal model of AD, these mice clearly provide a highly useful and manipulable experimental model of the AD process. Additional morphologic and neurochemical analyses of various transgenic mice of increasing age will further establish how closely the animals' disease resembles the AD pathologic process and in which ways it differs.

Assuming that studies of disease progression in DS and in transgenic mice are relevant to the mechanism of AD, one may postulate that the gradual accrual of Aβ peptides in the form of first diffuse and then fibrillar plaques may result in local cellular effects that include activation of microglial cells, reactive astrocytosis, and alterations of nearby axons and dendrites (Figure 10.2). The extent to which these cytotoxic events derive from properties of the aggregated Aβ protein itself or from the numerous Aβ-associated proteins that have been detected in plaques is yet unclear. These associated polypeptides, some of which have been referred to as pathologic chaperones because of their putative role in enhancing the aggregation, deposition, and toxicity of Aβ, include the normally secreted proteins, $alpha_1$-antichymotrypsin, apo E, serum amyloid P component, basement membrane–associated HSPG, and various components of the classic complement pathway. Activated microglia, which become associated with maturing plaques, are capable of releasing a number of well-characterized cytokines that can, in turn, stimulate local astrocytes to release yet other proteins, including $alpha_1$-antichymotrypsin and apo E. The serum amyloid P protein, which is associated with all forms of central and peripheral amyloid deposits, is not expressed in the brain and thus must come to the plaque via passage across the blood-brain bar-

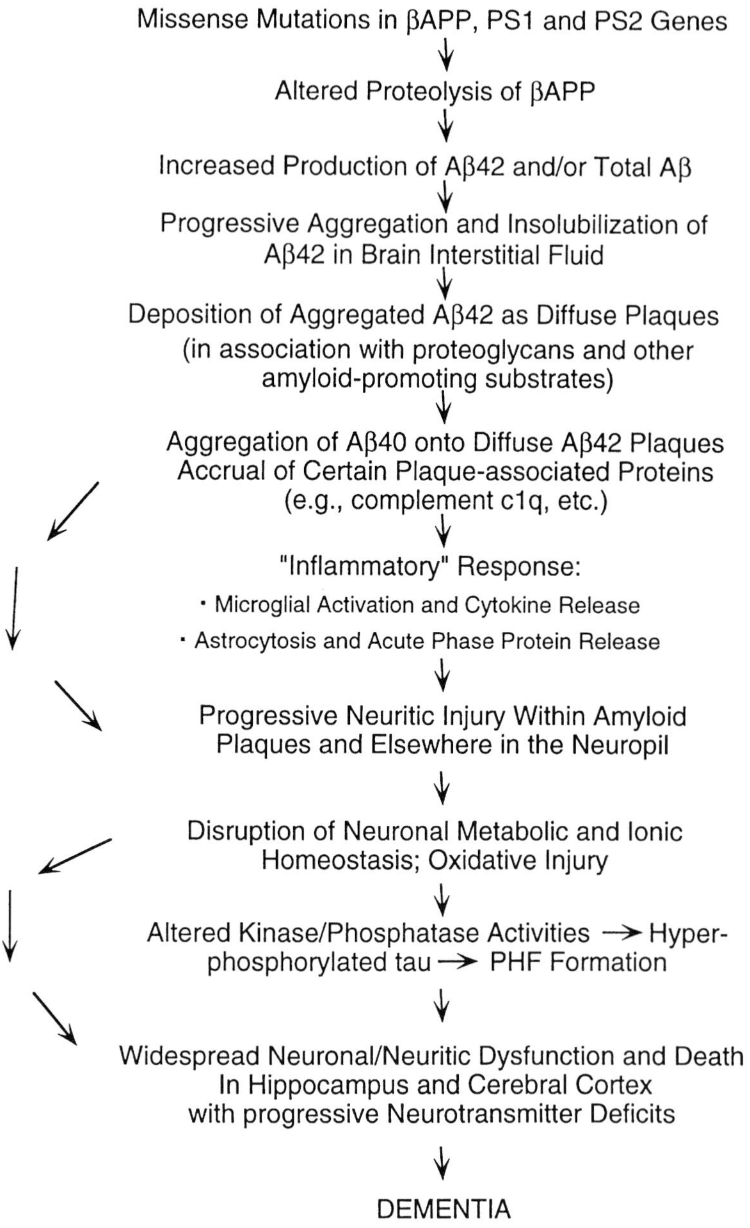

Figure 10.2 A hypothetical sequence of the molecular pathogenesis of familial forms of Alzheimer's disease. (Aβ = beta-amyloid; APP = amyloid precursor protein; PS = presenilin; PHF = paired helical filaments.)

rier [128]. To what extent other circulating molecules (including Aβ itself) breach the barrier to contribute to the pathologic changes is unclear.

It can be concluded that many proteins potentially capable of exerting biological activity on surrounding neurons and glia accumulate within the amyloid plaque. We thus face an embarrassment of riches in terms of potential effectors of AD cytopathology. At exactly which point axons and dendrites in the vicinity, as well as their cell bodies of origin, undergo an activation of kinases, deactivation of phosphatases, or both, that result in the hyperphosphorylation of *tau* proteins underlying tangle formation is difficult to say [129,130]. In all probability, the multiple molecular and cellular alterations found in AD cortex develop at varying rates but in reasonable proximity to each other. Biochemical and morphologic changes can presumably occur in cortical and subcortical neurons and their processes that are not directly associated with amyloid deposits. Subcortical neurons in regions such as the cholinergic nucleus basalis of Meynert, the noradrenergic locus ceruleus, and the serotoninergic median raphe nuclei, the axons of which all project into plaque-rich cortical areas, often show shrinkage, neurofibrillary tangle formation, and cell loss. The complex array of plaque-associated and non–plaque-associated cytopathology one observes by the end stage of AD may ultimately be very difficult to order into a precise sequence of temporal evolution.

The fact that neurofibrillary tangles arise in a variety of etiologically unrelated diseases in the absence of Aβ deposits suggests that they represent a response of neurons to a range of insults and are not specific for the amyloidotic process. The same may also be true of the *tau*-positive neuropil threads in the cortex, which can also occur in certain other degenerative diseases bearing tangles but lacking amyloid. On the other hand, the neuritic plaque, with its severe astrocytic and microglial cytopathology, is more specific for AD and DS. The observation that abundant Aβ deposits can be found in some cognitively normal elderly subjects, theoretically arguing against an important role for amyloid deposition, can be countered by pointing out that the vast majority of these deposits are of the diffuse type, lacking neuritic and glial alteration. This fact presumably explains why they are not associated with clinical dysfunction. A rough analogy could be made to clinically silent fatty streaks of cholesterol in the vasculature; as presumed precursors to clinically important atherosclerotic lesions, their abundance alone does not correlate precisely with disease symptoms, as is the case for diffuse plaques. On the other hand, the total number and density of diffuse and neuritic plaques are usually far higher in AD patients than in age-matched normal subjects [131], just as the extent of cholesterol-rich plaques of all types is often higher in patients with symptomatic atherosclerotic cardiovascular disease than in those free of symptoms.

The multiple neurotransmitter alterations in AD brain tissues that began to be uncovered in the late 1970s are now known to include several monoaminergic and neuropeptide deficiencies beyond the loss of cholinergic function that was first described. In the context of the complex, multicellular pathologic cascade discussed above, it comes as no surprise that AD does not affect a single neurotransmitter system. Indeed, morphologic studies have demonstrated that any one amyloid-bearing neuritic plaque may contain altered neurites derived from neurons of multiple neurotransmitter specificities. These considerations provide one explanation for the general lack of robust symptomatic improvement in patients given cholinergic replacement therapy such as acetylcholinesterase inhibitors.

Based on the foregoing reasoning, one can provide a flowchart that describes a hypothetical sequence of changes underlying the development of clinical dementia in familial forms of AD (see Figure 10.2). Clearly, this kind of scheme is speculative, but a number of the elements of the temporal sequence can clearly be justified on the basis of the published information reviewed in this chapter. Whether there are forms of AD in which the cerebral accumulation of Aβ and the gradual formation of particulate Aβ deposits (diffuse plaques) followed by filamentous amyloid deposits (neuritic plaques) are merely late secondary or tertiary events remains to be seen. No compelling evidence for such a scenario has arisen.

EVIDENCE OF A CENTRAL ROLE FOR PROGRESSIVE BETA-AMYLOID ACCUMULATION IN ALZHEIMER'S DISEASE PREDICTS SEVERAL NOVEL THERAPEUTIC STRATEGIES

A truism of biomedical science is that the development of therapies expected to slow or arrest the progression of a disease requires as detailed an understanding of the molecular pathogenesis as possible. The tools for screening a wide array of compounds for possible efficacy in AD are already in hand and include cell culture systems and the transgenic mouse models. Moreover, there is an array of potential therapeutic targets. Among these, the inhibition of Aβ secretion from neuronal and non-neuronal cells is being actively pursued. One way this can be accomplished is by designing specific inhibitors of the beta- and gamma-secretases after these proteases are definitively identified and cloned. There may be other ways of lowering Aβ production, however, that do not involve direct inhibition of these enzymes. In any event, screening of cells that continuously secrete Aβ is well under way and should lead to the identification of compounds that act by a variety of mechanisms. One specific question regarding this approach relates to whether chronic treatment with cholinergic agonists will result in increased processing of APP molecules by the alpha-secretase pathway and thus significantly diminished production of Aβ [30,132]. Such a possibility can initially be examined in transgenic mice, in which both cerebral and CSF Aβ levels can be measured, but it must then be confirmed in treated patients by measuring CSF Aβ levels. A variety of other first messengers may turn out to be at least as effective as cholinergic agonists in shifting APP processing from the beta- to the alpha-secretase pathway.

A therapeutic approach that seems particularly attractive is to attempt to slow the aggregation of the secreted Aβ peptide into its fibrillar, putatively cytotoxic form. In vitro studies indicate that certain small molecules, including the amyloid-binding dye Congo red, can retard the aggregation of synthetic Aβ peptides into high-molecular-weight aggregates. Compounds that interfere with Aβ assembly into amyloid fibrils could act in the extracellular space of the brain and thus avoid interference with the metabolism of APP and other molecules inside cells. Full-length APP and its various metabolites, including APP_s and perhaps even Aβ, have normal functions, whereas the aggregated forms of Aβ that compose plaques are believed to represent solely pathologic moieties. Thus, interfering with Aβ aggregation, if it can be done in a selective fashion, could avoid effects on the metabolism of APP and other molecules. The transgenic mouse models, which have fibrillar amyloid plaques, should be a reasonable system in which to evaluate the efficacy and safety of such compounds.

Yet another therapeutic approach based on the growing understanding of presymptomatic events in AD is the use of anti-inflammatory drugs that could interfere in part with the microglial activation, cytokine release, and acute phase response that occur in maturing amyloid plaques. Epidemiologic evidence suggests that individuals who have been on nonsteroidal anti-inflammatory drugs may have a lower likelihood of developing the pathologic and clinical features of AD. One may assume that the inflammatory process that appears around amyloid plaques is sufficiently distinct from peripheral forms of inflammation that it will require specialized anti-inflammatory compounds, which could again be identified and characterized in transgenic mice.

The devastating impairment of higher cortical functions that characterizes AD must ultimately be attributed to profound neuronal dysfunction and degeneration. Therefore, a variety of neuroprotective strategies can be envisioned in this disorder. One relatively specific approach would be to attempt to design compounds that interfere with any altered signal transduction pathways that are proven to mediate the effects of extracellular amyloid filaments and their closely associated molecules on neuronal homeostasis. No single cell-surface receptor for Aβ in its monomeric or aggregated form, however, has yet been found to fully mediate the toxicity. Instead, present evidence predicts that aggregated Aβ, by chronically altering the milieu of the neuronal surface, may trigger dysfunction of several or many cell-surface molecules and subsequent inappropriate activation of more than one second messenger system. Agents that could hypothetically interfere with such a process could include compounds that coat the amyloid aggregates in a way that makes them "invisible" to the cell and molecules that inhibit a downstream effector pathway inside the neuron.

In addition to such approaches directed at the specific neurotoxic cascade putatively induced by amyloid, therapies could be applied that might be equally applicable to AD and to other neurodegenerative disorders. Such strategies might include the use of inhibitors of excitotoxicity, agents that block cellular calcium entry, free radical scavengers, and other antioxidant treatments. Evidence is mounting from in vitro studies that aggregated Aβ induces multiple features of oxidative injury in cultured neurons. Neurotrophic therapy is another general approach to retarding neurodegeneration that might also be applicable to AD. Besides the considerable technical hurdles that must be overcome to chronically deliver neurotrophic peptides to the appropriate sites in the brains of elderly subjects, however, at least two theoretical concerns arise. First, some indirect evidence from tissue culture studies suggests that nerve growth factor treatment can potentially augment APP expression and perhaps its turnover into Aβ, something that would presumably not be desirable on a long-term basis in AD patients. Second, evidence exists that an apparent trophic or sprouting response already occurs in many cortical and limbic neurons [133]. This observation suggests that upregulation of trophic influences may actually be contributing in part to neuronal dysfunction in the disease.

It has been assumed that it will take a long time to develop compounds that affect any of the therapeutic targets summarized above. But the rate of progress in elucidating the fundamental mechanism of the disease and, in particular, the pathogenic role of Aβ deposition is sufficiently high to expect more refined therapeutic targets to emerge in the next 2–4 years. It may be, for example, that beta- and gamma-secretase enzymes will be identified, cloned, and then characterized as to possible mechanisms of inhibition. Moreover, prototype inhibitors of the cellular production of Aβ or its subsequent fibrillogenesis could emerge in just the next few years. In any event, a number of therapies advocated for neurodegenerative diseases in general, such as antioxidants and neuronal calcium channel blockers, are already advancing in clinical trials in AD patients.

The combined power of genetics, molecular biology, and biochemistry have produced remarkable advances in our understanding of the causes and mechanisms of AD. Given the great prevalence of the disease, the personal tragedy it represents for the patients and their families, and the enormous societal costs, one can safely predict that even more intensive effort on the part of academic and pharmaceutical laboratories will be brought to bear on the problem in the months and years ahead. The outcome could be that AD becomes one of the early examples of the amelioration or even prevention of a major, fatal brain disorder based on a thorough understanding of its molecular mechanism.

REFERENCES

1. Kang J, Lemaire HG, Unterbeck A, et al. The precursor of Alzheimer's disease amyloid A4 protein resembles a cell-surface receptor. Nature 1987;325:733–736.
2. Goldgaber D, Lerman MI, McBridge OW, et al. Characterization and chromosomal localization of a cDNA encoding brain amyloid of Alzheimer's disease. Science 1987;235:877–880.
3. Tanzi RE, Gusella JF, Watkins PC, et al. Amyloid beta protein gene: cDNA, mRNA distribution, and genetic linkage near the Alzheimer locus. Science 1987;235:880–884.
4. Robakis NK, Ramakrishna N, Wolfe G, Wisniewski HM. Molecular cloning and characterization of a cDNA encoding the cerebrovascular and the neuritic plaque amyloid peptides. Proc Natl Acad Sci U S A 1987;84:4190–4194.
5. Glenner GG, Wong CW. Alzheimer's disease and Down's syndrome: sharing of a unique cerebrovascular amyloid fibril protein. Biochem Biophys Res Commun 1984;122:1131–1135.
6. Masters CL, Simms G, Weinman NA, et al. Amyloid plaque core protein in Alzheimer disease and Down syndrome. Proc Natl Acad Sci U S A 1985;82:4245–4249.
7. Selkoe DJ, Abraham CR, Podlisny MB, Duffy LK. Isolation of low-molecular-weight proteins from amyloid plaque fibers in Alzheimer's disease. J Neurochemistry 1986;146:1820–1834.
8. Gorevic P, Goni F, Pons-Estel B, et al. Isolation and partial characterization of neurofibrillary tangles and amyloid plaque cores in Alzheimer's disease: immunohistological studies. J Neuropathol Exp Neurol 1986;45:647–664.
9. van Nostrand WE, Wagner SL, Suzuki M, et al. Protease nexin-II, a potent anti-chymotrypsin, shows identity to amyloid beta-protein precursor. Nature 1989;341:546–549.
10. Sinha S, Dovey HF, Seubert P, et al. The protease inhibitory properties of the Alzheimer's beta-amyloid precursor protein. J Biol Chem 1990;265:8983–8985.
11. Smith RP, Higuchi DA, Broze GJ Jr. Platelet coagulation factor XIa-inhibitor, a form of Alzheimer amyloid precursor protein. Science 1990;248:1126–1128.
12. Joachim CL, Mori H, Selkoe DJ. Amyloid beta-protein deposition in tissues other than brain in Alzheimer's disease. Nature 1989;341:226–230.
13. Podlisny MB, Tolan D, Selkoe DJ. Homology of the amyloid beta protein precursor in monkey and human supports a primate model for beta amyloidosis in Alzheimer's disease. Am J Pathol 1991;138:1423–1435.
14. Rosen DR, Martin-Morris L, Luo L, White K. A Drosophila gene encoding a protein resembling the human beta-amyloid precursor protein. Proc Natl Acad Sci U S A 1989;86:2478–2482.
15. Daigle I, Li C. *Apl–1*, a *C. elegans* gene encoding a protein related to the human beta-amyloid protein precursor. Proc Natl Acad Sci U S A 1993;90:12045–12049.

16. Zheng H, Jiang M, Trumbauer ME, et al. Beta-amyloid precursor protein-deficient mice show reactive gliosis and decreased locomotor activity. Cell 1995;81:525–531.
17. Wasco W, Bupp K, Magendantz M, et al. Identification of a mouse brain cDNA that encodes a protein related to the Alzheimer disease-associated amyloid beta-protein precursor. Proc Natl Acad Sci U S A 1992;89:10758–10762.
18. Slunt HH, Thinakaran G, Von Koch C, et al. Expression of a ubiquitous, cross-reactive homologue of the mouse beta-amyloid precursor protein (APP). J Biol Chem 1994;269:2637–2644.
19. Greenberg S, Koo EH, Selkoe DJ, et al. Secreted beta-amyloid precursor protein stimulates mitogen-activated protein kinase and enhances *tau* phosphorylation. Proc Natl Acad Sci U S A 1994;91: 7104–7108.
20. Saitoh T, Sundsmo M, Roch JM, et al. Secreted form of amyloid beta-protein precursor is involved in the growth regulation of fibroblasts. Cell 1989;58:615–622.
21. Mattson M, Cheng B, Culwell A, et al. Evidence for excitoprotective and intraneuronal calcium-regulating roles for secreted forms of the beta-amyloid precursor protein. Neuron 1993;10:243–254.
22. Qiu WQ, Ferreira A, Miller C, et al. Cell-surface beta-amyloid precursor protein stimulates neurite outgrowth of hippocampal neurons in an isoform-dependent manner. J Neuroscience 1995;15:2157–2167.
23. Schubert D, Jin LW, Saitoh T, Cole G. The regulation of amyloid beta-protein precursor secretion and its modulatory role in cell adhesion. Neuron 1989;3:689–694.
24. Small DH, Nurcombe V, Reed G, et al. A heparin-binding domain in the amyloid protein precursor of Alzheimer's disease is involved in the regulation of neurite outgrowth. J Neuroscience 1994;14: 2117–2127.
25. Weidemann A, Konig G, Bunke D, et al. Identification, biogenesis and localization of precursors of Alzheimer's disease A4 amyloid protein. Cell 1989;57:115–126.
26. Oltersdorf T, Ward PJ, Henriksson T, et al. The Alzheimer amyloid precursor protein. Identification of a stable intermediate in the biosynthetic/degradative pathway. J Biol Chem 1990;265:4492–4497.
27. Hung AY, Selkoe DJ. Selective ectodomain phosphorylation and regulated cleavage of beta-amyloid precursor protein. EMBO J 1994;13:534–542.
28. Selkoe DJ, Podlisny MB, Joachim CL, et al. Beta-amyloid precursor protein of Alzheimer disease occurs as 110–135 kilodalton membrane-associated proteins in neural and nonneural tissues. Proc Natl Acad Sci U S A 1988;85:7341–7345.
29. Esch FS, Keim PS, Beattie EC, et al. Cleavage of amyloid beta-peptide during constitutive processing of its precursor. Science 1990;248:1122–1124.
30. Nitsch RM, Slack BE, Wurtman RJ, Growdon JH. Release of Alzheimer amyloid precursor derivatives stimulated by activation of muscarinic acetylcholine receptors. Science 1992;258:304–307.
31. Buxbaum JD, Oishi M, Chen HI, et al. Cholinergic agonists and interleukin 1 regulate processing and secretion of the Alzheimer b/A4 amyloid precursor protein. Proc Natl Acad Sci U S A 1992;89:3055–3059.
32. Nitsch RM, Farber SA, Growdon JH, Wurtman RJ. Release of amyloid beta-protein precursor derivatives by electrical depolarization of rat hippocampal slices. Proc Natl Acad Sci U S A 1993;90:5191–5193.
33. Haass C, Schlossmacher MG, Hung AY, et al. Amyloid beta-peptide is produced by cultured cells during normal metabolism. Nature 1992;359:322–325.
34. Seubert P, Vigo-Pelfrey C, Esch F, et al. Isolation and quantitation of soluble Alzheimer's beta-peptide from biological fluids. Nature 1992;359:325–327.
35. Shoji M, Golde TE, Ghiso J, et al. Production of the Alzheimer amyloid beta protein by normal proteolytic processing. Science 1992;258:126–129.
36. Selkoe DJ. Physiological production of the amyloid beta-protein and the mechanism of Alzheimer's disease. Trends Neurosci 1993;16:403–409.
37. Haass C, Hung AY, Schlossmacher MG, et al. Beta-amyloid peptide and a 3-kDa fragment are derived by distinct cellular mechanisms. J Biol Chem 1993;268:3021–3024.
38. Golde TE, Estus S, Younkin LH, et al. Processing of the amyloid protein precursor to potentially amyloidogenic carboxyl-terminal derivatives. Science 1992;255:728–730.
39. Haass C, Koo EH, Mellon A, et al. Targeting of cell-surface beta-amyloid precursor protein to lysosomes: alternative processing into amyloid-bearing fragments. Nature 1992;357:500–503.
40. Saido TC, Iwatsubo T, Mann DMA, et al. Dominant and differential deposition of distinct beta-amyloid peptide species, A beta N3(pE) in senile plaques. Neuron 1995;14:457–466.
41. Iwatsubo T, Odaka A, Suzuki N, et al. Visualization of A beta 42(43) and Aβ40 in senile plaques with end-specific Aβ monoclonals: evidence that an initially deposited species is Aβ42(43). Neuron 1995; 13:45–53.
42. Iwatsubo T, Mann DM, Odaka A, et al. Amyloid beta protein (A beta) deposition: A beta 42(43) precedes A beta 40 in Down syndrome. Ann Neurol 1995;37:294–299.

43. Lemere CA, Blustzjan JK, Yamaguchi H, et al. Sequence of deposition of heterogeneous amyloid beta-peptides and Apo E in Down syndrome: implications for initial events in amyloid plaque formation. Neurobiol Dis 1996;3:16–32.
44. Hilbich C, Kisters-Woike B, Reed J, et al. Aggregation and secondary structure of synthetic amyloid beta A4 peptides of Alzheimer's disease. J Mol Biol 1991;218:149–163.
45. Jarrett JT, Berger EP, Lansbury PT Jr. The carboxy terminus of the beta amyloid protein is critical for the seeding of amyloid formation: implications for the pathogenesis of Alzheimer's disease. Biochemistry 1993;32:4693–4697.
46. Citron M, Diehl TS, Gordon G, et al. Evidence that Aβ42 and Aβ40 are generated from the beta-amyloid precursor protein by different protease activities. Proc Natl Acad Sci U S A 1996;93: 13170–13175.
47. Klafki H-W, Abramowski D, Swoboda R, et al. The carboxyl termini of beta-amyloid peptides 1–40 and 1–42 are generated by distinct gamma-secretase activities. J Biol Chem 1996;271:28655–28659.
48. Koo EH, Squazzo S. Evidence that production and release of amyloid beta-protein involves the endocytic pathway. J Biol Chem 1994;269:17386–17389.
49. Perez RG, Squazzo SL, Koo EH. Enhanced release of amyloid beta-protein from Codon 670/671 "Swedish" mutant beta-amyloid precursor protein occurs in both secretory and endocytic pathways. J Biol Chem 1996;271:9100–9107.
50. Yamazaki T, Koo EH, Selkoe DJ. Trafficking of cell-surface amyloid beta-protein precursor. II. Endocytosis, recycling and lysosomal targeting detected by immunolocalization. J Cell Sci 1996;109: 999–1008.
51. Yamazaki T, Koo EH, Selkoe DJ. Multiple fates of cell-surface amyloid beta-protein precursor: secretion, endocytosis, recycling and lysosomal targeting. J Cell Sci 1996;109:999–1008.
52. Wild-Bode C, Yamazaki T, Capell A, et al. Intracellular generation and accumulation of amyloid beta-peptide terminating at amino acid 42. J Biol Chem 1997;272:16085–16088.
53. Xia W, Zhang J, Ostaszewski B, et al. Mutant presenilins increase the generation of the 42-residue amyloid beta-protein in the Golgi apparatus. J Biol Chem. (In press.)
54. Haass C, Lemere CA, Capell A, et al. Swedish mutation causes early-onset AD by beta-secretase cleavage within the secretory pathway. Nat Med 1995;1:1291–1296.
55. Koo EH, Sisodia SS, Archer DA, et al. Precursor of amyloid protein in Alzheimer's disease undergoes fast anterograde axonal transport. Proc Natl Acad Sci U S A 1990;87:1561–1565.
56. Yamazaki T, Selkoe DJ, Koo EH. Trafficking of cell surface beta-amyloid precursor protein: retrograde and transcytotic transport in cultured neurons. J Cell Biol 1995;129:431–442.
57. Ikin AF, Annaert WG, Takei K, et al. Alzheimer amyloid protein precursor is localized in nerve terminal preparations to Rab5-containing vesicular organelles distinct from those implicated in the synaptic vesicle pathway. J Biol Chem 1996;271:31783–31786.
58. Wertkin AM, Turner RS, Pleasure SJ, et al. Human neurons derived from a teratocarcinoma cell line express solely the 695-amino acid amyloid precursor protein and produce intracellular beta-amyloid or A4 peptides. Proc Natl Acad Sci U S A 1993;90:9513–9517.
59. Knauer MF, Soreghan B, Burdick D, et al. Intracellular accumulation and resistance to degradation of the Alzheimer amyloid A4/β protein. Proc Natl Acad Sci U S A 1992;89:7437–7441.
60. Kurochkin IV, Goto S. Alzheimer's beta-amyloid peptide specifically interacts with and is degraded by insulin degrading enzyme. FEBS Lett 1994;345:33–37.
61. McDermott JR, Gibson AM. Degradation of Alzheimer's beta-amyloid protein by human and rat brain peptidases: involvement of insulin-degrading enzyme. Biochem Res 1997;22:49–56.
62. Qiu WQ, Ye Z, Kholodenko D, et al. Degradation of amyloid beta-protein by a metalloprotease secreted by microglia and other neural and non-neural cells. J Biol Chem 1997;272:6641–6646.
63. Roher AE, Lowenson JD, Clarke S, et al. Structural alterations in the peptide backbone of beta-amyloid core protein may account for its deposition and stability in Alzheimer's disease. J Biol Chem 1993; 268:3072–3083.
64. Frucht SJ, Koo EH. Beta-amyloid protein is higher in Alzheimer's disease brains: description of a quantitative biochemical assay. J Neuropathol Exp Neurol 1993;52:640–647.
65. Yamaguchi H, Nakazato Y, Hirai S, Shoji M. Immunoelectron microscopic localization of amyloid beta-protein in the diffuse plaques of Alzheimer-type dementia. Brain Res 1990;508:320–324.
66. Harper JD, Wong SS, Lieber CM, Lansbury PT Jr. Observation of metastable Aβ amyloid protofibrils by atomic force microscopy. Chem Biol 1997;4:119–125.
67. Kuo YM, Emmerling MR, Vigo-Pelfrey C, et al. Water-soluble A beta (N-40, N-42) oligomers in normal and Alzheimer disease brains. J Biol Chem 1996;271:4077–4081.
68. Games D, Adams D, Alessandrini R, et al. Alzheimer-type neuropathology in transgenic mice overexpressing V717F beta-amyloid precursor protein. Nature 1995;373:523–527.

69. Hsiao K, Chapman P, Nilsen S, et al. Correlative memory deficits, Aβ elevation, and amyloid plaques in transgenic mice. Science 1996;274:99–102.
70. Johnson-Wood K, Lee M, Motter R, et al. Amyloid precursor protein processing and Aβ42 deposition in a transgenic mouse model of Alzheimer disease. Proc Natl Acad Sci U S A 1997;94: 1550–1555.
71. Snow AD, Mar H, Nochlin D, et al. The presence of heparan sulfate proteoglycans in the neuritic plaques and congophilic angiopathy in Alzheimer's disease. Am J Pathol 1988;133:456–463.
72. Snow AD, Mar H, Nochlin D, et al. Early accumulation of heparan sulfate in neurons and in the beta-amyloid protein containing lesions of Alzheimer's disease and Down's syndrome. Am J Pathol 1990; 137:1253–1270.
73. Maggio JE, Stimson ER, Ghilardi JR, et al. Reversible in vitro growth of Alzheimer's disease beta-amyloid plaques by deposition of labeled amyloid peptide. Proc Natl Acad Sci U S A 1992;89: 5462–5466.
74. Esler WP, Stimson ER, Ghilardi JR, et al. In vitro growth of Alzheimer's disease beta-amyloid plaques displays first-order kinetics. Biochemistry 1996;35:749–757.
75. Yamaguchi H, Yamazaki T, Lemere CA, et al. Beta amyloid is focally deposited within the outer basement membrane in the amyloid angiopathy of Alzheimer's disease. Am J Pathol 1992;141:249–259.
76. Miyakawa T, Shimoji A, Kuramoto R, Higuchi Y. The relationship between senile plaques and cerebral blood vessels in Alzheimer's disease and senile dementia: morphological mechanism of senile plaque production. Virchows Arch 1982;40:121–129.
77. Abraham CR, Selkoe DJ, Potter H. Immunochemical identification of the serine protease inhibitor, A1-antichymotrypsin in the brain amyloid deposits of Alzheimer's disease. Cell 1988;52:487–501.
78. Kalaria RN, Golde TE, Cohen ML, Younkin SG. Serum amyloid P in Alzheimer's disease. Ann N Y Acad Sci 1991;640:145–148.
79. Eikelenboom P, Stam FC. Immunoglobulins and complement factors in senile plaques: an immunoperoxidase study. Acta Neuropathol 1982;57:239–242.
80. Rogers J, Cooper NR, Websger S, et al. Complement activation by beta-amyloid in Alzheimer disease. Proc Natl Acad Sci U S A 1992;89:10016–10020.
81. Namba Y, Tomonaga M, Kawasaki H, et al. Apolipoprotein E immunoreactivity in cerebral deposits and neurofibrillary tangles in Alzheimer's disease and kuru plaque amyloid in Creutzfeldt-Jacob disease. Brain Res 1991;541:163–166.
82. Wisniewski T, Frangione B. Apolipoprotein E: a pathological chaperone protein in patients with cerebral and systemic amyloid. Neurosci Lett 1992;135:235–238.
83. Whitson JS, Selkoe DJ, Cotman CW. Amyloid beta protein enhances the survival of hippocampal neurons in vitro. Science 1989;243:1488–1490.
84. Yankner BA, Duffy LK, Kirschner DA. Neurotrophic and neurotoxic effects of amyloid beta protein: reversal by tachykinin neuropeptides. Science 1990;250:279–282.
85. Koo EH, Park L, Selkoe DJ. Amyloid beta-protein as a substrate interacts with extracellular matrix to promote neurite outgrowth. Proc Natl Acad Sci U S A 1993;90:4748–4752.
86. Pike CJ, Burdick D, Walencewicz AJ, et al. Neurodegeneration induced by beta-amyloid peptides in vitro: the role of peptide assembly state. J Neuroscience 1993;13:1676–1687.
87. Lorenzo A, Yankner B. Beta-amyloid neurotoxicity requires fibril formation and is inhibited by Congo red. Proc Natl Acad Sci U S A 1994;91:12243–12247.
88. Mattson MP, Cheng B, Davis D, et al. Beta-amyloid peptides destabilize calcium homeostasis and render human cortical neurons vulnerable to excitotoxicity. J Neuroscience 1992;12:379–389.
89. Hensley K, Carney JM, Mattson MP, et al. A model for beta-amyloid aggregation and neurotoxicity based on free radical generation by the peptide: relevance to Alzheimer disease. Proc Natl Acad Sci U S A 1994;91:3270–3274.
90. Behl C, Davis JB, Lesley R, Schubert D. Hydrogen peroxide mediates amyloid beta protein toxicity. Cell 1994;77:817–827.
91. El Khoury J, Hickman SE, Thomas CA, et al. Scavenger receptor-mediated adhesion of microglia to β-amyloid fibrils. Nature 1996;382:716–719.
92. Paresce DM, Ghosh RN, Maxfield FR. Microglial cells internalize aggregates of the Alzheimer's disease amyloid β-protein via a scavenger receptor. Neuron 1996;17:553–565.
93. Yan SD, Chen X, Fu J, et al. RAGE and amyloid-β peptide neurotoxicity in Alzheimer's disease. Nature 1996;382:685–691.
94. St George-Hyslop PH, Tanzi RE, Polinsky RJ, et al. The genetic defect causing familial Alzheimer's disease maps to chromosome 21. Science 1987;235:885–889.
95. Goate A, Chartier-Harlin MC, Mullan M, et al. Segregation of a missense mutation in the amyloid precursor protein gene with familial Alzheimer's disease. Nature 1991;349:704–706.

96. Selkoe DJ. Alzheimer's disease: genotypes, phenotypes, and treatments. Science 1997;275:630–631.
97. Strittmatter WJ, Saunders AM, Schmechel D, et al. Apolipoprotein E: high-avidity binding to beta-amyloid and increased frequency of type 4 allele in late-onset familial Alzheimer disease. Proc Natl Acad Sci U S A 1993;90:1977–1981.
98. Saunders AM, Strittmatter WJ, Schmechel D, et al. Association of apolipoprotein E allele epsilon 4 with late-onset familial and sporadic Alzheimer's disease. Neurology 1993;43:1467–1472.
99. Corder EH, Saunders AM, Risch NJ, et al. Protective effect of apolipoprotein E type 2 allele for late onset Alzheimer's disease. Nat Genet 1994;7:180–184.
100. Schmechel DE, Saunders AM, Strittmatter WJ, et al. Increased amyloid beta-peptide deposition in cerebral cortex as a consequence of apolipoprotein E gentoype in late-onset Alzheimer disease. Proc Natl Acad Sci U S A 1993;90:9649–9653.
101. Rebeck GW, Reiter JS, Strickland DK, Hyman BT. Apolipoprotein E in sporadic Alzheimer's disease: allelic variation and receptor interactions. Neuron 1993;11:575–580.
102. Hyman BT, West HL, Rebeck GW, et al. Quantitative analysis of senile plaques in Alzheimer's disease: observation of log–normal size distribution and molecular epidemiology of differences associated with apolipoprotein E genotype and trisomy 21 (Down syndrome). Proc Natl Acad Sci U S A 1995;92:3586–3590.
103. Polvikoski T, Sulkava R, Haltia M, et al. Apolipoprotein E, dementia, and cortical deposition of β-amyloid protein. N Engl J Med 1995;333:1242–1247.
104. Greenberg SM, Rebeck GW, Vonsattel JPG, et al. Apolipoprotein E ε4 and cerebral hemorrhage associated with amyloid angiopathy. Ann Neurol 1995;38:254–259.
105. Evans KC, Berger EP, Cho CG, et al. Apolipoprotein E is a kinetic but not a thermodynamic inhibitor of amyloid formation: implications for the pathogenesis and treatment of Alzheimer disease. Proc Natl Acad Sci U S A 1995;92:763–767.
106. Nathan BP, Bellosta S, Sanan DA, et al. Differential effects of apolipoprotein E3 and E4 on neuronal growth in vitro. Science 1994;264:850–852.
107. Roses AD, Einstein G, Gilbert J, et al. Morphological, biochemical, and genetic support for an apolipoprotein E effect on microtubular metabolism. Ann N Y Acad Sci 1996;777:146–157.
108. Sherrington R, Rogaev EI, Liang Y, et al. Cloning of a novel gene bearing missense mutations in early onset familial Alzheimer disease. Nature 1995;375:754–760.
109. Levy-Lahad E, Wasco W, Poorkaj P, et al. Candidate gene for the chromosome 1 familial Alzheimer's disease locus. Science 1995;269:973–977.
110. Rogaev EI, Sherrington R, Rogaeva EA, et al. Familial Alzheimer's disease in kindreds with missense mutations in a gene on chromosome 1 related to the Alzheimer's disease type 3 gene. Nature 1995; 376:775–778.
111. Levitan D, Greenwald I. Facilitation of lin-12–mediated signalling by *sel-12*, a *Caenorhabditis elegans* S182 Alzheimer's disease gene. Nature 1995;377:351–354.
112. Scheuner D, Eckman C, Jensen M, et al. Secreted amyloid β-protein similar to that in the senile plaques of Alzheimer's disease is increased in vivo by the presenilin 1 and 2 and APP mutations linked to familial Alzheimer's disease. Nature Med 1996;2:864–870.
113. Borchelt DR, Thinakaran G, Eckman CB, et al. Familial Alzheimer's disease–linked presenilin 1 variants elevate Aβ1–42/1–40 ratio in vitro and in vivo. Neuron 1996;17:1005–1013.
114. Citron M, Westaway D, Xia W, et al. Mutant presenilins of Alzheimer's disease increase production of 42-residue amyloid β-protein in both transfected cells and transgenic mice. Nature Med 1997;3:67–72.
115. Xia W, Zhang J, Kholodenko D, et al. Enhanced production and oligomerization of the 42-residue amyloid β-protein by Chinese hamster ovary cells stably expressing mutant presenilins. J Biol Chem 1997;272:7977–7982.
116. Lemere CA, Lopera F, Kosik KS, et al. The E280A presenilin 1 Alzheimer mutation produces increased Aβ42 deposition and severe cerebellar pathology. Nature Med 1996;2:1146–1148.
117. Duff K, Eckman C, Zehr C, et al. Increased amyloid Aβ42(43) in brains of mice expressing mutant presenilin 1. Nature 1996;383:710–713.
118. Xia W, Zhang J, Koo EH, Selkoe DJ. Interaction between amyloid precursor protein and presenilins in mammalian cells: implications for the pathogenesis of Alzheimer disease. Proc Natl Acad Sci U S A 1997;94:8208–8213.
119. Motter R, Vigo-Pelfrey C, Kholodenko D, et al. Reduction of beta-amyloid peptide 42 in the cerebrospinal fluid of patients with Alzheimer's disease. Ann Neurol 1995;38:643–648.
120. Kanai M, Matsubara E, Kawarabayashi T, et al. CSF tau and Aß1–40/42 in Alzheimer's disease. Neurobiol Dis 1996;17:S184.
121. Soininen H, Syrjanen S, Heinonen O, et al. Amyloid β-protein deposition in skin of patients with dementia [letter]. Lancet 1992;339:245.

122. Lemere C, Yamaguchi H, Joachim C, Selkoe D. Amyloid β-protein immunoreactivity in spleen, lymph node and other non-neural tissues using a new AbP antiserum. Neurosci Abstr 1991;17:1443.
123. Giaccone G, Tagliavini F, Linoli G, et al. Down patients: extracellular preamyloid deposits precede neuritic degeneration and senile plaques. Neurosci Lett 1989;97:232–238.
124. Mann DMA. Cerebral amyloidosis, aging and Alzheimer's disease: a contribution from studies on Down's syndrome. Neurobiol Aging 1989;10:397–399.
125. Querfurth HW, Wijsman EM, St. George-Hyslop PH, Selkoe DJ. βAPP mRNA transcription is increased in cultured fibroblasts from the familial Alzheimer's disease–1 family. Mol Brain Res 1995;28:319–337.
126. Masliah E, Sisk A, Mallory M, et al. Comparison of neurodegenerative pathology in transgenic mice overexpressing V717F β-amyloid precursor protein and Alzheimer's disease. J Neurosci 1996; 16:5795–5811.
127. Games D, Carr T, Guido T, et al. Progression of Alzheimer-type neuropathology in PDAPP717$_{V \to F}$ transgenic mice. Soc Neurosci Abstr 1995;21:258.
128. Kalaria RN. Serum amyloid P and related molecules associated with the acute-phase response in Alzheimer's disease. Res Immunol 1992;143:637–641.
129. Goedert M, Trojanowski JQ, Lee VMY. The Neurofibrillary Pathology of Alzheimer's Disease. In SB Prusiner (ed), The Molecular and Genetic Basis of Neurological Disease (2nd ed). Boston: Butterworth–Heinemann, 1996;613.
130. Lee VMY. Disruption of the cytoskeleton in Alzheimer's disease. Curr Opin Neurobiol 1995;5:663–668.
131. Cummings BJ, Cotman CW. Image analysis of β-amyloid load in Alzheimer's disease and relation to dementia severity. Lancet 1995;346:1524–1528.
132. Hung AY, Haass C, Nitsch RM, et al. Activation of protein kinase C inhibits cellular production of the amyloid β-protein. J Biol Chem 1993;268:22959–22962.
133. Ihara Y. Massive somatodendritic sprouting of cortical neurons in Alzheimer's disease. Brain Res 1988;459:138–144.

11 Molecular Pathology of Alzheimer's Disease: Neuronal Cytoskeletal Abnormalities

Christopher M. Clark, Douglas Ewbank,
Virginia M.-Y. Lee, and John Q. Trojanowski

Alzheimer's disease (AD) is a heterogeneous neurodegenerative dementia that produces progressive memory loss, changes in behavior and personality, and impairments in insight, judgment, executive function, praxis, and other cognitive functions. Pathologically it is defined by the presence of extensive neuron loss, numerous amyloid plaques, and abundant neurofibrillary tangles (NFTs) in selectively vulnerable regions of the brain (for recent reviews and more extensive citations, see references 1–6).

For the most part, the specific factors responsible for initiating the pathologic lesions of AD remain obscure. There is mounting evidence, however, that the causes are multiple and involve complex interactions. Figure 11.1 represents a schematic representation depicting the heterogeneous nature of this disorder.

For a few patients, the responsible factor is a mutation in one of three genes located on chromosome 21 (amyloid precursor protein gene [*APP*]), chromosome 14 (presenilin-1 gene [*PS1*]), or chromosome 1 (presenilin-2 gene [*PS2*]) [7–9; see Chapter 6]. Although additional gene mutations may yet be discovered that are independently capable of producing the pathologic change of AD, for the majority of patients, it is unlikely a single cause, genetic or environmental, will be identified. For most patients, the crucial determinant may be the presence of enough susceptibility factors to initiate one or more of the pathologic cascades that result in neuronal dysfunction, cell death, and dementia. These susceptibility (i.e., risk) factors may involve a combination of genetic and environmental factors, none of which are independently capable of causing the disease.

Whereas both NFTs and neuritic (senile) plaques with beta-amyloid cores are hallmark pathologic lesions of AD, it is the abundance of NFTs that more closely correlates with the severity of dementia [10–14]. Thus, pathologic changes in the neuronal cytoskeleton represent a core component of this neurodegenerative disease.

Formation of NFTs represents the end result of the breakdown of the microtubule component of the neuron cytoskeleton. Thus, understanding the role of the cytoskeleton in maintaining normal neuronal function and the various ways

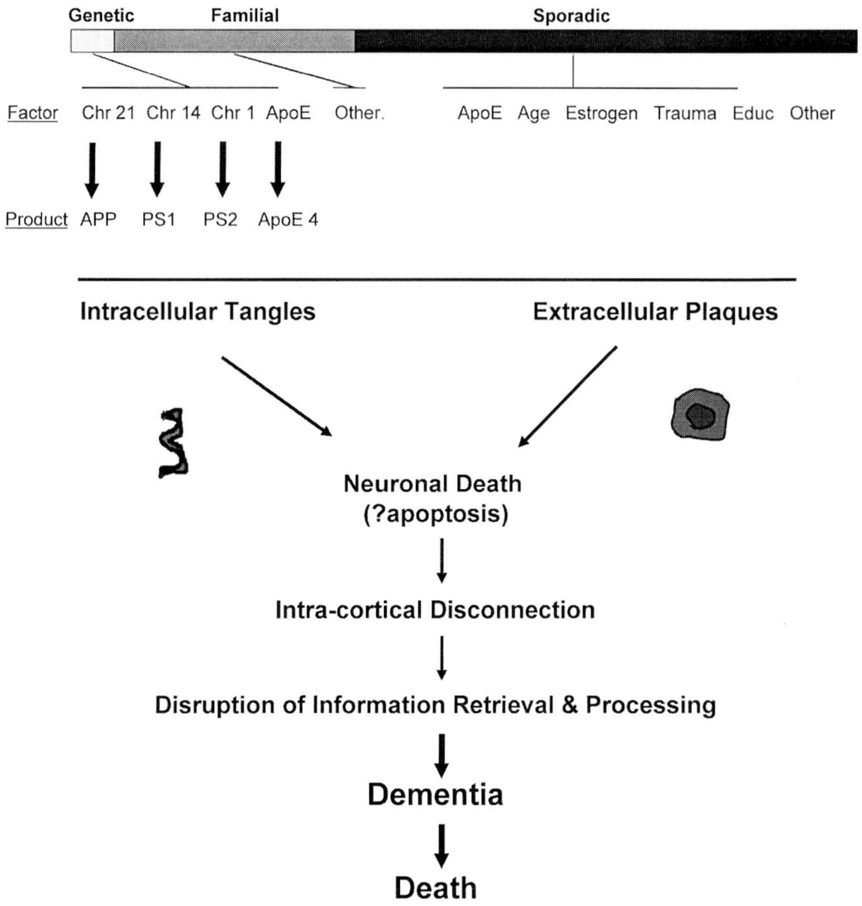

Figure 11.1 Schematic depicting the heterogeneous nature of Alzheimer's disease (AD). The bar represents an estimate of the proportion of AD that is genetic (i.e., due to a known gene mutation), familial (i.e., occurs in blood relatives more often than expected by chance alone), or sporadic. Factors depicted represent gene mutations to chromosomes 21, 14, and 1, known to be capable of causing AD, and other factors felt to increase the risk of AD. The products listed are the proteins (where known) produced by the factors. (Chr = chromosome; APP = amyloid precursor protein; PS1 = presenilin-1; PS2 = presenilin-2; ApoE = apolipoprotein E.)

cytoskeletal elements can be disrupted should provide key insights into the mechanisms by which this pathologic component of AD unfolds. This knowledge, in turn, should facilitate the development of new treatments capable of halting or slowing one of the pathologic cascades that leads to the destruction and death of the neuron. In addition, the identification of biochemical markers of cytoskeletal pathology in the cerebrospinal fluid (CSF) may provide a method to definitively recognize AD at its earliest stage, when it is most susceptible to treatment. Lastly, biochemical marker levels in the CSF may provide a convenient and reliable method to monitor disease progression and response to therapy.

NEURONAL CYTOSKELETON

The neuronal cytoskeleton consists of two major components: neurofilaments, which provide structural support and promote axonal and dendritic outgrowth, and microtubules (MTs), which are primarily involved in the transport of material between the cell body and its processes. In AD, the disruption of the MT system is associated with a hyperphosphorylation of the MT-associated protein *tau*. The end result is fragmentation and collapse of the MTs and the formation of *tau*-rich NFTs and dystrophic neurites.

MT pathology, however, is not the only cytoskeletal disruption seen in AD. Anywhere from 20–30% of AD patients also develop clinical signs of parkinsonism and have coexisting neurofilament pathology in the form of Lewy bodies (LBs), a pathologic hallmark of Parkinson's disease (PD) [15]. Thus, both components of the neuronal cytoskeleton can be involved in the clinical and pathologic spectrum of AD.

FUNCTIONAL ROLE OF *TAU* IN THE FORMATION AND STABILIZATION OF MICROTUBULES IN THE NEURON

Recognition of the role *tau* plays in the assembly and stabilization of MTs was first reported by Weingarten and colleagues [16] and has been the subject of several comprehensive reviews [1,17,18]. In the mature neuron, MTs are primarily found in the axons and dendrites. *tau* proteins are concentrated in neuronal axons, although they can also be detected in central nervous system (CNS) glia [19].

The details of how the multi-step assembly occurs and the methods by which it is controlled remain unclear.

The major role of the MT system is to facilitate transport of material between the cell body and the distal portions of its processes. Failure to maintain this two-way transport system leads to neuronal dysfunction and eventual death. There is mounting evidence that such a disruption of the MT-based transport system in neurons may be a major factor in the pathology of AD [20–23]. In addition to its role in facilitating intraneuronal transport, *tau* may also support the outgrowth of the axon and dendrites [24].

CNS *tau* is a family of small 55- to 64-kd proteins that are assembled from six alternatively spliced isoforms that are encoded by the same gene on chromosome 17 [25]. The isoforms are developmentally regulated with the fetal form expressed early in embryogenesis; all six isoforms (including the fetal form) can be found in adult human brains.

Each *tau* isoform contains either three or four consecutive MT-binding segments that are imperfect repeats of 31 or 32 amino acids (see references 1 and 26 for a review). The isoforms also differ with respect to the presence or absence of polypeptides, which are 29 or 58 amino acids in length, in the amino terminal third of the protein. In contrast to the MT-binding segments, the function of the amino terminal inserts is unknown. As a result of the alternative splicing of these inserts, CNS *tau* proteins range in size from 441 amino acids containing four repeated MT binding motifs and a 58–amino-acid long amino terminal insert to 352 amino acids containing three consecutive MT-binding repeats and

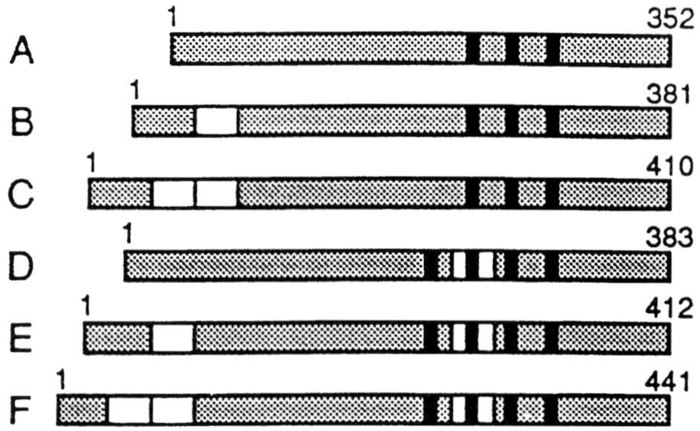

Figure 11.2 Schematic of the six isoforms of human adult *tau*. The number of amino acids for each isoform is noted at the carboxy end. The stippled areas indicate the regions that are common to all six isoforms. The white areas mark the location of the amino acid inserts that are used to distinguish among the isoforms. The black areas represent the tandem microtubule-binding repeats. Fetal brain contains only the 352–amino-acid isoform (A). Adult brain contains all six isoforms (A–F). (Adapted from M Goedert, JQ Trojanowski, VMY Lee. The Neurofibrillary Pathology of Alzheimer's Disease. In SB Prusiner [ed], The Molecular and Genetic Basis of Neurologic Disease (2nd ed). Boston: Butterworth–Heinemann, 1996;613.)

no amino terminal inserts (Figure 11.2). Fetal *tau* is the shortest of the six isoforms. All six isoforms contribute to the formation of both normal adult *tau* and the paired helical filament (PHF) *tau* found in AD.

In their normal functional state, *tau* proteins bind to MTs in a dynamic process as they facilitate polymerization of tubulin subunits into MTs and stabilize newly formed MTs [23,26–28]. They are present in neurons [20,29] and to a lesser extent in astrocytes and oligodendrocytes [19]. A larger isoform, sometimes called *big* tau, is found only in the peripheral nervous system [1,30].

tau Is the Basic Unit of the Neurofibrillary Tangle

NFTs are pathologically altered dysfunctional aggregates of *tau*. The aggregates are formed as a response to the accumulation of an excessive number of phosphate moieties on the *tau* protein. In this state, it is no longer able to promote the assembly and stability of MTs. The hyperphosphorylated *tau* dissociates from the MT, assumes a PHF configuration (20 nm in diameter with a twist having a periodicity of approximately 80 nm), and forms insoluble NFTs inside neuronal perikarya and similar aggregates in axons and dendrites (so-called dystrophic neurites or neuropil threads) (for recent reviews, see references 1, 4, and 31). Other cytoplasmic organelles, including RNA [32], become entrapped in the NFT, possibly contributing to the dysfunction status of the neuron and to its eventual death. In addition to accumulating within the cytoplasm of the neuron, remnants of NFTs are also found dispersed throughout the gray matter in the form of neuropil threads and clustered around extracellular deposits of amyloid. They can also be seen in the olfactory epithelium.

AD PHFs consist of CNS *tau* proteins that are abnormally phosphorylated (i.e., PHF*tau*), and it has been shown that full-length and truncated recombinant human *tau* will polymerize into PHF-like structures in vitro. Several serine (Ser) and threonine (Thr) residues were found to be abnormally phosphorylated in PHF*tau* relative to postmortem adult human CNS using monoclonal antibodies (e.g., T3P, AT8, Tau1, PHF1, AP422, AT270, AT180, 12E8) specific for defined domains in *tau* and mass spectrometry (e.g., Thr^{181}, Ser^{202}, Thr^{231}, Ser^{235}, Ser^{262}, Ser^{396}, Ser^{404}, Ser^{422}). Although early studies indicated that the major sites of abnormal phosphorylation in PHF*tau* were Ser-proline (Pro) or Thr-Pro sites, a reassessment of this issue using ion spray mass spectrometry led to the identification of 19 such sites in PHF*tau*, 10 of which were non–proline-directed. Furthermore, when fetal *tau* was examined, it was shown that the phosphorylation state of PHF*tau* partially recapitulated the phosphorylation state of fetal human and rat CNS *tau*. These findings prompted studies of rapidly isolated CNS *tau* proteins from human cortical brain biopsies and fresh samples of nonhuman primate and rodent brains, which indicated that freshly isolated adult CNS *tau* was phosphorylated at almost all of the same sites as PHF*tau*, albeit to a far lesser extent. Significantly, these studies demonstrated that at least one phosphate-dependent monoclonal anti-PHF*tau* antibody (i.e., AT100 or AT10) recognized a site unique to PHF*tau* (Figure 11.3).

Although some studies suggest that protein phosphatase PP2A and PP2B regulate the phosphorylation state of human CNS *tau* in a site-specific manner, whereas PP1 may not be involved, the role of phosphatases in the formation of PHF*tau* remains to be determined. Down-regulation or inactivation of one or more brain phosphatases could be involved in the conversion of normal *tau* into PHF*tau*. On the other hand, candidate proline-directed protein kinases (PDPKs) implicated in the phosphorylation of PHF*tau* include (1) mitogen-activated protein (MAP), or MAP kinases (also known as *extracellular signal–regulated kinases*); (2) glycogen synthase kinase-3; (3) PDPK; and (4) cyclin-dependent (CD) kinases CDK2 and CDK5. In addition, calcium-calmodulin–dependent protein kinase and cyclic adenosine monophosphate–dependent protein kinase phosphorylate normal *tau* in vitro but not at sites that are phosphorylated in PHF*tau*. Thus, several kinases and phosphatases may contribute to the onset and progression of AD. Further, proteoglycans and RNA may function as pathologic chaperones to augment PHF formation from *tau* [33,34].

Although understanding of the pathobiology of AD is fragmentary, the conversion of normal *tau* into PHF*tau* could lower the levels of MT-binding *tau*, destabilize MTs, disrupt axonal transport, and lead to the death of neurons in AD (Figure 11.4). Although still hypothetical, indirect support for this notion comes from studies of "tangle-only" familial and sporadic AD-like dementias that implicate PHF*tau* and tangles in neurodegenerative disease mechanisms independent of other lesions.

tau Is Involved in a Number of Neurodegenerative Diseases

NFTs are not unique to AD. Intraneuronal NFTs and tangle-like inclusions in glial cells are found in a number of seemingly unrelated neurodegenerative diseases (Table 11.1). In many respects, the abnormal *tau* in these disorders is similar to PHF*tau* in AD [35]. There are some differences, however, in the banding pattern

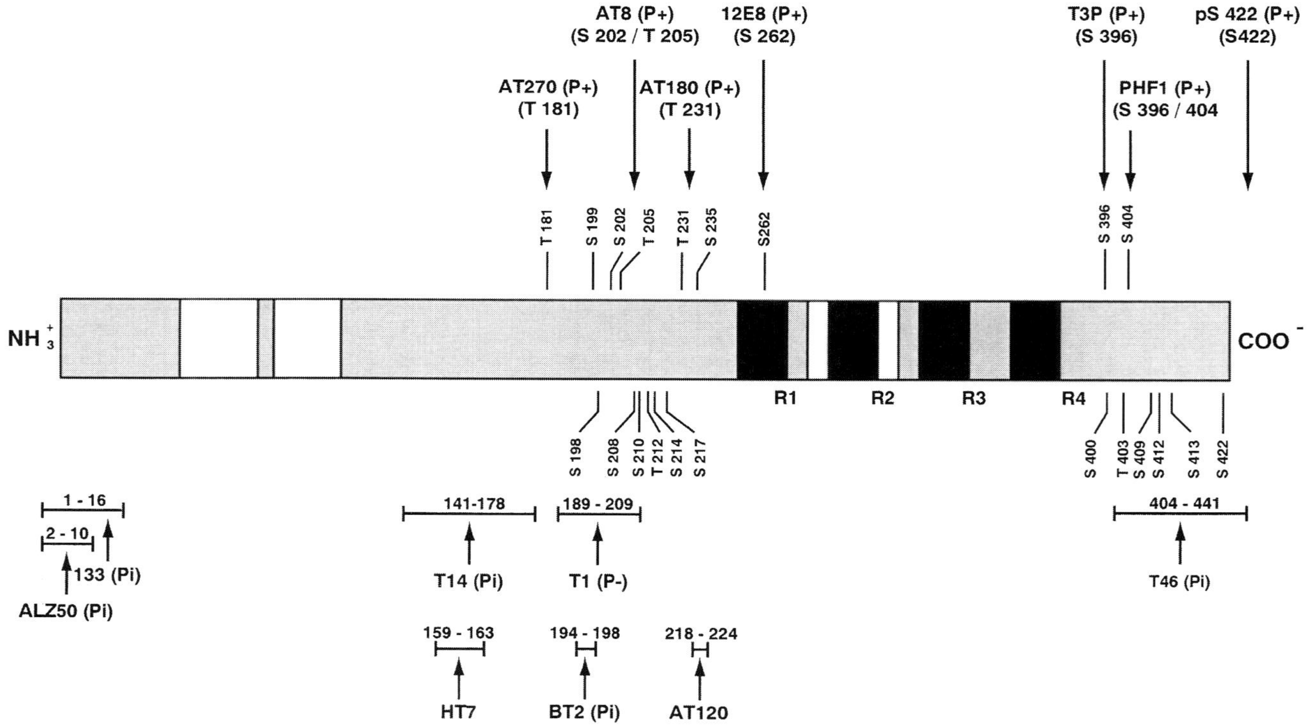

Figure 11.3 Schematic of the longest paired helical filament *tau* isoform indicating phosphorylation sites and monoclonal antibody recognition sites. The sites of phosphorylation and the location of epitopes recognized by various polyclonal and monoclonal antibodies are noted. The epitope for the phosphate-dependent monoclonal antibody AT10 is unknown. (T = threonine; S = serine; R1–R4 = microtubule-binding tandem repeats; P+ = requires presence of phosphate at epitope site; P– = requires absence of phosphate at epitope site; Pi = binds to epitope with or without presence of phosphate; NH_3^+ = amino terminal end; COO^- = carboxy terminal end.)

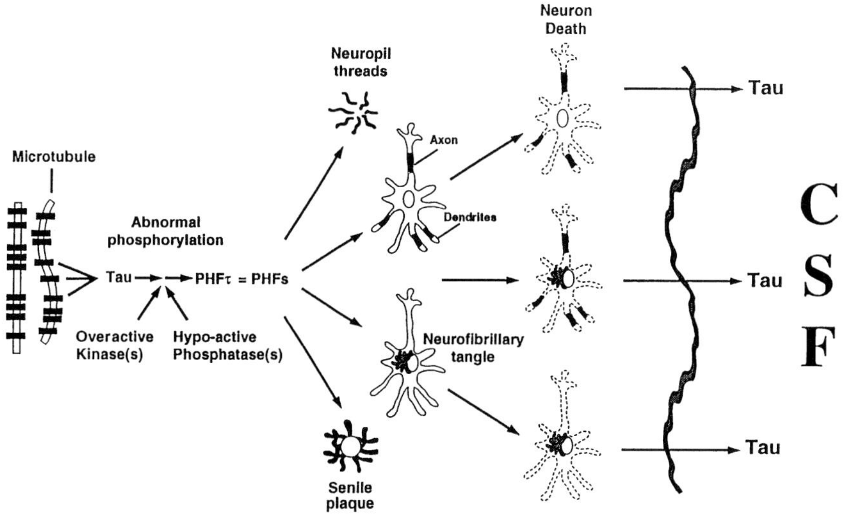

Figure 11.4 Schematic of *tau* breakdown. A hypothetical mechanism for the conversion of normal brain *tau* (*rectangles overlying two microtubules on the left*) into hyperphosphorylated *tau* (paired helical filament [PHF]*tau*). PHF*tau* is generated in neuronal perikarya and their processes as a consequence of overactivity or inappropriate activation of kinases(s), or hypoactivity or loss of phosphatase(s) that regulates the phosphorylation state of central nervous system *tau*. Filament formation may be augmented when the excess pool of unbound *tau* interacts with potential pathologic chaperones such as RNA or heparan sulfate proteoglycan. PHF*tau* then accumulates as filamentous aggregates in neuronal processes (i.e., neuropil threads [*top*]), in neuronal perikarya as neurofibrillary tangles (*middle*), and in dystrophic neurites associated with neuritic senile plaques (*bottom*). PHF*tau* loses the ability to bind MTs, and this could lead to the depolymerization of MTs, disruption of axonal transport, and dysfunction or degeneration of neurons in Alzheimer's disease. The accumulation of PHFs in neurons and dendrites could exacerbate this process by sequestering normal *tau* and by physically blocking the transport of proteins and organelles in neuronal perikarya, axons, and dendrites. The ultimate death of the neuron (*right*) is the culmination of this intracellular cascade of events. (CSF = cerebrospinal fluid.) (Reprinted with permission from JQ Trojanowski, CM Clark, ML Schmidt, et al. Implications of *tau*-Rich Neurofibrillary Lesions for the Pathobiology and Diagnosis of Alzheimer's Disease. In SH Appell [ed], Current Neurology. Chicago: Mosby–Year Book, 1996.)

of the PHF*tau* proteins in these other disorders, the reasons for which are unknown [1].

In each of these neurodegenerative conditions, the regional distribution of aggregates of abnormally hyperphosphorylated *tau* matches the major neuropathologic changes specific for the disorder and is consistent with the clinical pattern of impairment. Although the *tau* proteins in these disorders are phosphorylated at the same sites as PHF*tau* in AD, they differ in regional distribution and electrophoretic mobility [1,36,37]. Extensive neuron loss is a common element in each condition. Included among the diseases with prominent NFTs or

Table 11.1 Pathologic conditions associated with the presence of neurofibrillary tangles

Alzheimer's disease
Down syndrome
Pick's disease
Progressive supranuclear palsy
Multiple system atrophy
Dementia pugilistica
Inclusion body myositis
Gerstmann-Sträussler-Scheinker disease
Argyrophilic grain dementia
Amyotrophic lateral sclerosis–parkinsonism–dementia complex of Guam
Corticobasal degeneration
Niemann-Pick disease type C
Hallervorden-Spatz disease
Subacute sclerosing panencephalitis

tau-rich inclusions are Down syndrome (DS) [38,39], dementia pugilistica [40,41], inclusion body myositis [42], Gerstmann-Sträussler-Scheinker (GSS) disease [43–45], argyrophilic grain dementia [46,47], amyotrophic lateral sclerosis–parkinsonism–dementia complex of Guam (ALS/PDC) [48,49], Pick's disease [50,51], corticobasal degeneration (CBD) [52–55], progressive supranuclear palsy (PSP) [36,56,57], multiple system atrophy [58], Niemann-Pick disease type C [59,60], Hallervorden-Spatz disease [61], and subacute sclerosing panencephalitis [62,63].

In some of these diseases (i.e., DS, GSS, and ALS/PDC) the molecular weight characteristics of the abnormal *tau* proteins are similar to AD PHF*tau* [38,45,48]. In some of the others (PSP, CBD), the abnormal *tau* isoforms appear different on Western blot analysis [53,56]. Thus, although the hyperphosphorylation of *tau* in these other diseases resembles that of PHF*tau* in AD, both the manner in which this occurs and the resulting end product may differ in a disease-specific manner.

USE OF CEREBROSPINAL FLUID *TAU* AS A BIOCHEMICAL MARKER FOR THE CYTOSKELETAL PATHOLOGY OF ALZHEIMER'S DISEASE

For a definitive diagnosis of AD, a patient must have both the clinical documentation of a chronic progressive dementia and postmortem evidence of abundant senile plaques and NFTs in the brain [64]. The sensitivity of a clinical diagnosis of AD (i.e., how often a clinical diagnosis of AD will be confirmed at autopsy) is dependent on the expertise of the clinician and can vary from 77% for university-affiliated physicians (Table 11.2) to greater than 90% for clinicians working in an AD center clinic (C. M. Clark, unpublished data). Although diagnostic accuracy has improved markedly since the publication of the National Institute of Neurological and Communicative Disorders and Stroke/Alzheimer's Disease and Related Disorders Association consensus criteria [65], the development of disease-specific treatments has made the issue much more important than it may have been in the

Table 11.2 Sensitivity and specificity of a clinical diagnosis of Alzheimer's disease

	Pathologic diagnosis		
Clinical diagnosis	*Alzheimer's disease (AD)*	*Not AD*	*Total*
AD	54	10	64
Not AD	16	17	33
Total	70	27	97

Note: diagnostic sensitivity = 77%; diagnostic specificity = 63%; clinical false-positives = 16%; clinical false-negatives = 48%.

past. As a result, there is now a compelling need to develop a definitive diagnostic biochemical marker linked to the presence of AD-specific pathology. To be useful, the marker must be able to identify AD at its earliest stage, when the clinical diagnosis is most difficult; be able to distinguish AD from other dementing neurodegenerative disorders; and reliably identify subjects free of AD neuropathology.

The demonstration that hyperphosphorylated *tau* was the main constituent of PHFs and the knowledge that the severity of dementia correlated with the number of PHF*tau*-rich NFTs prompted efforts to measure CSF levels of *tau* by enzyme-linked immunosorbent assay (ELISA) in living AD patients. The potential relevance of a CSF *tau* ELISA strategy for developing an antemortem test for AD was not entirely evident from the initial studies. Attempts to compare the levels of CSF *tau*, irrespective of its phosphorylation state, in AD and different control populations, however, have yielded both promising and provocative results [66–79].

A major limitation of the studies evaluating the diagnostic utility of CSF *tau* is the lack of a pathologic confirmation of the diagnosis for the large majority of subjects studied. This means that for the most part, the quantitation of CSF *tau* is related to the clinical diagnosis of patients who have been evaluated at AD research centers. This complicates the interpretation of estimates of the sensitivity and specificity of tests based on CSF *tau*. For example, a true case of AD that exhibits high levels of CSF *tau* but is incorrectly diagnosed clinically is counted as a false-positive. Similarly, a case of dementia (e.g., Pick's disease or dementia with LBs) that does not show high levels of CSF *tau* but is incorrectly diagnosed clinically as AD is counted as a false-negative. Although the sensitivity of a clinical diagnosis of probable AD is quite high, the specificity (i.e., how often a pathologic examination confirms the absence of AD in a demented patient in whom the clinician has given a non-AD diagnosis) is not as good (see Table 11.2).

The use of clinical diagnoses is not a significant problem when comparing cases and controls from diagnostic categories that are easy to differentiate. For example, there is little overlap in CSF *tau* levels between probable AD cases and nondemented controls. The range of CSF *tau* levels in cases of other dementias, however, overlaps with both AD and nondemented controls. From a practical standpoint, this means that precise estimates of the ability of CSF *tau* measurements to distinguish between AD and conditions such as frontotemporal dementia (including Pick's disease) and dementia with LBs will have to await neuropathologic correlation (Figure 11.5).

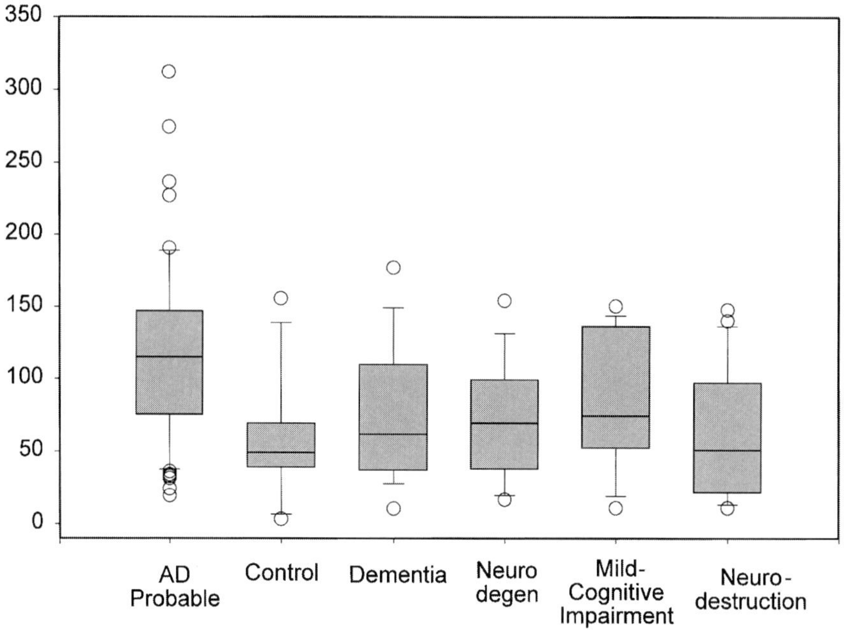

Figure 11.5 Cerebrospinal fluid *tau* levels by diagnostic category. The box contains *tau* values that fall within the twenty-fifth and seventy-fifth percentile. The line within the box marks the median value. The whiskers above and below the box indicate the ninetieth and tenth percentiles. Individual circles indicate points that fall outside the ninetieth and tenth percentiles. The numbers in parentheses indicate the number of subjects in each group. The probable Alzheimer's disease (AD) group (n = 61) met National Institute of Neurological and Communicative Disorders and Stroke/Alzheimer's Disease and Related Disorders Association criteria for probable AD, the control group (n = 14) contained cognitively normal subjects free of neurologic disease. The mild cognitive impairment group (n = 10) had memory loss but did not meet clinical criteria for dementia. The neurodestruction group (n = 22) included patients with cancer, infection, inflammation, and stroke. The neurodegenerative group (n = 13) included patients with frontotemporal dementia, diffuse Lewy body disease, corticobasal degeneration, Gerstmann-Sträussler-Scheinker syndrome, and Parkinson's disease. The dementia group (n = 12) contained patients for whom a specific diagnosis could not be established.

When receiver operating characteristic (ROC) curves are constructed comparing AD to all other types of dementia, the difficulties using CSF *tau* as a definitive diagnostic marker become even more clear. An ROC curve based on cases of probable AD and nondemented controls gives a respectable sensitivity of 82% and a specificity of 70% using a cutoff of 70 pg/ml (Figure 11.6A). When comparing possible AD cases with nondemented controls (Figure 11.6B) or AD cases with other dementing conditions (Figure 11.7), however, no easily identified sensitivity/specificity break points can be used to identify an appropriate cutoff value. In addition, the total area under the curve (a rough indicator of the robustness of the diagnostic marker) shrinks compared to that obtained using CSF *tau* levels to distinguish between AD patients and normal controls. Thus, the test is least likely to be informative in the clinical situation in which

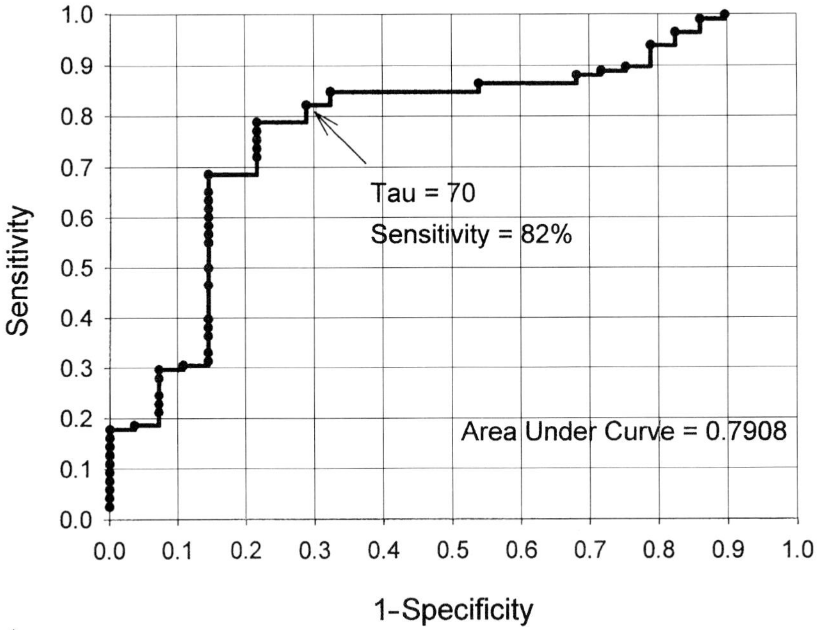

A

Figure 11.6 (A) Sensitivity and specificity of cerebrospinal fluid (CSF) *tau* in correctly classifying patients with a clinical diagnosis of probable Alzheimer's disease (AD) and cognitively normal control subjects. The arrow marks an arbitrary cutoff CSF *tau* value of 70 pg/ml that provides a sensitivity of 82% for the clinical diagnosis of probable AD.

it is most needed—distinguishing AD from other dementing conditions (see Figures 11.6 and 11.7).

This loss of diagnostic sensitivity and specificity is most likely due to a combination of clinical diagnostic inaccuracy and the possibility that the CSF *tau* level may be increased in neurodegenerative conditions other than AD. It is reasonable to assume that neuropathologic conditions that result in the death of *tau*-containing cells will have the potential to elevate CSF *tau* levels. Such an elevation in CSF *tau* has been demonstrated in large-volume stroke, encephalitis, and cancer. Although these are rarely confused with AD, there are other conditions in which dementia is a predominant feature that are difficult to distinguish clinically. Postmortem confirmation of clinical diagnosis is available for only a limited number of subjects. In our own small series of eight patients, only two of the four patients with AD had CSF *tau* levels that exceeded the ROC cutoff of 70 pg/ml. On the other hand, three of the four patients presenting with dementia symptoms that, at autopsy, were not related to AD had CSF *tau* values that exceeded 70 pg/ml.

The relationship of CSF *tau* to dementia severity has not been definitively settled. Although several reports suggest that the CSF *tau* level increases as cognitive function declines [76–78,80], other reports fail to find a correlation [66,69,70,74,75,79].

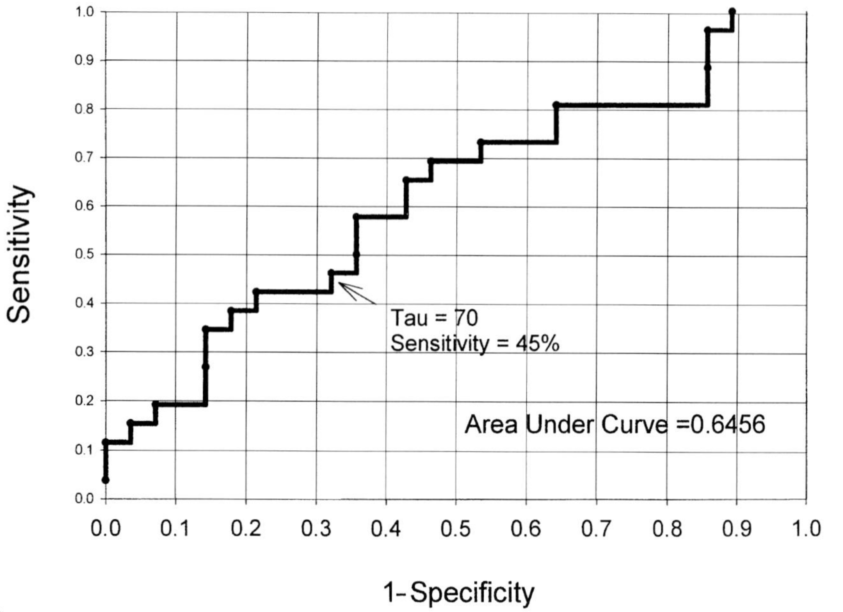

B

Figure 11.6 (continued) (B) Sensitivity and specificity of CSF *tau* in correctly classifying patients with a clinical diagnosis of possible AD and cognitively normal control subjects. The arrow marks an arbitrary cutoff CSF *tau* value of 70 pg/ml that provides a sensitivity of 45% for the diagnosis of possible AD.

The elevated CSF *tau* level is believed to reflect the destruction of neurons and other *tau*-containing cells in the brain, but this has never been demonstrated directly. In addition, the only published study that characterized spinal fluid *tau* failed to find intact, full-length protein [72]. If *tau* undergoes significant modification once it enters the CSF, the likelihood that *tau* can serve as a definitive diagnostic marker for AD will be reduced. Because CSF *tau* levels appear to be elevated early in the course of AD, however, it may serve as an early diagnostic marker in subjects whose symptoms are too mild to permit a definitive clinical diagnosis [70,81,82].

Thus, although CSF *tau* presently has only limited use in increasing the confidence level of a clinical diagnosis of AD, three main conclusions have come from these studies:

1. CSF *tau* levels are elevated in many but not all patients with a clinical diagnosis of probable AD.
2. Although not clearly correlated with disease severity, *tau* levels can be elevated in the earliest stages, when the symptoms are most mild [70].
3. AD is not the only neurodegenerative disease that can elevate CSF *tau* levels [67].

Despite the limitations imposed by the current assays, measurement of CSF *tau* has the potential to become an informative diagnostic procedure. To be clinically useful, the test must be modified so that it is better able to distinguish AD from

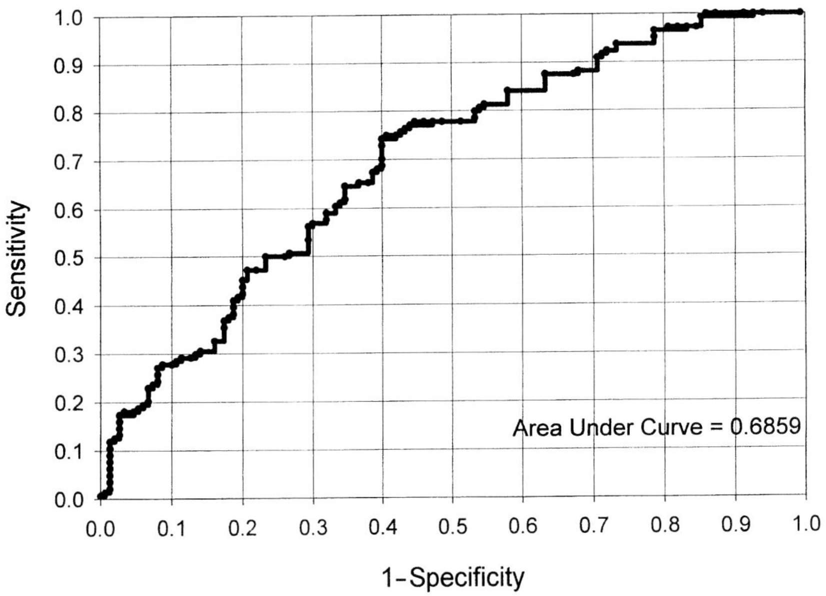

Figure 11.7 Sensitivity and specificity of cerebrospinal fluid (CSF) *tau* in correctly classifying patients with a clinical diagnosis of probable or possible Alzheimer's disease and non-Alzheimer's dementia. When these two groups are compared, there is no clear break point to indicate what CSF *tau* cutoff value should be used.

non-AD dementia, as well as very mild AD from age-related memory impairment. In addition, the test must do this with adequate sensitivity and specificity to warrant its use by general physicians. An AD diagnostic test with these characteristics would be helpful in making therapeutic decisions and in beginning to think about long-term issues at the earliest stage of the illness. If the marker were present in the presymptomatic stage, it would have the added benefit of accurately identifying at-risk subjects for whom treatments designed to delay the onset of clinical symptoms would be most appropriate. In addition, because hyperphosphorylation of *tau* is a relative "downstream" event in the AD pathologic cascade, quantitative measures could serve as a sensitive indicator of disease activity and thus a useful monitor of therapeutic efficacy.

NEUROFILAMENT PATHOLOGY IN ALZHEIMER'S DISEASE

Neurofilaments (NFs) are 10- to 12-nm intermediate filaments that extend from the perikaryon into the axons and dendrites of the neuron. They are composed of light (NFL), medium (NFM), and heavy (NFH) proteins. NFMs and NFHs give rise to side arm projections that help maintain the structural integrity of the cell. They represent one of the most prominent cytoskeletal organelles in large-diameter axons.

LBs are intraneuronal inclusions that represent pathologic aggregations of all three NF subunits. The filaments form a dense central core with a looser array of fibers radiating toward the periphery as the halo or corona of the LB. They differ from normal NFs in that they lack projecting side arms. Other components of the cell become entrapped in this filamentous network, including fragments of intracellular membranes and organelles [83]. Significantly, studies show that alpha-synuclein, which is mutated in familial PD [84], is a major component of LBs in sporadic PD and dementia with LBs [85]. When present in neocortex, LBs take on a less distinct morphology. They may lack the dense central core and surrounding corona characteristic of brain stem LBs and can be difficult to see with routine staining techniques. They are best visualized by antibodies that identify specific LB epitopes, and it is likely that alpha-synuclein antibodies will prove most effective in this regard [85].

Although most commonly associated with the pathologic changes of PD, LBs can be found in a variety of other neurodegenerative conditions, including AD. Often these AD patients have the typical extrapyramidal signs (EPSs) of parkinsonism—muscle rigidity, gait abnormalities, and postural instability [15]. This confluence of neurofilament cytoskeletal pathology (i.e., LBs) and classic AD cytoskeletal pathology (i.e., NFTs) can provide challenges to a clinician. When AD patients develop mild to moderate EPSs during the early or middle portion of their illness, they are often labeled as having the LB variant of AD [86,87]. In addition to the typical signs of parkinsonism, they may manifest psychosis and visual hallucinations as well as a more severe degree of cognitive impairment than AD patients matched for age and duration of illness [88,89]. Traditional PD medication rarely produces clinically meaningful improvement and may exacerbate the psychotic features. During life, however, it is sometimes difficult to distinguish patients who will turn out to have both AD lesions and LBs from patients with dementia who have LBs in their brain stem and neocortex as the sole pathologic finding (i.e., diffuse LB disease; see Chapter 3). So although clinical criteria have been proposed and validated for the premorbid diagnosis of diffuse LB disease [90,91], it was suggested that clinicians who suspect the presence of LBs in a non-PD patient with progressive dementia should use the diagnostic term *dementia with Lewy bodies* [13,92].

The pathologic cascade leading to the formation of LBs is not known. The subsequent entrapment of critical cellular proteins and organelles, however, may be a major factor contributing to neuronal dysfunction and eventual cell death. It is possible that as new antibodies (e.g., to alpha-synuclein) are developed that recognize previously unidentified epitopes, the breadth of LB pathology associated with these conditions will expand.

DIAGNOSTIC IMPLICATIONS OF NEUROFILAMENT CYTOSKELETAL PATHOLOGY IN ALZHEIMER'S DISEASE

At present there is no premorbid biochemical marker of AD-associated LB pathology. The development of a CSF assay that could reliably identify NF-related LB pathology in patients with AD, however, could provide a number of benefits. Chief among these would be the ability to prospectively identify patients destined to develop EPSs and psychotic features early in the course of their illness. This knowledge would facilitate the development of appropriate treatment approaches, such as avoiding the use of antipsychotic medications that block dopamine receptors. In addition, it would allow caregivers to anticipate the need to deal with gait and postural balance problems. Lastly, the identification of coexisting LB pathology in AD could enhance the methodology of clinical therapeutic trials by allowing assessment of the efficacy of new drugs with respect to the degree of NF and alpha-synuclein pathology.

THERAPEUTIC OPPORTUNITIES RELATED TO CYTOSKELETAL PATHOLOGY

Initial therapeutic attempts to improve cognitive function used acetylcholinesterase inhibitors to bolster interneuronal signal transmission. There was no evidence that the drugs (physostigmine, tacrine, donepezil, and metrifonate) influenced the underlying neurodegenerative process responsible for the symptoms. They were, however, associated with a modest, measurable effect on cognitive function and global improvement in a subset of patients [13,93–96]. The next therapeutic advance will most likely come from treatments that can delay the onset of symptoms in subjects at risk for AD or slow the rate of progression in patients in the earliest stages of the disease [97,98]. These treatment strategies will most likely involve a combination of risk factor reduction in susceptible individuals and the use of drugs to reduce the rate of AD-related neuron death (see Chapter 14). Drugs that intervene at any point along the AD cytoskeletal pathologic cascade may well play a key role in this therapeutic strategy.

The demonstration that both high-dose vitamin E and selegiline can increase the time of progression to major clinical milestones validates the legitimacy of a non–AD-specific neuroprotective therapeutic strategy [99]. Treatments targeting the Alzheimer-specific pathologic alterations in the neuronal cytoskeleton have the potential to be even more powerful. For example, it may be possible to preserve neuronal function and reduce the rate of neuron death with the discovery of drugs that could enhance the stability of the MT system, block the addition of excessive phosphate molecules to *tau*, remove phosphate residues from hyperphosphorylated *tau*, prevent the formation of NFTs, or enhance neuronal function in the face of accumulating PHFs.

A parallel logic exists for the development of successful treatments related to AD-associated LB pathology. Once the key pathologic events responsible for NF and alpha-synuclein aggregation and LB formation are known, it may be possible to develop specific drugs that can block or slow down the process. In addition to their efficacy in PD, these drugs should reduce the severity of EPSs and psychosis associated with the presence of LBs in the brain stem and cortex of patients with AD. In general, the development of drugs capable of accomplishing these goals will only occur with an improved understanding of the pathologic processes that disrupt these two components of the neuronal cytoskeleton.

CONCLUSION

Pathologic alteration of the neuronal cytoskeleton is associated with impaired cell function that ultimately results in the death of the neuron. Although disruption of MTs and the formation of NFTs by hyperphosphorylated *tau* is one of the hallmark lesions of AD, accumulation of NFs (and presumably alpha-synuclein) with subsequent formation of LBs also occurs in some patients and adds to the burden of dementia. There is no single cause yet identified that can initiate the pathologic cascades responsible for both lesions. Although there is no definitive evidence that genetic mutations involving the *APP*, *PS1*, or *PS2* genes are sufficient to induce NF pathology, one report showed that a novel *PS1* mutation (R269H) in a single case of early-onset AD was associated with an increase in the number of NFTs compared to that of AD patients with a similar duration of dementia [100].

The lack of a definitive link between the known disease-inducing genetic mutations and NFT pathology is consistent with the presumed heterogeneous nature of AD and the concept that the clinical expression of this particular neurodegenerative form of brain failure may involve a variable combination of "susceptibility genes," environmental stresses, and age-related changes. The initiating events and susceptibility risk factors (both genetic and nongenetic) for both *tau* and NF pathology may be quite different, but the end results have in common the intracellular aggregation of proteins, with sequestration of critical proteins and cellular organelles; disruption of normal cellular function; and ultimately, the death of the neuron. With a better understanding of the mechanisms responsible for these pathologic changes, it may be possible to identify additional risk factors for the disease, discover sensitive and specific diagnostic markers, and develop therapeutic agents directed at the basic molecular abnormalities in AD.

At the present time, abnormalities in *tau* phosphorylation appear to be a key factor in the disruption of the MT system and formation of NFTs. By the same token, identification of specific epitopes of *tau* in the CSF may prove to be a sensitive diagnostic marker of AD and provide an objective means of monitoring disease progression. Lastly, the most efficacious treatment strategies of the future may come from drugs targeting the pathologic changes that disrupt the integrity of the MT component of the neuronal cytoskeleton.

REFERENCES

1. Goedert M, Trojanowski JQ, Lee VMY. The Neurofibrillary Pathology of Alzheimer's Disease. In SB Prusiner (ed), The Molecular and Genetic Basis of Neurological Disease (2nd ed). Boston: Butterworth–Heinemann, 1996;613.
2. Golde TE, Younkin SG. Processing of the Amyloid β-Protein Precursor. In AM Goate, F Ashall (eds), Neuroscience Perspectives: Pathobiology of Alzheimer's Disease. London: Academic, 1995;115–144.
3. Johnson GVW, Jenkins SM. Tau protein in normal and Alzheimer's disease brain. Alzheimer Dis Rev 1996;138–154.
4. Lee VMY, Trojanowski JQ. Tau Proteins and Their Significance in the Pathobiology of Alzheimer's Disease. In AM Goate, F Marshall (eds), Neuroscience Perspectives: Pathobiology of Alzheimer's Disease. London: Academic, 1995;41–58.
5. Yankner BA. Mechanisms of neuronal degeneration in Alzheimer's disease. Neuron 1996;16: 921–932.

6. Yankner BA. New clues to Alzheimer's disease: unraveling the roles of amyloid and tau. Nature Medicine 1996;2:850–852.
7. Goate A, Chartier-Harlin MC, Mullan M, et al. Segregation of a missense mutation in the amyloid precursor protein gene with familial Alzheimer's disease. Nature 1991;349:704–706.
8. Levy-Lahad E, Wasco W, Poorkaj P, et al. Candidate gene for the chromosome 1 familial Alzheimer's disease locus. Science 1995;269:973–977.
9. Sherrington R, Rogaev EI, Liang Y, et al. Cloning of a gene bearing missense mutations in early-onset familial Alzheimer's disease. Nature 1995;375:754–760.
10. Arriagada PV, Growdon JH, Hedley-Whyte ET, Hyman BT. Neurofibrillary tangles but not senile plaques parallel duration and severity of Alzheimer's disease. Neurology 1992;42:631–639.
11. Bierer LM, Hof PR, Purohit DP, et al. Neocortical neurofibrillary tangles correlate with dementia severity in Alzheimer's disease. Arch Neurol 1995;52:81–88.
12. Dickson DW, Crystal HA, Bevona C, et al. Correlations of synaptic and pathological markers with cognition of the elderly. Neurobiol Aging 1995;16:285–298.
13. McKee AC, Kosik KS, Kowall NW. Neuritic pathology and dementia in Alzheimer's disease. Ann Neurol 1991;30:156–165.
14. Samuel WA, Henderson VW, Miller CA. Severity of dementia in Alzheimer disease and neurofibrillary tangles in multiple brain regions. Alzheimer Dis Assoc Disord 1991;5:1–11.
15. Hulette C, Mirra S, Wilkinson W, et al. The Consortium to Establish a Registry for Alzheimer's Disease (CERAD). Part IX. A prospective cliniconeuropathologic study of Parkinson's features in Alzheimer's disease. Neurology 1995;45:1991–1995.
16. Weingarten MD, Lockwood AH, Hwo SY, Kirschner MW. A protein factor essential for microtubule assembly. Proc Natl Acad Sci U S A 1975;72:1858–1862.
17. Kosik KS. The molecular and cellular biology of tau [review]. Brain Pathol 1993;3:39–43.
18. Mandelkow EM, Biernat J, Drewes G, et al. Microtubule-associated protein tau, paired helical filaments, and phosphorylation. Ann N Y Acad Sci 1993;695:209–216.
19. Chin SS, Goldman JE. Glial inclusions in CNS degenerative diseases. J Neuropathol Exp Neurol 1996;55:499–508.
20. Lee VM, Trojanowski JQ. The disordered neuronal cytoskeleton in Alzheimer's disease. Curr Opin Neurobiol 1992;2:653–656.
21. Trojanowski JQ, Schmidt ML, Otvos L Jr, et al. Vulnerability of the neuronal cytoskeleton in aging and Alzheimer disease: widespread involvement of all three major filament systems. Ann Rev Gerontol Geriat 1990;10:167–182.
22. Trojanowski JQ, Schmidt ML, Shin RW, et al. Altered tau and neurofilament proteins in neurodegenerative diseases: diagnostic implications for Alzheimer's disease and Lewy body dementias. Brain Pathol 1993;3:45–54.
23. Trojanowski JQ, Lee VM. Phosphorylation of neuronal cytoskeletal proteins in Alzheimer's disease and Lewy body dementias. Ann N Y Acad Sci 1994;747:92–109.
24. Shea TB, Beermann ML, Nixon RA, Fischer I. Microtubule-associated protein tau is required for axonal neurite elaboration by neuroblastoma cells. J Neurosci Res 1992;32:363–374.
25. Heutink P, Stevens M, Rizzu P, et al. Hereditary frontotemporal dementia is linked to chromosome 17q21–q22: a genetic and clinicopathological study of three Dutch families. Ann Neurol 1997;41: 150–159.
26. Goedert M. Tau protein and the neurofibrillary pathology of Alzheimer's disease. Ann N Y Acad Sci 1996;777:121–31.
27. Goode BL, Feinstein SC. Identification of a novel microtubule binding and assembly domain in the developmentally regulated inter-repeat region of tau. J Cell Biol 1994;124:769–782.
28. Matus A. Stiff microtubules and neuronal morphology. Trends Neurosci 1994;17:19–22.
29. Lee VM, Balin BJ, Otvos LJ, Trojanowski JQ. A68: a major subunit of paired helical filaments and derivatized forms of normal *tau*. Science 1991;251:675–678.
30. Trojanowski JQ, Lee MY. Phosphorylation of neuronal cytoskeletal proteins in Alzheimer's disease and Lewy body dementias. Ann N Y Acad Sci 1995;747:92–109.
31. Clark CM, Trojanowski JQ, Lee VMY. Neurofibrillary Tangles in Alzheimer's Disease: Clinical and Pathological Implications. In JD Brioni, MW Decker (eds). Pharmacological Treatment of Alzheimer's Disease: Molecular and Neurobiological Foundations. New York: Wiley-Liss, 1997;217–238.
32. Ginsberg SD, Crino PB, Lee VM, et al. Sequestration of RNA in Alzheimer's disease neurofibrillary tangles and senile plaques. Ann Neurol 1997;41:200–209.
33. Goedert M, Jakes R, Spillantini MG, et al. Assembly of microtubule-associated protein tau into Alzheimer-like filaments induced by sulphated glycosaminoglycans. Nature 1996;383:550–553.

34. Kampers T, Friedhoff P, Biernat J, et al. RNA stimulates aggregation of microtubule-associated protein tau into Alzheimer-like paired helical filaments. FEBS Lett 1996;399:344–349.
35. Iwatsubo T, Hasegawa M, Ihara Y. Neuronal and glial tau-positive inclusions in diverse neurologic diseases share common phosphorylation characteristics. Acta Neuropathol 1994;88:129–136.
36. Bancher C, Lassmann H, Budka H, et al. Neurofibrillary tangles in Alzheimer's disease and progressive supranuclear palsy: antigenic similarities and differences. Microtubule-associated protein tau antigenicity is prominent in all types of tangles. Acta Neuropathol 1987;74:39–46.
37. Schmidt ML, Huang R, Martin JA, et al. Neurofibrillary tangles in progressive supranuclear palsy contain the same epitopes identified in Alzheimer's disease PHF-tau. J Neuropathol Exp Neurol 1996; 55:534–539.
38. Flament S, Delacourte A, Mann DM. Phosphorylation of *tau* proteins: a major event during the process of neurofibrillary degeneration. A comparative study between Alzheimer's disease and Down's syndrome. Brain Res 1990;516:15–19.
39. Giaccone G, Tagliavini F, Linoli G, et al. Down patients: extracellular preamyloid deposits precede neuritic degeneration and senile plaques. Neurosci Lett 1989;97:232–238.
40. Allsop D, Haga S, Bruton C, et al. Neurofibrillary tangles in some cases of dementia pugilistica share antigens with amyloid beta-protein of Alzheimer's disease. Am J Pathol 1990;136:255–260.
41. Roberts GW, Allsop D, Bruton C. The occult aftermath of boxing. J Neurol Neurosurg Psychiatry 1990;53:373–378.
42. Askanas V, Engel WK, Bilak M, et al. Twisted tubulofilaments of inclusion body myositis muscle resemble paired helical filaments of Alzheimer brain and contain hyperphosphorylated tau. Am J Pathol 1994;144:177–187.
43. Ghetti B, Tagliavini F, Masters CL, et al. Gerstmann-Straussler-Scheinker disease. II. Neurofibrillary tangles and plaques with PrP-amyloid coexist in an affected family. Neurology 1989;39: 1453–1461.
44. Giaccone G, Tagliavini F, Verga L, et al. Neurofibrillary tangles of the Indiana kindred of Gerstmann-Straussler-Scheinker disease share antigenic determinants with those of Alzheimer disease. Brain Res 1990;530:325–329.
45. Tagliavini F, Giaccone G, Prelli F, et al. A68 is a component of paired helical filaments of Gerstmann-Straussler-Scheinker disease, Indiana kindred. Brain Res 1993;616:325–329.
46. Braak H, Braak E. Argyrophilic grains: characteristic pathology of cerebral cortex in cases of adult onset dementia without Alzheimer changes. Neurosci Lett 1987;76:124–127.
47. Itagaki S, McGeer PL, Akiyama H, et al. A case of adult-onset dementia with argyrophilic grains. Ann Neurol 1989;26:685–689.
48. Buee-Scherrer V, Buee L, Hof PR, et al. Neurofibrillary degeneration in amyotrophic lateral sclerosis/parkinsonism-dementia complex of Guam. Immunochemical characterization of tau proteins. Am J Pathol 1995;146:924–932.
49. Hof PR, Nimchinsky EA, Buee-Scherrer V, et al. Amyotrophic lateral sclerosis/parkinsonism-dementia complex of Guam: quantitative neuropathology, immunohistochemical analysis of neuronal vulnerability, and comparison with related neurodegenerative disorders. Acta Neuropathol 1994;88: 397–404.
50. Murayama S, Mori H, Ihara Y, Tomonaga M. Immunocytochemical and ultrastructural studies of Pick's disease. Ann Neurol 1990;27:394–405.
51. Perry G, Stewart D, Friedman R, et al. Filaments of Pick's bodies contain altered cytoskeletal elements. Am J Pathol 1987;127:559–568.
52. Feany MB, Dickson DW. Widespread cytoskeletal pathology characterizes corticobasal degeneration. Am J Pathol 1995;146:1388–1396.
53. Ksiezak-Reding H, Morgan K, Mattiace LA, et al. Ultrastructure and biochemical composition of paired helical filaments in corticobasal degeneration. Am J Pathol 1994;145:1496–1508.
54. Mori H, Nishimura M, Namba Y, Oda M. Corticobasal degeneration: a disease with widespread appearance of abnormal tau and neurofibrillary tangles, and its relation to progressive supranuclear palsy. Acta Neuropathol 1994;88:113–121.
55. Wakabayashi K, Oyanagi K, Makifuchi T, et al. Corticobasal degeneration: etiopathological significance of the cytoskeletal alterations. Acta Neuropathol 1994;87:545–553.
56. Flament S, Delacourte A, Verny M, et al. Abnormal *tau* proteins in progressive supranuclear palsy. Similarities and differences with the neurofibrillary degeneration of the Alzheimer type. Acta Neuropathol 1991;81:591–596.
57. Giaccone G, Tagliavini F, Street JS, et al. Progressive supranuclear palsy with hypertrophy of the olives. An immunocytochemical study of the cytoskeleton of argyrophilic neurons. Acta Neuropathol 1988;77:14–20.

58. Papp MI, Kahn JE, Lantos PL. Glial cytoplasmic inclusions in the CNS of patients with multiple system atrophy (striatonigral degeneration, olivopontocerebellar atrophy and Shy-Drager syndrome). J Neurol Sci 1989;94:79–100.
59. Love S, Bridges LR, Case CP. Neurofibrillary tangles in Niemann-Pick disease type C. Brain 1995;118:119–129.
60. Suzuki K, Parker CC, Pentchev PG, et al. Neurofibrillary tangles in Niemann-Pick disease type C. Acta Neuropathol 1995;89:227–238.
61. Eidelberg D, Sotrel A, Joachim C, et al. Adult onset Hallervorden-Spatz disease with neurofibrillary pathology. A discrete clinicopathological entity. Brain 1987;110:993–1013.
62. Mandybur TI, Nagpaul AS, Pappas Z, Niklowitz WJ. Alzheimer neurofibrillary change in subacute sclerosing panencephalitis. Ann Neurol 1977;1:103–107.
63. McQuaid S, Allen IV, McMahon J, Kirk J. Association of measles virus with neurofibrillary tangles in subacute sclerosing panencephalitis: a combined in situ hybridization and immunocytochemical investigation. Neuropathol Appl Neurobiol 1994;20:103–110.
64. The National Institute on Aging. Consensus Recommendations for the postmortem diagnosis of Alzheimer's disease. Neurobiol Aging 1997;18:1–3.
65. McKhann G, Drachman D, Folstein M, et al. Clinical diagnosis of Alzheimer's disease: report of the NINCDS-ADRDA Work Group under the auspices of Department of Health and Human Services Task Force on Alzheimer's Disease. Neurology 1984;34:939–944.
66. Arai H, Terajima M, Miura M, et al. Tau in cerebrospinal fluid: a potential diagnostic marker in Alzheimer's disease. Ann Neurol 1995;38:649–652.
67. Arai H, Morikawa Y, Higuchi M, et al. Cerebrospinal fluid tau levels in neurodegenerative diseases with distinct *tau*-related pathology. Biochem Biophys Res Commun 1997;236:262–264.
68. Blennow K, Wallin A, Agren H, et al. Tau protein in cerebrospinal fluid: a biochemical marker for axonal degeneration in Alzheimer disease? Mol Chem Neuropathol 1995;26:231–245.
69. Blomberg M, Jensen M, Basun H, et al. Increasing cerebrospinal fluid tau levels in a subgroup of Alzheimer patients with apolipoprotein E allele epsilon 4 during 14 months follow-up. Neurosci Lett 1996;214:163–166.
70. Galasko D, Clark C, Chang L, et al. Assessment of CSF levels of tau protein in mildly demented patients with Alzheimer's disease. Neurology 1997;48:632–635.
71. Jensen M, Basun H, Lannfelt L. Increased cerebrospinal fluid tau in patients with Alzheimer's disease. Neurosci Lett 1995;186:189–191.
72. Johnson GV, Seubert P, Cox TM, et al. The tau protein in human cerebrospinal fluid in Alzheimer's disease consists of proteolytically derived fragments. J Neurochem 1997;68:430–433.
73. Mori H, Hosoda K, Matsubara E, et al. Tau in cerebrospinal fluids: establishment of the sandwich ELISA with antibody specific to the repeat sequence in tau. Neurosci Lett 1995;186:181–183.
74. Munroe WA, Southwick PC, Chang L, et al. Tau protein in cerebrospinal fluid as an aid in the diagnosis of Alzheimer's disease. Ann Clin Lab Sci 1995;25:207–217.
75. Riemenschneider M, Buch K, Schmolke M, et al. Cerebrospinal protein tau is elevated in early Alzheimer's disease. Neurosci Lett 1996;212:209–211.
76. Rosler N, Wichart I, Bancher C, Jellinger KA. Tau protein and apolipoprotein E in CSF diagnostics of Alzheimer's disease: impact on non Alzheimer's dementia? J Neural Transm Suppl 1996;47:259–266.
77. Skoog I, Vanmechelen E, Andreasson LA, et al. A population-based study of tau protein and ubiquitin in cerebrospinal fluid in 85-year-olds: relation to severity of dementia and cerebral atrophy, but not to the apolipoprotein E4 allele. Neurodegeneration 1995;4:433–442.
78. Tato RE, Frank A, Hernanz A. Tau protein concentrations in cerebrospinal fluid of patients with dementia of the Alzheimer type. J Neurol Neurosurg Psychiatry 1995;59:280–283.
79. Vigo-Pelfrey C, Seubert P, Barbour R, et al. Elevation of microtubule-associated protein tau in the cerebrospinal fluid of patients with Alzheimer's disease. Neurology 1995;45:788–793.
80. Hock C, Golombowski S, Naser W, Muller-Spahn F. Increased levels of tau protein in cerebrospinal fluid of patients with Alzheimer's disease—correlation with degree of cognitive impairment. Ann Neurol 1995;37:414–415.
81. Arai H, Nakagawa T, Kosaka Y, et al. Elevated cerebrospinal fluid tau protein level as a predictor of dementia in memory-impaired individuals. Alzheimer Res 1997;3:211–213.
82. Terajima M, Arai H, Itabashi S, et al. Elevated cerebrospinal fluid tau levels: implications for the early diagnosis of Alzheimer's disease. J Am Geriatr Soc 1996;44:1012–1013.
83. Galvin JE, Lee VYL, Baba M, et al. Monoclonal antibodies to purified cortical Lewy bodies recognize the mid-size neurofilament subunit. Ann Neurol 1997;42:595–603.
84. Polymeropoulos MH, Lavedan C, Leroy E, et al. Mutation in the alpha-synuclein gene identified in families with Parkinson's disease. Science 1997;276:2045–2047.

85. Goedert M. The awakening of α-synuclein. Nature 1997;388:232–233.
86. Forstl H, Burns A, Luthert P, et al. The Lewy-body variant of Alzheimer's disease. Clinical and pathological findings. Br J Psychiatry 1993;162:385–392.
87. Hansen L, Salmon D, Galasko D, et al. The Lewy body variant of Alzheimer's disease: a clinical and pathologic entity. Neurology 1990;40:1–8.
88. Chui HC, Lyness SA, Sobel E, Schneider LS. Extrapyramidal signs and psychiatric symptoms predict faster cognitive decline in Alzheimer's disease. Arch Neurol 1994;51:676–681.
89. Clark CM, Ewbank D, Lerner A, et al. The relationship between extrapyramidal signs and cognitive performance in patients with Alzheimer's disease enrolled in the CERAD Study. Consortium to Establish a Registry for Alzheimer's Disease. Neurology 1997;49:70–75.
90. McKeith IG, Perry RH, Fairbairn AF, et al. Operational criteria for senile dementia of Lewy body type (SDLT). Psychol Med 1992;22:911–922.
91. McKeith IG, Fairbairn AF, Bothwell RA, et al. An evaluation of the predictive validity and inter-rater reliability of clinical diagnostic criteria for senile dementia of Lewy body type. Neurology 1994;44: 872–877.
92. Hansen LA, Samuel W. Criteria for Alzheimer's disease and the nosology of dementia with Lewy bodies. Neurology 1997;48:126–132.
93. Becker RE, Colliver JA, Markwell SJ, et al. Double-blind, placebo-controlled study of metrifonate, an acetylcholinesterase inhibitor, for Alzheimer disease. Alzheimer Dis Assoc Disord 1996;10:124–131.
94. Davis KL, Thal LJ, Gamzu ER, et al. A double-blind, placebo-controlled multicenter study of tacrine for Alzheimer's disease. The Tacrine Collaborative Study Group. N Engl J Med 1992;327:1253–1259.
95. Rogers SL, Friedhoff LT. The efficacy and safety of donepezil in patients with Alzheimer's disease: results of a US multicentre, randomized, double-blind, placebo-controlled trial. The Donepezil Study Group. Dementia 1996;7:293–303.
96. Ashford JW, Sherman KA, Kumar V. Advances in Alzheimer therapy: cholinesterase inhibitors. Neurobiol Aging 1989;10:99–105.
97. Khachaturian Z. The five-five, ten-ten plan for Alzheimer's disease. Neurobiol Aging 1992;13: 197–198.
98. Khachaturian ZS. Scientific opportunities for developing treatments for Alzheimer's disease: proceedings of Research Planning Workshop 1. Neurobiol Aging 1994;15(suppl 2):S11–S15.
99. Sano M, Ernesto C, Thomas RG, et al. A controlled trial of selegiline, alpha-tocopherol, or both as treatment for Alzheimer's disease. The Alzheimer's Disease Cooperative Study. N Engl J Med 1997; 336:1216–1222.
100. Gómez-Isla T, Wasco W, Pettingell WP, et al. A novel presenilin-1 mutation: increased beta-amyloid and neurofibrillary changes. Ann Neurol 1997;41:809–813.

12

Bioenergetics, Excitotoxicity, and Oxidative Injury in the Pathogenesis of Neurodegenerative Disease

M. Flint Beal

Neurodegenerative diseases are a heterogeneous group of illnesses with distinct clinical phenotypes and genetic etiologies. Dementia is a clinical hallmark of many of these diseases. The prototypical diseases are Alzheimer's disease (AD), Parkinson's disease (PD), Huntington's disease (HD), amyotrophic lateral sclerosis (ALS), and cerebellar degenerations. These illnesses are characterized by delayed insidious onset, often in middle or late life, and slowly progressive degeneration of circumscribed groups of neurons. Major advances in identifying genes associated with these disorders have been made since the mid-1990s. Identification of gene defects has led to the development of transgenic mouse models.

Despite these rapid and exciting advances, the biochemical mechanisms that contribute to neuron death in neurodegenerative diseases are still being elucidated. Our studies and those of others have focused attention on the potentially pivotal role of energy impairment and mitochondrial dysfunction. A fundamental defect in energy metabolism will have a number of deleterious consequences for the cell. These include impaired calcium buffering, secondary excitotoxicity, production of free radicals, activation of nitric oxide synthase (NOS), and activation of the mitochondrial permeability transition. These processes can then lead to cell death by either apoptosis or necrosis depending on the severity of the insult.

Research has provided evidence for both bioenergetic defects and mitochondrial genetic defects in several neurodegenerative diseases. The primary source of energy production within the cell is the mitochondria. Mitochondria contain the electron transport complexes that lead to the generation of adenosine triphosphate (ATP) (Figure 12.1). A secondary consequence is the generation of free radicals and oxidative damage. A role of oxidative damage in neurodegenerative diseases developed increasing credence after the discovery of point mutations in superoxide dismutase in association with familial ALS (FALS) [1]. This chapter reviews the substantial evidence for a role of oxidative damage in FALS and other neurodegenerative diseases.

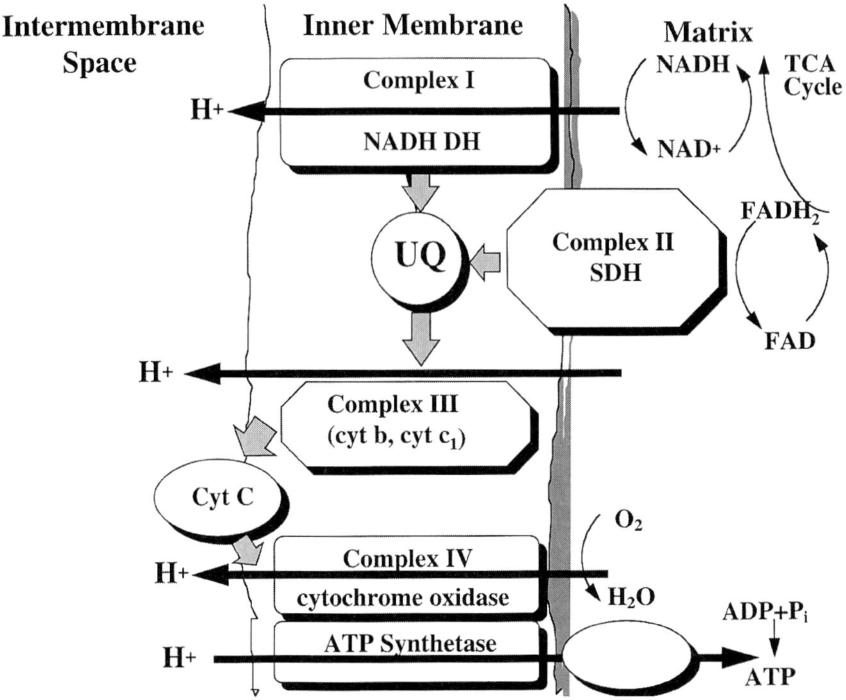

Figure 12.1 Diagram of the electron transport complexes in the inner mitochondrial membrane. (NADH DH = reduced nicotinamide adenine dinucleotide dehydrogenase; $FADH_2$ = reduced flavin adenine dinucleotide; SDH = succinate dehydrogenase; UQ = ubiquinone; cyt = cytochrome; TCA = tricarboxylic acid; ADP = adenosine diphosphate; P_i = inorganic phosphate; ATP = adenosine triphosphate.)

MITOCHONDRIA AND MECHANISMS OF CELL DEATH

Excitotoxicity

Excitotoxicity refers to cell death due to activation of excitatory amino acid receptors. Strong evidence has implicated excitotoxicity as a mechanism of cell death in acute neurologic illnesses, such as stroke, head trauma, and epilepsy. Due to convincing data in animal models, a number of studies of excitatory amino acid antagonists in stroke and head trauma are currently underway. The role of excitotoxicity in neurodegenerative disease is more circumstantial. In contrast to cerebral ischemia and brain trauma, there is little evidence that these diseases are associated with elevated glutamate concentrations, and searches for increased concentrations of other endogenous excitatory amino acid agonists have been unsuccessful.

The theory of excitotoxicity in neurodegenerative diseases was modified, therefore, and the expression *slow* (or *weak*) *excitotoxicity* was coined [2,3]. According to this theory, potential mechanisms capable of inducing excitotoxicity included genetic mutations leading to changes in the configuration of glutamate receptors or an impairment of energy metabolism allowing otherwise innocuous concentrations of glutamate to become toxic. The latter concept was initially verified by the in vitro studies of Novelli and colleagues [4]. Subsequent work in cultured chick retina provided evidence that impaired energy metabolism leads to partial neuronal depolarization allowing voltage-dependent *N*-methyl-D-aspartate (NMDA) excitatory amino acid receptors to be more easily activated [5,6]. The situation is more complex than originally appreciated because impaired energy metabolism enhances vulnerability to both NMDA and amino-3-hydroxy-5-methyl-4-isoxazole propionic acid (AMPA)/kainate agonists. This increased vulnerability is most likely due to effects of energy impairment on intracellular calcium buffering.

Cellular Calcium Buffering

A disruption of intracellular calcium homeostasis is a key mechanism in excitotoxicity, as originally pointed out by Choi [7]. Defective energy metabolism leads to activation of excitatory amino acid receptors and also impairs buffering of intracellular calcium. Therefore, a complex interplay between energy impairment and excitotoxicity exists. A direct relationship between elevations of intracellular calcium and eventual cell death has been difficult to establish, but two studies showed a good correlation between cell death and Ca^{2+} influx by the NMDA receptor [8,9]. Direct support comes from studies of cell-permeable Ca^{2+} chelators, which attenuate glutamate-induced increases in intracellular Ca^{2+} and neurotoxicity [10].

The source of the increases in intracellular calcium is important because elevations triggered by activation of NMDA receptors are much more toxic than those produced by activation of voltage-dependent Ca^{2+} channels [10]. This finding suggests a link between activation of NMDA receptors and damage to a sensitive cellular compartment such as the mitochondrion. Mitochondria play an important role in intracellular calcium buffering, particularly when there are large increases in intracellular calcium [11]. Mitochondria take up calcium through a voltage-driven Ca^{2+} uniporter and extrude Ca^{2+} through a Ca^{2+}/Na^{+} exchange [12]. Both transporters are dependent on the mitochondrial membrane potential. The uniporter shows half-maximal transport velocity at 10–100 mM Ca^{2+}, and V_{max} can be as high as 1,750 nmol/mg/min. The role of the uniporter, therefore, appears to be to sequester calcium as rapidly as possible when calcium concentration is high. Therefore, a reduction in mitochondrial membrane potential will lead to impaired calcium buffering in pathologic conditions as well as impaired calcium efflux from the mitochondria.

Production of Free Radicals

Substantial evidence links the production of free radicals to cell death by either apoptotic or necrotic mechanisms. Mitochondria are believed to be the most important intracellular source of free radicals. Mitochondria in state 4 generate 0.6–1.0 nmol H_2O_2/min/mg protein, accounting for approximately 2% of oxygen uptake under physiologic conditions [13]. The corresponding production of superoxide is estimated to be 2–3 nmol of $O_2^{\bullet}$/min/mg protein. The primary sites

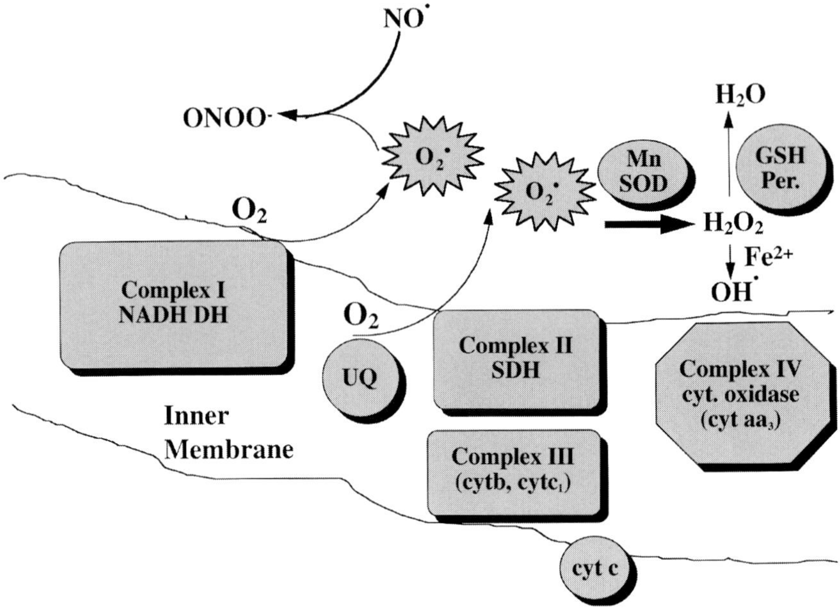

Figure 12.2 Sites of free radical production from mitochondria. The primary sites are complex I and ubiquinone (UQ), which lead to the generation of superoxide (O_2•). Superoxide can react with nitric oxide (NO•) to generate peroxynitrite ($ONOO^-$), or it can be detoxified by manganese SOD (MnSOD) and glutathione peroxidase (GSH Per). (NADH DH = reduced nicotinamide adenine dinucleotide dehydrogenase; SDH = succinate dehydrogenase; cyt = cytochrome; cyt aa_3 = cytochrome-*c* oxidase.)

of superoxide production are ubiquinone and reduced nicotinamide adenine dinucleotide (NADH) dehydrogenase (complex I) (Figure 12.2). Evidence favoring ubiquinone as a source is the finding that electrons are transferred one at a time to ubiquinone to form semi-ubiquinone radicals [14]. These radicals can then react with O_2 to form superoxide radicals. Administration of antimycin A, an inhibitor of complex III, results in increased mitochondrial hydrogen peroxide (H_2O_2) generation, presumably at the level of ubiquinone, and depletion of ubiquinone reduces H_2O_2 production [15,16].

Evidence favoring involvement of free radicals in cell death comes from studies showing that addition of exogenous H_2O_2, nitric oxide (NO), or oxidation-reduction (redox)–cycling quinone compounds leads to cell death in several systems [17–19]. Furthermore, depletion of the antioxidant glutathione renders cells vulnerable to oxidative stress-induced apoptosis [20,21]. Down-regulation of Cu/Zn superoxide dismutase leads to apoptotic cell death in both PC12 cells and spinal motor neurons [22,23]. NMDA-induced toxicity has been linked to mitochondrial superoxide generation in vitro [24–28]. Furthermore, we demonstrated that free radical spin-trapping compounds can attenuate excitotoxic cell death in vivo [29]. Both antioxidants as well as free radical scavenging enzymes can prevent cell death in vitro [30–32].

Nitric Oxide and Peroxynitrite

NO is a unique biological messenger molecule in the central nervous system [33]. It is an unusual transmitter because it is a free radical gas that is not stored in synaptic vesicles. It is generated from L-arginine by the enzyme NOS. A role of NO in excitotoxicity was originally reported by Dawson and colleagues [34]. They showed that toxicity was markedly attenuated after brief exposure of cultured cortical neurons to NMDA, direct inhibitors of NOS, and other compounds that modulate NOS activity, such as calmodulin antagonists, flavoprotein inhibitors, and reduced hemoglobin, which scavenges NO. Removal of arginine from the media also attenuated toxicity. Furthermore, pretreatment of cultures with quisqualate, which preferentially kills NOS neurons, blocked glutamate toxicity in both cultured striatal and cortical neurons [35]. These studies were extended by demonstrating that the cultured neurons from neuronal NOS (nNOS)–deficient mice are resistant to glutamate and NMDA-mediated excitotoxicity [36]. Interestingly, nNOS inhibitors protect against NMDA but not against AMPA or kainate toxicity, suggesting a link between activation of NMDA receptors and activation of NOS [34].

Studies with NOS inhibitors such as L-nitro-arginine in vivo yielded inconsistent results in protecting against ischemic brain damage, apparently due to nonselective inhibition of all NOS isoforms, including nNOS, endothelial NOS (eNOS), and inducible (macrophage) NOS (iNOS). Inhibition of eNOS leads to vasoconstriction, which may have deleterious effects in vivo by producing ischemia [37]. We used the relatively selective nNOS inhibitor 7-nitroindazole to show that it inhibits NMDA but not AMPA or kainate toxicity in vivo [29].

Although $NO^{\bullet}$ itself is a free radical, the critical mediator of $NO^{\bullet}$ toxicity appears to be peroxynitrite ($ONOO^-$), which is formed by the interaction of $NO^{\bullet}$ with $O_2^{\bullet}$ [38]. This reaction occurs at an extremely fast rate of 6.7×10^9 M^{-1}/sec^{-1}, which is essentially diffusion limited and does not require transition metals. Therefore, it depends on concentrations of superoxide and NO in the cell. $ONOO^-$ is relatively stable, with a half-life of 0.9 sec at physiologic pH. Therefore, it may be able to diffuse over several cell diameters to mediate cell damage. It can exist in an activated transitional state that acts in a "hydroxyl radical–like" manner, and it can also generate "nitronium-like" intermediates, which nitrate tyrosines, leading to the production of 3-nitrotyrosine, which is a useful biochemical marker of $ONOO^-$-mediated damage [39–41].

After administration of NMDA in vivo, we found increases in both markers of hydroxyl radical generation as well as 3-nitrotyrosine, consistent with involvement of $ONOO^-$ [29]. Furthermore, the increases were significantly attenuated by treatment with the nNOS inhibitor 7-nitroindazole.

The Mitochondrial Permeability Transition

Studies have provided strong evidence that activation of the mitochondrial permeability transition is involved in both necrotic and apoptotic cell death [42,43]. The mitochondrial permeability transition is an all or none alteration in the inner mitochondrial membrane enabling it to become nonselectively permeable to solutes of ≤1,500 d. The composition of the permeability transition pore is unknown, but evidence favors involvement of the adenine nucleotide transporter on the inner mitochondrial membrane and involvement of the voltage-dependent anion channel or the mitochondrial benzodiazepine receptor on the outer membrane.

The biochemistry and pharmacology of the mitochondrial transition pore have been extensively reviewed and its gating is complex [42,43]. A loss of mitochondrial membrane potential favors pore opening, whereas hyperpolarization favors pore closing. Elevated matrix calcium results in pore opening, and agents that inhibit calcium entry such as ruthenium red, an inhibitor of the voltage-driven Ca^{2+} uniporter, and calcium chelators favor pore closing. Matrix acidification favors pore closing, whereas matrix alkalization favors pore opening. Ligands of the adenine nucleotide translocator, such as atractyloside, pyridoxal phosphate, and acetyl coenzyme A favor pore opening, whereas adenosine diphosphate (ADP) and bongkrekic acid favor pore closing. A number of thiol-depleting agents and thiol-oxidizing agents favor pore opening, whereas thiol-reducing agents favor pore closing. Therefore, it is suggested that oxidation of thiols in an inner mitochondrial membrane protein may play a key role in the mitrochondrial transition pore. Consistent with this suggestion is the observation that a number of free radical–generating agents favor pore opening, whereas antioxidants favor pore closing. The redox state of pyridine nucleotides is also important because NADH and reduced nicotinamide-adenine dinucleotide phosphate (NADPH) favor pore closing, whereas NAD^+ and $NADP^+$ favor pore opening. The most consistent pharmacologic agent to modify the pore is cyclosporin A, which inhibits pore opening with high potency and selectivity. It is frequently used as the operational definition of the permeability transition, and its effects are mediated by interaction with a mitochondrial matrix cyclophilin [44].

The mitochondrial permeability transition results in a number of deleterious effects, including loss of the mitochondrial membrane potential, cessation of ATP synthesis, uncoupling of the respiratory chain, free radical generation, depletion of glutathione and NADH, and colloid-osmotic swelling of mitochondria. Inhibition of the mitochondrial permeability transition with cyclosporine attenuates excitotoxic cell death produced by both glutamate and NMDA [45,46]. Cyclosporine prevents immediate necrosis and delayed apoptosis after excitotoxic insults [47]. It also appears to play a key role in other forms of apoptotic cell death as discussed in the next section.

Apoptosis

Apoptosis refers to cell death that may be mediated by a genetic cell death program; this process has been best studied during development. It consists of cell death that occurs in the absence of cell and organelle swelling and in the absence of inflammation. A hallmark is chromatin clumping and cleavage of DNA by endonucleases. In the nematode *Caenorhabditis elegans*, specific genes involved have been cloned [48]. Genes *ced-3* and *ced-4* are necessary for cell death to occur, and *ced-9* protects cells from death. In mammals, *ced-9* corresponds to a family of proteins of which the prototype is bcl-2. Similarly ced-3, a cysteine protease, corresponds in mammals to a family of cysteine proteases formerly referred to as *interleukin-1b converting enzyme–like proteases*, but now called *caspases* [49]. Mammalian homologs for *ced-4* have recently been identified.

A growing body of evidence indicates that the mitochondrial permeability transition plays a critical role in induction of apoptotic cell death. In a wide variety of experimental systems, a loss of the mitochondrial membrane potential is among the earliest detectable events in cells induced to undergo apoptosis and usually precedes changes in other cellular compartments such as plasma membrane blebbing and nuclear chromatin condensation [50–56]. Furthermore, this view is supported by the observation that inhibitors of the permeability transition, such as cyclosporine and bongkrekic acid, prevent loss of the mitochondrial membrane potential and subsequent apoptotic events [57,58]. Protoporphyrin IX, which is a benzodiazepine receptor ligand that triggers the permeability transition, causes collapse of mitochondrial membrane potential and leads to apoptosis [58]. Similarly in cell free systems, atractyloside, an adenine nucleotide translocator ligand, induces the permeability transition and induces nuclear stigmata of apoptosis [57].

A release of two mitochondrial proteins has been linked to subsequent nuclear changes of apoptosis. Convincing evidence shows that release of cytochrome *c* may play a role [59]. Cell lysates purified from cells induced to undergo apoptosis with staurosporin contain cytochrome *c*, which in conjunction with dATP and an as yet unidentified cytosolic factor, activates caspase CPP32 and causes DNA fragmentation in isolated nuclei. In Fas-induced apoptosis, a loss of cytochrome *c* oxidase (COX) function is restored with exogenous cytochrome *c*, consistent with its release from mitochondria [60]. A second mitochondrial protein implicated is apoptosis-inducing factor (AIF), which originates from the membrane space and purifies as a 50-kd protease [61].

A role for bcl-2 in mitochondrial function was suggested by its localization, which includes the nucleus, the endoplasmic reticulum, and the outer mitochondrial membrane [62]. In cell free systems, a localization of bcl-2 to mitochondria is critical for its anti-apoptotic activity [63–65]. Studies show that bcl-2 prevents the release of cytochrome *c* and AIF in cells exposed to apoptotic-inducing stimuli. bcl-2 also has a number of other effects that modulate mitochondrial function. It enhances mitochondrial membrane potential, improves ATP-ADP ratios, potentiates maximal mitochondrial calcium uptake capacity, and protects against calcium-induced electron transport dysfunction; it also inhibits the mitochondrial permeability transition [57,66–69], has antioxidant activity, and prevents free radical generation [70–72]. The hierarchical relationship between mitochondrial events, bcl-2, and caspases is complex. However, bcl-2 appears to prevent release of mitochondrial components such as cytochrome *c* and AIF, which lead to caspase activity [73,74].

Bioenergetics and Aging

The most reliable and robust risk factor for neurodegenerative disease is normal aging. Normal aging is associated with the slow progressive development of physiologic deficits accompanied by a subtle degree of cognitive involvement. A leading theory as to the pathogenesis of aging is that it may arise from both mitochondrial dysfunction and increased free radical production [75,76]. Compelling evidence supporting this theory comes from studies of overexpression of the free radical scavenging enzymes Cu/Zn superoxide dismutase and catalase in fruit flies [77]. Overexpression of these enzymes increased longevity; increased functional activity and oxygen consumption; and decreased oxidative damage to protein, lipids, and DNA. Furthermore, caloric restriction, which consistently increases life span in experimental animals, is associated with reduced free radical generation and oxidative damage [78,79].

There is substantial evidence that mitochondrial function declines with age. This was studied in rat hepatocytes with direct measurements of the mitochondrial membrane potential [80]. These studies showed heterogeneity in mitochondrial membrane potential in old (20- to 28-month-old) rats as compared with young (3- to 5-month-old) rats. The older rats showed mitochondria with both a decline in mitochondrial membrane potential and an increase in free radical generation. We found a decline in activity of complex I and complex IV of the electron transport chain with normal aging in primate cortex [81].

It has been suggested that mitochondrial DNA (mtDNA) is more susceptible to oxidative damage and that it is repaired less efficiently. Studies of human fibroblasts treated with hydrogen peroxide showed threefold more damage to a fragment of mtDNA than to a fragment of nuclear DNA [82]. Furthermore, the mtDNA damage was much more persistent than nuclear DNA damage. A large number of studies showed that mtDNA deletions accumulate with normal aging in both animals and humans [75]. We found that there was a marked age-dependent accumulation of the oxidative DNA marker 8-hydroxy-2-deoxyguanosine in mtDNA isolated from human cerebral cortex [83].

An extremely interesting model of normal aging is accelerated aging, which occurs in prosimian primates [84]. These animals develop accelerated brain aging in early adult life characterized by gliosis and dystrophy of cholinergic axons at 10% of maximal life span and extensive cerebral amyloidosis starting at 50% of maximal life span. Consequently, these animals serve as a model for both accelerated aging and AD. These primates show mitochondrial abnormalities in the heart and proximal tubules by 1 year of age and, in the brain, degenerating mitochondrial profiles and axonal spheroids that are immunoreactive for manganese superoxide dismutase.

Cybrid Technology

A novel technique to investigate the role of mtDNA in disease processes was pioneered by King and Attardi [85]. This technique involves the transfer of mitochondria from living patients or cell lines to mitochondria-deficient cells (rho^0 cells) (Figure 12.3). Cell lines can be depleted of mtDNA by exposing them to low concentrations of ethidium bromide. Ethidium bromide is concentrated within mitochondria and intercalates into mtDNA at concentrations that inhibit replication of mitochondrial but not nuclear DNA. Exposed cells lose their mtDNA and assume an anaerobic phenotype. The cells become auxotrophic for uridine and pyruvate. Cybrids are cells formed by fusing mitochondria from a patient's platelets or other tissues with the rho^0 cells. Any cells that are not transformed are then eliminated by removing uridine and pyruvate from the media. Resulting cybrids enable determination of whether any observed defects in oxidative phosphorylation in a patient's tissues are attributable to alterations in

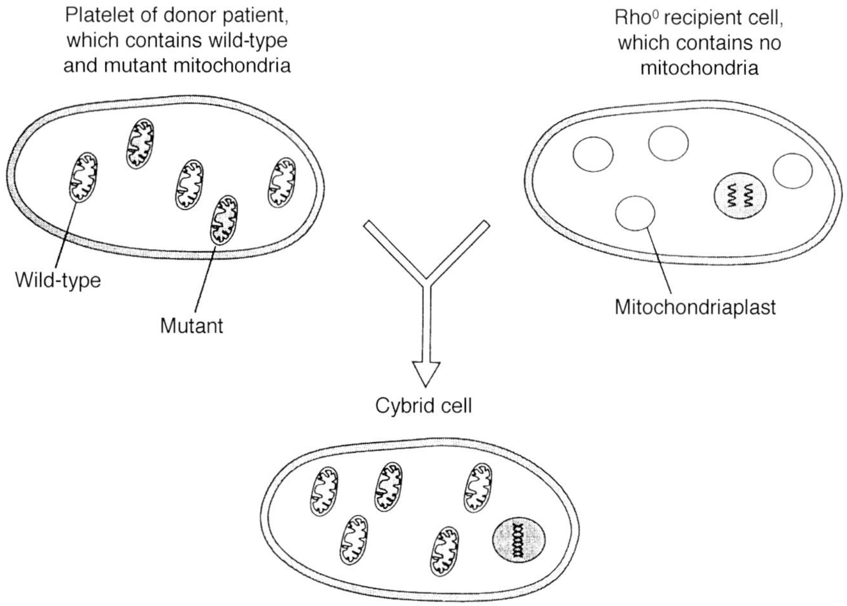

Figure 12.3 In the cybrid technique, mitochondria from a donor patient are transferred into a rho^0 recipient (mitochondrial DNA–free) cell. The resulting cybrid cell contains the patient's mitochondria in a new nuclear background. This technique may be used to determine whether observed defects in electron transport chain enzymes are attributable to mutations encoded by the donor patient's mitochondrial genome.

mtDNA, because the patient's mitochondria now function in the presence of a different nuclear genome.

Previous work demonstrated the usefulness of this technique in studying known mitochondrial disorders. It has been demonstrated that the mitochondrial defects that are associated with Leber's optic atrophy, Leigh's disease, MELAS syndrome (*m*itochondrial *e*ncephalopathy, *l*actic *a*cidosis, and *s*troke-like episodes), and MERRF syndrome (*m*yoclonus with *e*pilepsy and *r*agged-*r*ed *f*ibers) can be transferred from patients' platelets or fibroblasts into rho^0 cells [86–90]. After transfer of the mitochondria, these cell lines demonstrate defects in oxidative phosphorylation attributable to mtDNA mutations. This technique is, therefore, one of great potential usefulness in assessing the role of mtDNA defects in both normal aging and neurodegenerative diseases, including AD and PD. One study used the cybrid technology to obtain convincing evidence for mtDNA defects with normal aging in humans. Laderman and colleagues took mtDNA from fibroblasts of normal individuals aged 20 weeks to 103 years [91]. After transferring the mtDNA into rho^0 cells, the ensuing cybrid cell lines showed age-dependent decreases in oxygen consumption. There was also an age-dependent decrease in mtDNA content, but this did not correlate with oxygen consumption. These findings are consistent with the possibility that age-dependent accumulation of structural damage to the mitochondrial genome occurs in normal aging and has functional consequences.

NEURODEGENERATIVE DISEASES

Alzheimer's Disease

AD is the most common neurodegenerative disease. The most important risk factor is advancing age [92]. The illness occurs in a familial form, which is autosomal dominantly inherited, and as an apparently sporadic illness. Familial autosomal dominant AD accounts for approximately 5% of all cases (see Chapter 6). In the remaining apparently sporadic cases of AD, there is two and one-half- to threefold increased risk in families; however, there is no clear-cut pattern of inheritance. If mitochondrial defects play a role in this form of AD, one would expect that there would be evidence for maternal inheritance because the mitochondrial genome is inherited solely from the mother. Studies have suggested that indeed this is the case. These studies showed an increase in female to male ratio in the parental generation of AD probands [93,94]. In a group of families in which there was both an affected parent as well as at least two affected siblings, the ratio of mothers to fathers in the parental generation was 9 to 1 [94]. A sporadic inheritance pattern, familial association, and evidence for maternal transmission are therefore features that occur in both AD and known mitochondrial genetic diseases.

Evidence for metabolic defects in AD comes from a number of approaches. Studies using positron emission tomography (PET) have consistently shown reduced glucose metabolism in the temporoparietal regions of AD patients, which occurs quite early in the disease course (see Chapter 9). Furthermore, PET studies show increased oxygen utilization in comparison to glucose utilization [95]. This latter observation has been confirmed with direct measurements in arterial and jugular venous samples [96,97]. Abnormal glucose metabolism was also observed in brain biopsies and was interpreted as partial uncoupling of mitochondria [98]. Some studies using phosphorous magnetic resonance spectroscopy (MRS) have observed abnormalities in either phosphocreatine or P_i in AD patients as compared to elderly controls [99–101].

Initial studies of the electron transport enzymes in AD showed reduced complex IV activity in platelets [102]. This finding was initially contested but was subsequently confirmed in a follow-up study [103,104]. Three groups of authors including ours have reported that there is reduced COX activity in postmortem cerebral tissue of AD patients [105–107] (Figure 12-4). A study of highly purified mitochondria from AD brain tissue showed reduced catalytic activity yet normal amounts of cytochrome aa_3, suggesting that reduced complex IV activity is a consequence of abnormal catalytic activity rather than of decreased enzyme levels.

The cybrid technique has been used to demonstrate that the COX defects in AD appear to be encoded by mtDNA mutations in COX [108]. Research has found that COX defects can be transferred to cybrids from AD platelets and that the ensuing cybrid cell lines show markedly increased free radical production. Because there are three mtDNA-encoded subunits of COX, these were investigated for point mutations. The three mtDNA COX genes (*COX*) were sequenced from AD and cognitively normal age-matched controls. Polymorphisms were reported in the *COX1* and *COX2* genes that segregated with a majority of AD patients [108]. More recent work, however, has established that these polymorphisms are present in a nuclear pseudogene, which is a fragment of mitochondrial DNA incorporated

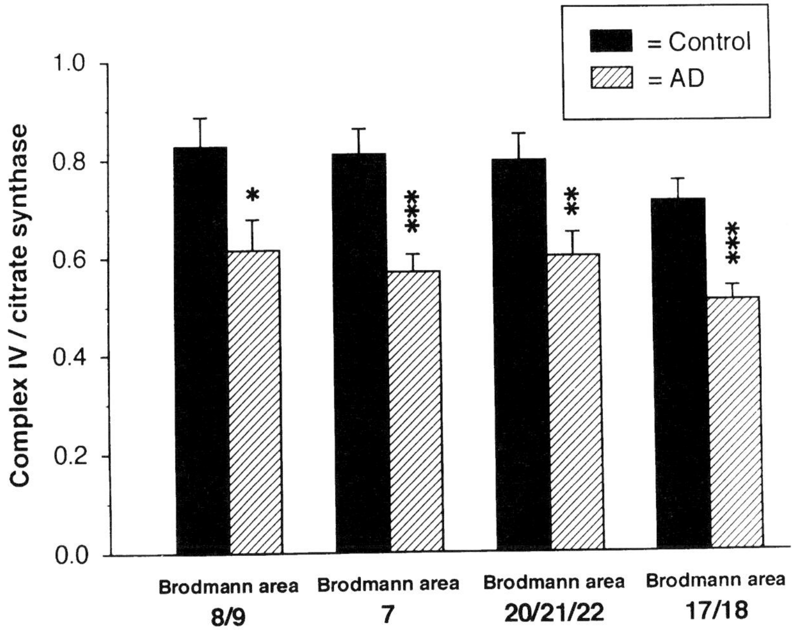

Figure 12.4 Cytochrome oxidase activity in four regions of Alzheimer's Disease (AD) cerebral cortex showing 25–30% reductions as compared with normal controls. (*P <.05; **P <.01; ***P <.001.)

into the nuclear genome early in evolution [109,110]. The cause of reduced COX activity in AD cybrids therefore requires further investigation.

The consequences of COX defects in the cybrid cell lines and intracellular calcium buffering have been examined. The AD cybrid shows elevated basal cytosolic calcium concentrations as well as enhanced sensitivity to inositol 1,4,5- triphosphate–mediated calcium release [111]. It also recovers more slowly from the increased calcium levels. These findings are consistent with earlier observations in AD fibroblasts [112–114]. They are also consistent with the finding of decreased calcium uptake in mitochondria from AD fibroblasts [115]. Impaired calcium buffering is also observed in fibroblasts from patients with the known mitochondrial disorder MELAS syndrome [116].

If mitochondrial defects truly play a central role in the pathogenesis of AD, then one might expect increased oxidative damage as a consequence. mtDNA might be expected to be particularly susceptible because it is located close to the inner mitochondrial membrane. Consistent with this possibility is a threefold increase in the 8-hydroxy-2-deoxyguanosine content of mtDNA in AD postmortem tissue as compared with age-matched controls [117]. In other studies, increased tissue concentrations of malondialdehyde and protein carbonyl groups have been reported [75,118]. Novel spin-trapping techniques showed increased oxidative damage to both lipids and proteins [119]. There is accumulating evidence for oxidative damage at the cellular level. Neurofibrillary tangle–bearing neurons show immunostaining with antibodies to advanced glycation end products, heme oxygenase-1, malondialdehyde, 4-hydroxynonenal, protein carbonyl groups, carbonylated neurofilaments, and 3-nitrotyrosine [120–128]. Interestingly, these antibodies tend to show increased staining in cell bodies and neurites rather than in senile plaques, suggesting an intracellular source of free radicals.

The pathologic hallmarks of AD are a deposition of amyloid in the form of senile plaques as well as the accumulation of neurofibrillary tangles in neurons. An impairment of COX activity with increased free radical production may play a role in both of these pathologic manifestations. There is evidence that impairment of COX in vitro leads to an increase in C-terminal fragments of the amyloid precursor protein, which contain the beta-amyloid (Aβ) peptide [129]. An increase in intracellular $A\beta_{1-42}$ was found after exposure of cultured guinea pig neurons to H_2O_2, and oxidative stress increased Aβ in mammalian lens tissue [130,131]. An increase in intracellular Aβ was also observed in cultured astrocytes from Down syndrome patients, whose cultured neurons and astrocytes generate free radicals [132]. Oxidative damage also leads to cross-linking and impaired solubility of Aβ, which could contribute to its deposition [133,134]. Preliminary evidence suggests that AD cybrids produce increased levels of cellular and extracellular Aβ, which correlate with decreases in COX activity [105].

An impairment of mitochondrial function and increased free radical production can contribute to both apoptotic and necrotic cell death. There is increasing evidence for the occurrence of apoptotic cell death in AD postmortem tissue [135,136]. Much of this evidence comes from studies demonstrating DNA strand breaks, although these cannot be considered absolutely specific for apoptosis. Oxidative injury has also been shown to lead to intramolecular cross-bridges and covalent bonds that could contribute to the generation of paired helical filaments [137,138].

Parkinson's Disease

A large body of evidence has implicated both mitochondrial dysfunction as well as increased free radical production in the pathogenesis of PD (see Chapter 4). Much of the interest was fostered by the development of an animal model of PD using the compound 1-methyl-4-phenyl-1,2,3,6-tetrahydropyridine (MPTP) [139]. This compound was associated with parkinsonism in humans and was subsequently shown to cause characteristic clinical and histopathologic features of PD in nonhuman primates. MPTP produces dopamine depletion and nigral cell loss in mice. It is converted to 1-methyl-4-phenylpyridinium (MPP^+) by monoamine oxidase B. MPP^+ is then taken up by the dopamine transporter and accumulates in mitochondria, where it inhibits complex I activity by binding reversibly to a site near the rotenone binding site. MPP^+ toxicity is associated with oxidative damage. Both MPP^+ in vitro and MPTP in vivo can induce apoptotic cell death [140].

The most consistent defect in oxidative phosphorylation in PD is reduced complex I activity [75]. Several studies have shown reduced complex I activity in the substantia nigra of PD brains but not in other brain regions, whereas three well-controlled studies showed reduced complex I activity in platelets from PD patients, including unmedicated patients [102,141,142]. We found that coenzyme Q_{10} (ubiquinone) levels are reduced in PD platelets, and this correlates with reduced complex I activity [143]. Some studies have shown reduced complex I activity in skeletal muscle and lymphocytes; however, this observation has been less consistent. A reduction in immunostaining for subunits of complex I and for alpha-ketoglutarate dehydrogenase has been shown in the substantia nigra of PD patients [144,145].

To investigate whether the observed complex I deficits were due to defects in mtDNA, the cybrid technique was applied to PD platelet mitochondria. After transfer of platelet mitochondria to produce cybrid cell lines, more complex I deficits were found in PD patients as compared with normal controls [146]. There was an increase in free radical production as well as increased vulnerability to apoptotic cell death. A transfer of complex I defects from PD platelet mitochondria to cybrids has also been found by Shapira and colleagues. Furthermore, the cybrid cell lines showed increased vulnerability to MPP^+, and they show impaired calcium buffering similar to the defects seen in AD cybrids [111].

If a mtDNA defect plays a role in the pathogenesis of PD, there should be some evidence for maternal inheritance. One study demonstrated that there was indeed evidence for maternal inheritance in certain families [147]. In five families in which a parent and multiple siblings had PD, the affected parent was the mother.

There is substantial evidence for oxidative damage in PD based on studies showing increases in both malondialdehyde and cholesterol ester hydroperoxides in the substantia nigra [148]. Furthermore, concentrations of 8-hydroxydeoxyguanosine (8-OHdG) are increased threefold to fourfold in the caudate and substantia nigra of PD patients [149]. An increase in 8-hydroxyguanine in the substantia nigra was confirmed, but other oxidative markers of DNA damage showed no changes [150]. A widespread increase in protein carbonyls in PD patient brains was also reported [151]. Reduced concentrations of glutathione are found in the substantia nigra of both PD patients and patients with incidental Lewy body disease [148,152,153], in which decreased glutathione may indicate a presymptomatic phase of PD. Increased nitrosyl complexes were found in PD patient substantia nigra [154]. Immunohistochemical studies showed increased 4-hydroxynonenal protein adducts, a marker of lipid peroxidation in substantia nigra neurons in PD patients [155]. Lastly, Lewy bodies stain with antibodies to heme oxygenase-1 and advanced glycation end products [156]. Despite good evidence for mitochondrial defects and oxidative damage, there is still no unequivocal evidence for apoptosis in PD [157,158].

Amyotrophic Lateral Sclerosis

ALS is a prototypical neurodegenerative disease of late life characterized by progressive muscle weakness, atrophy, and spasticity [159]. It leads to paralysis and death within 3–5 years of onset. The characteristic neuropathologic features are loss of anterior horn motor neurons and degeneration of the corticospinal tracts. In the motor neurons, abnormal accumulations of neurofilaments are found, as well as proximal axonal swelling [160]. Ninety percent of ALS cases are apparently sporadic, with no identifiable genetic or environmental risk factors. The remaining 10% of cases show familial inheritance (FALS). A major advance in the understanding of ALS was the identification of point mutations in the enzyme superoxide dismutase (SOD) in approximately 25% of patients who have FALS [1]. The illness in these families is inherited in an autosomal dominant fashion. More than 60 mutations have now been associated with the disease.

The observation that mutations in SOD cause familial ALS suggested that oxidative injury might be playing a role in its pathogenesis. The initial speculation that there might be a loss of function of the enzyme has not been borne out. A number of factors argue that the disease arises from an adverse gain of function from the mutant protein. These include the dominant inheritance pattern in FALS, the lack of correlation between enzyme activity and disease severity [161], and the observation that overexpression of the mutant enzyme in transgenic mice leads to motor neuron degeneration [162–164]. With rare exceptions, the mutations occur outside the active site of the enzyme: All mutations studied to date appear to alter the stability of the protein backbone and reduce the half-life of the molecule [165]. These changes may relax the conformation of the active channel, thereby allowing increased access of H_2O_2 or $ONOO^-$ to the active-site copper. This effect is predicted to increase generation of hydroxyl radicals or nitronium ions that can nitrate proteins [166]. Two in vitro studies show that SOD with two different familial ALS mutations generates increased amounts of hydroxyl radicals as compared to the amount produced by the wild-type molecule [167,168].

In sporadic ALS (SALS), there has been evidence to suggest impairment of energy metabolism. Reduced glucose metabolism has been observed in cerebral cortex of SALS patients using PET [169,170]. Although we did not find alterations in electron transport enzymes in SALS [171], heterogeneity in defects among patients could have obscured changes due to an averaging effect. Furthermore, abnormalities could be regionally specific or obscured by astrogliosis. Work using the cybrid technique showed the transfer of platelets from SALS patients into rho^0 cell lines was accompanied by mild decreases in complex I and IV activities, suggesting a defect encoded on the mitochondrial genome [146]. Furthermore, peripheral blood in lymphocytes from SALS patients shows increased cytosolic calcium and impaired responses to uncouplers of oxidative phosphorylation [172]. Ultrastructural studies of mitochondria and anterior horn cells from both FALS and SALS showed mitochondrial abnormalities [173–175]. Liver biopsy showed large mitochondria and intramitochondrial inclusions in SALS patients [176]. Mitochondria with abnormal protrusions were observed in a FALS patient who was later determined to have an *SOD1* mutation [175]. Studies of muscle biopsies of SALS patients show increased mitochondrial volume as well as increased calcium in the mitochondria [177]. There is evidence for oxidative damage in SALS patients. Protein carbonyl groups are increased in the motor cortex and spinal cord [171,178]. We measured concentrations of 3-nitrotyrosine and its major metabolite, 3-nitro-4-hydroxyphenylacetic acid, in the thoracic and lumbar spinal cord of both sporadic ALS and three FALS patients with *SOD* mutations [179]. Increased concentrations of both 3-nitrotyrosine and 3-nitro-4-hydroxyphenylacetic acid were found in both the sporadic and FALS patients. We also obtained evidence for oxidative damage at the cellular level. There was increased staining with antibodies to 3-nitrotyrosine, heme oxygenase-1, and malondialdehyde-modified protein in anterior horn cells of the spinal cord of SALS patients [180,181]. Similarly, there appears to be increased staining in the anterior horn cells of two FALS patients with *SOD1* mutations.

If mitochondrial dysfunction does indeed occur in ALS, it could contribute to the pathogenesis of the illness. One of the pathologic hallmarks is accumulation of neurofilaments. These can be cross-linked by oxidative damage. Furthermore, it has been speculated that 3-nitrotyrosine accumulation in the neurofilament light chain may impair normal aggregation of neurofilaments [166]. An energy defect may contribute to a slowing of axonal transport and thereby lead to accumulation of neurofilaments, which we observed in both SALS and FALS [160,173, 182]. A study of motor neurons in SALS patients showed an accumulation of mitochondria in proximal axons, a finding consistent with impaired axonal transport [173].

Huntington's Disease

The fundamental biochemical mechanism that underlies neuronal degeneration in HD is unknown. The gene defect consists of an expanded CAG repeat in a gene located on chromosome 4. The gene encodes the protein huntingtin, which is widely distributed in both peripheral tissues and in the central nervous system. Both the normal function of huntingtin and its role in the pathogenesis of neuronal degeneration in HD remain to be clarified. Evidence suggests that the disease mutation leads to a gain of function, causing cell type–specific neuronal degeneration predominantly in the striatum.

There is substantial evidence implicating defects in energy metabolism in HD. Decreased glucose metabolism using PET has been consistently shown in HD patients [75]. There also appears to be reduced glucose metabolism in some presymptomatic patients. We used proton MRS to demonstrate that there are elevated lactate concentrations in the occipital cortex and in the basal ganglia [183] (Figure 12.5). These increases occur in some but not all presymptomatic patients. There also appears to be increased lactate concentrations in both parietal and supplementary motor cortex. Other authors found increased lactate in frontal cortex as well as in occipital cortex and cerebellum [184,185]. We found a decrease in phosphocreatine to P_i ratio in resting gastrocnemius muscle of HD patients, providing evidence for a systemic defect in energy metabolism [186]. The latter observation is consistent with reports of progressive weight loss in HD patients despite increased caloric intake [187]. Cerebrospinal fluid (CSF) measurements show an increase in lactate to pyruvate ratios in HD subjects, which also may be indicative of an energy defect [186].

Prior studies examining enzymes of oxidative phosphorylation showed reduced succinate dehydrogenase activity [188,189]. One study showed a 55–60% decrease in complex II–III activity in HD caudate as well as a 33% decrease in complex IV activity [190]. We measured the enzymes of oxidative phosphorylation in the basal ganglia, two regions of cerebral cortex, and the cerebellum of HD patients [191]. Complex II–III activity was the most consistent deficit, with a reduction of 29% in the caudate and 67% in the putamen. Complex IV activity was also reduced 62% in the putamen but was spared in the caudate. Complex I activity and citrate synthase activities showed no changes. The finding of a decrease in complex II–III activity is of interest because an inherited defect in succinate dehydrogenase is associated with basal ganglia degeneration [192].

Results of studies of cultured fibroblasts from HD and control patients are consistent with a mitochondrial defect. Gutekunst and colleagues examined the consequence of calcium influx induced by ionomycin on mitochondrial membrane potential [193]. Normal fibroblasts showed depolarization followed by recovery,

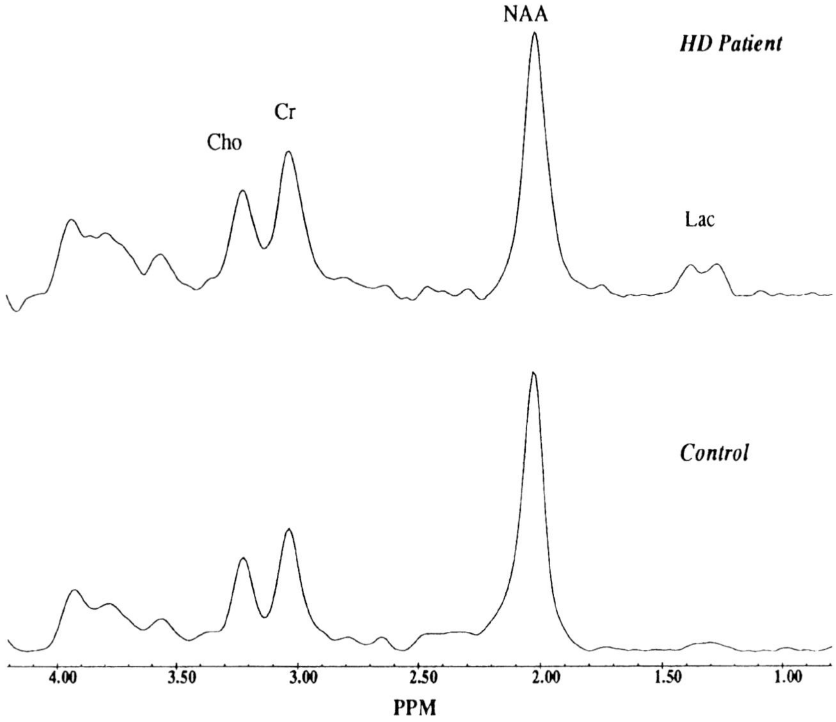

Figure 12.5 Comparison of proton magnetic resonance spectra from the occipital cortex in a patient with Huntington's disease (HD) and in a normal control. Spectra were processed with an exponential multiplication corresponding to a 3-Hz line-broadening (TR/TE/TM = 2,000/272/10). (Cho = choline; Cr = creatine; NAA = *N*-acetylaspartate; Lac = lactate; PPM = parts per million.)

but HD patient fibroblasts showed a failure to recover fully after the second application of ionomycin.

One proposed mechanism by which the HD gene defect could lead to impaired energy metabolism is by an interaction between huntingtin with glyceraldehyde-3-phosphate dehydrogenase (GAPDH), a critical component of the glycolytic pathway [194]. It was suggested that an increase in polyglutamine repeats in huntingtin could potentially inhibit this enzyme. We found that intrastriatal administration of the GAPDH inhibitor iodoacetate produces dose-dependent striatal excitotoxic lesions that correlate with inhibition of enzyme activity [195]. Our spectrophotometric assays of GAPDH activity in postmortem HD brain tissue, however, failed to show any significant differences compared to that in controls [191]. There are very few studies of oxidative damage in HD. In HD caudate, we found a significant 21% increase in 8-hydroxy-2-deoxyguanosine content in nuclear DNA [191]. In preliminary studies, we found a twofold significant increase in 8-OHdG content in mtDNA of HD parietal cortex. Initial immunohistochemical studies showed increased staining of striatal neurons of

HD patients with antibodies to heme oxygenase-1, 8-hydroxy-2-deoxyguanosine, and malondialdehyde-modified protein [196].

Animal models of neurologic diseases have proved useful in understanding pathogenesis. For instance, MPTP administration has been a dramatic success as a model of PD as discussed in the section on PD. We attempted to model HD with inhibitors of complex II–III function. One such inhibitor is 3-nitropropionic acid, which binds irreversibly to succinate dehydrogenase. Accidental ingestion of 3-nitropropionic acid in humans produces selective basal ganglia lesions and dystonia [197]. Systemic administration of 3-nitropropionic acid to nonhuman primates causes a movement disorder that closely resembles HD, with dystonia, choreiform movements, and loss of muscle tone [198]. Histologic evaluation shows basal ganglia degeneration with sparing of NADPH diaphorase interneurons, dendritic abnormalities in spiny neurons, and sparing of the nucleus accumbens. These striatal lesions are accompanied by both biochemical and histochemical evidence for increased oxidative damage.

Further evidence for a metabolic defect in HD comes from a transgenic animal model. Transgenic mice were bred by expressing a large number (130–140) of CAG repeats in exon 1 of the HD gene [199]. The mice develop normally for approximately 8 weeks, followed by onset of a movement disorder with tremors and subsequently seizures. The mice die at approximately 12 weeks of age. They do not show specific degeneration in the basal ganglia, but the brains appear small. A characteristic feature of these mice is a progressive weight loss starting at approximately 8 weeks of age despite increased caloric intake. This is consistent with observations in HD patients, who appear to have increased caloric expenditure [187].

Other Neurologic Diseases

A potential role of mitochondrial dysfunction in Friedreich's ataxia has been greatly strengthened by recent observations. Friedreich's ataxia is characterized by neurodegeneration and cardiomyopathy. The gene product was cloned and designated *frataxin*. Frataxin deficiency may occasionally be due to nonsense or missense point mutations, but the primary cause appears to be expansion of a polymorphic GAA trinucleotide repeat situated in the first intron of the corresponding gene on chromosome 9. This results in marked reduction in steady state level of mature frataxin mRNA. There appears to be a correlation between the regions of degeneration observed in the disease and sites of frataxin transcription, which is highest in the heart, spinal cord, and dorsal root ganglia. A gene from yeast is homologous to the human gene for frataxin protein [200]. This gene encodes a mitochondrial protein involved in iron homeostasis and respiratory function. Human frataxin was linked to green fluorescent protein and was shown to be a mitochondrial protein. These observations suggest that impaired function of this protein most likely leads to mitochondrial dysfunction in the ensuing disease process. It is also of interest that a Friedreich's ataxia–like syndrome with retinitis pigmentosa is caused by mutations in the alpha-tocopherol transfer protein [201]. This results in reduced concentrations of vitamin E. Neurologic symptoms include ataxia, dysarthria, hyporeflexia, and decreased proprioceptive and vibratory sensations. Because vitamin E is a well-characterized antioxidant, these findings suggest that oxidative injury can contribute to a phenotypic picture associated with Friedreich's ataxia.

Several cerebellar degenerations are also associated with an expansion of CAG repeats in proteins that have been designated *ataxins*. In spinocerebellar ataxia II, muscle biopsies show areas devoid of mitochondria or with focal accumulations as well as autophagic vacuoles that may contain mitochondria [202]. In spinocerebellar ataxia III (Machado-Joseph disease), there are abnormalities in ratios of CSF lactate to pyruvate, suggesting that there may be impaired energy metabolism [203]. A defect in platelet complex I activity was found in idiopathic dystonia [141,204]. Patients with Leber's optic atrophy with dystonia develop progressive basal ganglia degeneration. This illness has been demonstrated to be caused by a point mutation in the ND 6 subunit of complex I encoded on mtDNA [205].

THERAPEUTIC IMPLICATIONS

If a defect in energy metabolism underlies the pathogenesis of neurodegenerative diseases, then a reasonable therapeutic strategy would be to use compounds to improve mitochondrial function and thus compensate for disease-related defects. Coenzyme Q_{10} is an essential component of the electron transport chain, where it serves as an electron donor and acceptor. It is also a potent antioxidant, particularly in mitochondria. In vitro coenzyme Q_{10} protects against glutamate toxicity [206]. We demonstrated that coenzyme Q_{10} protects in a dose-dependent fashion against striatal lesions produced by the succinate dehydrogenase inhibitor malonate. It also protects against malonate-induced ATP depletions [207]. We also found that it protects against MPTP and 3-nitropropionic acid toxicity and obtained evidence that it prolongs survival in the transgenic mouse model of FALS (R. T. Matthews and M. F. Beal, unpublished data). Examination of its effects in HD patients showed that it produced significant 36% decreases in occipital cortex lactate concentrations as assessed by MRS [186]. After withdrawal of the coenzyme Q_{10} treatment, the lactate levels returned to baseline. In animal studies, coenzyme Q_{10} exerts additive effects with the NMDA antagonist MK-801 [208]. In view of these findings, a clinical trial has been started to examine the effects of coenzyme Q_{10} with or without an NMDA antagonist in the treatment of HD.

To the extent that oxidative damage contributes to neurodegenerative diseases, free radical scavengers might be useful in the treatment of these disorders. Free radical spin traps attenuate malonate, 3-nitropropionic acid, and MPTP neurotoxicity [209]. A critical mediator of oxidative damage may be $ONOO^-$ (see Nitric Oxide and Peroxynitrites, earlier). Mitochondrial dysfunction leads to increased $ONOO^-$ by increasing mitochondrial superoxide generation and raising cytosolic calcium levels, which then activate neuronal NOS. 7-Nitroindazole is a relatively selective neuronal NOS inhibitor. It dose-dependently blocks MPTP toxicity, and it also protects against both malonate and 3-nitropropionic acid toxicity [209,210]. Others also found that 7-nitroindazole protects against MPTP toxicity and extended our findings by showing that mice deficient in neuronal NOS due to genetic manipulation are resistant to MPTP toxicity [211]. We found profound neuroprotective effects against MPTP toxicity in baboons using 7-nitroindazole [212]. It prevented dopamine depletion, and loss of substantia nigra tyrosine hydroxylase–positive neurons, as well as the motor and cognitive deficits associated with MPTP toxicity in primates. We also demonstrated that another nNOS inhibitor, S-methylthiocitrulline protects against MPTP and malonate toxicity [195]. Mice deficient in neuronal NOS are resistant to MPP^+ toxicity as well as MPP^+-induced increases in 3-nitrotyrosine [213]. These findings raise the possibility that relatively selective NOS inhibitors might be useful in the treatment of neurodegenerative diseases.

Clinical findings using vitamin E to slow the progression of AD suggest that this is an effective therapeutic strategy [214] (see Chapter 13). Vitamin E or selegiline both slowed progression of AD as assessed by conversion to a higher clinical dementia rating score or by time to institutionalization. Epidemiologic findings that estrogen and anti-inflammatory drugs are also associated with a reduced incidence of AD could also be associated with the abilities of these compounds to inhibit free radical generation. Estrogens are known to have antioxidant effects, and anti-inflammatory agents could slow production of oxidants by microglial cells.

There is substantial evidence that neurotrophic factors protect against cell loss in animal models involving mitochondrial dysfunction [215]. Neurotrophic factors enhance the activities of free radical scavenging enzymes. They exert antioxidant effects in vivo. Other potentially useful therapeutic strategies are drugs that block glutamate release such as riluzole, which has been used in the treatment of ALS [216]. Direct-acting glutamate receptor antagonists acting at either the NMDA or AMPA site may also prove to be useful. These compounds are effective in blocking neurodegeneration produced by mitochondrial toxins in vivo.

CONCLUSION

Energy impairment leads to a complex series of interactions that involve excitotoxicity, impaired cellular calcium buffering, generation of free radicals, activation of NOS, activation of the mitochondrial permeability transition, and subsequent apoptotic or necrotic cell death. Evidence linking both AD and PD to mtDNA defects is increasing. The use of cybrid cell technology has greatly strengthened the evidence that mitochondrial defects play a fundamental role in these disease processes. There is also substantial evidence for oxidative damage in ALS. In HD, both animal models and direct assessment using MRS strongly suggest that there is indeed impaired energy metabolism as a consequence of the abnormal gene product. Recent evidence has linked Friedreich's ataxia to a mitochondrial protein associated with iron transport. If mitochondrial dysfunction and oxidative injury play a role in neurodegenerative diseases, then the prospects for a number of therapeutic interventions appear promising.

REFERENCES

1. Rosen DR, Siddique T, Patterson D, et al. Mutations in Cu/Zn superoxide dismutase gene are associated with familial amyotrophic lateral sclerosis. Nature 1993;362:59–62.
2. Beal MF. Does impairment of energy metabolism result in excitotoxic neuronal death in neurodegenerative illnesses? Ann Neurol 1992;31:119–130.

3. Albin RL, Greenamyre JT. Alternative excitotoxic hypotheses. Neurology 1992;42:733.
4. Novelli A, Reilly JA, Lysko PG, et al. Glutamate becomes neurotoxic via the *N*-methyl-D-aspartate receptor when intracellular energy levels are reduced. Brain Res 1988;451:205–212.
5. Zeevalk GD, Nicklas WJ. Chemically induced hypoglycemia and anoxia: relationship to glutamate receptor-mediated toxicity in retina. J Pharmacol Exp Ther 1990;253:1285–1292.
6. Zeevalk GD, Nicklas WJ. Mechanisms underlying initiation of excitotoxicity associated with metabolic inhibition. J Pharmacol Exp Ther 1991;257:870–878.
7. Choi DW. Ionic dependence of glutamate neurotoxicity. J Neurosci 1987;7:369–379.
8. Hartley A, Stone JM, Heron C, et al. Complex I inhibitors induced dose-dependent apoptosis in PC12 cells: relevance to Parkinson's disease. J Neurochem 1994;63:1987–1990.
9. Eimerl S, Schramm M. The quantity of calcium that appears to induce neuronal death. J Neurochem 1994;62:1223–1226.
10. Tymianski M, Wallace MC, Spigelman I, et al. Cell-permeant Ca^{2+} chelators reduce early excitotoxic and ischemic neuronal injury in vitro and in vivo. Neuron 1993;11:221–235.
11. Harrington J, Park YB, Babcock DF, et al. Dominant role of mitochondria in clearance of large Ca^{2+} loads from rat adrenal chromaffin cells. Neuron 1996;16:219–228.
12. Gunter TE, Gunter KK, Sheu SS, et al. Mitochondrial calcium transport: physiological and pathological relevance. Am J Physiol 1994;267:C313–C339.
13. Boveris A, Chance B. The mitochondrial generation of hydrogen peroxide. Biochem J 1973;134:707–716.
14. De Jong AMP, Albracht SPJ. Ubisemiquinones as obligatory intermediates in the electron transfer from NADH to ubiquinone. Eur J Biochem 1994;222:975–982.
15. Patole MS, Swaroop A, Ramasarma T. Generation of H_2O_2 in brain mitochondria. J Neurochem 1986;47:1–8.
16. Loschen G, Azzi A, Richter C, et al. Superoxide radicals as precursors of mitochondrial hydrogen peroxide. FEBS Lett 1974;42:68–72.
17. Hockenbery DM, Oltvai ZN, Yin XM, et al. Bcl-2 functions in an antioxidant pathway to prevent apoptosis. Cell 1993;75:241–251.
18. Albina JE, Cui S, Mateo RB, et al. Nitric oxide–mediated apoptosis in murine peritoneal macrophages. J Immunol 1993;150:5080–5085.
19. Dypbukt JM, Ankarcrona MMB, Sjoholm A, et al. Different prooxidant levels stimulate growth, trigger apoptosis, or produce necrosis of insulin-secreting RINm5F cells—the role of intracellular polyamines. J Biol Chem 1994;269:30553–30560.
20. Zhang Y, Marcillat O, Giulivi C, et al. The oxidative inactivation of mitochondrial electron transport chain components and ATPase. J Biol Chem 1990;265:16330–16336.
21. Fernandes RS, Cotter TG. Apoptosis and necrosis: intracellular levels of glutathione influence mode of cell death. Biochem Pharmacol 1994;48:675–681.
22. Rothstein JD, Bristol LA, Hosler B, et al. Chronic inhibition of superoxide dismutase produces apoptotic death of spinal neurons. Proc Natl Acad Sci U S A 1994;91:4155–4159.
23. Troy CM, Shelanski MI. Down-regulation of copper/zinc superoxide dismutase causes apoptotic death in PC12 neuronal cells. Proc Natl Acad Sci U S A 1994;91:6384–6387.
24. Bindokas VP, Jordan J, Lee CC, et al. Superoxide production in rat hippocampal neurons: selective imaging with hydroethidine. J Neurosci 1996;16:1324–1336.
25. Dugan LL, Sensi SL, Canzoniero LMT, et al. Mitochondrial production of reactive oxygen species in cortical neurons following exposure to *N*-methyl-D-aspartate. J Neurosci 1995;15:6377–6388.
26. Patel M, Day BJ, Crapo JD, et al. Requirement for superoxide in excitotoxic cell death. Neuron 1996; 16:345–355.
27. Reynolds IJ, Hastings TG. Glutamate induces the production of reactive oxygen species in cultured forebrain neurons following NMDA receptor activation. J Neurosci 1995;15:3318–3327.
28. Lafon-Cazal M, Pietri S, Culcasi M, et al. NMDA-dependent superoxide production and neurotoxicity. Nature 1993;364:535–537.
29. Schulz JB, Henshaw DR, Siwek D, et al. Involvement of free radicals in excitotoxicity in vivo. J Neurochem 1995;64:2239–2247.
30. Yue TL, Gu JL, Lysko PG, et al. Neuroprotective effects of phenyl-t-butyl-nitrone in gerbil global brain ischemia and in cultured rat cerebellar neurons. Brain Res 1992;574:193–197.
31. Monyer H, Hartley DM, Choi DW. 21-Aminosteroids attenuate excitotoxic neuronal injury in cortical cell cultures. Neuron 1990;5:121–126.
32. Chan PH, Chu L, Chen SF, et al. Attenuation of glutamate-induced neuronal swelling and toxicity in transgenic mice overexpressing human Cu/Zn-superoxide dismutase. Acta Neurochir 1990;51:245–247.
33. Dawson TM, Snyder SH. Gases as biologic messengers: nitric oxide and carbon monoxide in the brain. J Neurosci 1994;14:5147–5159.

34. Dawson VL, Dawson TM, London ED, et al. Nitric oxide mediates glutamate neurotoxicity in primary cortical cultures. Proc Natl Acad Sci U S A 1991;88:6368–6371.
35. Dawson TM, Steiner JP, Dawson VL, et al. Immunosuppressant FK506 enhances phosphorylation of nitric oxide synthase and protects against glutamate neurotoxicity. Proc Natl Acad Sci U S A 1993; 90:9808–9812.
36. Dawson VL, Kizushi VM, Huang PL, et al. Resistance to neurotoxicity in cortical cultures from neuronal nitric oxide synthase-deficient mice. J Neurosci 1996;16:2463–2478.
37. Huang Z, Huang PL, Panahian N, et al. Effects of cerebral ischemia in mice deficient in neuronal nitric oxide synthase. Science 1994;265:1883–1885.
38. Beckman JS, Crow JP. Pathological implications of nitric oxide superoxide and peroxynitrite formation. Biochem Soc Trans 1993;21:330–334.
39. Ischiropoulos H, Zhu L, Chen J, et al. Peroxynitrite-mediated tyrosine nitration catalyzed by superoxide dismutase. Arch Biochem Biophys 1992;298:431–437.
40. Crow JP, Spruell C, Chen J, et al. On the pH-dependent yield of hydroxyl radical products from peroxynitrite. Free Radic Biol Med 1994;16:331–338.
41. Beckman JS, Beckman TW, Chen J, et al. Apparent hydroxyl radical production by peroxynitrite: implications for endothelial injury from nitric oxide and superoxide. Proc Natl Acad Sci U S A 1990; 87:1620–1624.
42. Zoratti M, Szabo I. The mitochondrial permeability transition. Biochim Biophys Acta 1995;1241: 139–176.
43. Bernardi P, Broekemeier KM, Pfeiffer DR. Recent progress on regulation of the mitochondrial permeability transition pore; a cyclosporin-sensitive pore in the inner mitochondrial membrane. J Bioenerg Biomembr 1994;26:509–517.
44. Nicolli A, Basso E, Petronilli V, et al. Interactions of cyclophilin with the mitochondrial inner membrane and regulation of the permeability transition pore, a cyclosporin A-sensitive channel. J Biol Chem 1996;271:2185–2192.
45. Schinder AF, Olson EC, Spitzer NC, et al. Mitochondrial dysfunction is a primary event in glutamate neurotoxicity. J Neurosci 1996;16:6125–6133.
46. White RJ, Reynolds IJ. Mitochondria and Na^+/Ca^{2+} exchange buffer glutamate-induced calcium loads in cultured cortical neurons. J Neurosci 1995;15:1318–1328.
47. Ankarcrona M, Dypbukt JM, Orrenius S, et al. Calcineurin and mitochondrial function in glutamate-induced neuronal cell death. FEBS Lett 1996;394:321–324.
48. Shaham S, Horvitz HR. Developing caenorhabditis elegans neurons may contain both cell-death protective and killer activities. Genes Dev 1996;10:578–591.
49. Alnemri ES, Livingston DJ, Nicholson DW, et al. ICE/CED-3 protease nomenclature. Cell 1996;87:171.
50. Zamzami N, Marchetti P, Castedo M, et al. Sequential reduction of mitochondrial transmembrane potential and generation of reactive oxygen species in early programmed cell death. J Exp Med 1995; 182:367–377.
51. Zamzami N, Marchetti P, Castedo M, et al. Reduction in mitochondrial potential constitutes an early irreversible step of programmed lymphocyte death in vivo. J Exp Med 1995;181:1661–1672.
52. Petit PX, Lecoeur H, Zorn E, et al. Alterations in mitochondrial structure and function are early events of dexamethasone-induced thymocyte apoptosis. J Cell Biol 1995;130:157–167.
53. Castedo M, Hirsch T, Susin SA, et al. Sequential acquisition of mitochondrial and plasma membrane alterations during early lymphocyte apoptosis. J Immunol 1996;157:512–521.
54. Cossarizza A, Franceschi C, Monti D, et al. Protective effect of *N*-acetylcysteine in tumor necrosis factor-alpha–induced apoptosis in U937 cells: the role of mitochondria. Exp Cell Res 1995;220:232–240.
55. Deckwerth TL, Johnson EM. Temporal analysis of events associated with programmed cell death (apoptosis) of sympathetic neurons deprived of nerve growth factor (NGF). J Cell Biol 1993;123: 1207–1222.
56. Vayssiere JL, Petit PX, Risler Y, et al. Commitment to apoptosis is associated with changes in mitochondrial biogenesis and activity in cell lines conditionally immortalized with simian virus 40. Proc Natl Acad Sci U S A 1994;91:11752–11756.
57. Zamzami N, Susin SA, Marchetti P, et al. Mitochondrial control of nuclear apoptosis. J Exp Med 1996;183:1533–1544.
58. Marchetti P, Castedo M, Susin SA, et al. Mitochondrial permeability transition is a central coordinating event of apoptosis. J Exp Med 1996;184:1155–1160.
59. Liu X, Kim CN, Yang J, et al. Induction of apoptotic program in cell-free extracts: requirement for dATP and cytochrome *c*. Cell 1996;86:147–157.
60. Krippner A, Matsuno-Yagi A, Gottlieb RA, et al. Loss of function of cytochrome *c* in Jurkat cells undergoing Fas-mediated apoptosis. J Biol Chem 1996;271:21629–21636.

61. Susin SA, Zamzami N, Castedo M, et al. Bcl-2 inhibits the mitochondrial release of an apoptogenic protease. J Exp Med 1996;184:1331–1341.
62. Krajewski S, Tanaka S, Takayama S, et al. Investigations of the subcellular distribution of the bcl-2 oncoprotein: residence in the nuclear envelope, endoplasmic reticulum, and outer mitochondrial membrane. Cancer Res 1993;53:4701–4714.
63. Zhu W, Cowie A, Wasfy GW, et al. Bcl-2 mutants with restricted subcellular location reveal spatially distinct pathways for apoptosis in different cell types. EMBO J 1996;15:4130–4141.
64. Tanaka S, Salto K, Reed J. Structure-function analysis of the apoptosis-suppressing bcl-2 oncoprotein: substitution of a heterologous transmembrane domain restores function to truncated bcl-2 proteins. J Biol Chem 1993;268:10920–10926.
65. Nguyen M, Branton P, Walton P, et al. Role of membrane anchor domain of bcl-2 in suppression of apoptosis caused by E1B-defective adenovirus. J Biol Chem 1994;269:16521–16524.
66. Batty G, Miyashita T, Williamson JR, et al. Apoptosis induced by withdrawal of interleukin-3 (H-3) and an H-3-dependent hematopoietic cell line is associated with repartitioning of intracellular calcium and is blocked by enforced Bcl-2 oncoprotein production. J Biol Chem 1993;268:6511–6519.
67. Hennet T, Bertoni G, Richter C, et al. Expression of Bcl-2 protein enhances the survival of mouse fibrosarcoid cells in tumor necrosis factor-mediated cytotoxicity. Cancer Res 1993;53:1456–1460.
68. Murphy AN, Bredesen DE, Cortopassi G, et al. Bcl-2 potentiates the maximal calcium uptake capacity of neural cell mitochondria. Proc Natl Acad Sci U S A 1996;93:9893–9898.
69. Smets LA, Van der Berg J, Acton D, et al. BCL-2 expression and mitochondrial activity in leukemic cells with different sensitivity to glucocorticoid-induced apoptosis. Blood 1994;84:1613–1619.
70. Kane DJ, Sarafian TA, Anton R, et al. Bcl-2 inhibition of neural death: decreased generation of reactive oxygen species. Science 1993;262:1274–1277.
71. Hockenbery DM, Oltvai ZN, Yin XM, et al. Bcl-2 functions in an antioxidant pathway to prevent apoptosis. Cell 1993;75:241–251.
72. Myers KM, Fiskum G, Liu Y, et al. Bcl-2 protects neural cells from cyanide/aglycemia-induced lipid oxidation, mitochondrial injury, and loss of viability. J Neurochem 1995;65:2432–2440.
73. Chinnaiyan AM, Orth K, O'Rourke K, et al. Molecular ordering of the cell death pathway. J Biol Chem 1996;271:4573–4576.
74. Boulakia C, Chen G, Ng FWH, et al. Bcl-2 and adenovirus E1B 19 kDa protein prevent E1A-induced processing of CPP32 and cleavage of poly(ADP-ribose) polymerase. Oncogene 1996;12:29–36.
75. Beal MF. Aging, energy and oxidative stress in neurodegenerative diseases. Ann Neurol 1995;38:357–366.
76. Shigenaga MK, Hagen TM, Ames BN. Oxidative damage and mitochondrial decay in aging. Proc Natl Acad Sci U S A 1994;91:10771–10778.
77. Orr WC, Sohal RS. Extension of life-span by overexpression of superoxide dismutase and catalase in *Drosophila melanogaster*. Science 1994;263:1128–1130.
78. Kaneko T, Tahara S, Matsuo M. Retarding effect of dietary restriction on the accumulation of 8-hydroxy-2'-deoxyguanosine in organs of Fischer 344 rats during aging. Free Radic Biol Med 1997; 23:76–81.
79. Sohal RS, Weindruch R. Oxidative stress, caloric restriction, and aging. Science 1996;273:59–63.
80. Hagen TM, Yowe DL, Bartholomew JC, et al. Mitochondrial decay in hepatocytes from old rats: membrane potential declines, heterogeneity and oxidants increase. Proc Natl Acad Sci U S A 1997; 94:3064–3069.
81. Bowling AC, Mutisya E, Walker LC, et al. Age-dependent impairment of mitochondrial function in primate brain. J Neurochem 1993;60:1964–1967.
82. Yakes FM, Van Houten B. Mitochondrial DNA damage is more extensive and persists longer than nuclear DNA damage in human cells following oxidative stress. Proc Natl Acad Sci U S A 1997;94: 514–519.
83. Mecocci P, MacGarvey U, Kaufman AE, et al. Oxidative damage to mitochondrial DNA shows marked age-dependent increases in human brain. Ann Neurol 1993;34:609–616.
84. Schmechel DE, Burkhart DS, Ange R, et al. Cholinergic axonal dystrophy and mitochondrial pathology in prosimian primates. Exp Neurol 1996;142:111–127.
85. King MP, Attardi G. Human cells lacking mtDNA: repopulation with exogenous mitochondria by complementation. Science 1989;246:500–503.
86. Enriquez JA, Chomyn A, Attardi G. MtDNA mutation in MERRF syndrome causes defective aminoacylation of tRNA (Lys) and premature translation termination. Nature Genet 1995;10:47–55.
87. Hofhaus G, Johns DR, Hurko O, et al. Respiration and growth defects in transmitochondrial cell lines carrying the 11778 mutation associated with Leber's hereditary optic neuropathy. J Biol Chem 1996;271:13155–13161.

88. Jun AS, Trounce IA, Brown MD, et al. Use of transmitochondrial cybrids to assign a complex I defect to the mitochondrial DNA-encoded NADH dehydrogenase subunit 6 gene mutation at nucleotide pari 14459 that causes Leber hereditary optic neuropathy and dystonia. Mol Cell Biol 1996;16:771–777.
89. King MP, Koga Y, Davidson M, Schon EA. Defects in mitochondrial protein synthesis and respiratory chain activity segregate with the tRNA(Leu(UUR)) mutation associated with mitochondrial myopathy, encephalopathy, lactic acidosis, and strokelike episodes. Mol Cell Biol 1992;12:480–490.
90. Trounce I, Neill S, Wallace DC. Cytoplasmic transfer of mtDNA nt 8993 T→G (ATP6) point mutation associated with Leigh syndrome into mtDNA-less cells demonstrates cosegregation with a decrease in state III respiration and ADP/O ratio. Proc Natl Acad Sci U S A 1994;91:8334–8338.
91. Laderman KA, Penny JR, Mazzucchelli F, et al. Aging-dependent functional alterations of mitochondrial DNA (mtDNA) from human fibroblasts transferred into mtDNA-less cells. J Biol Chem 1996;271:15891–15897.
92. Evans DA, Funkenstein HH, Albert MS, et al. Prevalence of Alzheimer's disease in a community population of older persons. JAMA 1989;262:2551–2556.
93. Duara R, Lopez-Alberola RF, Barker WW, et al. A comparison of familial and sporadic Alzheimer's disease. Neurology 1993;43:1377–1384.
94. Edland SD, Silverman JM, Peskind ER, et al. Increased risk of dementia in mothers of Alzheimer's disease cases: evidence for maternal inheritance. Neurology 1996;47:254–256.
95. Fukuyama H, Ogawa M, Yamauchi H, et al. Altered cerebral energy metabolism in Alzheimer's disease: a PET study. J Nucl Med 1994;35:1–6.
96. Ogawa M, Fukuyama H, Ouchi Y, et al. Altered energy metabolism in Alzheimer's disease. J Neurol Sci 1996;139:78–82.
97. Hoyer S. Intermediary metabolism disturbance in AD/SDAT and its relation to molecular events. Prog Neuropsychopharmacol Biol Psychiatry 1993;17:199–228.
98. Sims NR, Finegan JM, Blass JP, et al. Mitochondrial function in brain tissue in primary degenerative dementia. Brain Res 1987;436:30–38.
99. Smith MA, Rudnicka-Nawrot M, Richey PL, et al. Carbonyl-related posttranslational modification of neurofilament protein in the neurofibrillary pathology of Alzheimer's disease. J Neurochem 1995;64:2660–2666.
100. Pettegrew JW, Klunk WE, Kanal E, et al. Changes in brain membrane phospholipid and high-energy phosphate metabolism precede dementia. Neurobiol Aging 1995;16:973–975.
101. Brown GG, Levine SR, Gorell JM, et al. In vivo ^{31}P NMR profiles of Alzheimer disease and multiple subcortical infarct dementia. Neurology 1989;39:1423–1427.
102. Parker WD Jr, Boyson SJ, Parks JK. Abnormalities of the electron transport chain in idiopathic Parkinson's disease. Ann Neurol 1989;26:719–723.
103. Van Zuylen AJ, Bosman GJ, Ruitenbeek W, et al. No evidence for reduced thrombocyte cytochrome oxidase activity in Alzheimer's disease. Neurology 1992;42:1246–1247.
104. Parker WD, Parks J, Filley CM, et al. Electron transport chain defects in Alzheimer's disease brain. Neurology 1994;44:1090–1096.
105. Parker WD, Davis RE. Primary Mitochondrial DNA Defects as a Causative Event in Alzheimer's Disease. In MF Beal, N Howell, I Bodis-Wollner (eds), Mitochondria and Free Radicals in Neurodegenerative Diseases. New York: Wiley-Liss, 1997;319–333.
106. Mutisya EM, Bowling AC, Beal MF. Cortical cytochrome oxidase activity is reduced in Alzheimer's disease. J Neurochem 1994;63:2179–2184.
107. Kish SJ, Bergeron C, Rajput A, et al. Brain cytochrome oxidase in Alzheimer's disease. J Neurochem 1992;59:776–779.
108. Davis RE, Miller S, Hermstadt C, et al. Mutations in mitochondrial cytochrome *c* oxidase genes segregate with late-onset Alzheimer's disease. Proc Natl Acad Sci U S A 1997;94:4526–4531.
109. Hirano M, Shtilbans A, Mayeux R, et al. Apparent mtDNA heteroplasmy in Alzheimer's disease patients and in normals due to PCR amplification of nucleus-embedded mtDNA pseudogenes. Proc Natl Acad Sci U S A 1997;94:14894–14899.
110. Wallace DC, Stugard C, Murdock D, et al. Ancient mtDNA sequences in the human nuclear genome: a potential source of errors in identifying pathogenic mutations. Proc Natl Acad Sci U S A 1997; 94:14900–14905.
111. Sheehan JP, Swerdlow RH, Miller SW, et al. Calcium homeostasis and reactive oxygen species production in cells transformed by mitochondria from individuals with sporadic Alzheimer's disease. J Neurosci 1997;17:4612–4622.
112. Ito E, Kotaro O, Etcheberrigaray R, et al. Internal Ca^{2+} mobilization is altered in fibroblasts from patients with Alzheimer disease. Proc Natl Acad Sci U S A 1994;91:534–538.

113. Huang HM, Toral-Barza L, Thaler H, et al. Inositol phosphates and intracellular calcium after bradykinin stimulation in fibroblasts from young, normal aged and Alzheimer donors. Neurobiol Aging 1991;12:469–473.
114. Gibson GE, Zhang H, Toral-Barza L, et al. Calcium stores in cultured fibroblasts and their changes with Alzheimer's disease. Biochim Biophys Acta 1996;1316:71–77.
115. Kumar U, Dunlop D, Richardson JC. Mitochondria from Alzheimer's fibroblasts show decreased uptake of calcium and increased sensitivity to free radicals. Life Sci 1994;54:1855–1860.
116. Moudy AM, Handran SD, Goldberg MP, et al. Abnormal calcium homeostasis and mitochondrial polarization in a human encephalomyopathy. Proc Natl Acad Sci U S A 1995;92:729–733.
117. Mecocci P, MacGarvey U, Beal MF. Oxidative damage to mitochondrial DNA is increased in Alzheimer's disease. Ann Neurol 1994;36:747–751.
118. Lyras L, Cairns NJ, Jenner A, et al. An assessment of oxidative damage to proteins, lipids, and DNA in brain from patients with Alzheimer's disease. J Neurochem 1997;68:2061–2069.
119. Hensley K, Hall N, Subramaniam R, et al. Brain regional correspondence between Alzheimer's disease histopathology and biomarkers of protein oxidation. J Neurochem 1995;65:2146–2156.
120. Smith CD, Pettigrew LC, Avison MJ, et al. Frontal lobe phosphorus metabolism and neuropsychological function in aging and in Alzheimer's disease. Ann Neurol 1995;38:194–201.
121. Smith MA, Perry G, Richey PL, et al. Oxidative damage in Alzheimer's. Nature 1996;382:120–121.
122. Smith MA, Kutty RK, Richey PL, et al. Heme oxygenase-1 is associated with the neurofibrillary pathology of Alzheimer's disease. Am J Pathol 1994;145:42–47.
123. Smith MA, Richey Harris PL, Sayre LM, et al. Widespread peroxynitrite-mediated damage in Alzheimer's disease. J Neurosci 1997;17:2653–2657.
124. Yan SD, Chen X, Schmidt AM, et al. Glycated *tau* protein in Alzheimer disease: a mechanism for induction of oxidant stress. Proc Natl Acad Sci U S A 1994;91:7787–7791.
125. Good PF, Werner P, Hsu A, et al. Evidence for neuronal oxidative damage in Alzheimer's disease. Am J Pathol 1996;149:21–28.
126. Premkumar DRD, Smith MA, Richey PL, et al. Induction of heme oxygenase-1 mRNA and protein in neocortex and cerebral vessels in Alzheimer's disease. J Neurochem 1995;65:1399–1402.
127. Sayre LM, Zelasko DA, Harris PLR, et al. 4-Hydroxynonenal-derived advanced lipid peroxidation end products are increased in Alzheimer's disease. J Neurochem 1997;68:2092–2097.
128. Schipper HM, Cisse S, Stopa EG. Expression of heme oxygenase-1 in the senescent and Alzheimer-diseased brain. Ann Neurol 1995;37:758–768.
129. Gabuzda D, Busciglio J, Chen LB, et al. Inhibition of energy metabolism alters the processing of amyloid precursor protein and induces a potentially amyloidogenic derivative. J Biol Chem 1994;269: 13623–13628.
130. Frederikse PH, Garland D, Zigler JS, et al. Oxidative stress increases production of β-amyloid (Aβ) in mammalian lenses, and Aβ has toxic effects on lens epithelial cells. J Biol Chem 1996;271:10169–10174.
131. Ohyagi Y, Younkin SG. Hydrogen peroxide induces Aβ accumulation in neurons. Soc Neurosci Abst 1996;22:1207.
132. Busciglio J, Yankner BA. Apoptosis and increased generation of reactive oxygen species in Down's syndrome neurons in vitro. Nature 1995;378:776–779.
133. Dyrks T, Dyrks E, Masters CL, et al. Amyloidogenicity of rodent and human βA4 sequences. FEBS Lett 1993;324:231–236.
134. Dyrks T, Dyrks E, Hartmann T, et al. Amyloidogenicity of βA4 and βA4-bearing amyloid protein precursor fragments by metal-catalyzed oxidation. J Biol Chem 1992;267:18210–18217.
135. Su JH, Satou T, Anderson AJ, et al. Up-regulation of Bcl-2 is associated with neuronal DNA damage in Alzheimer's disease. Neuroreport 1996;7:437–440.
136. Su JH, Deng G, Cotman CW. Bax protein expression is increased in Alzheimer's brain: correlations with DNA damage, Bcl-2 expression, and brain pathology. J Neuropathol Exp Neurol 1997;56:86–93.
137. Troncoso JC, Sukhov RR, Kawas CH, et al. In situ labeling of dying cortical neurons in normal aging and in Alzheimer's disease: correlations with senile plaques and disease progression. J Neuropathol Exp Neurol 1996;55:1134–1142.
138. Schweers O, Mandelkow EM, Biernat J, Mandelkow E. Oxidation of cysteine-322 in the repeat domain of microtubule-associated protein *tau* controls the in vitro assembly of paired helical filaments. Proc Natl Acad Sci U S A 1995;92:8463–8467.
139. Bloem BR, Irwin I, Buruma OJS, et al. The MPTP model: versatile contributions to the treatment of idiopathic Parkinson's disease. J Neurol Sci 1990;97:273–293.
140. Tatton NA, Kish SJ. In situ detection of apoptotic nuclei in the substantia nigra compacta of 1-methyl-4-phenyl-1,2,3,6-tetrahydropyridine-treated mice using terminal deoxynucleotidyl transferase labelling and acridine orange staining. Neuroscience 1997;77:1037–1048.

141. Benecke R, Strumper P, Weiss H. Electron transfer complex I defect in idiopathic dystonia. Ann Neurol 1992;32:683–686.
142. Haas RH, Nasirian F, Nakano K, et al. Low platelet mitochondrial complex I and complex II/III activity in early untreated Parkinson's disease. Ann Neurol 1995;37:714–722.
143. Schults CW, Haas RH, Passov D, et al. Coenzyme Q_{10} is reduced in mitochondria from parkinsonian patients. Ann Neurol 1997;42:261–264.
144. Mizuno Y, Matuda S, Yoshino H, et al. An immunohistochemical study on α-ketoglutarate dehydrogenase complex in Parkinson's disease. Ann Neurol 1994;35:204–210.
145. Hattori N, Tanaka M, Ozawa T, et al. Immunohistochemical studies on complexes I, II, III and IV of mitochondria in Parkinson's disease. Ann Neurol 1991;30:563–571.
146. Swerdlow RH, Parks JK, Miller SW, et al. Origin and functional consequences of the complex I defect in Parkinson's disease. Ann Neurol 1996;40:663–671.
147. Wooten GF, Currie LJ, Bennett JP, et al. Maternal inheritance in Parkinson's disease. Ann Neurol 1997;41:265–268.
148. Dexter DT, Sian J, Rose S, et al. Indices of oxidative stress and mitochondrial function in individuals with incidental Lewy body disease. Ann Neurol 1994;35:38–44.
149. Sanchez-Ramos JR, Overvik E, Ames BN. A marker of oxyradical-mediated DNA damage (8-hydroxy-2'deoxyguanosine) is increased in nigro-striatum of Parkinson's disease brain. Neurodegeneration 1994;3:197–204.
150. Alam ZI, Jenner A, Daniel SE, et al. Oxidative DNA damage in the Parkinsonian brain: an apparent selective increase in 8-hydroxyguanine levels in substantia nigra. J Neurochem 1997;69: 1196–1203.
151. Alam ZI, Daniel SE, Lees AJ, et al. A generalised increase in protein carbonyls in the brain in Parkinson's but not incidental Lewy body disease. J Neurochem 1997;69:1326–1329.
152. Sofic E, Lange KW, Jellinger K, et al. Reduced and oxidized glutathione in the substantia nigra of patients with Parkinson's disease. Neurosci Lett 1992;142:128–130.
153. Sian J, Dexter DT, Lees AJ, et al. Alterations in glutathione levels in Parkinson's disease and other neurodegenerative disorders affecting basal ganglia. Ann Neurol 1994;36:348–355.
154. Shergill JK, Cammack R, Cooper CE, et al. Detection of nitrosyl complexes in human substantia nigra, in relation to Parkinson's disease. Biochem Biophys Res Commun 1996;228:298–305.
155. Yoritaka A, Hattori N, Uchida K, et al. Immunohistochemical detection of 4-hydroxynonenal protein adducts in Parkinson's disease. Proc Natl Acad Sci U S A 1996;93:2696–2701.
156. Castellani R, Smith MA, Richey PL, et al. Glycoxidation and oxidative stress in Parkinson disease and diffuse Lewy body disease. Brain Res 1996;737:195–200.
157. Mochizuki H, Imai H, Endo K, et al. Iron accumulation in the substantia nigra of 1-methyl-4-phenyl-1,2,3,6-tetrahydropyridine (MPTP)-induced hemiparkinsonian monkeys. Neurosci Lett 1994; 168:251–253.
158. Kosel S, Egensperger R, Mehraein P, et al. No association of mutations at nucleotide 5460 of mitochondrial NADH dehydrogenase with Alzheimer's disease. Biochem Biophys Res Commun 1994; 203:745–749.
159. Browne SE, Bowling AC, MacGarvey U, et al. Oxidative DNA damage and impaired mitochondrial metabolism in Huntington's disease. Soc Neurosci Abst 1995;21:489.
160. Rouleau GA, Clark AW, Rooke K, et al. SOD1 mutation is associated with accumulation of neurofilaments in amyotrophic lateral sclerosis. Ann Neurol 1996;39:128–131.
161. Bowling AC, Barkowski EE, McKenna-Yasek D, et al. Superoxide dismutase concentration and activity in familial amyotrophic lateral sclerosis. J Neurochem 1995;64:2366–2369.
162. Ripps ME, Huntley GW, Hof PR, et al. Transgenic mice expressing an altered murine superoxide dismutase gene provide an animal model of amyotrophic lateral sclerosis. Proc Natl Acad Sci U S A 1995;92:689–693.
163. Wong PC, Pardo CA, Borchelt DR, et al. An adverse property of a familial ALS-linked SOD1 mutation causes motor neuron disease characterized by vacuolar degeneration of mitochondria. Neuron 1995;14:1105–1116.
164. Gurney ME, Pu H, Chiu AY, et al. Motor neuron degeneration in mice that express a human Cu,Zn superoxide dismutase mutation. Science 1994;264:1772–1775.
165. Borchelt DR, Lee MK, Slunt HS, et al. Superoxide dismutase 1 with mutations linked to familial amyotrophic lateral sclerosis possesses significant activity. Proc Natl Acad Sci U S A 1994;91: 8292–8296.
166. Beckman JS, Carson M, Smith CD, et al. ALS, SOD and peroxynitrite. Nature 1993;364:584.
167. Wiedau-Pazos M, Goto JJ, Rabizadeh S, et al. Altered reactivity of superoxide dismutase in familial amyotrophic lateral sclerosis. Science 1996;271:515–518.

168. Yim MB, Kang JH, Yim HS, et al. A gain-of-function of an amyotrophic lateral sclerosis-associated Cu,Zn-superoxide dismutase mutant: an enhancement of free radical formation due to a decrease in K_m for hydrogen peroxide. Proc Natl Acad Sci U S A 1996;93:5709–5714.
169. Hatazawa J, Brooks RA, Dalakas MC, et al. Cortical motor-sensory hypometabolism in amyotrophic lateral sclerosis: a PET study. J Comput Assist Tomogr 1988;12:630–636.
170. Dalakas MC, Hatazawa J, Brooks RA, et al. Lowered cerebral glucose utilization in amyotrophic lateral sclerosis. Ann Neurol 1987;22:580–586.
171. Bowling AC, Schulz JB, Brown JRH, et al. Superoxide dismutase activity, oxidative damage, and mitochondrial energy metabolism in familial and sporadic amyotrophic lateral sclerosis. J Neurochem 1993;61:2322–2325.
172. Curti D, Malaspina A, Facchetti G, et al. Amyotrophic lateral sclerosis: oxidative energy metabolism and calcium homeostasis in peripheral blood lymphocytes. Neurology 1996;47:1060–1064.
173. Sasaki S, Iwata M. Ultrastructural study of synapses in the anterior horn neurons of patients with amyotrophic lateral sclerosis. Neurosci Lett 1996;204:53–56.
174. Sasaki S, Maruyama S, Yamane K, et al. Ultrastructure of swollen proximal axons of anterior horn neurons in motor neuron disease. J Neurol Sci 1990;97:233–240.
175. Hirano A. Cytopathology in amyotrophic lateral sclerosis. Adv Neurol 1991;56:91–101.
176. Masui Y, Mozai T, Kakehi K. Functional and morphometric study of the liver in motor neuron disease. J Neurol 1985;232:15–19.
177. Siklos L, Engelhardt J, Harati Y, et al. Ultrastructural evidence for altered calcium in motor nerve terminals in amyotrophic lateral sclerosis. Ann Neurol 1996;39:203–219.
178. Shaw PJ, Ince PG, Falkous G, et al. Oxidative damage to protein in sporadic motor neuron disease spinal cord. Ann Neurol 1995;38:691–695.
179. Beal MF, Ferrante RJ, Browne SE, et al. Increased 3-nitrotyrosine in both sporadic and familial amyotrophic lateral sclerosis. Ann Neurol 1997;42:644–654.
180. Ferrante RJ, Shinobu LA, Schulz JB, et al. Increased 3-nitrotyrosine and oxidative damage in mice with a human copper/zinc superoxide dismutase mutation. Ann Neurol 1997;42:326–334.
181. Beal MF. Oxidative damage in neurodegenerative diseases. Neuroscientist 1997;3:21–27.
182. Shibata N, Hirano A, Kobayashi M, et al. Intense superoxide dismutase-1 immunoreactivity in intracytoplasmic hyaline inclusions of familial amyotrophic lateral sclerosis with posterior column involvement. J Neuropathol Exp Neurol 1996;55:481–490.
183. Jenkins B, Koroshetz W, Beal MF, et al. Evidence for an energy metabolism defect in Huntington's disease using localized proton spectroscopy. Neurology 1993;43:2689–2695.
184. Harms L, Meierkord H, Timm G, et al. Decreased *N*-acetyl-aspartate/choline ratio and increased lactate in the frontal lobe of patients with Huntington's disease: a proton magnetic resonance spectroscopy study. J Neurol Neurosurg Psych 1997;62:27–30.
185. Martin WRW, Hanstock C, Hodder J, et al. Brain energy metabolism in Huntington's disease measured with in vivo proton magnetic resonance spectroscopy. Ann Neurol 1996;40:538.
186. Koroshetz WJ, Jenkins BG, Rosen BR, et al. Energy metabolism defects in Huntington's disease and possible therapy with coenzyme Q_{10}. Ann Neurol 1997;41:160–165.
187. O'Brien CF, Miller C, Goldblatt D, et al. Extraneural metabolism in early Huntington's disease. Ann Neurol 1990;28:300–301.
188. Stahl WL, Swanson PD. Biochemical abnormalities in Huntington's chorea brains. Neurology 1974;24:813–819.
189. Butterworth J, Yates CM, Reynolds GP. Distribution of phosphate-activated glutaminase, succinic dehydrogenase, pyruvate dehydrogenase and γ-glutamyl transpeptidase in post-mortem brain from Huntington's disease and agonal cases. J Neurol Sci 1985;67:161–171.
190. Gu M, Gash MT, Mann VM, et al. Mitochondrial defect in Huntington's disease caudate nucleus. Ann Neurol 1996;39:385–389.
191. Browne SE, Bowling AC, MacGarvey U, et al. Oxidative damage and metabolic dysfunction in Huntington's disease: selective vulnerability of the basal ganglia. Ann Neurol 1997;41:646–653.
192. Bourgeron T, Rustin P, Chretien D, et al. Mutation of a nuclear succinate dehydrogenase gene results in mitochondrial respiratory chain deficiency. Nature Genet 1995;11:144–149.
193. Gutekunst CA, Peng TI, Whaley WL, et al. Mitochondrial calcium homeostasis in Huntington's disease fibroblasts. Soc Neurosci Abst 1996;22:227.
194. Burke JR, Enghild JJ, Martin ME, et al. Huntingtin and DRPLA proteins selectively interact with the enzyme GAPDH. Nature Med 1996;2:347–350.
195. Matthews RT, Yang L, Beal MF. S-Methylthiocitrulline, a neuronal nitric oxide synthase inhibitor, protects against malonate and MPTP neurotoxicity. Exp Neurol 1997;143:282–286.

196. Ferrante RJ, Kowall NW, Hersch SM, et al. Immunohistochemical localization of markers for oxidative injury in Huntington's disease. Soc Neurosci Abst 1996;22:227.
197. Ludolph A, Seelig M, Ludolph A, et al. 3-Nitropropionic acid: exogenous animal neurotoxin and possible human striatal toxin. Can J Neurol Sci 1992;18:492–498.
198. Brouillet E, Hantraye P, Ferrante RJ, et al. Chronic mitochondrial energy impairment produces selective striatal degeneration and abnormal choreiform movements in primates. Proc Natl Acad Sci U S A 1995;92:7105–7109.
199. Mangiarini L, Sathasivam K, Seller M, et al. Exon 1 of the HD gene with an expanded CAG repeat is sufficient to cause a progressive neurological phenotype in transgenic mice. Cell 1996;87: 493–506.
200. Babcock M, de Silva D, Oaks R, et al. Regulation of mitochondrial iron accumulation by Yfh1p, a putative homolog of frataxin. Science 1997;276:1709–1712.
201. Yokota T, Shiojiri T, Gotoda T, et al. Friedreich-like ataxia with retinitis pigmentosa caused by the His ^{101}Gln mutation of the α-tocopherol transfer protein gene. Ann Neurol 1997;41:826–832.
202. Forsgren L, Libelius R, Holmberg M, et al. Muscle morphology and mitochondrial investigations of a family with autosomal dominant cerebellar ataxia and retinal degeneration mapped to chromosome 3p12–p21.1. J Neurol Sci 1996;144:91–98.
203. Matsuishi T, Sakai T, Naito E, et al. Elevated cerebrospinal fluid lactate/pyruvate ratio in Machado-Joseph disease. Acta Neurol Scand 1996;93:72–75.
204. Schapira AHV, Warner T, Gash MT, et al. Complex I function in familial and sporadic dystonia. Ann Neurol 1997;41:556–559.
205. Jun AS, Brown MD, Wallace DC. A mitochondrial DNA mutation at nucleotide pair 14459 of the NADH dehydrogenase subunit 6 gene associated with maternally inherited Leber hereditary optic neuropathy and dystonia. Proc Natl Acad Sci U S A 1994;91:6206–6210.
206. Favit A, Nicoletti F, Scapagnini U, et al. Ubiquinone protects cultured neurons against spontaneous and excitotoxin-induced degeneration. J Cereb Blood Flow Metab 1992;12:638–645.
207. Beal MF, Henshaw R, Jenkins BG, et al. Coenzyme Q_{10} and nicotinamide block striatal lesions produced by the mitochondrial toxin malonate. Ann Neurol 1994;36:882–888.
208. Schulz JB, Matthews RT, Henshaw DR, et al. Neuroprotective strategies for treatment of lesions produced by mitochondrial toxins: implications for neurodegenerative diseases. Neuroscience 1996;71: 1043–1048.
209. Schulz JB, Matthews RT, Muqit MMK, et al. Inhibition of neuronal nitric oxide synthase by 7-nitroindazole protects against MPTP-induced neurotoxicity in mice. J Neurochem 1995;64:936–939.
210. Schulz JB, Matthews RT, Jenkins BG, et al. Blockade of neuronal nitric oxide synthase protects against excitotoxicity in vivo. J Neurosci 1995;15:8419–8429.
211. Przedborski S, Jackon-Lewis V, Yokoyama R, et al. Role of neuronal nitric oxide in 1-methyl-4-phenyl-1,2,3,6-tetrahydropyridine (MPTP)-induced dopaminergic neurotoxicity. Proc Natl Acad Sci U S A 1996;93:4565–4571.
212. Hantraye P, Brouillet E, Ferrante R, et al. Inhibition of neuronal nitric oxide synthase prevents MPTP-induced parkinsonism in baboons. Nature Med 1996;2:1017–1021.
213. Matthews RT, Beal MF, Fallon J, et al. MPP+ induced substantia nigra degeneration is attenuated in nNOS knockout mice. Neurobiol Dis 1997;4:114–121.
214. Sano M, Ernesto C, Thomas RG, et al. A controlled trial of selegiline, alpha-tocopherol, or both as treatment for Alzheimer's disease. N Engl J Med 1997;336:1216–1222.
215. Kirschner PB, Jenkins BG, Schulz JB, et al. NGF, BDNF and NT-5, but not NT3 protect against MPP^+ toxicity and oxidative stress in neonatal animals. Brain Res 1996;713:178–185.
216. Bensimon G, Lacomblez L, Meininger V, et al. A controlled trial of riluzole in amyotrophic lateral sclerosis. N Engl J Med 1994;330:585–591

III

Treatment of the Dementias

13
Current Pharmacologic Treatments for Dementia

Harry Allen and Alistair Burns

The pharmacologic treatment of dementia aims at two broad targets: neuropsychological deficits (predominantly memory disorders) and neuropsychiatric features (such as affective disorders, paranoid ideas, delusions, misidentifications, aggression, and agitation). This chapter reviews critically

1. Drugs that have been licensed to treat the cognitive deficits of Alzheimer's disease (AD)
2. Drugs that have been given in an attempt to treat cognitive deficits and have been shown to be safe with varying degrees of efficacy
3. Drugs that are currently available for the control of neuropsychiatric features of dementia, including vascular dementia (VaD) and Lewy body dementia

TREATMENT OF COGNITIVE DEFICITS IN ALZHEIMER'S DISEASE

There is a theoretical distinction between treatments that provide symptomatic improvement and those with predominantly a stabilizing action. For many drugs, however, it is impossible to reduce their mechanism of action exclusively to one of these categories.

Design of Trials

With the increasing number of drugs undergoing safety and efficacy trials in dementia in general and AD in particular, guidelines have been developed in an attempt to encapsulate the important features of trial design [1]. Accurate diagnosis of the dementia syndrome (excluding depression and delirium) and of the cause of the syndrome (e.g., AD, VaD) are essential and require adherence to standardized criteria. The main domains in which efficacy should be indepen-

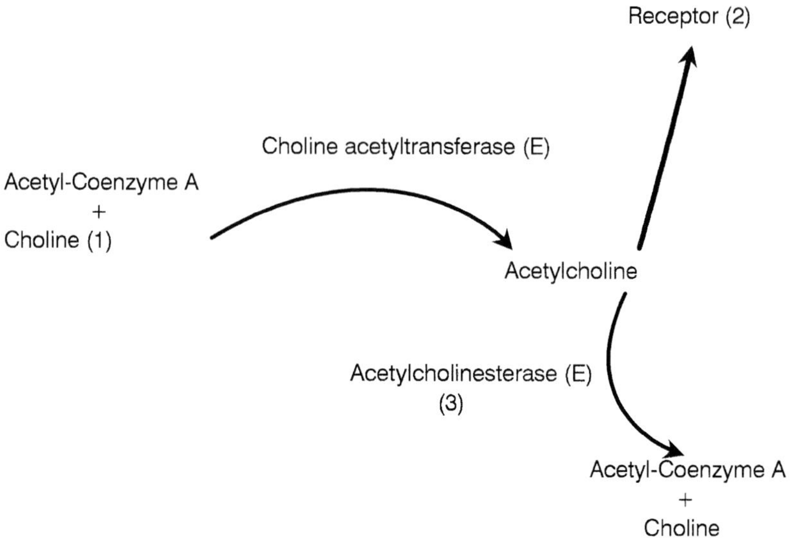

Figure 13.1 Possible approaches to increasing acetylcholine activity. (E = enzyme; 1 = precursor loading; 2 = receptor agonists; 3 = cholinesterase inhibition.)

dently assessed are cognition, activities of daily living, and global clinical response with defined primary outcome variables, at least one of which should be cognition. Measurement should be made using valid instruments that are applicable across cultures and include observer-rated components and objective measures of cognitive function. Ratings of the overall severity of dementia should be available (e.g., using the Clinical Dementia Rating Scale [2]) and the dimension of quality of life considered. Controlled clinical trials to demonstrate efficacy and monitor adverse effects should be at least 6 months long, preferably 1 year. There should be an attempt to collect information that will allow subgroups to be identified who may have a different response to the treatment and may address the issue of predicting who best is helped by a particular drug (e.g., apolipoprotein status, severity of dementia, presence of vascular disease or Lewy body features).

Cholinergic Neurotransmission

The cholinergic hypothesis of AD is based on a large body of evidence showing that deficits in acetylcholine and related enzymes are deficient in patients with AD [3–5], which can be related to the clinical signs of the disease, especially memory dysfunction. There are three approaches to raising the levels of acetylcholine (Figure 13.1):

1. Substrate loading—increasing precursors of acetylcholine in the form of choline (as lecithin) or acetyl coenzyme A. Results with choline and lecithin in

isolation have been disappointing [6], but lecithin has been used with modest success in combination with anticholinesterases such as tacrine [7]. Acetyl-L-carnitine is structurally related to acetylcholine and has a number of actions, including reduction of oxidized radicals and increased uptake and release of acetylcholine. It may act as a precursor to acetyl coenzyme A. Two studies have shown the superiority of this drug over placebo in the treatment of AD [8,9].

2. Direct receptor action—muscarinic cholinergic receptors belong to the family of G protein receptors and are the prominent type of acetylcholine receptor in the brain. Different subtypes have differing functional activities and anatomic distributions, and whereas some studies with muscarinic agonists have produced disappointing results [10], a number of M_1 agonist drugs are in development.

Nicotinic receptors are the major mediator of cholinergic neurotransmission at the neuromuscular junction. Their role in the brain is not clear, although they are probably involved in the reinforcing actions of nicotine in tobacco smoke, and people who smoke have been reported to have a reduced risk of developing AD [11].

3. Anticholinesterases (acetylcholinesterase inhibitors)—most success in the symptomatic improvement of the cognitive defects of AD has been achieved with this class of drugs, which inhibit the enzyme responsible for the breakdown of acetylcholine. Physostigmine improves memory in some patients [12], but the short half-life, narrow therapeutic index, and poor oral absorption of the compound has made it unsuitable for clinical use. Tetrahydroaminoacridine (THA, tacrine, or Cognex) was the first drug to become available for the treatment of mild to moderate AD. Doubts about the clinical efficacy of tacrine resulted from methodologic problems in the initial study by Summers and colleagues, published in 1986 [13]. Subsequent studies [7,14–16] showed definite benefit of the drug over placebo in tests of cognitive function and global ratings of dementia by caregivers and independent clinicians. Response to tacrine is variable, and only 20–30% of patients show a positive response, with a placebo response in up to 20% of patients. Up to half of the patients were withdrawn from studies due to adverse events, including gastrointestinal effects (nausea, vomiting, diarrhea, loss of appetite), aggression and irritability, skin rashes, and headaches. Elevated levels of the liver enzyme alanine transaminase [17] occurred in approximately 40% of patients. In 25% of subjects, the level was raised to three times the normal level, a dose-related effect and one that reverses following cessation of tacrine.

Rivastigmine (Exelon) is a carbamate acetylcholinesterase inhibitor, and initial trials have suggested efficacy in ameliorating cognitive decline over 6 months at a starting dose of 3 mg twice a day, which is safe and produces only mild transient gastrointestinal side effects [18]. Other drugs in development include the anticholinesterases metrifonate [19] and galanthamine [20] and M_1 agonists such as milameline and SB202026 (Memric) [21].

Donepezil

Donepezil hydrochloride (E2020, Aricept) is a piperidine-based anticholinesterase (tacrine is acridine-based) with specificity for brain acetylcholinesterase. One hundred and sixty-one patients took part in an initial study comparing placebo and donepezil (in doses of 1, 3, or 5 mg) for 12 weeks [22]. Tests of cognitive function showed that only 11% of patients taking 5 mg of the medicine showed a decline over the trial period compared to 20% of patients on placebo. A self-rated quality of life assessment also showed improvement in those taking active drug. Memory improvement (as measured by the Alzheimer's Disease Assessment Scale [23]) correlated with red cell cholinesterase activity. Those patients taking donepezil had no more adverse effects compared to placebo, and any side effects were largely understandable in terms of peripheral anticholinesterase actions (e.g., gastrointestinal disturbance). Two further studies have been carried out in the United States and one in Europe; published results of the 26-week double-blind placebo-controlled trial [24] confirm a positive clinical effect for the drug in terms of cognitive function and the Clinician's Interview-Based Impression of Change [25]. Trials suggest that the improvement in cognitive function in patients on donepezil over 6 months is of the same magnitude as the deterioration occurring over the same period.

Prescribing Donepezil

Donepezil is now licensed for the symptomatic treatment of mild to moderate AD, defined in terms of the inclusion criteria of the clinical trials as a score on the Mini-Mental State Examination (MMSE) [26] of 10–26 or a Clinical Dementia Rating Scale score of 1 or 2. The starting dose is 5 mg with the option to increase after 28 days to 10 mg to minimize the emergence of side effects which are greater with the higher dose. Monitoring of the response is recommended by serial assessments of cognitive scores (using, for example, the MMSE). No guidelines indicate when the drug should be stopped, but probably the best criterion for cessation of treatment is lack of efficacy. A patient who shows a deterioration of the order of magnitude expected had they not been on the drug (approximately 3 points on the MMSE per year) should discontinue use. More realistically, when significant end points of the disease have been reached, such as institutionalization or deterioration leading to loss of independence, it would be reasonable to stop the medication. The difficulties in stopping the drug should not be underestimated, and even moderate cognitive decline can be taken as a reason for continuing the drug in the absence of knowing what the patient would have been like otherwise. Further deterioration (sometimes precipitous) after discontinuation (as has been described with tacrine) may further complicate the picture, and pressure to restart the medication placed on the physician by the patient's family or caregivers can sometimes be irresistible.

Conclusion

The cholinergic approach offers the only currently available treatment strategy to ameliorate the symptoms of AD. Drugs are effective in producing a modest improvement in cognitive function, clearly superior to that of placebo. The evidence to date is that such drugs are only effective in the mild or moderate stages of the disease and the effects of long-term treatment are unknown. The lack of side effects would logically make donepezil the drug of first choice in view of the liver toxicity of tacrine. Second-generation anticholinesterases are being developed, as well as direct muscarinic agonists, and trials of combination therapy with

Table 13.1 Noncholinergic approaches to the treatment of Alzheimer's disease

Stabilization	*Symptomatic*	*Others*
Antioxidant vitamins	Vasodilators	Mitochondrial enhancers
Anti-inflammatory agents	Calcium channel blockers	Enhanced phospholipid synthesis/reduced neuronal membrane degradation
Monoamine oxidase B inhibitors	Neuroendocrine (e.g., estrogen, thyrotropin-releasing hormone)	Nootropics
Metal chelation	Anti-inflammatory agents	Angiotensin
Nerve growth factor	Monoamine oxidase B inhibitors	Psychostimulants
Neurotransmitter replacement		

these two drug classes are planned. Although cholinergic treatments for AD have been directed at reversing the cholinergic deficit, evidence suggests that muscarinic-induced increased protein kinase C activity may alter amyloid precursor protein metabolism and *tau* phosphorylation, both of which are clearly implicated in the pathogenesis of AD [27].

Noncholinergic Approaches

Noncholinergic Neurotransmitter Systems

Neither treatment with noradrenergic receptor agonists [28] nor with selective serotonin reuptake inhibitors (SSRIs) has been successful in altering cognitive function, but they ameliorate the noncognitive signs and symptoms of the disease. It has been suggested [29] that citalopram, one of the newer SSRIs, may be of some benefit in AD, but the evidence suggests that it is helpful in relieving symptoms of irritability, anxiety, and restlessness rather than having any significant effect on cognitive function per se. Drugs acting on the dopamine system have also been investigated, and of these, selegiline has shown the most promise with both cognitive and noncognitive effects (Table 13.1) [30,31].

Antioxidant Vitamins

Both vitamins E and C have antioxidant potential, and in vitro evidence exists that vitamin C can reduce amyloid protein aggregation and vitamin E may attenuate cholinergic loss in animal studies [32]. In the best clinical study of antioxidants to date, Sano and colleagues [33] reported that vitamin E and selegiline, alone and in combination, slowed the progression of AD. The study was a prospective, double-blind, placebo-controlled, randomized multicenter trial that examined the progress of 341 patients to defined end points of disease—loss of ability to carry out two of three activities of daily living (i.e., eating, grooming, using the toilet), progression to severe dementia (as defined by the Clinical Dementia Rating Scale), institutionalization, or death. After covarying for initial cognitive score, selegiline alone (10 mg per day), vitamin E (2,000 IU per day), or a combination of the two significantly delayed time to progression to the end points, but no additional benefit was conferred by the combination. As vitamin E is available over the counter, many physicians now recommend taking it as a preventative strategy for AD. Further studies are needed to confirm these results.

Anti-Inflammatory Agents

The finding in some case-control studies that the presence of arthritis was protective against AD could be explained by the taking of nonsteroidal anti-inflammatory agents [34]. Circumstantial evidence suggests that autoimmune inflammatory mechanisms may have a role in the causation of AD [35], the hypothesis being that the inflammatory process is the primary event, so drugs that inhibit the inflammatory response may ameliorate symptoms and delay progression. A twin study [36] confirmed the protective effect of corticosteroids and adrenocorticotropic hormone (ACTH) but not of nonsteroidal anti-inflammatory agents and aspirin. Indomethacin in a dose of 100–150 mg per day has been shown to be effective in reducing cognitive decline in AD [37] over 6 months, but this class of drugs is associated with significant, often gastrointestinal, side effects.

Monoamine Oxidase Inhibitors

The rationale for the treatment of AD with monoamine oxidase inhibitors (MAOIs) is that they stimulate the *N*-methyl-D-aspartate receptor, the glutamate receptor subtype involved in long-term potentiation of postsynaptic neurons, a hypothesized mechanism for memory formation. They also inhibit noradrenaline and dopamine degradation in the presynaptic terminal, leading to a net increase in neurotransmitter concentration. MAOI-B activity increases with age and in AD [38]. Milacemide, both an MAOI-B inhibitor and glycine pro-drug, has been found to be ineffective in the treatment of AD [39]. However, selegiline has been found to be effective in controlling behavioral disturbances in AD [30], in adding to the therapeutic efficacy of anticholinesterases [31], and, alone or in combination with vitamin E, of ameliorating the disease course in AD and Parkinson's disease [33,40].

Estrogen

Estrogen can have a number of effects on the brain [41]: It stimulates cholinergic markers, reverses glucocorticoid damage, increases cerebral blood flow, prevents neuronal atrophy, and acts synergistically with nerve growth factors. Epidemiologic evidence suggests that estrogen protects against the development of AD [42–44], with odds ratios predicting protection of 0.33, 0.40, and 0.46, respectively. In a study by Henderson and colleagues [42], patients with AD taking estrogen were less cognitively impaired than those not taking estrogen. The beneficial effects on memory of estrogen supplementation have been suggested by some studies [45] but not others [46]. An open-label study found that four of seven patients with AD improved slightly on mental test scores with 2 mg of estrogen daily [47]. Further clinical trials using current rigorous methods are needed to address the question of whether estrogen is effective in AD. The additive effects of estrogen on the response to tacrine has also been noted [48].

Calcium Channel Blockers

Intracellular calcium levels are raised in AD [49] and may contribute to excitotoxic neuronal death (Chapter 12). Drugs that block cellular calcium channels, used for the treatment of cardiac arrhythmias and hypertension, affect membrane permeability by blocking intracellular influx of calcium. This observation prompted speculation that calcium channel blockers might prevent neurodegeneration and therefore be useful in treating dementia. A postmarketing surveillance survey on some 4,000 patients who received nimodipine (90 mg per day) suggested benefit over placebo [50], with the effect being both for primary dementia of the Alzheimer type and VaD [51]. Further evidence is needed before the prescription of these agents is recommended.

Nerve Growth Factor

The selective vulnerability of cholinergic neurons in AD and the fact that they express nerve growth factor led to the hypothesis that prevention of further nucleus basalis degeneration might be achieved by the administration of nerve growth factor [52]. Early support for this theory came from Seiger and colleagues [53], who reported a single patient with AD whose episodic memory improved postinfusion of nerve growth factor with demonstrable changes in positron emission tomography, single photon emission tomography, and electroencephalogram (EEG). Side effects of the treatment (e.g., meningeal irritation and fibrosis as a result of the need for intraventricular administration) have stalled subsequent development of the treatment. Nerve growth factor studies, however, may provide information on mechanisms underlying AD and may be of use in understanding the process of normal aging [54].

Metal Chelation

The implication of aluminum in the causation of AD has prompted trials of metal chelation. One study, which has yet to be replicated, used the trivalent iron chelator desferrioxamine [55]. This was administered intramuscularly twice daily, 5 days a week, for 24 months and compared to oral placebo and no treatment. The injected group had a significant reduction (approximately 50%) in the rate of decline in daily living skills.

Vasodilators

The best known drug in this category is a combination of ergoloid mesylates (Hydergine). A large number of trials have been carried out suggesting improvements in symptoms such as confusion and depression, but many have used flawed methodology. Schneider and Olin [56] carried out a meta-analysis of trials of the drug in which the following criteria were satisfied: randomized, placebo-controlled, double-blind parallel group studies with defined outcome measures and sufficient sample sizes to compute effect size. One-third of 151 identified trials satisfied these criteria. The findings were that Hydergine was more effective than placebo in terms of improvements in global ratings of dementia and composite neuropsychological measures. Efficacy of the drug was associated with VaD, doses of more than 4 mg per day, and being an inpatient at the time of the study (possibly improving compliance). The case for the prescription of Hydergine remains to be made conclusively, although it is licensed for the treatment of "idiopathic decline in memory" by the U.S. Food and Drug Administration and appears as a treatment for mild to moderate dementia in the British National Formulary.

Other Drugs

Other drugs form a heterogeneous group of compounds from which there is usually a rationale for their prescription and some evidence that they have some effect in AD. Nootropic drugs act in a variety of ways, including stimulation of acetylcholine synthesis and release. Trials have been disappointing with results like "ineffective in reducing cognitive impairment" (oxiracetam [57]), "unlikely to confer symptomatic benefit" (pramiracetam [58]), and "might slow the progression of cognitive deterioration" (piracetam [59]). There is no evidence to support the effectiveness of the following drugs: naloxone (an opioid antagonist that might reverse opioid-induced amnesia [60]), thiamine [61], ACTH, vasopressin, phospholipids, psychostimulants, or angiotensin-converting enzyme inhibitors (trials pending on the latter) [62,63].

Conclusions

What is the clinician to do when faced with this bewildering array of medications, all of which are said to have some beneficial effect in treating the cognitive impairments of AD? With the vast majority of these drugs, the effect size is modest. Some of the study designs are less than ideal, with small numbers of patients. The evidence is lacking (with the exception of the anticholinesterases) that any single drug or group of drugs is effective in the treatment of dementia in general or AD in particular. Even with use of the acetylcholinesterase inhibitors, however, not all patients improve, and the magnitude of response is generally modest in those who do respond. Muscarinic agonists have produced promising preliminary results. For prophylaxis, vitamin E and selegiline may delay the progression of the disease, whereas estrogen and anti-inflammatory agents may protect against its development. Vitamin E is unique because it can be bought without prescription; both it and selegiline may delay end points of the disease but do not appear to improve cognitive test scores. For the present, anticholinesterases represent the best therapeutic option.

PHARMACOLOGIC TREATMENTS OF NONCOGNITIVE FEATURES OF DEMENTIA

Dementia presents most often with memory problems; however, patients can present with mood disturbance, personality changes, or psychotic symptoms such as delusions and hallucinations. These noncognitive features are important because they cause significant distress to patients and caregivers, and are often one of the main reasons for a patient with dementia being admitted to institutional care [64–67].

Depressive Symptoms

We all have an idea of what depressive symptoms are. The temporary feeling of being fed up, irritable, tired, and unmotivated is a common enough experience in life. In psychiatric terms, depressive symptoms become significant when a minimum duration and a less easily defined minimum severity are reached. Psychological symptoms such as low mood, guilty ideas, lack of interest in normal activities, loss of sense of humor, poor concentration, or suicidal ideas can occur in patients with dementia.

Many of these symptoms depend for their expression on retained language ability. As AD progresses and temporoparietal lobe damage becomes more extensive, language disturbance is a more common feature. Therefore, too great a dependence on complaints of depressed mood may lead the clinician to overlook depressive symptoms in moderate and severe dementia.

Vegetative or biological symptoms of depression are less dependent on verbal skills for their expression and therefore may play a very significant part in the diagnosis of depression in dementia. Sleep disturbance (typically, waking earlier than an individual's normal waking time), loss of enjoyment of food, weight loss, or a variation in mood with improvement as the day goes by can be seen.

Studies that describe depressive symptoms in dementia often group patients who have some of the above symptoms separately from those who have sufficient symptoms to meet diagnostic criteria for depressive illness. Various criteria are used to determine the syndrome of depression. One example is the *Diagnostic and Statistical Manual of Mental Disorders* (4th ed) (*DSM-IV*) [68]. In this diagnostic system, a minimum duration of 2 weeks is required for the depressive symptoms. In addition to this duration criterion, the patient must have at least five out of nine listed possible symptoms of depression (the severity criterion).

As dementia progresses, depression can manifest in a variety of ways. Aggression, wandering, agitation, dependency, importuning, or "clinging" behaviors can all be symptoms of depression, particularly in the dementia sufferer. In our experience, these symptoms may have a diurnal variation and improve in the afternoon or evening.

There have been many reports of the frequency of these symptoms and syndromes in AD. A weighted mean prevalence rate for studies using the National Institute of Neurological and Communicative Disorders and Stroke–Alzheimer's Disease and Related Disorders Association criteria [69] for symptoms of depression is 30.4% and for the syndrome of depression is 19.1% [70].

Treatment of Depressive Symptoms

The detection of the presence of depression in the setting of dementia depends primarily on the history and mental state examination of the patient. This examination should include, where possible, an interview with a relative or caregiver. Patients with dementia often minimize or forget their symptoms, and the informant interview enables the clinician to better determine the details of affective, cognitive, and behavioral symptoms. This was demonstrated by Mackenzie and Robiner [71] who found that interviewing a patient's family and friends increased the detection of depressive symptoms by more than 300%. It is possible that a family's reports of depressive symptoms may be biased by their own feelings of stress from looking after the patient.

There are many symptoms that are common to both depression and dementia—for example, loss of interest, decreased energy, psychomotor retardation or agitation, disturbed sleep, and loss of appetite. In dementia, these symptoms may have their origin in an awareness of cognitive problems and consequent unwillingness to interact socially, or perhaps in more severe dementia, a disturbance of diurnal rhythm. When the history reveals the development of *new* symptoms such as these, however, the clinical suspicion of depression must be heightened.

There is no shortcut to the diagnosis of depression. Diagnostic interviews can help in the organization of the assessment of the patient, but tend to err on the side of overinclusiveness. Rating scales abound, but there is simply no substitute for a thorough clinical interview. We would endorse, however, the use of rating scales for the assessment of change in the severity of a patient's depression. Some scales in common usage in this area have a bias for symptoms that are common in physical illnesses [72], whereas other scales rely on the retention of verbal abilities for completion [73]. No scale can help rate depression in dementia across the whole range of dementia severity.

Many advances in structural and functional neuroimaging have been made, but no test can help the clinician make a positive diagnosis of depression as distinct from dementia. EEG, dexamethasone suppression test, and scanning [74] serve more to demonstrate the overlap between early dementia and depression in late life than to distinguish them. There are some disadvantages to trying too hard to exclude those who have no depressive symptoms because it may be better to give a treatment trial of antidepressants for a limited period.

When the interview is completed, the clinician is faced with deciding whether to treat pharmacologically. There is little evidence to guide the clinician in this choice when the patient has AD [75]. Examination of several groups of medically ill patients has shown that when autonomic symptoms of depression are present, depressed mood is also likely to be present [76,77]. The conclusion is that if the syndrome of major depression is present, treatment should be initiated. Conversely, if the patient is in good spirits and there is nothing from the clinical evaluation to indicate a depressive disorder, antidepressant treatment is not warranted [78].

Selecting Treatment

The choice of antidepressants has grown significantly. These are grouped into three main categories: the tricyclics (e.g., amitriptyline, imipramine, and dothiepin) and related drugs; SSRIs (e.g., fluoxetine, sertraline, paroxetine, and citalopram); and the MAOIs. Other drugs that cannot be classified within these three groups are also available and are considered individually.

Tricyclics

The often quoted double-blind placebo-controlled study by Reifler and colleagues [78] showed that AD patients who also meet *DSM-III* [79] criteria for depression showed an improvement in their depressive symptoms after treatment with imipramine. A similar improvement, however, was seen in those patients treated with placebo [78]. The authors speculated that the 8-week duration of the study was too short. Other open-label studies have shown similar results and advised the use of low doses and careful monitoring [80].

The need for caution lies in the sensitivity of the elderly patient, and particularly the AD patient, to anticholinergic side effects [81]. Further, it is counterproductive to block cholinergic neurotransmission in AD patients who may be receiving cholinomimetic drugs to improve cognition. As there is growing evidence that depression in the elderly requires long-term treatment [82], there are few reasons for choosing a tricyclic antidepressant in this patient group [82]. One reason in mild AD is if there has been previous experience of a good response to a tricyclic. If the dementia is more severe, and there is perhaps an even greater sensitivity to anticholinergic side effects, drugs with such effects should be avoided as a first choice. When the depressive symptoms are severe enough to merit a subcategorization of melancholia [68] (greater emphasis on vegetative symptoms), the evidence about the potency of SSRIs is conflicting [83,84]. The conclusion so far is to try tricyclics as a second choice in these patients and to select those with the least anticholinergic effects.

Selective Serotonin Reuptake Inhibitors

There is almost as little double-blind, placebo-controlled trial evidence for the efficacy of SSRIs in treating depression in dementia as there is for the use of tricyclics. Two studies of the use of citalopram in this patient group were conducted [85,86]. Both studies were short (4–6 weeks of double-blind phase) and both included patients with mild depressive symptoms. The results favored citalopram in both studies. The results in patients with more severe depressive symptoms, however, were not significant at the 5% level.

The SSRIs have the advantage that they do not have the anticholinergic side effects of the tricyclics. This means that their use does not involve the potential for impairing cognitive function. They are not without side effects, however. Analysis of dropout rates has shown conflicting results [87,88]. These studies are not specific for the elderly, and the balance of tolerability may be more conclusively toward SSRIs in the older patient. Some reports link certain antidepressants with unusual side effects: sertraline with extrapyramidal side effects [89], and fluoxetine with both extrapyramidal side effects and visual hallucinations [89,90].

Table 13.2 Relative strengths* of side effects for a selection of antidepressants

Drug	*Anticholinergic*	*Antihistaminic*	*Adrenergic*
Amitriptyline	5	5	5
Imipramine	4	2	5
Lofepramine	1–2	1	1
Trazodone	0	3	1
Fluoxetine	0	0	0–1
Paroxetine	0	0	0
Moclobemide	0	0	0

*Numbers 0–5 indicate relative effect on an arbitrary scale; higher number indicates greater effect.
Source: Adapted from RC Baldwin. Depressive Illness. In R Jacoby, C Oppenheimer (eds), Psychiatry in the Elderly. Oxford: Oxford University Press, 1997;536–573.

Other Treatment Options

Lofepramine seems to combine some of the advantages of potency compared to the older tricyclics and perhaps the SSRIs [91,92]. It has less of the anticholinergic properties of the other tricyclics, and fewer cardiac effects, which may be an advantage in the elderly (Table 13.2).

Moclobemide is a reversible inhibitor of MAO-A. Its relative lack of anticholinergic side effects makes it a potentially suitable antidepressant in AD patients and an open-label study has shown promising results [93]. The relative lack of a tyramine (cheese) reaction makes the use of this drug less of a risk in patients with memory problems.

It would be fair to say that most antidepressants in the treatment of depression in dementia, far from having a proven past, have an unblemished future. Whichever drug is chosen, it would be prudent to start at a low dose, sometimes even less than the manufacturer's recommended starting dose, and to increase slowly to tolerance. The treatment of depressive symptoms in dementia cannot be rushed, and a trial of 8 weeks at tolerance dose would be considered adequate.

In cases in which drug treatment has failed, electroconvulsive therapy (ECT) may be considered. Dementia is not a contraindication to ECT [94]. Some clinicians prefer a shorter course using bilateral ECT, whereas others prefer a longer unilateral course with less postictal memory loss. Modern ECT machines allow titration of dosage and should therefore ensure an adequate seizure.

Psychotic Symptoms

Delusions are beliefs that are usually false (the reasoning is false if not the actual belief) and are held in clear consciousness, out of keeping with cultural norms, and in the face of logical argument. Distinction must be made from ideas that may be generated out of memory impairment and that might have a paranoid edge to them but that are accepted by the patient as being false when a correct explanation is given. These ideas would not have been held with delusional intensity. The weighted mean prevalence rate of delusions in AD is 29.6% [70].

Hallucinations are percepts in the absence of appropriate stimuli. They may be in any of the five sensory modalities. In AD, the weighted mean prevalence rate for all hallucinations is 18.6% [70]. Auditory hallucinations occur at approximately 50–70% the rate of visual hallucinations.

Misidentification phenomena occur when a percept (often visual) is incorrectly identified. For example, a patient may believe that a television personality actually lives in his or her house and he or she may prepare meals for that person (prevalence rate: 10–15%) [70]. Reduplication phenomena occur when the patient states that a person or object has been duplicated.

Treatment of Psychotic Symptoms

Psychotic symptoms do not always require treatment. In other circumstances, treatment may not simply be indicated but may be a matter of urgency. Delusions or hallucinations that are distressing to the patient as shown by comments, fearful behavior, or perhaps pushing caregivers away because the patient believes that he or she is going to be harmed may require treatment if reassurance and a calm approach do not help. It may not be appropriate or helpful to treat the mild paranoid symptoms of the lifelong loner in the hope that he or she may attend a day center. When beliefs interfere with self-care, social interaction, or participation in activities, particularly when the symptoms cause a change in behavior, treatment should be considered. If symptoms cause patients to put themselves or others in danger, then urgent treatment may be indicated [95].

Environmental changes may help in psychotic symptoms, but the options are often limited. An example is when a patient demonstrates the mirror sign—a failure to recognize his or her own reflection. By itself this symptom is usually not a problem, but when the reflection is recognized as a threatening or persecutory character, the simple expedient of removing the household mirrors from easy view can avoid the need for medication.

Selecting Treatment

Neuroleptics are used in the treatment of noncognitive features in dementia in two broad symptom groups: symptoms of a psychotic nature (delusions, hallucinations, misidentifications, reduplications) and symptoms of a behavioral nature (aggression, agitation). As with depression, a thorough assessment is necessary before considering treatment options.

The choice of neuroleptic for the treatment of psychotic symptoms in a patient with dementia is the same as for the nondemented elderly patient. In both cases, the clinician is guided by personal experience, preference, and the side effect profile of the available alternatives. Low-potency antipsychotics (thioridazine, promazine) are more likely to cause sedation and anticholinergic side effects [96], but high-potency antipsychotics (haloperidol, trifluoperazine) have a greater tendency to cause parkinsonian symptoms and akathisia. No antipsychotic has consistently been shown to have a superior effect in treating these symptoms in the elderly. Start with very small doses and titrate upward in small increments every

3–4 days according to clinical response. There is some justification for the use of atypical neuroleptics in the elderly (e.g., clozapine, olanzapine, risperidone, sertindole, quetiapine), which have fewer extrapyramidal side effects but can still cause significant sedation and postural hypotension, symptoms that can be dangerous in the elderly.

Stopping treatment is as important as starting it, particularly in the elderly population, in which polypharmacy is common. Psychotic symptoms are often transient in dementia [97], and a trial of discontinuing the antipsychotic should be considered when the behavior is stabilized.

Behavioral Symptoms

It is preferable to discuss behavioral symptoms in a purely descriptive way rather than to speculate on the cognitive abilities or psychotic experiences of the patient. Hope and Patel [98] categorized behavioral changes in dementia into six types: aggression, activity disturbances, changes in eating behavior, disturbances of diurnal rhythm, sexual behavior, and other miscellaneous behavioral disturbances that do not fit into the other five categories.

Aggressive behavior is an overt nonaccidental delivery of noxious stimuli to another organism, object, or self [98]. It can be verbal or physical but can also appear in the form of passive resistance. Activity disturbances are a broad category that includes various types of wandering, purposeless behavior, or agitation [70]. There is no generally accepted definition of this type of behavior. Changes in eating behavior can lead to increases or decreases in quantity of nutrients consumed, which may be reflected in changes in weight. Patients may also consume non-nutritious materials such as feces or soil. Disturbances of diurnal rhythm are often particularly poorly tolerated by caregivers [99]. Patients may wake during the night more often and for longer periods [98]. They may sleep during the day, which leads to further difficulties in initiating sleep at night. In the latter stages of dementia, the diurnal rhythm can be grossly disturbed [98]. Disturbances of sexual activity can include inappropriate sexual comments, suggestions, or actions such as physical contact, self-exposure, or masturbation. A variety of other less well characterized behaviors (e.g., hiding objects, obsessional traits, picking at clothing) have been described, and they may contribute to the burden of caring for the patient with dementia.

Treatment of Behavioral Symptoms

The consequences of disruptive behaviors for the patient may include decreased quality of care due to physical restraints, alienation, and labeling, and also a decreased quality of life due to exclusion from social activities [100]. Assessment of behavioral changes before starting pharmacologic treatment is essential. The physical state of the patient must be examined. Conditions such as infections, metabolic disturbances, hypoxia, hyper- or hypoglycemia, dehydration, pain, or constipation may cause delirium. The patient may be agitated, aggressive, or fearful at night, which may lead to requests for medication by caregivers. The clinician should attempt to resolve the medical problems appropriately before instituting further pharmacologic intervention, while remembering that the medication the patient is already taking may be the cause of the behavior.

The ability of the patient to receive and process sensory information may be impaired. Sight or hearing loss may reduce the patient's ability to understand his or her surroundings and lead to disorientation and wandering. Excessive noise or changes in routine may provoke verbal or physical aggression. A move to a residential or nursing home can be a potent cause of behavioral symptoms.

Other psychiatric complaints may be the cause of behavioral changes in dementia. Depression may present in many ways, including morning aggression or wandering, resistance to caregiving, and insomnia. Anxiety or psychotic states as described above can be present, and so the clinician must bear these in mind when assessing the agitated patient.

Selecting Treatment

Specific symptoms should be identified and the effect of the intervention should be monitored with the use of charts on which caregivers may rate the frequency and severity of the symptom. Medication should be given for limited periods only, preferably with a review date set at the start of a treatment trial. Behavioral symptoms tend to be more persistent than depressive or psychotic symptoms, but Devanand and colleagues [97] showed that although more than 90% of 235 patients had some behavioral disturbance on at least one occasion during a 2-year study, less than 50% had symptoms at all four 6-month assessments.

There have been no consistent reports that certain symptoms respond to specific medications. Strategies for drug selection have been proposed [101] but have not yet been validated. As many of these drugs do not have the control of agitation or aggression as a licensed indication, specific consent may have to be sought from next of kin and their use discussed in multidisciplinary meetings.

Several reviews of the trial literature on the use of neuroleptics in the treatment of behavioral changes have been conducted [102–104]. Tune and colleagues [102] reported that a variety of symptoms responded to neuroleptics, including agitation, anxiety, overactivity, and restlessness. Studying the effect of discontinuing medication [105] has shown that neuroleptics have an effect in treating these symptoms, but that for many patients, symptoms did not return [106]. In a meta-analysis, Schneider and associates [103] showed that the use of neuroleptics could lead to an improvement in symptoms for 18% of agitated patients. Although neuroleptics are consistently more effective than placebo, the effect size is small and not correlated with dosage. Therefore, there seems little advantage to increasing the dose in most patients.

No consistent evidence shows any one neuroleptic to be superior to another, and so the choice is governed by the side effect profile, personal choice, and experience. As with the antidepressants, there are newer antipsychotic medications available that have not yet been tried in controlled trials. Case reports [107,108] have suggested that risperidone may improve aggression in association with psychosis in dementia.

Other Treatment Options

Benzodiazepines

Benzodiazepines have been used in the management of behavioral disturbances in dementia since they were first available. Reviews have suggested that anxiety, tension, and agitation can be diminished [109,110]. The comparative studies, however, tend to show that neuroleptics are probably superior [109–111]. Care must be taken in the use of benzodiazepines. There are problems with the addictive potential and with the tendency to cause acute confusional states. Short-acting benzodiazepines (e.g., oxazepam) are preferable to those that have persistent metabolites (e.g., diazepam).

Buspirone

Buspirone is a serotonin-partial agonist [112], and some case reports [113] show improvements in symptoms with its use. A pilot placebo-controlled trial (10 patients), however, showed no effect of buspirone at what would be considered to be an anxiolytic dose [114].

Lithium

Schneider and Sobin [104] reviewed the use of lithium and found little evidence of a beneficial effect. In various case reports, the drug was used to treat hypomania, depression, agitation, and sleep disturbance. The reviewers concluded that most patients did not respond favorably to lithium, and they pointed out that elderly patients may be particularly sensitive to side effects at usual therapeutic doses.

Propranolol

Beta-blockers are effective in controlling aggression, and several case reports and open-label trials support this [110,115]. Cardiovascular and respiratory side effects may limit the usefulness of these drugs in the elderly.

Anticonvulsants

The most studied anticonvulsant in this area is carbamazepine. Numerous case reports and open studies have suggested a beneficial effect on agitation, rage, and fighting [104,111,116–118]. A small (six patients), double-blind crossover trial showed a reduction in aggression [119].

Trazodone

Case reports show an improvement in symptoms of head banging, screaming, and agitation [120] with use of trazodone, but it is likely that these results are due to the particularly sedative effect of the drug, rather than to antidepressant effects.

Conclusions

The fact that so many psychoactive drugs have been tried in the treatment of noncognitive symptoms indicates a lack of reliable efficacy of any individual drug. The drugs are effective, but often side effects are the limiting factor in their prescription. No evidence suggests that antidepressants are less effective in the depression associated with dementia than in depression in the absence of cognitive impairment. Similarly, neuroleptic drugs are effective in controlling delusions in patients with dementia in the same way as in schizophrenia. The use of any of these drugs in elderly people with dementia should be planned both in terms of starting and, more importantly, stopping therapy. The clinician should determine the aim of therapy beforehand and set a review date so that an ineffective treatment is not prolonged.

VASCULAR DEMENTIA

That prevention is better than a cure is true both for AD and VaD, but at least there are recognizable and sometimes treatable risk factors for the development of dementia due to vascular causes (Chapter 15). Advancing age, male gender, hypertension, diabetes mellitus, atrial fibrillation, congestive heart failure, coronary heart disease, cigarette smoking, peripheral vascular disease, and stroke are associated with a greater risk of VaD [121]. Moroney and colleagues [122] showed that patients who had strokes complicated by global cerebral hypoxic or ischemic conditions such as seizures, sepsis, cardiac arrhythmias, or congestive cardiac failure were at more than four times greater risk of developing dementia within 5 years than those who had uncomplicated strokes. What is not clear is how much the risks can be reduced by aggressive treatment of these conditions.

Calcium antagonists, especially nimodipine, have been tried in vascular dementia. The rationale is that the final common pathway for the multifactorial process that leads to dementia is partly mediated by an increase in intracellular calcium. This rise in intracellular calcium activates enzymes such as kinases, phospholipases, and endonucleases, which promote cell death. Reduction in the influx of calcium may protect the cell from damage. In a review of seven studies of the effect of nimodipine, Marler and colleagues [123] reported that there were some improvements, but that these were not consistent and may have been greater in noncognitive features such as depression.

Pentoxifylline increases red blood cell deformability and has been shown to slow the progression of dementia in clinical trials [124]. Propentofylline is a xanthine derivative that has neuroprotective properties by inhibiting glutamate release, calcium accumulation, and free radical formation. Long-term studies have suggested that it may result in an improvement in cognitive function [124].

LEWY BODY DEMENTIA

The clinical syndrome of Lewy body dementia is characterized by an illness with a fluctuating course punctuated by periods of behavioral disturbance and psychotic experiences. Parkinsonian features are also present [125]. Because of the marked disturbances seen, patients are often prescribed neuroleptic drugs to control agitation or hallucinations. Sensitivity to neuroleptics is a recognized consequence of neuroleptic prescription [126]. McKeith and colleagues [125] found that although the proportion of patients who had Lewy body dementia and who were prescribed neuroleptics was similar, eight of 14 patients deteriorated rapidly either after a first dose of neuroleptic or after an increase in dose. This prompted the U.K. Committee on Safety of Medicine to state that "if neuroleptic medications are used in elderly patients with dementia, very low doses should be given with cautious titration against the clinical state. Particular care should be taken in patients with features of the newly described Lewy body dementia because sudden life threatening deterioration may occur" [127]. Neuroleptic sensitivity in Lewy body dementia seems to relate to loss of neurons in the substantia nigra with impairment of the compensatory upregulation in postsynaptic D_2 receptors in the striatum [128,129]. D_2-receptor blockade by neuroleptics, therefore, is enough to impair the system to produce extrapyramidal effects, and other drugs will potentially be of more practical use in the treatment of Lewy body dementia. Initial results with novel antipsychotics such as risperidone and clozapine are promising, the blockade of the 5-hydroxytryptamine receptor, subtype 2 (5-HT_2) of the former explaining the relatively low extrapyramidal side effect profile. Antiparkinsonian treatments disrupt the acetylcholine-noradrenaline balance, and reducing this medication would be a logical first step in the treatment of noncognitive disorders. Anticholinesterases are a logical treatment for the condition in view of the profound cholinergic defect, the response of patients with Lewy body dementia to tacrine [130], and the beneficial effects of physostigmine on deluded patients with AD [131]. To avoid extrapyramidal side effects completely, sedation with benzodiazepines or chlormethiazole may be effective, and ondansetron (a 5-HT_3 antagonist) has been described as improving psychotic symptoms in Parkinson's disease. Unconfirmed reports suggest that antiepileptic drugs may be of benefit. Depression should be treated in the usual way, theoretically with SSRIs because the anticholinergic effects of tricyclic drugs may exacerbate cognitive impairment.

CONCLUSION

There have been promising results for many of the drugs discussed in this chapter, but none has been developed into a proven effective specifically licensed agent. Clinicians would do well to be cautious in choosing such agents in response to pressure from patients and relatives eager to try anything that may help. The bias in reporting positive findings inevitably skews the literature at this stage in the development of antidementia therapies.

REFERENCES

1. Committee for Proprietary Medicinal Products (ed). Note for Guidance on Medicinal Products in the Treatment of Alzheimer's Disease. London: The European Agency for the Evaluation of Medicinal Products, 1997.
2. Hughes C, Berg L, Danziger W, et al. A new clinical scale for the staging of dementia. Br J Psychiatry 1982;140:566–572.

3. Whitehouse P, Price D, Strubble R, et al. Alzheimer's disease and senile dementia: loss of neurons in the basal forebrain. Science 1982;215:1237–1239.
4. Bowen DM, Smith CB, White P, Davison AN. Neurotransmitter-related enzymes and indices of hypoxia in senile dementia and other abiotrophies. Brain 1976;99:495–496.
5. Rossor MN, Iversen LL, Reynolds GP, et al. Neurochemical characteristics of early and late onset types of Alzheimer's disease. BMJ 1984;288:961–964.
6. Little A, Levy R, Chuaqui KP, Hand D. A double-blind, placebo controlled trial of high-dose lecithin in Alzheimer's disease. J Neurol Neurosurg Psychiatry 1985;48:736–742.
7. Eagger SA, Levy R, Sahakian BJ. Tacrine in Alzheimer's disease. Lancet 1991;337:989–992.
8. Livingston GA, Sax KB, McClenahan Z, et al. Acetyl-L-carnitine in dementia. Int J Geriatr Psychiatry 1991;6:853–860.
9. Sano M, Bell K, Cote L, et al. Double-blind parallel design pilot study of acetyl levocarnitine in patients with Alzheimer's disease. Arch Neurol 1992;49:1137–1141.
10. Spiegel R, Azcona A, Wettstein A. First Results with RS86, an Orally Active Muscarinic Agonist in Healthy Subjects and in Patients with Dementia. In R Wurtman, S Corkin, J Growdon (eds), Alzheimer's Disease: Advances in Basic Research and Therapy. Cambridge, MA: Centre for Brain Sciences and Metabolism Charitable Trust, 1987;391–405.
11. van Duijn C, Hofman A. Relation between nicotine intake and Alzheimer's disease. BMJ 1991; 302:149–154.
12. Thal LJ. Oral physostigmine and lecithin improve memory in Alzheimer's disease. Ann Neurol 1983; 13:491–496.
13. Summers WK, Majovski LV, Marsh GM, et al. Oral tetrahydroaminoacridine in long-term treatment of senile dementia, Alzheimer type. N Engl J Med 1986;315:1241–1245.
14. Wilcock G, Surmon D, Scott N, et al. An evaluation of the efficacy and safety of THA without lecithin in the treatment of Alzheimer's disease. Age Ageing 1993;22:316–324.
15. Farlow M, Gracon SI, Hershey LA, et al. A controlled trial of tacrine in Alzheimer's disease. JAMA 1992;268:2523–2529.
16. Davis KL, Thal LJ, Gamzu ER, et al. A double-blind placebo-controlled multicenter study of tacrine. N Engl J Med 1992;327:1253–1259.
17. Watkins P, Zimmerman H, Knapp M, et al. Hepatotoxic effects of tacrine administration in patients with Alzheimer's disease. JAMA 1994;271:992–998.
18. Anand R, Gharabaw G, Enz A. Efficacy and safety results of the early phase studies with Exelon in Alzheimer's disease. J Drug Develop Clin Prac 1996;8:1–8.
19. Cummings J, Bieber F, Mas J, et al. Metrifonate in Alzheimer's Disease. In K Iqbal, B Winblab, T Mishimura, et al. (eds), Alzheimer's Disease: Biology, Diagnosis and Therapeutics. Chichester, UK: Wiley, 1997;665–670.
20. Wilcock G, Wilkinson D. Galantamine Hydrobromine: Interim Results of a Group Comparative Placebo-Controlled Study of Efficacy and Safety in Patients with a Diagnosis of Senile Dementia of the Alzheimer Type. In K Iqbal, B Winblab, T Mishimura, et al. (eds), Alzheimer's Disease: Biology, Diagnosis and Therapeutics. Chichester, UK: Wiley, 1997;661–664.
21. Kumar R, Orgogozo J. Efficacy and Safety of SB 202026 as a Symptomatic Treatment for Alzheimer's Disease. In K Iqbal, B Winblab, T Mishimura, et al. (eds), Alzheimer's Disease: Biology, Diagnosis and Therapeutics. Chichester, UK: Wiley, 1997;677–686.
22. Rogers SL, Friedhoff LT, and the Donepezil Study Group. The efficacy and safety of donepezil in patients with Alzheimer's disease. Dementia 1996;7:293–303.
23. Rosen WG, Mohs RC, Davis KL. A new rating scale for Alzheimer's disease. Am J Psychiatry 1984;141:1356–1364.
24. Rogers SL, Farlow MR, Doody RS, et al. A 24-week, double-blind, placebo-controlled trial of donepezil in patients with Alzheimer's disease. Neurology 1998;50:136–145.
25. Boothby H. Measuring Change in Dementia: The Reliability of Clinical Global Assessments. In R Levy, R Howard (eds), Developments in Dementia and Functional Disorders in the Elderly. London: Wrightson Biomedical Publishing, 1995;97–102.
26. Folstein MF, Folstein S, McHugh P. Mini-mental state. A practical method for grading the cognitive state of patients for the clinician. J Psychiatry Res 1975;12:189–198.
27. Lovestone S. Muscarinic therapies in Alzheimer's disease; from palliative treatments to disease modification. Intl J Psychiatry Clin Prac 1997;1:15–20.
28. Knesevic S, Bogdanovic N, Spilich G, Chundy D. Pharmacological Treatment of Alzheimer's Dementia: A Review. In I Kostovic, S Knezevic, H Wisniewski, GJ Spilich (eds), Neurodevelopment, Ageing and Cognition. Boston: Birkhauser, 1992;384–394.
29. Gottfries CG. Use of citalopram in syndromes related to 5-HT disturbance. Rev Comtemp Pharmacother 1995;6:307–313.

30. Tariot PN, Cohen RM, Sunderland T, et al. L-Deprenyl in Alzheimer's disease. Preliminary evidence for behavioural change with monoamine oxidase B inhibition. Arch Gen Psychiatry 1987;44:427–433.
31. Schneider LS, Olin JT, Pawluczyk S. A double-blind crossover pilot study of L-deprenyl (selegiline) combined with cholinesterase inhibitor in Alzheimer's disease. Am J Psychiatry 1993;150:321–323.
32. Maneesub Y, Sanvarinda Y, Govitrapong P. Partial restoration of choline acetyltransferase activities in ageing and AF64A lesioned rat brains by vitamin E. Neurochem Int 1993;22:487–491.
33. Sano M, Ernesto C, Thomas RG, et al. A controlled trial of selegiline, alpha-tocopherol, or both as treatment for Alzheimer's disease. N Engl J Med 1997;336:1216–1247.
34. Andersen K, Launer LJ, Ott A, et al. Do nonsteroidal anti-inflammatory drugs decrease the risk for Alzheimer's disease? The Rotterdam study. Neurology 1995;45:1441–1445.
35. Aisen PS, Davis KL. Inflammatory mechanisms in Alzheimer's disease: implications for therapy. Am J Psychiatry 1994;151:1105–1113.
36. Breitner JCS, Gau BA, Welch KA, et al. Inverse association of anti-inflammatory treatments and Alzheimer's disease. Initial results of a co-twin control study. Neurology 1994;44:227–231.
37. Rogers J, Kirby LC, Hempelman SR, et al. Clinical trial of indomethacin in Alzheimer's disease. Neurology 1993;43:1609–1611.
38. Alexopoulos GS, Lieberman KW, Young RC. Platelet MAO activity in primary degenerative dementia. Am J Psychiatry 1984;141:97–99.
39. Dysken MW, Mendels J, LeWitt P, et al. Milacemide: a placebo-controlled study in senile dementia of the Alzheimer type. J Am Geriatr Soc 1992;40:503–506.
40. Parkinson Study Group. Effects of tocopherol and deprenyl on the progression of disability in early Parkinson's disease. N Engl J Med 1993;328:176–183.
41. Burns A, Murphy D. Protection against Alzheimer's disease? [editorial]. Lancet 1996;348:420–421.
42. Henderson B, Pagnini-Hill A, Emaneuel C, et al. Oestrogen replacement therapy in older women. Arch Neurol 1994;51:896–900.
43. Tang M, Jacobs D, Stern Y, et al. Effect of oestrogen during menopause on risk and age at onset of Alzheimer's disease. Lancet 1996;348:429–432.
44. Kawas C, Resnick S, Morrison A, et al. A prospective study of estrogen replacement therapy and the risk of developing Alzheimer's disease. Neurology 1997;48:1517–1521.
45. Robinson D, Freidman L, Marcus R, et al. Oestrogen replacement therapy and memory in older women. J Am Geriatr Soc 1994;42:919–922.
46. Barrett-Connor E, Silverstein D. Oestrogen replacement therapy and cognitive function in older women. JAMA 1993;269:2639–2641.
47. Fillit H, Weinreg H, Cholst I, et al. Observations in a preliminary open trial of estradiol therapy for senile dementia-Alzheimer's type. Psychoneuroendocrinology 1986;11:337–345.
48. Schneider LS, Farlow MR, Henderson VW, Pogoda JM. Effects of estrogen replacement therapy on response to tacrine in patients with Alzheimer's disease. Neurology 1996;46:1580–1584.
49. Petersen C, Golman J. Alterations in calcium uptake in cultured skin fibroblasts from patients with Alzheimer's disease. N Engl J Med 1985;312:1063–1065.
50. Bernhardt T, Köbler J, Erzigeit H. Deficinia da funao cerebral na idade avanada: nimodipina utilizada em clinica geral. Eur J Clin Res 1997;7:205–215.
51. Ban T, Morey L, Agulia E, et al. Nimodopine in the treatment of old age dementias. Prog Neuropsychopharmacol Biol Psychiatry 1990;14:525–551.
52. Koliatsos VE, Clatterbuck RE, Nauta HJ, et al. Human nerve growth factor prevents degeneration of basal forebrain cholinergic neurons in primates. Ann Neurol 1991;30:831–840.
53. Seiger A, Nordbert A, von Holst H, et al. Intracranial infusion of purified nerve growth factor to an Alzheimer patient: the first attempt of a possible future treatment strategy. Behav Brain Res 1993;57:255–261.
54. Wilcock GK. Nerve Growth Factor and Other Experimental Approaches. In R Levy, R Howard, A Burns (eds), Treatment and Care in Old Age Psychiatry. London: Wrightson Biomedical Publishing, 1993;3–10.
55. Crapper McLachlan DR, Dalton AJ, Kruck TPA, et al. Intramuscular desferrioxamine in patients with Alzheimer's disease. Lancet 1991;337:1304–1308.
56. Schneider LS, Olin JT. Overview of clinical trials of Hydergine in dementia. Arch Neurol 1994;51:787–792.
57. Green RC, Goldstein FC, Auchus AP, et al. Treatment trial of oxiracetam in Alzheimer's disease. Arch Neurol 1992;49:1135–1136.
58. Claus JJ, Ludwig C, Mohr E, et al. Nootropic drugs in Alzheimer's disease. Neurology 1991;41:570–574.
59. Croisile B, Trillet MD, Fodarai J, et al. Long-term and high-dose piracetam treatment of Alzheimer's disease. Neurology 1993;43:301–305.

60. Henderson VW, Robert E, Wimer C, et al. Multicentre trial of naloxone in Alzheimer's disease. Ann Neurol 1989;25:404–406.
61. Nolan KA, Black RS, Sheu KFR, et al. A trial of thiamine in Alzheimer's disease. Arch Neurol 1991; 48:81–83.
62. Gray J, Gauthier S. Stabilization Strategies under Development. In S Gautier (ed), Clinical Diagnosis and Management in Alzheimer's Disease. London: M Dunitz, 1996;261–268.
63. Feldman H, Gracon S. AD Symptomatic Drugs under Development. In S Gautier (ed), Clinical Diagnosis and Management in Alzheimer's Disease. London: M Dunitz, 1996;239–260.
64. Rabins PV, Mace NL, Lucas MJ. The impact of dementia on the family. JAMA 1982;248:333–335.
65. Margo JL, Robinson JR, Corea S. Referrals to a psychiatric service from old people's homes. Br J Psychiatry 1980;136:396–401.
66. Steele C, Rovner BW, Chase GA, Folstein MF. Psychiatric symptoms and nursing home placement of patients with Alzheimer's disease. Am J Psychiatry 1990;147:1049–1051.
67. Glosser G, Wexler D, Balmelli M. Physicians' and families' perspectives on the medical management of dementia. J Am Geriatr Soc 1985;33:383–391.
68. American Psychiatric Association. Diagnostic and Statistical Manual of Mental Disorders (4th ed). Washington, DC: American Psychiatric Association, 1994.
69. McKhann G, Drachman DA, Folstein MF, et al. Clinical diagnosis of Alzheimer's disease: report of the NINCDS-ADRDA Work Group under the auspices of Department of Health and Human Services task force on Alzheimer's disease. Neurology 1984;34:939–944.
70. Allen NHP, Burns AB. The non-cognitive features of dementia. Rev Clin Gerontol 1995;5:57–75.
71. Mackenzie TB, Robiner WN. Differences between patient and family assessments of depression in Alzheimer's disease. Am J Psychiatry 1990;147:377–378.
72. Hamilton M. A rating scale for depression. J Neurol Neurosurg Psychiatry 1960;23:56–62.
73. Montgomery S, Åsberg M. A new depression scale designed to be sensitive to change. Br J Psychiatry 1979;134:381–382.
74. Emery VO, Oxman TE. Update on the dementia spectrum of depression. Am J Psychiatry 1992;149: 305–317.
75. Jones BN, Reifler BV. Depression coexisting with dementia. Med Clin North Am 1994;78:823–840.
76. Starkstein SE, Preziosi TJ, Forrester AW, Robinson RG. Specificity of affective and autonomic symptoms of depression in Parkinson's disease. J Neurol Neurosurg Psychiatry 1990;53:869–873.
77. Federoff JP, Starkstein SE, Parikh RM, et al. Are depressive symptoms non-specific in patients with acute stroke? Am J Psychiatry 1991;148:1172–1176.
78. Reifler BV, Teri L, Raskind MA, et al. A double-blind trial of a tricyclic antidepressant in Alzheimer's patients with and without depression. Am J Psychiatry 1989;146:45–49.
79. American Psychiatric Association. Diagnostic and Statistical Manual of Mental Disorders (3rd ed). Washington, DC: American Psychiatric Association, 1980.
80. Teri L, Reifler BV, Vieth RC, et al. Imipramine in the treatment of depression in Alzheimer's disease: impact on cognition. J Gerontol 1991;46:372–377.
81. Sunderland T, Tariot PN, Cohen RM, et al. Anticholinergic sensitivity in patients with dementia of the Alzheimer type and age-matched controls. Arch Gen Psychiatry 1987;44:418–426.
82. Old Age Depression Interest Group. How long should the elderly take antidepressants? A double-blind placebo-controlled study of continuation/prophylaxis therapy with dothiepin. Br J Psychiatry 1993;162:175–182.
83. Hale AS, Stokes PE. The Utility of Serotonin Reuptake Inhibitors in Endogenous and Severe Depression. In HL Freeman (ed), The Uses of Fluoxetine in Clinical Practice. London: Royal Society of Medicine, 1991;15–25.
84. Roose SP, Glassman AH, Attia E, Woodring S. Comparative efficacy of selective serotonin reuptake inhibitors and tricyclics in the treatment of melancholia. Am J Psychiatry 1994;151:1735–1739.
85. Nyth AL, Gottfries CG, Lyby K, et al. A controlled multicenter clinical study of citalopram and placebo in elderly depressed patients with and without dementia. Acta Psychiatry Scand 1992;86: 138–145.
86. Nyth AL, Gottfries CG. The clinical efficacy of citalopram in treatment of emotional disturbances in dementia disorders. A Nordic multicentre study. Br J Psychiatry 1990;157:894–901.
87. Montgomery SA, Henry J, McDonald G, et al. Selective serotonin reuptake inhibitors: meta-analysis of discontinuation rates. Int Clin Psychopharmacol 1994;9:47–53.
88. Anderson I. Lessons to be learned from meta-analyses of newer versus older antidepressants. Adv Psychiatric Treat 1997;3:58–63.
89. Gormley N, Watters L, Lawlor BA. Extrapyramidal side effects in elderly patients exposed to selective serotonin reuptake inhibitors. Hum Psychopharmacol 1997;12:139–143.

90. Omar SJ, Robinson D, Davies HD, et al. Fluoxetine and visual hallucinations in dementia. Biol Psychiatry 1995;38:556–558.
91. Kerihuel JC, Dreyfus JF. Meta-analyses of the efficacy and tolerability of the tricyclic antidepressant lofepramine. J Int Med Res 1991;19:183–201.
92. Anderson IM, Tomenson BM. The efficacy of selective serotonin reuptake inhibitors in depression: a meta-analysis of studies against tricyclic antidepressants. J Psychopharmacol 1994;8:238–249.
93. Postma JU, Vranesci D. Moclobemide in the treatment of depression in demented geriatric patients. Acta Ther 1985;11:1–4.
94. Nelson JP, Rosenberg DR. ECT treatment of demented elderly patients with major depression: a retrospective study of efficacy and safety. Convuls Ther 1991;7:157–165.
95. Peisah C, Brodaty H. Practical guidelines for the treatment of behavioural complications of dementia. Med J Aust 1994;161:558–563.
96. Loebel JP, Leibovici A. The management of other psychiatric states. Med Clin North Am 1994;78: 841–859.
97. Devanand DP, Jacobs DM, Tang Ming-X, et al. The course of psychopathology in mild to moderate Alzheimer's disease. Arch of Gen Psychiatry 1997;54:257–263.
98. Hope RA, Patel V. Assessment of Behavioural Phenomena in Dementia. In A Burns (ed), Ageing and Dementia: A Methodological Approach. London: Edward Arnold, 1993;221–236.
99. Sanford JRA. Tolerance of debility in elderly dependants by supporters at home: its significance for hospital practice. BMJ 1975;3:471–473.
100. Beck CK, Shue VM. Interventions for treating disruptive behaviour in demented elderly people. Nurs Clin North Am 1994;29:143–155.
101. Ahmed I. Pharmacologic treatment of behavioral symptoms of Alzheimer's dementia. A review and a possible strategy. Clin Gerontol 1995;16:3–16.
102. Tune LE, Steele C, Cooper T. Neuroleptic drugs in the management of behavioral symptoms of Alzheimer's disease. Psychiatry Clin North Am 1991;14:353–373.
103. Schneider LS, Pollock VE, Lyness SA. A metaanalysis of controlled trials of neuroleptic treatment in dementia. J Am Geriatr Soc 1990;38:553–563.
104. Schneider LS, Sobin P. Treatment for Psychiatric Symptoms and Behavioural Disturbances in Dementia. In A Burns, R Levy (eds), Dementia. London: Chapman and Hall Medical, 1993;519–540.
105. Barton R, Hurst L. Unnecessary use of tranquilizers in elderly patients. Br J Psychiatry 1966;112: 989–990.
106. Raskind MA, Risse SC, Lampe TH. Dementia and antipsychotic drugs. J Clin Psychiatry 1987;48(suppl 5):16–18.
107. Jeanblanc W, Battey Davis Y. Risperidone for treating dementia-associated aggression. Am J Psychiatry 1995;152:1239.
108. Raheja RK, Bharwani I, Penetrante AE. Efficacy of risperidone for behavioural disorders in the elderly: a clinical observation. J Geriatr Psychiatry Neurol 1995;8:159–161.
109. Stern RG, Duffelmeyer ME, Zemishlani Z, Davidson M. The use of benzodiazepines in the management of behavioural symptoms in demented patients. Psychiatry Clin North Am 1991;14:375–384.
110. Risse SC, Barnes R. Pharmacologic treatment of agitation associated with dementia. J Am Geriatr Soc 1986;34:368–376.
111. Wragg RE, Jeste DV. Neuroleptics and alternative treatments. Management of behavioural symptoms and psychosis in Alzheimer's disease and related conditions. Psychiatry Clin North Am 1988;11: 195–213.
112. Hoyer D. Functional correlates of serotonin $5\text{-}HT_1$ recognition sites. J Recept Res 1986;8:59–81.
113. Colenda CC. Buspirone in the treatment of agitated dementia patient. Lancet 1988;2:1169.
114. Lawlor BA, Radcliffe J, Molchan SE, et al. A pilot placebo-controlled study of trazodone and buspirone in Alzheimer disease. Int J Geriatr Psychiatry 1994;9:55–59.
115. Petrie WM, Ban TA. Propranolol in organic agitation. Lancet 1981;1:324.
116. Lemke MR. Effect of carbamazepine on agitation in Alzheimer's inpatients refractory to neuroleptics. J Clin Psychiatry 1995;56:354–357.
117. Lemke MR. Effect of carbamazepine on agitation and emotional lability associated with severe dementia. Eur J Psychiatry 1995;10:259–262.
118. Sky AJ, Grossberg GT. The use of psychotropic medication in the management of problem behaviors in the patient with Alzheimer's disease. Med Clin North Am 1994;78:811–822.
119. Cooney C, Mortimer A, Smith A, et al. Carbamazepine use in aggressive behaviour associated with senile dementia. Int J Geriatr Psychiatry 1996;11:901–905.
120. Greenwald B, Marin D, Silverman SM. Serotonergic treatment of screaming and banging in dementia [letter]. Lancet 1986;2:1464–1465.

121. Skoog I. Risk factors for vascular dementia: a review. Dementia 1994;5:137–144.
122. Moroney JT, Bagiella E, Desmond DW, et al. Risk factors for incident dementia after stroke. Role of hypoxic and ischemic disorders. Stroke 1996;27:1283–1289.
123. Marler JR, Kozloff RC, Kunitz SC. The NINDS Approach to Vascular Dementia and the Ongoing Nimodipine Clinical Trial. In I Prohovnik, J Wade, S Knezevic, et al. (eds), Vascular Dementia. Chichester, UK: Wiley, 1996;313–329.
124. Knezevic S, Labs KH, Kittner B, et al. The Treatment of Vascular Dementia: Problems and Prospects. In I Prohovnik, J Wade, S Knezevic, et al. (eds), Vascular Dementia. Chichester, UK: Wiley, 1996; 301–312.
125. McKeith IG, Perry RH, Fairburn AF, et al. Operational criteria for senile dementia of Lewy body type (SDLT). Psychol Med 1992;22:911–922.
126. McKeith I, Fairburn A, Perry R, et al. Neuroleptic sensitivity in patients with senile dementia of Lewy body type. BMJ 1992;305:673–678.
127. Committee on Safety of Medicines. Neuroleptic sensitivity in patients with dementia. Curr Probl Pharmacovigilance 1994;20:6.
128. Piggott MA, Perry EK, McKeith IG, et al. Dopamine D_2 receptor in demented patients with severe neuroleptic sensitivity. Lancet 1994;343:1044–1045.
129. McKeith I, Fairburn A, Harrison R. Management of the Non-Cognitive Symptoms of Lewy Body Dementia. In RH Perry, IG McKeith, E Perry (eds), Dementia with Lewy Bodies. Cambridge: Cambridge University Press, 1996;381–396.
130. Eagger S, Harvey R. Clinical Heterogeneity in Dementia: Responders to Cholinergic Therapy. In RH Perry, IG McKeith, E Perry (eds), Dementia with Lewy Bodies. Cambridge: Cambridge University Press, 1996;425–438.
131. Cummings JL, Gorman DG, Shapira J. Physostigmine ameliorates the delusions of Alzheimer's disease. Biol Psychiatry 1993;33:536–541.

14
The Future of Drug Therapy in Alzheimer's Disease

Peter J. Whitehouse

The future of drug treatment in Alzheimer's disease (AD) will depend on advances in basic science and the efficiency of technology transfer from laboratory to clinic. The receptiveness of patients to take such treatments, families to give them, and health care systems to pay for them, however, are also key issues. This chapter focuses on the rapid changes at these interfaces between science and society. Current approaches to treatment are discussed in Chapter 13. Reviews of relevant basic science are featured in Chapters 6, 7, 10, 11, and 12.

Public pressure to find more effective interventions is the social and financial energy behind neuroscience, technology transfer, and reimbursements. Such pressure depends on the perception of the magnitude of the problem of dementia worldwide and the clarity of consensus concerning therapeutic goals. Thus, this chapter begins with broader considerations of epidemiology and ethics that help explain the social motivation to develop more effective treatments for dementia.

EPIDEMIOLOGY OF DEMENTIA

An analysis of the age-based stratification of human populations on the earth, including the rapidity with which such demographics are changing, is frightening [1]. Western Europe, particularly Scandinavia, leads in the aging of its nations' population. Resulting strains on health and social systems are evident as these countries race to enhance the productivity of their younger generations to keep their countries competitive in an international market while maintaining a social commitment to the elderly.

Epidemiologic studies conducted in these countries and others around the world reveal that the incidence and prevalence of a variety of dementias are relatively comparable. AD is identified as the most common cause of cognitive impairment in the elderly, with vascular dementia, stroke, and mixed dementia (i.e., both AD and vascular dementia) close behind. The most rapidly growing segment of the populations of fully industrialized countries are individuals over the age of 85 years, who are at most risk for dementia. Some studies in the United States suggest that the chance of having significant cognitive impairment is almost 50% at that age [2]. Other degenerative dementias, such as Lewy body dementia and frontal lobe dementia, are now known to contribute much more to the pool of individuals with dementia than was previously suspected.

Perhaps the most profound implications of global aging are seen in Asian countries [1]. Epidemiologic data from these countries are not as extensive as those in Western Europe and North America, but rates of dementia appear similar. Compared to people in North America and Europe, some Asians may be more prone to hypertension, and vascular dementia has thus been thought to be relatively more common in Japan, China, and perhaps Korea. Nevertheless, high rates of dementia, which are most likely due to AD, will accompany aging in these Asian countries as well as in Europe and North America.

The most dramatic aspect of epidemiology in the Pacific countries is the rapidity with which their demographics are changing. In 1945, the average life expectancy in Japan was the same as that in Europe at the turn of the century, yet the Japanese now have the longest life expectancy in the world. Japan's population is aging five times more rapidly than Western Europe, and China and India's populations are aging even faster than Japan's [1]. A more rapid rate of aging does not allow time for medical and social services to adapt to the needs of older individuals. Moreover, because older individuals have more illnesses and often chronic diseases, which require care over longer periods of time, health care costs will increase. The problem may be most acute in China, where not only is the rate of aging high, but successful birth control programs have also been put into effect. The "one child per couple" rule will lead to a phenomenally low dependency ratio—that is, a low number of younger individuals in the workforce compared to those who are retired and are no longer directly contributing to the gross national product of the country.

Other cultural factors are at work in Asia that will affect care available to the elderly. More women are entering the workforce, so they are not providing as much unpaid care. Patterns of housing are changing, as are social attitudes toward the elderly, who have been traditionally revered in Asian cultures.

As global communication systems permit even greater exchange of cultural beliefs and social data, the world will be able to share the most phenomenal demographic change that has yet occurred: the dramatic aging of the world's populations. This drastic change will require fundamental rethinking of the economic, social, and health systems in all countries around the globe.

The needs of patients with dementia will be at the forefront of creating this revolution in health care. Not only is dementia one of the most common diseases of the elderly, it is also one of the most frightening. Moreover, dementia, by definition, creates cognitive impairment, making the patient more dependent on society than do illnesses that produce solely physical infirmity. Because of this tremendous "age wave" affecting the world and the frequency with which older individuals are affected by dementia, there seems to be little question that the problem of dementia will create increasing social concern in the next millennium.

THERAPEUTIC ETHICS AND GOALS

It seems clear that the problem of dementia will grow and that social attention will focus more on this problem, but it is less clear how different cultures will perceive the situation and react to it. In the United States and much of Western Europe, the dominant model of AD is one of a medical disease with strong genetic components that can be cured (or at least significantly better treated than at present) once the abnormal genes have been identified, the proteins produced by those genes found, and the cascade of pathogenetic events understood well enough that drugs can correct the fundamental abnormalities [3]. Cultural and social factors concerning the phenomenology of dementia are minimized in this model. In other countries, attitudes toward cognitive impairment in the elderly are more complex, with cultural factors playing a dominant role. Although many medical systems in the Third World are being influenced by Western models, it is still widely believed that cognitive impairment is a common and even expected accompaniment of normal aging. Thus, either because of different and, perhaps, stronger cultural traditions, or because of lack of access to Western medical knowledge and models of disease, peoples of the world view dementia in quite different ways.

Just as the goals of medicine are being re-examined internationally [4–7], attitudes toward diseases of the elderly need to be critically examined in the United States and Western Europe. In these countries, particularly the United States, medicine has been dominated by technology and has focused on finding a cure for diseases rather than providing care. One gets the impression that the goal in U.S. medicine is to help people live forever. The focus of U.S. medical care on the individual, with autonomy as the dominant ethical principle, is being challenged and tested in relation to community health problems of enormous scope, including the aging of the population. In the future, public rather than individual health will achieve more emphasis [8]. There will be a greater focus on quality of life rather than quantity of life. Reconsideration of the therapeutic goals in dementia will lead to some reconsiderations of the purpose of health care systems [9–11].

Little attention has been paid to the therapeutic goals in AD beyond that of finding a cure. In this chapter, the goals considered are symptomatic improvement and alteration of disease course. Ultimately, alteration of disease course involves either preventing the disease or stopping it once it has started, or at least slowing deterioration of the patient's cognitive impairment [12]. Too often, the lofty goal of cure, which may be unrealistic in any reasonable time for planning systems of care, has prevented examination of more realistic goals that might be achieved in the short term. Moreover, a focus on biological interventions tends to minimize the need to think systematically about care for the patient using a biopsychosocial model. The hegemony of overly simplistic biological approaches is not desirable.

Fundamental changes are occurring in health care systems around the world. The diseases of the elderly are requiring medical professionals to look at the artificial distinction between medical and social care. The goals of treating chronic disease are different from those for treating acute disease. The goals of treating individuals who are near the end of life are different from those for individuals who are nearer the beginning of life [13]. To date, the implications of chronic diseases like AD have received little recognition because most of the focus is on the acute care system, particularly its cost. The development of internal markets in the United Kingdom and the development of managed care in the United States represent similar trends, in which organizations of providers are becoming responsible for groups of patients in a capitated fashion. The focus on evidence-based medicine and outcomes research will continue to challenge health care providers to document the impact of interventions on quality of life [14,15]. When we recognize that we cannot have two systems of care, acute and long-term, then the integration of care systems will lead to more complex but it is hoped seamless systems of care that can follow patients with chronic diseases over the long course of illness. Common models of care, financing, and information processing will integrate these systems.

Perhaps the most critical area of public discourse to watch in monitoring the evolution of values in health care systems is attitudes and laws concerning physician-assisted suicide and euthanasia [16]. Changes in clinical practice and occasionally the law have occurred in countries such as the Netherlands, Australia, and the United States. It is likely that discussion about the definition of life and attitudes toward its ending will be as contentious as the issue of abortion has been [17]. To date, dementia has been essentially precluded from this debate, because so far it has been accepted that patients must be judged mentally competent before they can participate in any kind of physician-assisted suicide or active euthanasia decision. How will we deal with the demented patient in a health care system that values quality of life and permits individuals more control over death? If I write an advance directive about euthanasia when I am competent, will my family and health care providers honor it if I become demented? Do I want to consume society's resources when I am severely impaired?

A number of other ethical issues will be critical to drug development in the future [7]. Attention to the process of informed consent [18] in research with patients with cognitive impairment is increasing. Conflicts of interest between academics and industry need to be identified and managed [19]. In ethical deliberations, attention to the quality of the communication [20] and engagement of a wide group of participants in the discourse, including affected individuals, are key issues [21]. The appropriate use of genetic testing for diagnosis and perhaps to predict responsiveness to drugs is still an active topic of discussion [22,23]. One such issue that requires more public discussion is the appropriate use of placebos in drug trials now that several compounds are being approved [24]. Moreover, what weight of evidence is required to recommend use of a compound such as vitamin E [25,26]? Should we maintain our standard of two well-controlled trials, or under some circumstances could epidemiologic and retrospective data contribute to the approval process? Attention to these ethical issues will be important so that the environment in which drug development proceeds maintains an atmosphere of sincerity and trust.

HISTORY OF ALZHEIMER'S DISEASE DRUG DEVELOPMENT

Through the centuries, numerous medications, herbs, and other biological products have been used to treat older patients with cognitive impairment. The development of drugs to treat AD parallels the identification of the clinicopathologic entity as the principal cause of dementia, particularly in Western countries.

Before this time, a major focus had been the development of medications to serve as general cerebral metabolic enhancers or vasodilators. The latter approach was based on the notion that vascular causes (e.g., low blood flow to the brain) were the principal reason for cognitive impairment in the elderly. Thus, the modern era began with the identification of degenerative dementia, particularly AD, as the most common problem and the beginning of biological studies of the disease that went beyond descriptive neuropathologic studies.

In the 1960s, a loss of acetylcholinesterase was identified in the brains of patients with AD, but this marker is not specific for cholinergic neurons. In the middle and late 1970s, it became clear that a profound loss of choline acetyltransferase, a marker for cholinergic neurotransmitter systems, was perhaps the most characteristic and consistent neurotransmitter deficiency [27]. It had been known before this observation that drugs with anticholinergic properties could in fact cause delirium and memory impairment in human beings as well as in animals.

The next step in understanding the biological basis of cognitive impairment in dementia occurred when the neurons in the septum, diagonal band, and nucleus basal of Meynert (collectively called *basal forebrain*) were identified as the source of the cholinergic innervation of telencephalic structures [28]. The identification of the cholinergic basal forebrain system enabled lesion studies in animals and animal testing of medications. Moreover, early studies identified that physostigmine might have some brief and modest benefits in patients with the disease. It took considerable time before drugs that had better pharmacokinetic properties (i.e., longer half-lives) were developed, permitting studies that demonstrated their efficacy in dementia. Some drugs, such as donepezil and rivastigmine, were developed de novo. Others, such as tacrine and metrifonate, had been used medically for other purposes [29].

Evidence that tacrine benefits patients with dementia was discovered in parallel with a set of guidelines from the U.S. Food and Drug Administration (FDA) concerning what would constitute an adequate application for approval [30]. After several new drug applications were submitted to the FDA, tacrine was approved based on findings that it had statistically significant positive effects on both an objective psychometric test (Alzheimer Disease Assessment Scale) and a measure of clinical meaningfulness (Clinician's Interview-Based Impression of Change).

This history is notable for the long gap between the identification of the biological abnormality and of the development of a medication that was approved. Moreover, it highlights that the focus has been exclusively on the development of drugs to improve cognition. Noncognitive (behavioral) symptoms have been ignored, and little attention has been paid to whether a drug could alter the course of a disease rather than just provide symptomatic benefit. Thus, the development of the first medications approved for dementia illustrate the important interactions between basic biology, technology transfer, and the social acceptance of therapeutic goals.

FUTURE OF ALZHEIMER'S DISEASE DRUG DEVELOPMENT

The biological opportunities of developing more effective medications for dementia are commonly divided into three time periods: short term, intermediate term, and long term [31]. In the short term, we expect to have drugs that will improve the symptoms in patients with dementia based on an understanding of the neural populations affected in the disease and their associated neurotransmitters. In the intermediate term, we hope to have medications that will actually enhance the health of neurons at risk in the disease and therefore slow progression of disease. Our ultimate goal is to understand pathogenesis well enough to develop more targeted approaches to blocking the pathogenetic cascade that leads to cell death.

Short-Term Approaches

A number of neurotransmitter systems have been characterized as damaged in AD, but the principal focus continues to be on the cholinergic system. It is likely that in the next several years a number of other cholinesterase inhibitors will be approved that will provide modest benefits to patients in terms of improved attention and memory. More attention should also be paid to other cognitive abilities—for example, executive dysfunction that may predict need for supervision and health care services [32]. Second-generation cholinergic drugs include selective muscarinic and nicotinic cholinergic agonists. Researchers hope that by developing M_1-selective cholinergic agonists we can improve the effect of cholinergic drugs on cognition and minimize side effects. Phase II studies of several muscarinic agonists, including xanomeline, memric (SB 202026), and melameline (CI-979), suggest that these drugs have some limited efficacy. Unfortunately, whether appropriate dosages can be found that achieve appropriate efficacy and also minimize side effects is unclear. The same can be said for cholinergic channel or nicotinic agonists. Nicotine does appear to have some positive effects on cognition, but it remains to be seen whether side effects can be minimized by developing receptor-selective drugs.

Cholinergic drugs account for the majority of drugs that are currently in Phase II or Phase III trials. One exception is propentofylline, which has some positive effects on both AD and vascular dementia. Its mechanism is unclear, but it may work through mitochondrial metabolism or adenosine. This drug also offers some hope for slowing progression of disease or at least providing some sustained effects after the drug is stopped. Drugs acting on other neurotransmitter systems, such as noradrenalin and serotonin, are also under study.

Intermediate Approaches

In the intermediate term, we need to understand more about the viability of normal nerve cell populations. The pivotal discovery was that nerve growth factor (NGF) is important for the survival of cholinergic basal forebrain neurons, even in adults. Intraventricular NGF has shown some effects on cognition, but unfortunately a remarkably consistent and rather severe side effect profile has also emerged, at least for mouse NGF. Thus, some companies are trying to develop NGF-receptor agonists to avoid the necessity for intraventricular administration of a protein. Other growth factors may also play a role in AD.

A variety of basic science studies suggest that inflammation of an atypical nature may play a role in the pathogenesis of AD [33]. Studies of nonsteroidal anti-inflammatory agents and corticosteroids are underway. Epidemiologic data suggest that exposure to such inflammatory agents may be associated with a reduced risk of dementia [34].

A variety of compounds, including propentofylline; calcium channel blockers, such as nimodipine; and even nicotine [35] have been claimed to slow progression of AD. For example, nicotine appears to protect against amyloid toxicity in cell culture. This finding is even more intriguing when one notes that a number of epidemiologic studies have suggested that smokers are less likely than nonsmokers to develop AD. Thus, the evidence for drugs that may affect neuronal viability come from both laboratory studies and epidemiologic studies in which protective factors have been identified.

Estrogen receptors are present in cholinergic basal forebrain neurons, and estrogen has been shown to improve cognition in healthy older women and in small studies of AD patients. Epidemiologic studies suggest that it may in fact prevent or delay the onset of cognitive impairment in older women. Some trials of estrogen are underway [36].

Free radical damage is also presumed to play a role in AD [37], and recently vitamin E was shown to delay nursing home placement, to slow the progression of AD, and even delay death [25,26]. Problems with the study design limit its interpretation, but it deserves follow-up with studies of other free radical scavengers and antioxidants.

Long-Term Approaches

If we are to prevent or cure AD, we will have to understand the specific pathogenetic mechanisms. Here the focus has been principally on amyloid (see Chapter 10), which appears to be toxic, particularly in the fibrillar form. This view is controversial, but it seems that preventing formation of amyloid and increasing its clearance may be effective early therapy. The apolipoprotein E (*APOE*) allele *ε2* may be protective against AD, and we now know for certain that the *APOE-ε4* allele is a risk factor for AD. Thus, another approach would be to identify compounds that can mimic *APOE-ε2* and transfer the protective effect. Neurofibrillary tangles are clearly associated with neural populations at risk for death (see Chapter 11). The formation of neurofibrillary tangles may involve critical steps, such as the phosphorylation of *tau*. Drugs that interfere with this phosphorylation may prevent the intracellular tangle formation from contributing to cell death.

ADVANCED TECHNOLOGY IN ALZHEIMER'S DISEASE DRUG DEVELOPMENT

Advanced technology will permit us to bring basic science discoveries into the laboratory and develop candidate drugs more rapidly. Many pharmaceutical companies are investing heavily, often in collaborative endeavors into genomics. Large-scale genomics sequencing is exemplified by the Human Genome Project, which is working to generate a physical map of genes involved in human diseases and identify the mechanisms of control of gene expression. This will permit the development of target molecules for drug candidates. As this genetic knowledge is gained, bioinformatics will become increasingly important; that is, information about biological systems and genes will need to be organized into large databases that can be searched and cross-referenced.

A second major advance is combinatorial chemistry. Here the focus is on the identification and screening of lead drug candidates. These procedures can be highly automated, permitting large numbers of compounds to be produced and screened. Both parallel synthesis and combinatorial synthesis are being used. In parallel synthesis, 100 to 10,000 compounds are produced in a single reaction step. Quantitative biological data can be obtained, making this approach useful for lead optimization—that is, the selection of drug candidates that are worth further study. Combinatorial synthesis produces libraries of 100,000 or more members, although in smaller amounts than the parallel process does.

The power of creating such large numbers of compounds is realized only when the compounds can be screened quickly for initial biological effects. The gel diffusion method is one example of the translation from combinatorial chemistry to combinatorial screening. The beads produced by combinatorial chemistry are placed in gels, which are infiltrated with enzymes or other chemicals to allow examination of the activity of the compounds. Once candidates have been identified by these screening assays, they can be brought forward into more complex biological systems, including cell cultures and eventually live animals, to screen for properties that are more directly tied to therapeutic effects.

CHANGES IN THE PHARMACEUTICAL RESEARCH ENVIRONMENT

Pharmaceutical companies are under unrelenting financial pressure for a variety of reasons. In the United States, an estimated 60 million people are enrolled in health maintenance organizations, of which approximately 75% have controlled drug formularies. Furthermore, most drugs lose perhaps 50% of their market share when their generic equivalents become available. Most remarkably, it has been estimated that a single day of delay in putting a drug on the market costs a company over a million dollars in sales [38].

As a result, pharmaceutical companies are reorganizing their clinical research enterprises. Many more companies are outsourcing their clinical trials to clinical research organizations (CROs) or other trial management organizations. It has been reported that the involvement of CROs increased from one out of four projects to more than one out of two projects between 1993 and 1996 [38]. New CROs are consolidating into larger firms or into niche players. Moreover, novel forms of trial management organizations are being developed. Much effort is being devoted to improving the patient recruitment process, as this step is critical to rapid trial launching. Thus, some trial management organizations are contracting with sites to provide rapid availability of patients; direct contact with patient groups may also be a trend to watch in the future.

Another force at work is the globalization of drug development, which is discussed in more detail in the section on Globalization of Drug Development below. Major roadblocks to global approval of drugs have been the various regulatory mechanisms in different countries and the difficulties that companies have in organizing their activities on a global basis. Concern has arisen that U.S. researchers may be losing Phase II studies to Europe because of the perception in the industry that there are greater impediments to performing these studies in the United States. On the other hand, in trials of dementia, there is a sense that U.S. investigators can conduct trials with higher reliability and validity.

Across all levels of clinical drug review (the company, the trial sites, and the FDA itself) there is increased pressure for faster and better performance. The FDA's Prescription Drug User Fee Act of 1992 has improved the speed of the approval process: In 1996, the FDA approved 46 new drugs and 37 new medical devices, compared with 26 drugs and 27 devices in the previous year. In this environment, the traditional dominance of academic medical centers as sites for trials will increasingly be challenged, and academic centers have begun to organize to protect themselves. An example is the University Hospital Consortium, which has approximately 70 academic center members. To proceed successfully, academic centers will have to develop better marketing, quicker review by institutional review boards and legal counsel, better use of information system technology, and better quality assurance programs. In general, they must demonstrate their ability to meet study deadlines with lower costs.

Changes in the Health Care System

This section reviews the broad changes that are occurring in health care systems and describes the response of the pharmaceutical industry to these changes. Although health care systems are changing in different ways in different countries, due to economic and cultural pressures, some generalizations can be made about industrialized countries in which a significant percentage of citizens are older than 65 years of age.

A principal driving force behind health care changes is that cost (as a percentage of gross national product spent on health) is rising in many countries, particularly the United States. Reducing the bottom line is often the dominant motivator for change. Closely tied, and even more important in the long run, is a focus on outcomes research and evidence-based medicine. It makes no sense to talk about the cost of the health care intervention without having some knowledge of whether it works and to what extent. Thus, organizations that produce health care products will more frequently be asked to justify their products in terms of their cost-benefit ratios, using pharmacoeconomic studies. Renewed attention has been paid to such issues in the treatment of dementia [10,11,39].

The response to these pressures for efficiency has been to develop more closely integrated health care systems. In the United States, one response to the need for change has been to move to capitation—that is, a set price per individual in the health care system per year rather than fee-for-service. With this change, the incentives for providing health care are reversed 180 degrees. In a fee-for-service environment there is little disincentive to diminish the number of services provided. In a capitation system, one tries to minimize the use of expensive services and emphasize prevention and patient education.

Thus, in general, there is a focus on improving efficiencies through developing integrated health care systems. Systems can be integrated in different ways, but attention needs to be paid to elements such as care pathways, information systems, and financial reimbursement. For a system to be integrated, care plans must be shared among different providers in the system. Moreover, financial remuneration often is the glue that binds the providers together. A second glue is information systems, which provide system-wide financial and patient care data.

As these integrated systems form and the roles of health care providers change, an increasing emphasis is placed on primary care providers, who are perceived to be less costly than specialists. Primary care providers frequently include not only physicians but also nurses and other health professionals, sometimes practicing as interdisciplinary teams.

Even so, little attention has been given to integrating acute care and chronic care [40]. This is particularly important for the elderly, because their health problems tend to be best viewed as biopsychosocial rather than purely medical. In many countries, the provision of acute medical care for the elderly is separated from the provision of lifelong care for chronic diseases such as dementia. We frequently see poor coordination between hospitals and nursing homes, with community services in a battleground between them. Efforts to integrate acute care and chronic care are being spearheaded by groups such as the National Chronic Care Consortium in the United States. In the United Kingdom, attempts are being made to link health and social services at a local level. Such changes in the health care system are affecting patients with AD and their families, although little is known about their experiences.

As innovative integrated systems are developed, patients with dementia will be viewed as an important population to target. They can become a driving force in the delivery of more innovative health care programs in communities and institutions. In the United States, for example, more than 20% of nursing homes now have special care units for dementia, even though the evidence of their effectiveness is not yet available [41,42]. Special care units have also been developed in many other countries that are facing increasing numbers of patients who require institutionalization.

Health care reform is creating great opportunities as well as concerns for pharmaceutical companies. Like health care providers, pharmaceutical companies need to demonstrate that their products have value. This will require demonstration of effectiveness in large populations of patients, rather than in carefully controlled Phase III trial environments. For patients with dementia, pharmaceutical companies will need to demonstrate the impact of their products on activities of daily living, quality of life, and use of health care services.

Pharmaceutical companies are recognizing that they can no longer view themselves as isolated giants connected to the health care system only by the flow of pills and dollars. Thus, companies are investing in horizontal and vertical integration. Horizontal integration, through consolidation into megamultinational corporations, is designed to increase efficiencies and abilities to deal with the global market. Vertical integration, such as buying pharmaceutical benefit managers and relating to large health care systems, is expected to tie the companies more directly to health care systems.

Companies are also investing in disease-state management, recognizing that the integration of medications into provision of health care will be increasingly important. For example, in the United States, Warner Lambert Parke-Davis (Morris Plains, NJ) and Eisai, Inc. (Teaneck, NJ); and Pfizer, Inc. (New York, NY) recognize the virtues of providing services to patients, families, and physicians, and offer access through toll-free phone numbers. In the near future, with numerous cholinesterase inhibitors approaching the market with similar biological and clinical effects, competition may be based more on information marketing and educational products than on the medications themselves.

As the process of conducting clinical trials changes, opportunities for pharmaceutical companies to collaborate with integrated health care systems will expand. These health care systems will care for large populations of patients and will have extensive information systems, so they will be helpful to pharmaceutical companies in conducting large-scale trials. We may find changes in the traditional distinctions among Phase I to Phase IV. Pharmacoeconomic data will likely be included in early phases. More use of limited approvals may be made, with requirements to collect more data in Phase IV. Currently, in the United States and Europe, the approval process usually requires two pivotal randomized control trials, but the dominance of randomized control studies as the only requirement for approval is being reviewed. Do we always need two independent studies for approval? Could epidemiologic data affect the decision?

GLOBALIZATION OF DRUG DEVELOPMENT

An increasingly important component in the success of pharmaceutical companies will be how efficiently medications can be developed on a worldwide basis. To accomplish this, pharmaceutical companies will need to work with academics and regulators to ensure greater harmonization of efforts in collecting data to support new drug applications in different regulatory bodies. The International Working Group on Harmonization of Dementia Drug Guidelines has been operating now for almost 3 years, developing position papers on various clinical trial designs [43–46]. Subcommittees have prepared reports dealing with outcome measures, such as objective psychometric tests, activities of daily living, and quality of life. Moreover, serious attention has been given to determining which trial designs can demonstrate that a drug improves behavior, slows progression of disease, or even prevents dementia. Finally, consideration has been given to some of the cultural and ethical issues that profoundly affect attitudes toward medications and drug studies in different countries. The aim of this group is to support a global effort to develop drugs for dementia more efficiently by establishing principles for drug development that can be adopted in many different countries. This effort is respectful of local variations in culture and ethical attitudes toward such topics as conflict of interest and informed consent. At the same time, however, it recognizes that more could be done to help the global community of investigators, companies, and regulators working for the betterment of patients who are affected by dementia around the world.

CONCLUSION

The process of drug development in AD is the focal point of major rapid changes. Basic science discoveries combined with epidemiologic observations are opening up vast realms of intellectual inquiry that may lead to more effective therapies. The development of more integrated health care systems offers tremendous hope for improved care for patients with dementia and their families. The integration of biological and psychosocial interventions in a more comprehensive model of care will be a tremendous challenge, but the future for this endeavor looks bright. The academic, government, and industry commitments to developing more effective therapies for dementia are real.

Despite this vast array of opportunities, or perhaps because of it, careful, critical thought combined with social dialogue is also necessary. We must continue to ask questions about what we are trying to accomplish. Fostering academic careers, producing dollars for pharmaceutical companies, and getting elected again are secondary goals. The principal goal for all concerned is more cost-effective medications for patients with dementia. Yet as we consider the state of dementia drug development, it is increasingly important to consider this goal within the broader framework of aging. Most patients with dementia are elderly and have other medical and social problems. The treatment of dementia must be embedded in a larger social response to changing demographics. In addition, we must be aware that health priorities will shift. Although the health priorities of the elderly should remain high, we must not neglect other populations of potential patients in our population, particularly the young, who after all will be called on to be productive workers in a world in which more elderly patients with dementia will need to be supported.

REFERENCES

1. U.S. Bureau of the Census. Current Population Reports, Series P95/92-2: Population and Health Transitions. Washington, DC: U.S. Government Printing Office, 1992.
2. Evans DA, Funkenstein HH, Albert MS, et al. Prevalence of Alzheimer's disease in a community population of older persons: higher than previously reported. JAMA 1989;262:2551–2556.
3. Whitehouse PJ. Genesis of Alzheimer's disease. Neurology 1997;48(suppl 7):1–6.
4. International Group Leaders. The goals of medicine: setting new priorities. Hastings Center Report 1996;26(suppl 6):S1–S27.
5. Institute of Medicine 25th Anniversary Symposium. 20/20 Vision: Health in the 21st Century. Washington, DC: National Academy Press, 1996.
6. Donaldson MS, Yordy KD, Lohr KN, Vanselow NA (eds). Primary Care: America's Health in a New Era. Washington, DC: National Academy Press, 1996.
7. Binstock R, Post SG, Whitehouse PJ (eds). Dementia and Aging: Ethics, Values and Policy Choices. Baltimore: Johns Hopkins University Press, 1992.
8. Whitehouse PJ. Deep bioethics now for a liveable future. (In preparation.)
9. U.S. Department of Health and Human Services, Public Health Services. A report to Congress of the advisory panel on Alzheimer's disease and related dementias: acute and long-term care services. National Institutes of Health, National Institute on Aging. 1996.
10. Whitehouse PJ, Rabins PV. Quality of life and dementia [editorial]. Alzheimer Dis Assoc Disord 1992;6:135–138.
11. The World Health Organization Quality of Life assessment (WHOQOL): position paper from the World Health Organization. Soc Sci Med, 1995;41:1403–1409.
12. Whitehouse PJ (ed). Slowing progress of Alzheimer's disease. Alzheimer Dis Assoc Disord 1997; 11(suppl 5).
13. Whitehouse PJ, Post SG, Sachs GA. Dementia care at the end of life: empirical research and international collaboration. Alzheimer Dis Assoc Disord 1996;10:3–4.
14. Whitehouse PJ. Defining and measuring outcomes in research on Alzheimer's disease and related chronic conditions: an interdisciplinary communication and collaborative challenge. J Mental Health Aging 1996;2:151–152.

15. Whitehouse PJ, Smyth KA, Maslow K. Outcomes research in Alzheimer's disease. Alzheimer Dis Assoc Disord 1997;11(suppl 6).
16. Post SG, Whitehouse PJ. The Moral Basis for Limiting Treatment: Hospice and Advanced Progressive Dementia. A Hurley, L Volicer (eds). (In press.)
17. Dworkin R. Life's Dominion: An Argument about Abortion, Euthanasia, and Individual Freedom. New York: Vintage Books, 1994.
18. High DM, Post SG, Whitehouse PJ. Ethical and legal issues in Alzheimer disease research. Introduction. Alzheimer Dis Assoc Disord 1994;8(suppl 4):1–4.
19. Kodish E, Murray T, Whitehouse PJ. Conflict of interest in university-industry research relationships: realities, politics, and values. Academ Med 1996;71:1287–1290.
20. Post SG, Ripich DN, Whitehouse PJ. Discourse ethics: research, dementia, and communication. Alzheimer Dis Assoc Disord 1994;8(suppl 4):58–65.
21. Post SG, Whitehouse PJ. Fairhill guidelines on ethics of the care of people with Alzheimer's disease: a clinical summary. J Am Geriatr Soc 1995;43:1423–1429.
22. Eastwood R, Amaducci L, Brayne C, et al. The challenge of the dementias. Writing Committee, Lancet conference 1996. Lancet 1996;347:1303–1307.
23. Post S, Whitehouse P, Binstock R, et al. The clinical introduction of genetic testing for Alzheimer's disease. JAMA 1997;277:832–836.
24. Karlawish J, Whitehouse PJ. Are placebos appropriate in dementia trials in a post donepezil era? (In preparation.)
25. Sano M, Ernesto C, Thomas RG, et al. A controlled trial of selegiline and alpha-tocopherol or both as treatment for Alzheimer's disease. N Engl J Med 1997;336:1216–1222.
26. Sano M, Ernesto C, Klauber MR, et al. Rationale and design of a multicenter study of selegiline and alpha-tocopherol in the treatment of Alzheimer's disease using novel clinical outcomes. Alzheimer's Disease Cooperative Study. Alzheimer Dis Assoc Disord 1996;10:132–140.
27. Price DL, Whitehouse PJ, Struble RG. Cellular pathology in Alzheimer's and Parkinson's disease. Trends Neurosci 1986;9:29–33.
28. Whitehouse PJ, Price DL, Struble RG, et al. Alzheimer's disease and senile dementia: loss of neurons in the basal forebrain. Science 1982;215:1237–1239.
29. Whitehouse PJ, Geldmacher DS. Pharmacotherapy of Alzheimer's Disease. In R Friedland (ed), Clinics in Geriatric Medicine, vol 10. Philadelphia: Saunders, 1994;339–350.
30. Davis KL, Thal LJ, Gamzu ER, et al. A double-blind, placebo-controlled multicenter study of tacrine for Alzheimer's disease. The Tacrine Collaborative Study Group. N Engl J Med 1992;327: 1253–1259.
31. Whitehouse PJ. Future prospects for Alzheimer's disease therapy: ethical and policy issues for the international community. Acta Neurol Scand 1996;165(suppl):145–149.
32. Patterson M, Mack J, Geldmacher D, Whitehouse P. Executive functions and Alzheimer's disease: problems and prospects. Eur J Neurol 1996;3:5–15.
33. McGeer PL, Schulzer M, McGeer EG. Arthritis and anti-inflammatory agents as possible protective factors for Alzheimer's disease: a review of 17 epidemiological studies. Neurology 1996;47: 425–432.
34. Kawas C, Resnick S, Morrison A, et al. A prospective study of estrogen replacement therapy and the risk of developing Alzheimer's disease: The Baltimore Longitudinal Study of Aging. Am Acad Neurol 1997;48:1517–1521.
35. van Duijn CM, Havekes LM, Van Broeckhoven C, et al. Apolipoprotein E genotype and association between smoking and early onset Alzheimer's disease. BMJ 1995;310:627–631.
36. Henderson B, Pagnini-Hill A, Emaneuel C, et al. Oestrogen replacement therapy in older women. Arch Neurol 1994;51:896–900.
37. Smith MA, Sayre LM, Monnier VM, Perry G. Radical AGEing in Alzheimer's disease. Trends Neurosci 1995;18:172–176.
38. Lightfoot G, Moench E, Adelgass J, et al. ARCP white paper on future trends: their impact on sponsors, CROs and investigative sites. A report of the ACRP Future Trends Committee. Monitor 1997;1–11.
39. Whitehouse PJ, Orgogozo JM, Becker RE, et al. Quality-of-life assessment in dementia drug development. Position paper from the International Working Group on Harmonization of Dementia Drug Guidelines. Alzheimer Dis Assoc Disord 1997;11(suppl 3):56–60.
40. Evashwick CJ, Weiss LJ (eds). Managing the Continuum of Care. Rockville, MD: Aspen, 1987.
41. Martin RJ, Gwyther LP, Whitehouse PJ. Special care unit research: ethical issues. Alzheimer Dis Assoc Disord 1994;8:S360–S367.
42. Holmes D, Ory M, Teresi J. Dementia special care: overview of research, policy, and practice. Alzheimer Dis Assoc Disord 1994;8(suppl 1):S5–S13.

43. Whitehouse PJ. The International Working Group on Harmonization of Dementia Drug Guidelines: past, present, and future. Alzheimer Dis Assoc Disord 1997;11(suppl 3):2–5.
44. Whitehouse PJ, Sciulli C, Mason R. Dementia drug development: use of information systems to harmonize global drug development. Psychopharmacol Bull 1997;33:129–133.
45. Whitehouse PJ (ed). Report of the International Working Group on Harmonization of Dementia Drug Guidelines. Alzheimer Dis Assoc Disord 1997;11(suppl 3).
46. De Wolf P. The Pharmaceutical Industry: Towards One Single Market? In HW de Jong (ed), The Structure of European Industry. Netherlands: Kluwer Academic Publishers, 1993;237–271.

IV
Questions and Controversies

Introduction

John H. Growdon and Martin N. Rossor

In the practice of clinical medicine, there are more uncertainties than certainties. It is preferable to confront these ambiguous areas and explicitly examine them rather than perpetuate beliefs that are poorly documented. Part IV includes three chapters that address unresolved questions and controversies.

In Chapter 15, Dr. Helena Chui responds to the editors' question, Does vascular dementia exist? She summarizes the biases that prompted this question: (1) Vascular dementia is rarely encountered in the clinical units or in the brain banks of centers that specialize in the care of patients with dementia; (2) as opposed to Alzheimer's disease (AD), there is no consistent vascular dementia phenotype; and (3) it is freqently stated that vascular dementia is simply a matter of strokes, although in fact, many demented individuals with strokes have coexisting AD. Dr. Chui then discusses each point directly and urges freedom from the narrow constraints of dementia concepts that are inherent in the AD model. She documents the biases that hide vascular dementia from clinicians that specialize in dementia. She points out that many different causes, lesion types, and areas of tissue damage can cause vascular dementia, just as many different types of lesions can produce dementia from neurodegenerative causes. Just as AD, Pick's disease, and Huntington's disease are not lumped together in a category called *neurodegenerative dementia*, so it is necessary to admit the plurality of vascular dementia phenotypes. From a mechanistic point of view, Dr. Chui emphasizes emerging evidence that chronic ischemia, alone or in concert with other factors that by themselves may be insufficient to cause damage, can trigger neuronal dysfunction and death. This line of investigation opens new prospects of treatment and emphasizes prevention of dementia by minimizing risk factors for ischemia as well as acute stroke.

In Chapter 16, Dr. Karen Ritchie addresses the vexing question, Is AD just old age? In the past, discussions centered on this question have been more philosophical than scientific. With Dr. Ritchie's chapter, however, it is clear that the tenor of the discussions will change as more experimental data accrue. Shall we view AD as the inevitable albeit unfortunate end result of normal aging, or is AD a disease process superimposed on the aging process? In the chapter's terminology, is AD age dependent or age related? As Dr. Ritchie points out, the answers to these and other corollary questions have enormous biological, medical, and societal implications. On balance, she seems to favor the disease medical model, as do her editors.

The final chapter, Controversies in the Classification of Focal Lobar Atrophies, by Drs. David Neary, David Mann, and Julie Snowden, deals with the nosology of diseases characterized by frontotemporal degeneration. As such, this chapter is really a displaced discussion from Part I. The authors offer their interpretation of how frontal lobe dementia and Pick's disease both fit under the broad diagnostic category of frontotemporal lobar degeneration. According to their view, the topography of cortical atrophy and neuronal loss predicts the clinical symptoms and signs of dementia better than the specific underlying histopathologic changes.

15
Rethinking Vascular Dementia: Moving from Myth to Mechanism

Helena Chang Chui

THE PROBLEM

Vascular dementia (VaD) may be broadly defined as multifaceted cognitive decline that results from cerebrovascular injury to brain regions important for memory, cognition, and behavior. Few would argue that such a scenario commonly occurs. Yet skepticism remains about whether vascular dementia exists as a reliably identifiable entity. Recent titles allude to this skepticism: *Vascular and Multi-Infarct Dementia: Do They Exist?* [1]; *Vascular Dementia Is Underdiagnosed* [2]; *Vascular Dementia Is Overdiagnosed* [3]; *The Decline and Resurgence of Vascular Dementia* [4]; *New Criteria for the Diagnosis of Vascular Dementia: Do We Know Enough Yet?* [5]; *Vascular Dementia: A Radical Redefinition* [6]; *The Dubious Disease* [7]. Vascular dementia continues to provoke controversy.

VaD is surrounded by many problems related to heterogeneity, relevance, prevalence, and uniqueness. First, there is no consistent phenotype, because strokes can strike any region of the brain (the location problem). Second, it is difficult to link causally a stroke to dementia and exclude the possibility that Alzheimer disease (AD) is lurking somewhere in the background (the causality problem). Third, research centers for AD and related disorders rarely see vascular dementia (the sampling problem). Finally, there are doubts that the study of VaD differs from stroke (the significance problem). In 1968, Fisher said that "vascular dementia is a matter of strokes, large and small" [8]. In 1993, Drachman concluded that "from a therapeutic and preventative viewpoint, stroke and stroke-related vascular dementia do not differ" [5]. Thus, the young clinical investigator with an interest in the second most common cause of dementia is apparently faced with a messy set of problems of little basic import.

This work was supported by grants from the National Institute on Aging (1P01 AG12435 and 1P50 AG05142) and the California Department of Health Services.

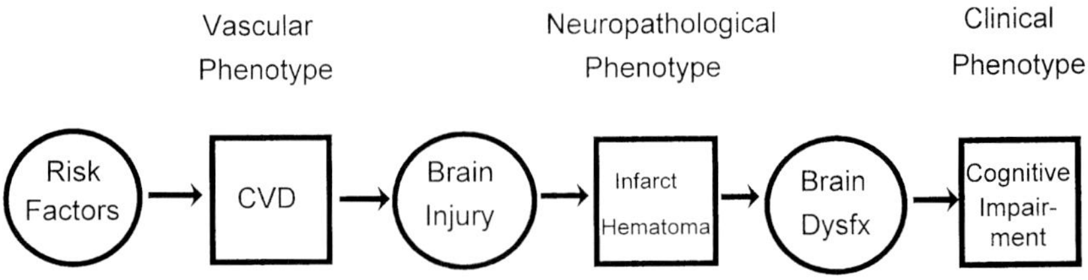

Figure 15.1 Sequence of steps leading from risk factors to cognitive impairment. (CVD = cerebrovascular disease; Dysfx = dysfunction.)

In this chapter, we return to the beginning to rethink the concept and the problems. Rudimentary questions are posed: What are we doing? Where are we? How did we get here? What has happened? Where should we be going? Key issues become clearer when focus is shifted from an attempt to find a mythical common phenotype to the underlying mechanisms that cause brain injury. Mechanisms of brain injury operating over a period of years, rather than hours, remain a needed, but relatively neglected field of inquiry. A shift from phenotype to mechanism promises, in the end, to lead the way to better patient outcomes.

WHAT ARE WE DOING?

Cognitive impairment results from dysfunction of neurons subserving cognition. The relation between risk factors, cerebrovascular disease (CVD), brain injury, and VaD can be viewed as a series of boxes, each holding a large number of possibilities. Risk factors may lead to CVD, CVD may lead to brain injury, and brain injury may lead to VaD. VaD results only when risk factors contribute to produce CVD that is sufficiently severe to effect cerebral injury. Further, that injury must be strategically located and sufficiently severe and lasting to meaningfully impair cognition (Figure 15.1).

A number of risk factors for CVD have been identified, some modifiable (e.g., hypertension, diabetes mellitus), some nonmodifiable (e.g., age, sex, race, heredity) (Table 15.1). There are numerous forms of cardiovascular disease: affecting the heart (e.g., atrial fibrillation, endocarditis), vasculature (e.g., atherosclerosis, arteriolosclerosis, amyloid angiopathy [9,10]), or blood content (e.g., anemia, hypoxia, hypoglycemia). Distinct vascular-related mechanisms leading to brain injury (e.g., ischemia, hemorrhage, or anoxia), and innumerable sites and combinations of sites of brain injury (e.g., cortical association areas, subcortical loops, deep white matter) are possible, resulting in dramatic variations in clinical phenotype (e.g., amnesia, aphasia, abulia, hemiparesis, hemisensory loss). To say the least, there are many steps and possible paths from initial risk to clinical phenotype.

It is worthwhile to note that the diagnosis and prevention of VaD focus on opposite ends of this spectrum. The determination that dementia results from vascular disease requires, first, demonstration of cerebrovascular brain injury and, second, assessment of the lesion's strategic impact on cognition. In contrast,

Table 15.1 The spectrum of vascular dementia

Risk factors	*Vascular phenotype: cerebrovascular disease (CVD)*	*Distribution*	*Mechanism of brain injury*	*Neuropathologic phenotype*	*Location/ neural network*	*Clinical phenotype: syndrome*
Modifiable	Cerebrovascular	Single artery	Ischemia	Infarction	Limbic-dien-	Multi-infarct
Hypertension	Atherosclerosis	Large artery	*Acute*	"Incomplete"	cephalic	dementia
Hyperglycemia	Arteriolosclerosis	Small arteriole	Thrombosis	infarction	memory	Strategic infarct
Hyperlipidemia	Amyloid	Capillary	Embolism	Hematoma	system	dementia
(apolipoproteins)	Angiopathy	Border zone	*Chronic*	Neuronal loss	Multimodal	Lacunar state
Smoking	Vasculitis	Large arteries	Hypoperfusion	with gliosis	association	Binswanger's
Obesity	Tortuosity	Small arterioles	Hemorrhage		areas	disease
Nonmodifiable	Anomaly	Capillaries	Leaky BBB		Corticobasal	
Age	Cardiac	Vein	Anoxia		ganglia–thala-	
Gender	Atrial fibrillation				mocortical	
(estrogen)	Endocarditis				loops	
Race	Myopathy				Deep white matter	
Heredity	Mural thrombus				connections	
CADASIL	Blood content					
HCHWA-D	Hypoglycemia					
HCHWA-I	Hypoxemia					
	Hemoglobinopathy					
	Coagulopathy					

CADASIL = cerebral autosomal dominant arteriopathy with subcortical infarcts and leukoencephalopathy; HCHWA-D = hereditary cerebral hemorrhage with amyloidosis, Dutch type; HCHWA-I = hereditary cerebral hemorrhage with amyloidosis, Icelandic type; BBB = blood-brain barrier.

prevention of VaD does not depend on either demonstration of injury or specific location of injury. We can choose the side on which we wish to start our approach.

Presently, the relation between vascular brain injury and dementia seems best understood in terms of the site and size of injury within neural networks that subserve cognition and behavior. At times, a dementia syndrome may result from a single strategically placed lesion. In some individuals, a single paramedian arterial branch supplies both anteromedial thalamic regions. Occlusion of the paramedian artery in these cases leads to bilateral infarction of the dorsomedial nucleus and the mammillothalamic tracts [11], disconnecting the prefrontal executive and limbic-diencephalic memory systems. Similarly, an infarct in the inferior genu of the internal capsule may strategically disrupt the inferior and medial thalamic peduncles carrying thalamocortical fibers related to cognition and memory [12,13].

A common fallacy in studies of VaD has been to ignore critical features in the sequence of causative events (see Table 15.1). For example, early clinicopathologic studies of VaD examined volume of injury without considering location. Tomlinson and colleagues [14] reported that greater than 50 cc of softening was found in 32% of the demented patients compared to 7% of controls, whereas more than 100 cc of softening was found in 18% of dementia patients but in none of the controls. The volume of softening may vary widely among dementia patients (from <1 to 229 cc) [15]. Other studies have examined location with regard to arterial distribution [16] but not necessarily in relation to cognitive network. Thus, correlations between volume of injury and severity of cognitive impairment have been found but are weak.

The study of VaD emphasizes memory and thinking problems, particularly the interface between cerebrovascular brain injury and cognitive systems of the brain. What can we learn about brain-behavior relationships from the consequences of stroke? What sites of injury are more likely to be associated with cognitive impairment or dementia? Are the effects of repeated or multiple brain injury additive or multiplicative? On the behavioral side of the spectrum, these legitimate questions remain of interest, particularly given recent advances in behavioral and functional imaging. In this chapter, however, we review a broader set of questions and approaches. Our primary purpose as clinicians is to improve the outcome and quality of life of our patients. For this reason, we must be willing to consider alternatives and, if necessary, move on.

WHERE ARE WE?

Hospital-Based Series

The ratio of AD to VaD is approximately 5 to 1 in hospital-based dementia clinics. A review of seven clinical series of patients with dementia (n = 689) showed the most common diagnosis by far to be primary degenerative dementia (47%); a diagnosis of VaD was made in only 9% of patients [17]. This ratio is significantly higher than found in community-based surveys (see the section on Community-Based Surveys, later). Referral bias represents the most likely explanation. Patients with strokes tend to go to stroke clinics rather than to memory clinics.

As expected, the prevalence of dementia among patients hospitalized with stroke is much higher. Based on performance on the Wechsler Adult Intelligence Scale, 56.3% of 71 patients hospitalized with stroke were diagnosed with dementia [18]. Tatemichi and colleagues [19] examined 726 patients with acute ischemic stroke and judged 15.9% to be demented. In a separate series of 251 stroke patients studied 3 months after acute infarction, Tatemichi and colleagues [20] diagnosed dementia in 26.8% based on modified *Diagnostic and Statistical Manual of Mental Disorders* (3rd ed)—Revised (*DSM-IIIR*) criteria. Similarly, Suzuki and colleagues [21] found dementia in 27.2% of 136 patients and Pohjasvaara and associates [22] found dementia in 20% of 486 patients hospitalized with stroke. Thus, dementia is common after stroke, occurring in one-fourth to one-third of cases.

Autopsy Series

In a series of 50 autopsied cases of dementia, Tomlinson and colleagues [14] ascribed an arteriosclerotic cause in 18%. In a review of eight autopsy series, O'Brien [2] noted that "at least one-third of all patients with dementia have a significant vascular component." Mirsen and Hachinski [23] reviewed three autopsy series and classified 15–19% with pure VaD and 9–18% with mixed dementia. Among the first 106 autopsies of patients enrolled in the Consortium to Establish a Registry for Alzheimer Disease (CERAD) with a clinical diagnosis of AD, 87% showed histologic changes confirming a diagnosis of AD [24]. Vascular lesions of varying nature and size, however, were also present in 21%. The proportion of cases with mixed vascular and primary neuronal pathologies has been noted to increase with age. VaD was diagnosed in 15% of patients dying younger than age 70 years and in 22.5% of patients dying older than age 70 years [25]. Thus, data from hospital autopsy series indicate that vascular disease contributes to dementia in approximately one-fourth to one-third of cases.

Community-Based Surveys

In a meta-analysis of 47 dementia studies reported between 1945 and 1985, Jorm and colleagues [26] noted that the overall prevalence of dementia increased exponentially with age, doubling every 5.1 years. In two community surveys of persons older than age 85 years, dementia was found in nearly 30% [27,28]. In Europe and the United States, AD was approximately twice as common as VaD, whereas in Japan and Russia, the proportions were reversed [26]. These patterns hold up in recent reviews [27]. In community surveys of individuals over the age of 65 years [29–40] (Table 15.2), the overall prevalence rate for dementia is approximately 4.5%. In Western nations, the prevalence rate for AD is approximately 2.6% and the rate for VaD is 1.5%. In Asia, particularly Japan, the rates and the proportions are reversed: approximately 2.2% are due to VaD and 1% to AD. In a 30-year complete community surveillance of Hisayama, Japan, dementia was diagnosed in 5.4% (n = 48) of 887 subjects [40]. Pathologic verification was available in half of the dementia cases (n = 24). VaD was diagnosed in 50% and AD in 25%. CVD poses a major threat to cognitive well-being throughout the global community; in some countries it is the most common cause of dementia.

Table 15.2 Prevalence of vascular dementia and Alzheimer's disease in population-based surveys

First author	*Year*	*Location*	*Sample size*	*Dementia severity*	*Lower age limit*	*Dementia prevalence*	*VaD prevalence*	*AD prevalence*	*Mixed (AD and VaD)*	*Other*
Europe and the United States										
Kay [31]	1964	Newcastle, UK	309	sev	65	4.9	2.60 (53.1%)	1.30 (26.5%)	–	20.4%
Broe [32]	1976	Glasgow, UK	808	mild-sev	65	8.1	1.84 (22.7%)	5.77 (71.2%)	–	6.1%
Mölsa [33]	1982	Turku, Finland	19,482	mod-sev	65	2.0	0.72 (36.1%)	1.04 (51.8%)	–	12.1%
Gurland [34]	1983	London	396	mod-sev	65	2.3	0.26 (11.1%)	2.04 (88.9%)	–	0%
Gurland [34]	1983	New York	445	mod-sev	65	4.9	0.68 (13.9%)	3.79 (77.3%)	21.3%	9.1%
Sulkava [35]	1985	Finland	8,000	sev	65	6.7	2.68 (40.0%)	3.64 (54.4%)	–	5.6%
Folstein [36]	1985	Baltimore	3,481	sev	65	6.1	2.80 (45.9%)	2.00 (32.8%)	–	30.0%
Schoenberg [37]	1985	Copiah County, MS	4,503	sev	65	2.2	0.33 (15.0%)	1.21 (55.0%)	–	–
Mean						4.6	1.49	2.60	–	–
Asia										
Hasegawa [38]	1979	Tokyo	4,716	mild-sev	65	4.5	2.70 (59.9%)	1.16 (25.8%)	–	14.3%
Karasawa [39]	1982	Tokyo	4,502	mild-sev	65	4.6	1.67 (36.4%)	0.58 (12.6%)	–	51.0%
Hasegawa [40]	1984	Kanagawa, Japan	1,507	mild-sev	65	4.8	1.99 (41.4%)	1.17 (24.3%)	–	34.3%
Li [41]	1989	Beijing	1,090	mod-sev	65	1.8	1.03 (57.1%)	0.39 (21.4%)	7.1%	14.3%
Ueda [42]	1992	Hisayama, Japan	887	mild-sev	65	6.7	3.35 (50.0%)	1.68 (25.0%)	14.6%	10.4%
Mean						4.5	2.15	0.99	–	–

VaD = vascular dementia; AD = Alzheimer's disease; mod = moderate; sev = severe.

Source: Adapted from TK Tatemichi, N Sacktor, R Mayeux. Dementia Associated with Cerebrovascular Disease, Other Degenerative Diseases, and Metabolic Disorders. In RD Terry, R Katzman, K Bick (eds), Alzheimer's Disease. New York: Raven Press, 1994;123.

HOW DID WE GET HERE?

Several biases exert undue influence over current conceptualization, diagnosis, and treatment of VaD. We have labeled these (1) *categorical bias*, (2) *Alzheimer bias*, and (3) *acute ischemia bias*. Our own bias is that these perspectives have become counterproductive.

Categorical Bias

The very label *VaD* implies several distinct categories: demented versus nondemented and vascular versus nonvascular. Categorical approaches work well as long as the categories are distinct and widely separated. Categories work for cataclysmic events (e.g., trauma or stroke), but less well for slow multifactorial degenerative processes (e.g., AD, chronic ischemia, or mixed degenerative/vascular injury). A diagnosis of dementia forces us to make an arbitrary or operational cutoff. This allows us to communicate with each other but creates a mythical reality.

The distinction between vascular and nonvascular can also prove problematic. Because AD and CVD are both highly prevalent disorders that increase exponentially with age, mixed pathologies would be expected to occur frequently and to increase with age. To a variable extent, the deposition of amyloid is accelerated in blood vessels as well as brain parenchyma [41]. Furthermore, ultrastructural studies in AD cases demonstrate consistent morphologic changes in the microvasculature [42]. In our own series of 26 consecutive patients with neuropathologically confirmed AD [43], moderate to severe atherosclerosis was found in 54%, arteriolosclerosis in 23%, and cerebral amyloid angiopathy in 81%. Lacunar infarcts were found in 15% and hemorrhages in 12%. Unsuspected microinfarcts, often multiple, were discovered in 53% of cases. When there is so much overlap, it may be more accurate to characterize, rather than categorize, the contributions of neurodegenerative and vascular pathologies to cognitive impairment.

Several studies suggest that vascular and Alzheimer-type pathologies interact in an additive or multiplicative fashion. Tomlinson and colleagues [14] observed that some patients with dementia showed both softenings and senile plaques, but neither the softenings nor the plaques alone were greater in demented patients than in nondemented patients. Similarly, among patients with abundant senile plaques and some neurofibrillary tangles, the presence of lacunar infarcts in the subcortical gray and white matter was associated with poorer cognitive function and a higher prevalence of dementia [44]. Quantitative rather than categorical approaches are required to better understand the complex interactions between mixed pathologies.

Alzheimer Bias

Our concept of dementia is heavily influenced by AD. Beyond the formal criteria embodied in *DSM-IIIR* and *DSM-IV* [45,46] (i.e., memory plus other cognitive loss, sufficiently severe to interfere with everyday occupational and social functioning, in clear consciousness), we subconsciously associate dementia with a global process, usually including lack of insight or awareness—such as occurs in AD. It is not clinical practice to diagnose dementia for a patient with a large middle cerebral artery (MCA) stroke or even a small left angular gyrus stroke, even though a computerized algorithm for *DSM-III* criteria would result in a diagnosis of dementia. We do not consistently practice what we have put on paper.

Clinicians often seem to expect a consistent phenotype for VaD. This approach has proved useful in the characterization of AD and other degenerative dementias. In these disorders, specific populations of neurons show selective vulnerability (e.g., limbic, paralimbic, and multimodal association cortices are particularly vulnerable to neurofibrillary degeneration). Degeneration of these neurons produces a fairly characteristic phenotype (i.e., early amnesia, followed by aphasia and apraxia in AD). Experience with neurodegenerative disorders, however, does not necessarily generalize to other types of dementias.

Although a general pattern may be discerned for lacunar state, thalamic dementia, and Binswanger's disease, there is no characteristic phenotype for VaD as a whole. Vascular disease may strike anywhere in the brain. Textbook descriptions [47], as well as the ischemia score [48], have suggested that emotional incontinence, preservation of personality, or epileptic seizures are characteristic of multi-infarct dementia (MID). Clinicopathologic studies, however, do not indicate that these features can reliably differentiate between AD and MID [49]. A characteristic behavioral pattern for VaD is a myth. Fortunately, phenotype is not relevant for primary prevention and secondary protection. Hence, we should not be bothered by heterogeneity of phenotype.

Anti–Chronic Ischemia Bias

Ischemia is the most common vascular mechanism leading to brain injury. Ischemia occurs when blood flow is inadequate to provide the essential substrates (e.g., oxygen and glucose) to support cell metabolism. The relationship between cerebral blood flow (CBF) and cell dysfunction is determined by (1) specific oxygen and glucose requirements of individual cells; (2) local CBF, assuming normal blood content; and (3) duration of hypoperfusion. Energy requirements are higher for neurons than for glia. CBF is lowest in the periventricular and deep white matter, regions that are perfused by long, small, penetrating end-arterioles with no collaterals [50,51]. Thus, the deep white matter is most susceptible to ischemia when there is either an acute systemic drop in blood pressure (acute hypotension) or widespread small vessel arteriopathy (e.g., arteriosclerosis associated with chronic hypertension [52] or cerebral autosomal dominant arteriopathy with subcortical infarcts and leukoencephalopathy [CADASIL] [53]). The threshold for ischemic injury differs depending on the duration of diminished blood flow. In one experimental study, neuronal damage was similar when CBF was reduced below 5 ml/100 g/min for 20 minutes or below 15 ml/100 g/min for 80 minutes [54]. Little is known about neuronal viability when ischemia lasts for years, which is the relevant time frame in the setting of a slowly progressive dementia.

Several physiologic stages are associated with progressive reduction in cerebral perfusion pressure [55,56]. Initially, autoregulatory responses maintain blood flow by inducing vasodilation and increasing blood volume. Once autoregulatory reserve is exhausted, CBF falls. Nonetheless, for a time, cerebral oxygen metabolism is maintained by increasing the fraction of oxygen extracted from blood. Thus, in settings of acute ischemia, increased oxygen extraction fraction (OEF) is taken as a sign of incipient ischemia, indicating that CBF is no longer sufficient by itself to maintain oxygen metabolism.

$$\text{Regional cerebral metabolic rate for oxygen } (\text{rCMRO}_2) = \text{OEF} \times \text{arterial oxygen content} \times \text{regional CBF}$$

If perfusion pressure continues to decline, oxygen metabolism can no longer be maintained. First neuronal dysfunction, then irreversible death occur. The oxygen requirement of infarcted tissue is low. Thus, increased OEF occurs transiently during a critical period of incipient ischemia and then disappears.

Since the 1880s, two different pathogenetic mechanisms have been proposed for ischemic VaD: chronic ischemia and multiple acute infarcts. Binswanger [57] and Alzheimer [58–60] described several dementing disorders associated with CVD: encephalitis subcorticalis chronica progressiva (which later became known as *Binswanger's disease*) and postapoplectic dementia (which later became MID). Pathologically, "incomplete softening" from chronic ischemia due to arteriosclerotic disease of the small vessels was differentiated from "colliquation necrosis" due to acute infarction.

The pendulum subsequently swayed. Initially, the arteriosclerosis/chronic ischemia school was popular. Alzheimer believed that cerebral arteriosclerosis caused both atrophy and dementia [58]. Kinnier Wilson [61] stated, "Apart from gross vascular lesions, haemorrhagic or occluding, a degenerative state of cerebral blood-vessels, if severe and widespread enough, often induces symptoms of a non-specific yet definite kind, not abruptly like a 'stroke' but in a gradual and insidious way." Purves-Stewart and Worster-Drought [62] noted that CVD leads to "neuronic decay," a major cause of presenile and senile dementia. The *DSM-I* [63] definition for VaD was chronic brain syndrome associated with cerebral arteriosclerosis; the *DSM-II* [64] diagnosis was psychosis with cerebral arteriosclerosis.

In the 1970s, a conceptual shift occurred away from arteriosclerosis of the blood vessels and toward multiple infarcts of the brain. In 1968, the term *multi-infarct dementia* was coined, and dementia due to chronic ischemia was said to be rare [8]. Hachinski and colleagues [48] observed that whereas the proportion of gray matter was equally reduced in VaD and degenerative dementia, perfusion was only diminished in VaD. Using the intra-arterial 133 xenon clearance method, however, no reduction was noted in hypocapnic reactivity in either group. Therefore, Hachinski and colleagues concluded that low flow in VaD represented decreased metabolism secondary to infarction, rather than primary vascular insufficiency. That is, VaD is due to multiple infarcts, not chronic ischemia [48,65]. Subsequently, Frackowiak and colleagues [66] found a modest decrease in CBF using positron emission tomography (PET) in patients with MID or AD but no significant increase in OEF to indicate ischemia. Meguro and colleagues [67] found no significant differences in OEF or rCMRO_2 in patients with mild to moderate leukoaraiosis, although in this study metabolic data were obtained only in gray and not white matter. Both the *DSM-III* [45] definition of MID and the *DSM-IV* [46] definition of dementia of the vascular type presume acute infarction to be the mechanism underlying VaD. If chronic ischemia does not exist, then we agree with Drachman [5] who concludes that VaD equals the cumulative effects of acute strokes: The primary prevention and secondary treatment of VaD becomes equivalent to that of stroke.

Experimental and clinical data suggest that the situation may be more complex. Experimental reduction of CBF to 30–60% for 1–3 months in rats [68,69] and gerbils [70–73] produces behavioral impairment and patchy loss of neurons in the hippocampus, striatum, and cerebral cortex. By 8–12 weeks of reduced CBF, both Kudoh and colleagues [73] and Hattori and associates [74] observed alterations of the white matter, including demyelination and gliosis. CBF in these animals, although reduced, remained well above the thresholds associated with tissue injury in acute ischemia models, suggesting that the threshold for cerebral injury differs depending on the time frame. The threshold appears to be higher when the period of hypoperfusion is prolonged. These studies affirm the plausibility of chronic ischemic injury.

Clinical data suggest that decreased blood flow in patients with VaD may reflect, at least in part, compromised vascular reserve—not simply a secondary accommodation to decreased metabolic requirements of infarcted tissue. Rogers and colleagues [75] noted that decreases in CBF preceded the onset of dementia in patients with multiple infarcts but followed the onset in patients with AD. Using $H_2{}^{15}O$ PET, Kuwabara and colleagues [76] confirmed comparable reductions in resting CBF in patients with dementia of the Alzheimer and Binswanger types (25% decrease) but found significant impairment in vasoreactivity to hypercapnia only among the vascular patients (Binswanger group = +1.8%; AD group = +5.7%). These studies suggest that clinical states of chronic or repeated hypoperfusion probably do occur.

Evidence of increased OEF continues to be sought as specific evidence of ongoing ischemia. In patients with severe carotid stenosis, decreased CBF and a trend toward increased OEF was observed in the anterior border zone [77]. Neuropsychological status was not reported in these patients. Yao and colleagues [78] studied eight hypertensive patients with severe confluent leukoaraiosis, with and without dementia, compared with seven normal controls. In the demented patients compared with controls, CBF and $rCMRO_2$, measured using ^{15}O PET, were reduced by 20–30% in gray matter and 30–40% in white matter. In the nondemented patients with leukoaraiosis, no significant changes in CBF and $rCMRO_2$ levels in gray matter were seen, but a 30% decline in CBF and a 130% increase in OEF was found in the white matter. Thus, evidence of ischemia—namely increased OEF—was associated with leukoaraiosis before the development of more globally decreased blood flow and cognitive impairment.

Finally, clinical data suggest that chronic hypoperfusion can lead to ischemic brain injury in the absence of frank infarction. In patients with carotid occlusion, Yamauchi and colleagues [79] observed hyperintensities in the basal ganglia and white matter, progressive atrophy of the corpus callosum, and reduction of oxygen metabolism, without evidence of infarction. Taken as a whole, demonstrations of decreased vascular reserve, increased OEF, and progressive atrophy without infarction urge re-evaluation of chronic ischemia as a valid mechanism for brain injury.

WHAT HAS HAPPENED?

Conceptualization

The change in terminology from MID to VaD was intended to recognize that several vascular mechanisms and many vascular diseases may lead to dementia. Patients with small-vessel disease are not the same as those with cardioembolic strokes or major vessel occlusive disease. White matter changes are more likely to occur in patients with chronic hypertension than in patients with atrial fibrillation. Patients with recurrent lobar hemorrhages should not be treated with anticoagulation drugs. From the point of view of nosology, VaD is akin to neurodegenerative dementia—highly heterogeneous. In practice, however, we are not fully conscious of or committed to the plurality of VaD. We do not expect all neurodegenerative disorders to share similar neuropsychological profiles, metabolic patterns, or responses to treatment. We do not see papers describing the neuropsychological profile of neurodegenerative dementias with Huntington's disease, Parkinson's disease, Alzheimer's disease, and Pick's disease all lumped together. Yet this remains common practice with VaD.

Current diagnostic criteria for VaD contribute, unfortunately, to this confusion. Contemporary criteria tend to lump multiple types of VaD together and favor acute over chronic mechanisms. Thus, it should come as no surprise that epidemiologic, neuropsychological, and treatment studies also tend to lump VaD together. Indeed, in a critical review of the literature regarding dementia associated with stroke, Gorelick [80] concluded that although many of the cardiovascular disease risk factors are logical antecedents, age was the only factor that could be considered a well-documented risk factor. The ε4 allele of the apolipoprotein E gene (*APOE-ε4*) is a well-established risk factor for AD, but its relationship to VaD has been inconsistent [81]. The significance of *APOE-ε4* in patients with VaD is likely to remain obscure until an intermediate hypothesis can be formulated and tested (e.g., Is *APOE-ε4* a risk factor for atherosclerosis?) Methods for subject selection must go beyond current diagnostic criteria to clearly identify what mechanistic subtype of VaD is being studied. Failing this, clear results are likely to remain elusive.

Diagnosis

The choice of diagnostic criteria influences the estimates of incidence and prevalence. In patients hospitalized for stroke, Tatemichi and colleagues [82] applied three definitions of dementia and found three corresponding prevalence rates (27.5%, 30.3%, 41.4%). Also, in a sample of hospitalized stroke patients, Pohjasvaara and associates [22] applied five different definitions of dementia and reported prevalence rates ranging from 6.0% to 25.5%. In a community study of persons older than 85 years, Skoog and colleagues [27] noted that the proportion of cases attributed to VaD ranged from 12.9% to 47.0%, depending on the definition used. In our multicenter study of a series of case vignettes, the proportion of cases diagnosed with VaD ranged from 5% using the National Institute of Neurological and Communicative Disorders and Stroke–Association Internationale pour la Recherche et l'Enseignement en Neurosciences (NINDS-AIREN) criteria [83] to 25% using the modified Hachinski Ischemia Score (HIS) [49] or *DSM-IV* criteria [46] (H. Chui and colleagues, unpublished observations).

As a general rule, current criteria for VaD (Table 15.3) (HIS [48], *DSM-IV* [46], NINDS-AIREN [83], Alzheimer's Disease Diagnostic and Treatment Center [ADDTC] criteria [84], and *International Classification of Diseases* [10th ed.] [*ICD-10*] [85]) share similar characteristics and, arguably, limitations. These criteria are (1) categorical, (2) conservative, and (3) weak in their delineation of subtypes. They have similar degrees of inter-rater reliability [86] but differ in sensitivity and specificity. These distinctions are reviewed below, as they may be useful in selecting criteria for practice or research.

Categorical

Endless hours could be spent debating where to draw the line between demented and nondemented. Which cognitive domains must be affected (e.g., memory impairment plus some other cognitive impairment [*DSM-IIIR*] [45] or any combination of multifaceted cognitive impairment) [84,87]? How many cognitive domains must be affected (e.g., two [83] or three [87])? How severe must the cognitive impairment be (e.g., 1 or 2 standard deviations below the norm, sufficiently severe to interfere with everyday social and occupational functioning [45], or severe enough to interfere with one's customary affairs of life [84])? In principle, any operational definition will serve equally well, although each investigator may have a particular preference. In 1994, the Canadian Research Consortium for Clinical Cognitive Research reviewed the state of diagnostic criteria for VaD and concluded that "no one set of criteria is demonstrably superior to another" [88].

Magnetic resonance imaging (MRI) greatly facilitates the determination of whether vascular parenchymal injury is present or absent. Many investigators would argue about the pathophysiologic significance of white matter signal hyperintensities. Some would point out that microinfarcts are below the MRI detection threshold. For the most part, however, imaging goes a long way in helping us categorize patients as having vascular or nonvascular dementia. Again, the main dilemma lies in determining whether there is a primary neurodegenerative process as well. When the classification schema is categorical, identification of an overlap group is inherently problematic. Diagnostic criteria to distinguish pure AD from pure MID do not perform well in identifying cases in which AD and MID occur together.

Conservative

When one considers the potential spectrum of acute and chronic ischemia and multifactorial cases, current diagnostic criteria are conservative. Few of the criteria delineate a place for chronic ischemia (see Table 15.3). This contrasts with the relatively liberal criteria for AD. In clinical practice, AD is considered a possibility unless a clear reason excludes it. In neuropathologic practice, AD is diagnosed based on widespread neuritic plaques, absent neurofibrillary tangles (CERAD), with fewer lesions required in more elderly persons [89,90]. Thus, when applied together, current clinical diagnostic criteria tend to overestimate AD and underestimate VaD.

Table 15.3 Comparison of some clinical criteria for vascular dementia

	Definition of dementia			*Mechanism of brain injury*				
Criteria	*Memory impairment*	*Cognitive impairment*	*Cerebrovascular disease*	*Acute ischemia*	*Chronic ischemia*	*Hemorrhage*	*Structural neuroimaging*	*Causal relationship*
HIS	NS	NS	Atherosclerosis	Yes	No	No	No	No
DSM-IV	Yes	One other	NS	Yes	NS	Yes	No	Yes
NINDS-AIREN	Yes	Two other	NS	Yes	NS	Yes	Yes	Yes
ADDTC	No	"Not single narrow category"	NS	Yes	Yes	No	Yes	Yes
ICD-10	Yes	Two other	NS	Yes	NS	Yes	No	Yes

NS = not specified; HIS = Hachinski Ischemia Score; *DSM-IV* = *Diagnostic and Statistical Manual of Mental Disorders* (4th ed); NINDS-AIREN = National Institute of Neurological and Communicative Disorders and Stroke/Association Internationale pour la Recherche et l'Enseignement en Neurosciences; ADDTC = Alzheimer Disease Diagnostic and Treatment Center criteria; *ICD-10* = *International Classification of Diseases* (10th ed).

Other criteria for VaD (ADDTC [84], NINDS-AIREN [83]) are even more conservative, as they also require evidence for a causal relation between stroke and dementia (see Table 15.3). In a patient who presents with an acute stroke and a slowly progressive dementia, this stipulation reduces the likelihood of missing a diagnosis and subsequent treatment of the patient as though he or she had AD. Although this is a logical requirement for the diagnosis of VaD per se, it is ironically less relevant for its treatment. The objective of primary and secondary prevention is to reduce vascular brain injury, regardless of location and clinical presentation. The requirement for a demonstrable causal relationship between stroke and dementia challenges our understanding of brain-behavior relationships but may lead to missed treatment opportunities. Such criteria may be going in the wrong direction.

Inadequate Delineation of Subtype

In general, current diagnostic criteria for VaD do not provide a consistent framework for identifying subtypes. The HIS [48] and the ADDTC criteria [84] are directed at the ischemic subtype of VaD. Of these, only the ADDTC criteria recognize chronic as well as acute ischemic mechanisms, but this is not apparent from the basic categories (probable, possible, and definite ischemic vascular dementia). Bennett and colleagues [91] proposed criteria specifically for the Binswanger subtype of chronic ischemic VaD. Subtypes are identified by NINDS-AIREN based on location: cortical, subcortical, and thalamic. *ICD-10* [85] identifies several subtypes of VaD (i.e., acute onset, multi-infarct, subcortical, mixed cortical and subcortical), but the divisions are not based on a consistent conceptual framework; type of onset, number of lesions, and location of lesions are mixed together as classifiers. A consistent subclassification schema is needed to reduce confusion and inform treatment.

Reliability

Results were obtained for a study of inter-rater reliability of the diagnosis of dementia, AD, and VaD (H. Chui and colleagues, unpublished observations). Twenty-five case vignettes were prepared in a standardized clinical format including results of laboratory, neuropsychological, and neuroimaging studies. Clinical diagnoses were made for each case at seven ADDTCs in California using standardized coding sheets for several published criteria for dementia ($n = 4$), AD ($n = 2$), and VaD ($n = 5$). Inter-rater reliability was highest for the diagnosis of dementia ($\kappa = 0.65$–0.74) and fairly good for the diagnosis of AD ($\kappa = 0.4$–0.56) and VaD ($\kappa = 0.42$–0.65). Thus, criteria for VaD can be applied reliably across independent centers.

Validity

Validity of clinical diagnosis is measured against a designated gold standard. For a diagnosis of AD, the traditional gold standard is the demonstration of neurofibrillary tangles and senile plaques, widely distributed throughout cerebral cortex. Detection of these lesions requires microscopic examination of appropriately stained brain tissue. Neither of these lesions is specific to AD—each may occur in elderly persons with normal cognition or in other neurodegenerative disorders. Neither of these lesions is thought to represent the earliest signs of the disease. Arbitrary age-related cutoffs for lesion numbers have served to operationalize the diagnosis of definite AD [89, 90]. Thus, the designation of these histopathologic findings as the gold standard for AD refers more to their historic role, rather than their specificity or primacy.

Neuropathologic studies are also important for VaD but for different reasons. To confirm the presence of vascular lesions greater than 2 mm in diameter, there is no need to wait for postmortem brain tissue. As with demyelinating lesions in multiple sclerosis, vascular brain injury is readily visible by modern structural neuroimaging (e.g., computed tomography or MRI). Furthermore, neuropathology does not elucidate whether there was a causal relationship between a vascular lesion and dementia. Nonetheless, autopsy is still required to identify some types of vascular pathology (e.g., cerebral amyloid angiopathy or tortuosity) and to detect microscopic vascular and Alzheimer pathologies. The neuropathologic examination is essential in sorting out mixed pathologies.

Clinicopathologic correlations illustrate the value of autopsy data. Victoroff and colleagues [92] reported 196 cases evaluated at one of seven ADDTCs. The clinical diagnosis of AD was based on National Institute of Neurological and Communicative Disorders and Stroke–Alzheimer's Disease and Related Disorders Association criteria for AD; however, no standardized criteria were used across the centers for the clinical diagnosis of VaD. Of the 116 cases clinically diagnosed with AD, 100 (86%) had Alzheimer-type pathology, but 20 (17%) had unexpected cerebral infarcts (this included large and small infarcts but not microinfarcts). Using the pathologic findings as the gold standard, the clinical diagnosis of AD showed a relatively high sensitivity of 89% but a low specificity of 37%. Of the 11 patients clinically diagnosed with VaD, five (46%) had CVD pathology (two of these had Alzheimer-type pathology as well as infarcts). Six patients (54%) did not have CVD (four had Alzheimer-type and two had Lewy body pathology). Finally, of the 19 patients clinically diagnosed as mixed AD/VaD, only four (21%) revealed mixed AD/VaD pathology; nine had AD pathology without CVD, two had CVD without AD pathology, and four had neither AD or CVD pathology. Thus, apparently straightforward cases often show mixed pathology, whereas cases with suspected mixed AD/VaD pathology often turn up with something else.

At the present time, there are limited data regarding the sensitivity and specificity of the more recently published criteria for VaD. Prospective clinicopathologic correlations show the HIS to be fairly sensitive and specific for the differentiation of pure AD and MID (approximately 70–80%), but relatively insensitive to the presence of mixed disease (17–50%) (for review, see Chui [18]). A meta-analysis [93] of 262 pathologically verified cases (163 AD, 60 MID, 39 mixed AD and MID [MIX]) showed significant group differences in mean ischemic scores (AD = 3.1 ± 2.5; MID = 10.5 ± 4.2; MIX = 7.4 ± 5.2). AD and MID were best discriminated by stepwise deterioration, fluctuating course, hypertension, atherosclerosis, and focal neurologic symptoms. Very few items distinguished MIX from either MID or AD. Thus, an HIS ischemic score of 5 or 6 was 92% sensitive but only 18% specific for a diagnosis of MIX.

In a collaborative study among several California ADDTCs, the sensitivity and specificity of the HIS, as well as the *DSM-IV*, ADDTC, and NINDS-AIREN were examined using the "final diagnosis" as the gold standard (H. Chui and colleagues, unpublished observations). The final diagnoses for 25 case vignettes were based on prospective follow-up (mean duration = 4.4 years ± 2.5; range = 1–10 years), as well as from autopsy data (available in 56% of cases). The final diagnoses were distributed as follows: 20% nondemented, 16% AD, 16% VaD, 8% MIX, 40% other dementias. In general, the criteria for VaD showed low to moderate sensitivity but high specificity. The *DSM-IV* and ADDTC criteria showed moderate sensitivity (52% and 50%, respectively) and high specificity (83% and 89%, respectively). The HIS was less sensitive (31% for the original HIS; 38% for the modified HIS), but still very specific (92% for the original HIS; 79% for the modified HIS). The NINDS-AIREN criteria were by far the least sensitive (17%) although the most specific (97%). Thus, currently used criteria for VaD differ greatly in sensitivity.

Treatment

Randomized, double-blind, placebo-controlled trials have been conducted for a wide variety of compounds in patients with VaD. Experience with these drugs has been reviewed [94,95]. Alkaloid derivatives, such as a combination of ergoloid mesylates (Hydergine) and nicergoline, have been used because of their vasoactive and metabolic activating effects [96,97]. Vinca alkaloids (e.g., vincamine, vinburine, vinpocetine) increase CBF, activate cerebral metabolism, and modulate neurotransmitter release [98,99]. Similarly, piracetam and its analogues (aniracetam, etiracetam, oxiracetam, and pramiracetam) appear to enhance cerebral metabolism and modulate neurotransmitter functions [100–103]. Pentoxifylline increases red cell deformability, decreases blood viscosity, inhibits platelet aggregation and thrombus formation, and suppresses leukocyte adhesion [104–106]. Propentofylline has similar hemorrheologic properties but also some neuroprotective effects, including inhibition of excessive glutamate release, calcium accumulation, and free radical formation [94]. Calcium channel antagonists (e.g., nimodipine) exert a neuroprotective effect in acute experimental ischemia [95]. Many of the compounds studied so far have shown only moderate benefit, often of similar magnitude in AD as well as VaD patients, suggesting that their mode of action may be common to both types of dementia or a nonspecific form of tertiary amelioration.

Pharmacologic trials for VaD have generally targeted phenotype (i.e., dementia) without clearly defining the mechanism by which improvement is expected to occur and selecting subjects accordingly. As mentioned previously in the section on Inadequate Delineation of Subtype, current diagnostic criteria are not sufficiently rigorous or informative in this regard. For example, a drug may be chosen because of its rheologic properties (e.g., pentoxifylline) without attempting to select patients with microcirculatory defects. Similarly, a drug may be studied for its neurotransmitter effects (e.g., bromocriptine) without selecting those patients that are likely to have this defect. Or a drug may be studied because of its protective effects in acute experimental ischemia without attempting to select patients with ongoing ischemia. A classification schema that emphasizes mechanism may clarify the relation between pharmacologic rationale and subject selection.

Unless one's target is ongoing ischemia and its possible interactions with other mechanisms of neuronal injury, the prevention and treatment of VaD is essentially the same as the prevention and treatment of stroke [5]. Expecting improved cognition in MID is akin to seeking motor recovery from hemiparesis following a completed MCA stroke. No effective drug treatment has been found. On the other hand, the prevention of further cognitive decline in MID is akin to preventing recurrent transient ischemic attacks or infarcts. Indeed, Meyer and colleagues [107,108] found that 325 mg of aspirin, administered daily, improved or stabilized decline in cerebral perfusion and cognition in patients with MID. Many of the treatments being developed for acute stroke are also likely to reduce the burden of VaD.

WHERE SHOULD WE GO?

Classification

Despite the limitations discussed in the section on Categorical Bias, a categorical approach (i.e., diagnosis) is likely to remain a necessity in clinical practice. Patient and payor seek diagnoses. Notwithstanding, changes can be made to bring diagnosis into closer alignment with cause and treatment. We can classify VaD based on pathogenetic mechanism(s) and risk factors, as well as on phenotype. We propose a multilevel classification schema that addresses risk factors (primary prevention), mechanism (secondary prevention), and functional impairment (tertiary amelioration) (Table 15.4). This method readily accommodates multifactorial contributions to brain injury. This classification schema could be used in a variety of ways. For example, one could start with phenotype (tertiary amelioration), specify cause (secondary prevention), and finally list major risk factors (primary prevention). Accordingly, a patient previously diagnosed with MID would be classified as having dementia, due to acute ischemic brain injury as a result of hypertension and atrial fibrillation. A patient formerly diagnosed with Binswanger's disease [109,110] would be classified as dementia, due to acute and chronic ischemic brain injury as a result of hypertension. A patient with mixed dementia would be classified as having dementia due to (1) acute ischemic vascular injury due to hypertension and to (2) sporadic AD. In this way, the major functional impairments, as well as opportunities for treatment, would be systematically highlighted.

We agree with Hachinski [6] that emphasis should be placed on the early recognition of cognitive impairment due to CVD, long before it becomes severe multifaceted cognitive impairment or dementia. Hachinski has suggested that VaD be redefined as *vascular cognitive impairment* to heighten our sensitivity for early detection and treatment. Arguably, this shift in emphasis is equally pertinent to other causes of dementia, such as AD, Pick's disease, or hypothyroidism. Furthermore, whereas catching a patient with early cognitive impairment is better than waiting until there is dementia, it is, in a sense, still too late. The proposed classification scheme uses cognitive impairment rather than dementia as the primary functional impairment category. The scheme could be readily applied to other causes of dementia. Finally, this system of classification acknowledges vas-

Table 15.4 Classification of vascular brain injury based on treatment strategy

- Primary prevention: risk factor reduction—identify by risk factors
  - Hypertension
  - Hyperglycemia
  - Hyperlipidemia
  - Atrial fibrillation
- Secondary prevention: classify by proximate mechanistic cause
  - Ischemic vascular brain injury
    - Acute
      - Atherosclerosis
      - Arteriosclerosis
      - Cardioembolism
      - Vasculitis
    - Chronic
      - Arteriosclerosis
      - Atherosclerosis
      - Cerebral amyloid angiopathy
      - Systemic hypotension
      - Cerebral autosomal dominant arteriosclerotic subcortical infarcts and leukoencephalopathy (CADASIL)
  - Hemorrhagic vascular brain injury; due to
    - Hypertension
    - Vascular anomaly
      - Arteriovenous malformation
      - Aneurysm
    - Cerebral amyloid angiopathy
      - Sporadic
      - Hereditary cerebral amyloid angiopathy with hemorrhage (HCAWH): Dutch type, Icelandic type
      - With Alzheimer's disease
- Tertiary amelioration: classify by symptoms (e.g., ischemic vascular brain injury with . . .)
  - Cognitive impairment (e.g., amnesia, aphasia, neglect, dementia)
  - Affective disorder (e.g., depression, irritability, anxiety, abulia, apathy)
  - Behavioral disorder (e.g., hyperactivity, agitation)
  - Motor impairment (e.g., hemiparesis, extrapyramidal)
  - Sensory impairment (e.g., hemianopia, hemianesthesia)

cular brain injury irrespective of phenotype and identifies risk factors even before there is brain injury.

Treatment

Treatment must have an explicitly defined purpose and target (Table 15.5) to guide research design and subject selection. If our objective is primary prevention, we must define the risk factor and associated type of CVD. The primary outcome measure would be the rate of worsening of CVD, not VaD, a phenotype that appears only if several intermediate steps fall into a certain path that may have little to do with the intervention. For example, we may wish to determine if the

Table 15.5 Possible treatment strategies for vascular brain injury leading to dementia

Treatment strategy		*Mechanism of injury*		
		Hemorrhage	*Acute ischemia*	*Chronic ischemia*
Primary prevention	Manage or reduce risk factors	Management of hypertension Discontinue alcohol	Management of: Hypertension Hyperglycemia Hyperlipidemia Vasospasm Vasculitis Discontinue smoking	Management of hypertension
	Avoid proximate cause		Antiplatelet therapy Anticoagulation	Improve rheology (?)
Secondary prevention/ protection	Neuroprotection	Excitatory amino acid (AA) antagonism (?)	Thrombolysis Excitatory AA antagonism (?) Ca^{++} channel blockers (?) Antioxidants (?)	Excitatory AA antagonism (?) Ca^{++} channel blockers (?) Antioxidants (?)
Tertiary amelioration	Symptomatic treatment Caregiver support Functional rehabilitation	Neurotrophic factors (?)	Neurotrophic factors (?)	Neurotrophic factors (?)

administration of estrogen in postmenopausal women will decrease the rate of atherosclerosis, as measured by the rate of thickening of the carotid intima.

If the purpose is secondary prevention of acute ischemic injury, the clinical trial must be set up in a longitudinal fashion to look for significant differences in the rate of incident stroke or functional decline. This design might be analogous to the beta-interferon trials for relapsing-remitting multiple sclerosis, in which the primary outcome measure was relapse-free interval and global disability [111]. If our purpose is secondary prevention of chronic ischemia, the clinical design would be analogous to clinical trials for chronic progressive multiple sclerosis. Subjects would need to be selected according to the goals of the study.

If secondary neuroprotection for acute ischemia is intended, participation in acute stroke trials may be an option (after the addition of cognitive outcome measures). If secondary protection for chronic ischemia is the target, study patients must be selected based on the likelihood of ongoing ischemia. If our aim is tertiary amelioration, some of the same symptomatic treatments developed for AD, including antidepressants, neuroleptics, and even anticholinesterase inhibitors, may be used.

Similar pathogenetic processes underlie coronary vascular disease and CVD. Many of the interventions for acute stroke (e.g., thrombolytic therapy) have capitalized on developments and experience in the cardiac lab. Strategies to protect neurons from acute ischemia (e.g., *N*-methyl-D-aspartate [NMDA] or α-amino-3-hydroxy-5-methyl-4-isoxazole proprionic acid [AMPA] antagonists) may be effective in settings of multiple infarcts or chronic hypoperfusion. The cost-effectiveness of these new developments in cardiology and stroke for patients with VaD should be systematically assessed.

Other Research Priorities

Several features define a unique field of inquiry for clinicians who are interested in VaD, as opposed to acute stroke. First, the relevant time frame spans years, rather than hours. Second, a variety of mixed pathologies are often at play. Third, as people get older, the variability between them increases. This section describes several important areas for basic and clinical research.

Experimental Models of Chronic Ischemia

The field of acute stroke has been greatly influenced by information obtained from cell culture and animal models. A number of cytotoxic mechanisms have been identified, including excitotoxicity [112], oxidative injury [113], and apoptosis [114]. A variety of neuroprotective strategies have been suggested, and new drugs have been tested in animal models [115–117] and in some human clinical trials [118].

Comparable studies are greatly needed in brains that are hypoperfused over longer periods. Studies thus far have largely been conducted in Japan. Experimental studies in rats or gerbils have demonstrated the injurious effects of chronic low flow states on brain and behavior (for review, see reference 119). In the future, these models may help to clarify the sequence of molecular and neurochemical changes in chronic ischemia, the effects of mild but repeated ischemia [120,121], interactions between ischemia and other pathologies (e.g., beta-amyloidosis), and the effects of candidate neuroprotective drugs.

Neural Networks

At the present time, the relations between vascular brain injury and dementia seem best understood in terms of the locus(i) of injury within neural networks that subserve cognition and behavior. For example, localization of lesions within the context of parallel cortico–basal ganglia–thalamocortical networks [122,123] explains how lesions widely separated in space may lead to similar prefrontal behavioral syndromes [124,125]. The study of vascular lesions has contributed greatly to our understanding of brain-behavior relations in the past. The ability to integrate structural and functional data, not only for an individual case but also among groups of patients, provides new and powerful tools for this endeavor.

Quantitative Modeling of Complex Pathologic and Host Variables

Alternative approaches other than categorical diagnoses should be developed to describe slowly progressive, multifactorial processes. Quantitative models would use continuous variables to describe the severity of injury for each pathogenetic mechanism (e.g., size of acute versus chronic ischemic vascular brain injury, numbers of neurofibrillary tangles and senile plaques, synaptic density) as well as their interactions. Ideally, these models would incorporate the moderating effects of lesion location, host reserve, and regenerative responses. The ability to generate in vivo data, either directly or indirectly, is greatly enhanced by structural, functional, and biochemical imaging tools, although we are likely to remain dependent on neuropathology for certain types of information.

In conclusion, it is time to rethink our approach to VaD. While attending to the needs of our patients, we must consider how they got there; we must relinquish our need for a mythical archetype and return to basic mechanisms, including those operating over longer periods.

REFERENCES

1. Marshall J. Vascular and Multi-Infarct Dementia. Do They Exist? In JS Meyer, H Lechner, J Marshall, JF Toole (eds), Vascular and Multi-Infarct Dementia. New York: Futura, 1988;1–3.
2. O'Brien MD. Vascular dementia is underdiagnosed. Arch Neurol 1988;45:797–798.
3. Brust JCM. Vascular dementia is overdiagnosed. Arch Neurol 1988;7:799–801.
4. Hachinski VC. The decline and resurgence of vascular dementia. Can Med Assoc J 1990;142:107–111.
5. Drachman DA. New criteria for the diagnosis of vascular dementia: do we know enough yet? Neurology 1993;43:243–245.
6. Hachinski VC. Vascular dementia: a radical redefinition. Dementia 1994;5:130–132.
7. Prohovnik I, Wade J, Knezevic S, et al. The Dubious Disease. In Vascular Dementia: Current Concepts. New York: Wiley, 1996;ix–xiii.
8. Fisher CM. Dementia in Cerebrovascular Disease. In JF Toole, RG Siekert, JP Whisnant (eds), Cerebral Vascular Diseases: Sixth Conference. New York: Grune-Stratton, 1968;232–236.

9. Wattendorff AR, Bots GTAM, Went LN, Endtz LJ. Familial cerebral amyloid angiopathy presenting as recurrent cerebral haemorrhage. J Neurol Sci 1982;55:121–135.
10. Gudmundsson G, Hallgrímsson J, Jónasson TA, Bjarnason O. Hereditary cerebral hemorrhage with amyloidosis. Brain 1972;95:387–404.
11. Bogousslavsky J, Regli F, Uske A. Thalamic infarcts: clinical syndrome, etiology and prognosis. Neurology 1988;38:837–848.
12. Tatemichi T, Desmond DW, Prohovnik I, et al. Confusion and memory loss from capsular genu infarction: a thalamocortical disconnection syndrome? Neurology 1992;42:1966–1979.
13. Tatemichi TK, Desmond DW, Prohovnik I. Strategic infarcts in vascular dementia: a clinical and brain imaging experience. Drug Res 1995;45:371–385.
14. Tomlinson BE, Blessed G, Roth M. Observations on the brains of demented old people. J Neurol Sci 1970;11:205–242.
15. Erkinjuntti T, Haltia M, Palo J, et al. Accuracy of the clincial diagnosis of vascular dementia: a prospective clinical and post-mortem neuropathological study. J Neurol Neurosurg Psychiatry 1988:51:1037–1044.
16. Tatemichi T, Desmond DW, Paik M, et al. Clinical determinant of dementia related to stroke. Ann Neurol 1993;33:568–575.
17. Chui HC. Dementia: a review emphasizing clinicopathologic correlation and brain-behavior relationships. Arch Neurology 1989;46:806–814.
18. Ladurner G, Iliff LD, Lechner H. Clinical factors associated with dementia in ischemic stroke. J Neurol Neurosurg Psychiatry 1982;45:97–101.
19. Tatemichi T, Foulkes MA, Mohr JP, et al. Dementia in stroke survivors in the Stroke Data Bank cohort. Prevalence, incidence, risk factors, and computed tomographic findings. Stroke 1990;21:858–866.
20. Tatemichi T, Desmond DW, Mayeux R, et al. Dementia after stroke: baseline frequency, risks, and clinical features in a hospitalized cohort. Neurology 1992;42:1185–1193.
21. Suzuki K, Kutsuzawa T, Nakajima K, Hatano S. Epidemiology of Vascular Dementia and Stroke in Akita, Japan. In A Hartmann, W Kuchinski, S Hoyer (eds), Cerebral Ischemia and Dementia. New York: Springer-Verlag, 1991;16–24.
22. Pojasvaara T, Erkinjuntti T, Vataja R, Kaste M. Dementia three months after stroke: baseline frequency and effect of different definitions of dementia in the Helskinki stroke aging memory study (SAM) cohort. Stroke 1997;28:785–792.
23. Mirsen T, Hachinski V. The Epidemiology and Classification of Vascular and Multi-Infarct Dementia. In JS Meyer, H Lechner, J Marshall, JF Toole (eds), Vascular and Multi-Infarct Dementia. New York: Futura, 1988;61–76.
24. Gearing M, Mirra SS, Hedreen JC, et al. The Consortium to Establish a Registry for Alzheimer's Disease (CERAD). Part X. Neuropathology confirmation of the clinical diagnosis of Alzheimer's disease. Neurology 1995;45:461–466.
25. Katzman R, Lasker B, Bernstein N. Advances in the Diagnosis of Dementia: Accuracy of Diagnosis and Consequences of Misdiagnosis of Disorders Causing Dementia. In RD Terry (ed), Aging and Dementia. New York: Raven Press, 1988;17–62.
26. Jorm AF, Korten AE, Henderson AS. The prevalence of dementia: a quantitative integration of the literature. Acta Pyschiatr Scand 1987;76:465–479.
27. Skoog I, Nilsson L, Palmertz B, et al. A population-based study of dementia in 85-year-olds. N Engl J Med 1993;328:153–158.
28. Ebly EM, Parhad IM, Hogan DB, Fung TS. Prevalence and types of dementia in the very old: results from the Canadian Study of Health and Aging. Neurology 1994;44:1593–1600.
29. Kay DWK, Beamish P, Roth M. Old age mental disorders in Newcastle upon Tyne. Part I: a study of prevalence. Br J Psychiatry 1964;110:146–158.
30. Broe GA, Akhatar AJ, Andrews GR, et al. Neurological disorders in the elderly at home. J Neurol Neurosurg Psychiatry 1976;39:362–366.
31. Mölsa PK, Marttila RJ, Rinne UK. Epidemiology of dementia in a Finnish population. Acta Neurol Scand 1982;86:541–552.
32. Gurland B, Copeland J, Kuriansky J, et al. The Mind and Mood in Aging. London: Croom Helm,1983.
33. Sulkava R, Wikstrom J, Aromaa A, et al. Prevalence of severe dementia in Finland. Neurology 1985;35:1025–1029.
34. Folstein M, Anthony JC, Parhad I, et al. The meaning of cognitive impairment in the elderly. J Am Geriatr Soc 1985;33:228–235.
35. Schoenberg BS, Anderson DW, Haerer AF. Severe dementia: prevalence and clinical features in a biracial US population. Arch Neurol 1985;42:740–742.
36. Hasegawa K. Aspects of community health care of the elderly in Japan. Int J Ment Health 1979;8:36–49.

37. Karasawa K, Kawashima K, Kasahara H. Epidemiological Study of the Senile in Tokyo Metropolitan Area. In Proceedings of the World Psychiatric Association Regional Symposium. Tokyo: Japanese Society for Psychiatry and Neurology, 1982;285–289.
38. Hasegawa K, Homma A, Sato H, et al. The prevalence study of age-related dementia in the community (Japanese). Geriatr Psychiatry 1984;1:94–105.
39. Li G, Shen YC, Chen CH, et al. An epidemiological survey of age-related dementia in an urban area of Beijing. Acta Psychiatr Scand 1989;79:557–563.
40. Ueda K, Kawano H, Hasuo Y, Fugishima M. Prevalence and etiology of dementia in a Japanese community. Stroke 1992;23:798–803.
41. Vinters HV. Cerebral amyloid angiopathy: a critical review. Stroke 1987;18:311–324.
42. Perlmutter LS, Chui HC. Microangiopathy in the vascular basement membrane: a review. Brain Res Bull 1990;24:677–686.
43. Chui H, Zhang Q, Victoroff J, Zaias B. Differentiating Alzheimer Disease and Vascular Dementia: Reframing the Question. In R Becker, E Giacobini (eds), Alzheimer Disease: From Molecular Biology to Therapy. Boston: Birkhäuser, 1996;13–17.
44. Snowden DA, Greiner LH, Mortimer JA, et al. Brain infarction and the clinical expression of Alzheimer disease: the nun study. JAMA 1997;277:813–817.
45. American Psychiatric Association. Diagnostic and Statistical Manual of Mental Disorders (3rd ed). Washington, DC: American Psychiatric Association, 1980.
46. American Psychiatric Association. Diagnostic and Statistical Manual of Mental Disorders (4th ed). Washington, DC: American Psychiatric Association, 1994.
47. Roth M. The natural history of mental disorder in old age. J Ment Sci 1955;101:281–301.
48. Hachinski VC, Iliff LD, Zilkha E, et al. Cerebral blood flow in dementia. Arch Neurol 1975;32: 632–637.
49. Rosen WG, Terry RD, Fuld PA, et al. Pathological verification of ischemic score in differentiation of dementias. Ann Neurol 1979;7:486–488.
50. de Reuck J. The human periventricular arterial blood supply and the anatomy of cerebral infarctions. Eur Neurol 1971;5:321–334.
51. Moody DM, Bell MA, Challa VR. Features of the cerebral vascular pattern that predict vulnerability to perfusion or oxygenation deficiency: an anatomic study. Am J Neuroradiol 1990;11:431–439.
52. Pantoni L, Garcia JH. Pathogenesis of leukoaraiosis. Stroke 1997;28:652–659.
53. Tournier-Lasserve E, Joutel A, Melki J, et al. Cerebral autosomal dominant arteriopathy with subcortical infarcts and leukoencephalopathy maps to chromosome 19q12. Nat Genet 1993;3: 256–259.
54. Heiss WD. Flow thresholds of functional and morphological damage of brain tissue. Stroke 1983;14: 329–331.
55. Strandgaard S, Paulson OB. Regulation of cerebral blood flow in health and disease. J Cardiovasc Pharmacol 1992;19:S89–S93.
56. Powers WJ. Hemodynamics and metabolism in ischemic cerebrovascular disease. Neurologic Clinics 1992;10:31–48.
57. Binswanger O. Die Abgrenzung der allgemeinen progressiven Paralyse. Berl Klin Wochenschr 1894;31:1102–1105, 1137–1139.
58. Alzheimer A. Die arterioskerotische Atrophie de Gehirns. Allg Z Psychiatr 1895;51:809–811.
59. Alzheimer A. Neure Arbeiten über die Dementia senilis und die auf atheromatöser Gefässerkrankung basierenden Gehirnkrankenheiten. Monatsshr Psychiatr Neurol 1989;3:101–115.
60. Alzheimer A. Die Seelenstörungen auf arteioskerotischer Grundlage. Allg Z Psychiatr 1902;59:695–711.
61. Kinnier Wilson SA. Neurology. London: Butterworths, 1940.
62. Purves-Stewart J, Worster-Drought C. The Psychoneuroses and Psychoses. In The Diagnosis of Nervous Diseases. London: Edward Arnold, 1952;740–742.
63. American Psychiatric Association. Diagnostic and Statistical Manual of Mental Disorders (1st ed). Washington, DC: American Psychiatric Association, 1952.
64. American Psychiatric Association. Diagnostic and Statistical Manual of Mental Disorders (2nd ed). Washington, DC: American Psychiatric Association, 1968.
65. Hachinski VC, Lassen NA, Marshall J. Multi-infarct dementia. A cause of mental deterioration in the elderly. Lancet 1974;2:207–210.
66. Frackowiak RS, Pozzilli C, Legg NJ, et al. Regional cerebral oxygen supply and utilization in dementia. Brain 1981;104:753–778.
67. Meguro K, Hatazawa J, Yamaguchi T, et al. Cerebral circulation and oxygen metabolism associated with subclinical periventricular hyperintensity as shown by magnetic resonance imaging. Ann Neurol 1990;28:378–383.

68. de la Torre JC, Fortin T, Park GAS, et al. Chronic cerebrovascular insufficiency induces dementia-like deficits in aged rats. Brain Res 1992;582:186–195.
69. de la Torre JC, Fortin S, Park GA, et al. Brain blood flow restoration "rescues" chronically damaged rat CA1 neurons. Brain Res 1993;623:6–15.
70. Naritomi H, Sasaki M, Kanashiro M, et al. Experimental approaches to vascular dementia. Recent Adv Cardiovasc Dis 1990;11(suppl 1):61–68.
71. Naritomi H. Experimental basis of multi-infarct dementia: memory impairments in rodent models of ischemia. Alzheimer Dis Assoc Disord 1991;2:103–111.
72. Kudoh T, Tada K, Takeda M, Nishimura T. Learning impairment and microtubule-associated protein 2 decrease in gerbils under chronic cerebral hypoperfusion. Stroke 1990;21:1205–1209.
73. Kudoh T, Takeda M, Tanimukai S, Nashimura T. Neuropathologic changes in the gerbil brain after chronic hypoperfusion. Stroke 1993;24:259–265.
74. Hattori H, Takeda M, Kudo T, et al. Cumulative white matter changes in the gerbil brain under chronic cerebral hypoperfusion. Acta Neuropathol 1992;84:437–442.
75. Rogers RL, Meyer JS, Mortel KF, et al. Decreased cerebral blood flow precedes multi-infarct dementia, but follows senile dementia of the Alzheimer type. Neurology 1986;36:1–6.
76. Kuwubara Y, Ichiya Y, Otsuka M, et al. Cerebrovascular responsiveness to hypercapnia in Alzheimer's dementia and vascular dementia of the Binswanger type. Stroke 1992;23:594–598.
77. Leblanc R, Yamamoto L, Tyler JL, et al. Borderzone ischemia. Ann Neurol 1987;22:797–813.
78. Yao H, Sadoshima S, Kuwabara Y, et al. Cerebral blood flow and oxygen metabolism in patients with vascular dementia of the Binswanger type. Stroke 1990;21:1694–1699.
79. Yamauchi H, Fukuyama H, Ouchi Y, et al. Progression of callosal atrophy with deterioration of cerebral oxygen metabolism after carotid artery occlusion. J Cereb Blood Flow Metab 1995;15(suppl 1):S677.
80. Gorelick PB. Status of risk factors for dementia associated with stroke. Stroke 1997;28:459–463.
81. Slooter AJC, Tang MX, van Duijn CM, et al. Apolipoprotein E ε4 and the risk of dementia with stroke. A population-based investigation. JAMA 1997;277:818–821.
82. Tatemichi TK, Desmond DW, Stern Y, et al. Prevalence of dementia after stroke depends on diagnostic criteria. Neurology 1992;42(suppl 3):413.
83. Román GC, Tatemichi TK, Erkinjuntti T, et al. Vascular dementia: diagnostic criteria for research studies. Report of the NINDS-AIREN International Workshop. Neurology 1993;43:250–260.
84. Chui HC, Victoroff JI, Margolin D, et al. Criteria for the diagnosis of ischemic vascular dementia proposed by the State of California Alzheimer's Disease Diagnostic and Treatment Centers. Neurology 1992;42:473–480.
85. World Health Organization. Mental and Behavioral Disorders: Diagnostic Criteria for Research. In The International Classification of Diseases (10th ed). Geneva: World Health Organization, 1993;36–40.
86. Verhey FRJ, Lodder J, Rozendaal N, Jolles J. Comparison of seven sets of criteria used for the diagnosis of vascular dementia. Neuroepidemiology 1996;15:166–172.
87. Cummings JL, Benson DF. Dementia: A Clinical Approach (2nd ed). Boston: Butterworth–Heinemann, 1992.
88. Rockwood K, Parhad I, Hachinski V, et al. Diagnosis of vascular dementia: Consortium of Canadian Centres for Clinical Cognitive Research consensus statement. Can J Neurol Sci 1994;21:358–364.
89. Khachaturian Z. Diagnosis of Alzheimer's disease. Arch Neurol 1985;42:1097–1105.
90. Mirra SS, Heyman A, McKeel D, et al. The Consortium to Establish a Registry for Alzheimer's Disease (CERAD). Part II: standardization of the neuropathological assessment of Alzheimer's disease. Neurology 1991;41:479–486.
91. Bennett DA, Wilson RS, Gilley DW, Fox JH. Clinical diagnosis of Binswanger's disease. J Neurol Neurosurg Psychiatry 1990;53:961–965.
92. Victoroff J, Mack WJ, Lyness S, Chui HC. Multicenter clinicopathological correlation in dementia. Am J Psychiatry 1995;152:1476–1484.
93. Tatemichi TK, Moroney J, Bagiella E, et al. Meta-analysis of the Hachinski Ischemia Score in pathologically-verified dementias. Neurology 1995;45:A239.
94. Knezevic S, Labs KH, Kittner B, et al. The Treatment of Vascular Dementia: Problems and Prospects. In I Prohovnik, J Wade, S Knezevic, et al. (eds), Vascular Dementia: Current Concepts. New York: Wiley, 1996;301–312.
95. Marler JR, Kozloff RC, Kunitz SC. The NINDS Approach to Vascular Dementia and the Ongoing Nimodipine Clinical Trial. In I Prohovnik, J Wade, S Knezevic, et al. (eds), Vascular Dementia: Current Concepts. New York: Wiley, 1996;313–329.
96. Schneider LS, Olin JT. Overview of clinical trials of hydergine in dementia. Arch Neurol 1994;51:787–798.

97. Battaglia A, Bruni G, Ardia A, Sacchetti G. Nicergoline in mild to moderate dementia: a multicenter, double-blind, placebo-controlled study. J Am Geriatr Soc 1989;37:295–302.
98. Nicholson CS. Pharmacology of nootropics and metabolically active compounds in relation to their use in dementia. Psychopharmacology 1990;101:147–159.
99. Hindmarch I, Fuchs HH, Erzigkeit J. Efficacy and tolerance of vinpocetine in ambulant patients suffering from mild to moderate organic psychosyndromes. Int Clin Psychopharmacol 1991;6:31–43.
100. Vernon MW, Sorkin EM. Piracetam: an overview of its pharmacological properties and its therapeutic use in senile cognitive disorders. Drugs Aging 1991;1:7–35.
101. Baumel B, Eisner L, Karukin M, et al. Oxiracetam in the treatment of multi-infarct dementia. Prog Neuropsychopharmacol Biol Psychiatry 1989;13:673–682.
102. Villardita C, Grioli S, Lomeo C, et al. Clinical studies with oxiracetam in patients with dementia of the Alzheimer type and multi-infarct dementia of mild to moderate degree. Neuropsychobiology 1992;25:24–28.
103. Bottini G, Vallar G, Cappa S, et al. Oxiracetam in dementia: a double-blind, placebo-controlled study. Acta Neurol Scand 1992;86:237–241.
104. Black RS, Barclay LL, Nolan KA. Pentoxifylline in cerebrovascular dementia. J Am Geriatr Soc 1992;40:237–244.
105. Blume J, Ruhlmann KU, de la Haye R, Rettig K. Treatment of chronic cerebrovascular disease in elderly patients with pentoxifylline. J Med 1992;23:417–432.
106. Folnegovic-Smalc V, et al. The European Pentoxifylline Multi-Infarct Dementia Trial (EPMID) Study. Fourth Meeting of the European Neurological Society, Barcelona, Spain. June 1994.
107. Meyer JS, Rogers RL, McClintic K, Mortel KF. Controlled clinical trial of daily aspirin therapy in multi-infarct dementia. Stroke 1988;19:148.
108. Meyer JS, Roger RL, McClinitic K, et al. Randomized clinical trial of daily aspirin therapy in multi-infarct dementia: a pilot study. J Am Geriatr Soc 1989;37:549–555.
109. Caplan LR, Schoene WC. Clinical features of subcortical arteriosclerotic encephalopathy (Binswanger disease). Neurology 1978;28:1206–1215.
110. Caplan LR. Binswanger's disease—revisited. Neurology 1995;45:626–633.
111. The IFNB Multiple Sclerosis Study Group. Interferon beta-1b is effective in relapsing-remitting multiple sclerosis. I. Clinical results of a multicenter, randomized, double-blind, placebo-controlled trial. Neurology 1993;43:655–661.
112. Choi DW. Excitotoxic cell death. J Neurobiol 1992;23:1261–1276.
113. Samdani AF, Dawson TM, Dawson VL. Nitric oxide synthase in models of focal ischemia. Stroke 1997;28:1283–1288.
114. MacManus JP, Buchan AM, Hill IE, et al. Global ischemia can cause DNA fragmentation indicative of apoptosis in rat brain. Neurosci Lett 1993;164:89–92.
115. Davis S, Helfaer MA, Traystman RJ, Hurn PD. Parallel antioxidant and antiexcitotoxic therapy improves outcome after incomplete global ischemia in dogs. Stroke 1997;28:198–205.
116. Haseldonckx M, Van Reempts J, Van de Ven M, et al. Protection with lubeluzole against delayed ischemic brain damage in rats. Stroke 1997;28:428–432.
117. Lo EH, Pierce AR, Mandeville JB, Rosen BR. Neuroprotection with NBQX in rat focal cerebral ischemia. Effects on ADC probability distribution functions and diffusion-perfusion relationships. Stroke 1997;28:439–447.
118. Grotta J, Clark W, Coull B, et al. Safety and tolerability of the glutamate antagonist CGS 19755 (Selfotel) in patients with acute ischemic stroke. Results of a phase IIa randomized trial. Stroke 1995;26:602–605.
119. Naritomi H. Experimental Approaches to Vascular Dementia. In I Prohovnik, J Wade, S Knezevic, et al. (eds), Vascular Dementia: Current Concepts. New York: Wiley, 1996;29–39.
120. Kitagawa K, Matsumoto M, Tagaya M, et al. "Ischemic tolerance" phenomenon found in the brain. Brain Res 1990;528:21–24.
121. Li JY, Ueda H, Seiyama A, et al. A near-infrared spectroscopic study of cerebral ischemia and ischemic tolerance in gerbils. Stroke 1997;28:1451–1457.
122. Alexander GE, Crutcher MD. Functional architecture of basal ganglia circuits: neural substrates of parallel processing. Trends Neurosci 1990;13(7):266–271.
123. Alexander GE, DeLong MR, Strick PL. Parallel organization of functionally segregated circuits linking basal ganglia and cortex. Annu Rev Neurosci 1986;9:357–381.
124. Cummings JL. Frontal-subcortical circuits and human behavior. Arch Neurol 1993;50:873–880.
125. Chui HC, Willis L. Vascular Diseases of the Frontal Lobes. In BL Miller, JL Cummings (eds), Frontal Lobes. New York: Guilford Press, 1998.

16
Is Alzheimer's Disease Just Old Age?

Karen Ritchie

Conceptual assumptions concerning both the aging process and its associated impairments have an impact not only on the directions selected for future research but also on everyday clinical practice. In particular, the question of whether progressive cognitive loss is a normal aspect of human development or a pathology to be treated is of central importance in our understanding of the place of the dementias within the health system. In a research context, it raises the issue of whether separate etiologic factors from those determining biological aging should be sought, and in clinical practice, it underlies the decision to provide either palliative care or active therapeutic intervention. This chapter discusses the two issues central to this debate: (1) What is normal aging? and (2) Is senile dementia the endpoint of a normal aging process?

THE NORMAL ELDERLY

The social response to aging is ambiguous. Age criteria are commonly applied in our society for access to positions of responsibility and decision making; wisdom is generally considered an attribute of older rather than of younger adults. At the same time, aging is characterized as a process of progressive disintegration and loss of physical and mental abilities for which the clinical response is essentially palliative and the social response to withdraw responsibility. As Regan suggests to King Lear in Shakespeare's *King Lear*,

> O Sir, you are old
> Nature in you stands on the very verge
> Of her confine. You should be ruled and led
> By some discretion that discerns your state
> Better than yourself

Although the loss of physical and mental abilities with age appears to be an inevitable consequence of accumulated biological stress and perhaps even, as many theorists maintain, the biological programming of senescence at a cellular level [1], the more pertinent issue to be addressed here is to differentiate which changes observed at higher ages are actually due to an inevitable aging process and which are due to disease. A distinction has been made in this regard by Brody and Schneider [2] between "age-related" and "age-dependent" disorders to distinguish diseases that have a high prevalence with age within a subgroup of elderly individuals from those that are the result of the aging process itself and are thus universal should the person live long enough. As an age-dependent disease is also semantically an age-related disease, the alternative terminology of *age-related* and *aging-related disorders* has been suggested [3]. From the point of view of the epidemiologist, age-related disorders have a higher incidence in a vulnerable subgroup of the elderly population for all or part of the senescent period but unlike aging-related disorders, incidence rates do not necessarily increase proportionally to biological aging.

This dual model is in fact rather difficult to apply in practice. For example, incidence rates of diseases such as certain cancers, which increase in the 50s and decrease in the 70s, may be considered age related, but as Forbes and Thompson [4] have pointed out, although all individuals will not contract cancer even if they live a very long time, its appearance in some genetically vulnerable individuals may be triggered by the aging process. Kohn [5] has proposed a probably more satisfactory three-dimensional model distinguishing (1) diseases whose incidence increases with age (2) diseases which are in themselves aging processes, and (3) diseases that have more serious consequences with increasing age.

Difficulty in applying conceptual models of the relationship of age to disease is related in part to limits in present knowledge. The notion of what is biologically "normal" aging is consistently being challenged. Reviewing the present debate over normal values of blood pressure and blood sugar levels, and whether the values justifying treatment should be age adjusted, Manton [6] concludes that "such an age criterion is tending to disappear, suggesting that the 'normal' state for the elderly is not necessarily very different than [that] for younger persons." Manton makes the point that even changes in biological functions once considered to constitute in themselves markers of the aging process are progressively being reassigned to the category of treatable pathology rather than that of normal aging. An example of this is resting cardiac output, which is now considered not to decline significantly with age when latent cardiac disease is screened out; no significant difference has been found between healthy 30 year olds and 80 year olds.

Overall, the normal health expectancy of elderly populations is being set at increasingly higher levels. This can most clearly be seen in the examination of population health trends over several decades. Contrary to Kramer's [7] prediction, based on national health surveys, that increases in life expectancy would be accompanied by a pandemic of illnesses and their associated disabilities, repeat calculations of health expectancy over a 30-year period in Europe, Australia, the United States, Canada, and Japan suggest that although life expectancy has increased, the number of years of life expectancy without disability has remained constant. Levels of severe physical and mental disability show an evolution in parallel with increases in life expectancy, thus producing a state of "dynamic equilibrium" [8] in which the prevalence of chronic diseases increases with the fall in mortality but the prevalent states are less severe [9]. These findings together suggest that the period of poor health associated with aging and preceding death is being pushed upward to higher ages, and the consequences of poor health on everyday functioning is less severe.

It would thus seem that the normal aging process may be a far less catastrophic process than once believed, although elderly populations may nonetheless have high rates of morbidity. Normal health (not to be confused with "average" health) in the elderly may thus be construed as being on the one hand not greatly different from that of younger populations but increasingly rare with age. Such a conclusion would have two important corollaries: First, in a research context, normal functioning cannot be taken to be the average performance of all elderly persons in an age cohort, and second, in a clinical context, many disorders of the elderly are probably undertreated due to an incorrect assumption that they are "normal for the person's age." The latter point is demonstrated by two unpublished observations made by the author.

Fifth-year medical students have been noted to change their diagnosis and treatment strategy if the age of a patient in a case example is altered from 40 years to 80 years, even though the presenting symptoms remain the same. In addition, a high number of cases of essential tremor/extrapyramidal signs in our longitudinal study of cerebral aging [10] were found to be untreated because their general practitioners felt it normal for old people to tremble. Undertreatment of mental disorder, particularly depression, in elderly populations has also been reported elsewhere to be due to a failure to differentiate pathology and normal aging processes [11].

AGING AND COGNITIVE FUNCTIONING

At a biological level, a certain number of aging-related changes in the central nervous system appear to be universal and independent of disease processes. Progressive cortical involution, characterized by neuronal shrinking and loss, enlargement of the ventricles, and loss of dendritic branches and synaptic connections, appears to commence in the 60s, producing an average loss in cerebral weight of approximately 2% per decade [12]. This process is not uniform, with the greatest loss occurring by the ninth decade in the region of the hippocampus, amygdala, and locus coeruleus. It should be noted, however, that age-related cortical loss appears to be far less significant when initial cerebral capacity is taken into account [13].

Studies of cognitive functioning in elderly individuals generally support biological observations, and it has been consistently demonstrated that older adults perform more poorly than younger adults on a wide range of intellectual abilities, in particular on tasks related to limbic system functioning. Deficits are seen particularly on tasks involving analysis of visual stimuli [14,15], attentional abilities as measured by a dichotomous listening paradigm [16,17], and secondary memory for events, or episodic memory [17–19]. On the other hand, short-term, or working, memory and semantic abilities appear to remain relatively stable when results are compared across cohorts and sensory impairments are taken into account [17,20,21].

It is important to note that longitudinal studies of cognitive functioning have demonstrated that much of the difference observed in cognitive functioning between old and young individuals may be attributed to cohort or generation differences, rather than to the aging process [22–24]. The 20-year follow-up study by Schaie and Willis demonstrates quite different results when cross-sectional and longitudinal analyses are compared. Long-term follow-up of individuals, rather than comparison of age cohorts, demonstrates that until the eighth decade, elderly individuals show relative stability across time. This study not only suggests that age-group comparisons may overestimate age-related cognitive decline, but also points to evolution in cognitive functioning. That is, elderly individuals today are performing better than those from the previous generation due probably to factors such as improved health care, nutrition, and education. It may also be an artifact of the greater familiarity of more recent generations with the concept of cognitive testing.

Applying cluster analysis techniques to changing cognitive abilities in a normal elderly population, it was found that 397 elderly persons with subclinical cognitive impairment showed five separate patterns of cognitive impairment across time [23]. Two groups were found to be at high risk for Alzheimer's disease (AD), one group had high rates of depressive symptomatology, one group had a high incidence of acute physical illness, and one group (approximately 10%) showed stability over time. This latter group appear to best represent normal aging, and it is argued that stricter criteria should be applied in the selection of normal groups in studies of cognitive aging and dementia. Above all, results demonstrate the great heterogeneity seen in patterns of cognitive aging and the confounding effects of undiagnosed neuropathology. Examining almost any aspect of cognitive performance in an elderly population, one can see that standard deviations broaden widely with age, thus making it difficult statistically to characterize cognitive performance at a given age and thus establish cutoff points for clinical intervention. This point brings us to the central theme of this discussion: differentiating normal aging processes from the senile dementias.

Generally speaking, two conceptual frameworks have evolved to explain the wide range of individual differences seen in cognitive performance in the elderly, which may range from those showing no change to the catastrophic progressive deterioration seen in the dementias. The first may be described as the cognitive psychology or normative model that makes no distinction between sick and well populations but rather proposes a continuum along a normal distribution from "successful aging," which involves very little loss of function, to the senile dementias (Figure 16.1). Between these two extremes, different degrees of more common forms of cognitive impairment may be differentiated. A number of nosologic categories have been proposed to describe these intermediary stages; *benign senescent forgetfulness* [25] and *age-associated memory impairment* (AAMI) [26] both describe, for example, mild nonpathologic cognitive difficulties related to the normal aging process. The former is defined by reference to elderly persons of the same age and the latter by comparison with young adult performance. The World Health Organization has also introduced the concept of *mild cognitive disorder* into *The International Classification of Diseases* [27] to cover subjective complaints of low-grade, nonprogressive cognitive difficulties that are secondary to a physical disorder.

The dichotomous medical model, which makes a clear distinction between "well" and "ill" populations, provides an alternative conceptual framework. In this case, normal cognitive aging, which may include benign senescent forgetfulness

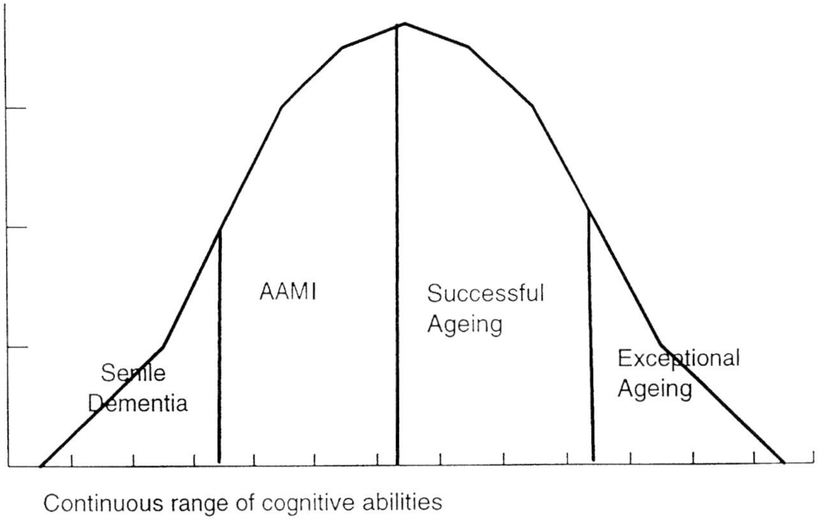

Figure 16.1 Frequency distribution of differing degrees of cognitive impairment according to a continuum, or psychological, model. (AAMI = age-associated memory impairment.)

and AAMI, is clearly differentiated from the senile dementias. Mild cognitive disorder is construed as a pathology secondary to a nondementing disorder that may overlap with normal aging if its course is temporary or fluctuating. Overlap may occur between ill and well populations only in cases in which diagnosis is uncertain or symptomatology has not yet reached clinical levels (Figure 16.2).

The principal difference between these two conceptualizations of cognitive disorder is that adherents of the continuum hypothesis determine the limits for senile dementia by fixing a cutoff point along a continuous range of cognitive decline that may vary according both to the degree to which the cognitive impairment is tolerated by the individual and his or her social context. The dementias are considered to be the endpoint in the normal process of cerebral aging, which we shall all develop if we live long enough. Adherents of the medical model emphasize that dementia involves a pathologic process related to etiologic factors different from those involved in normal aging, although there may be interaction with aging-related processes. Evidence for whether dementia should be construed within a continuum or medical model is the subject of the final section of this discussion. The debate centers on AD as the most common of the senile dementias.

EVIDENCE FOR THE CONCEPTUALIZATION OF ALZHEIMER'S DISEASE AS AN ACCELERATION OF NORMAL CEREBRAL AGING

A number of compelling arguments exist in favor of conceptualizing AD according to the continuum model. At a biological level, senile plaques and neurofibril-

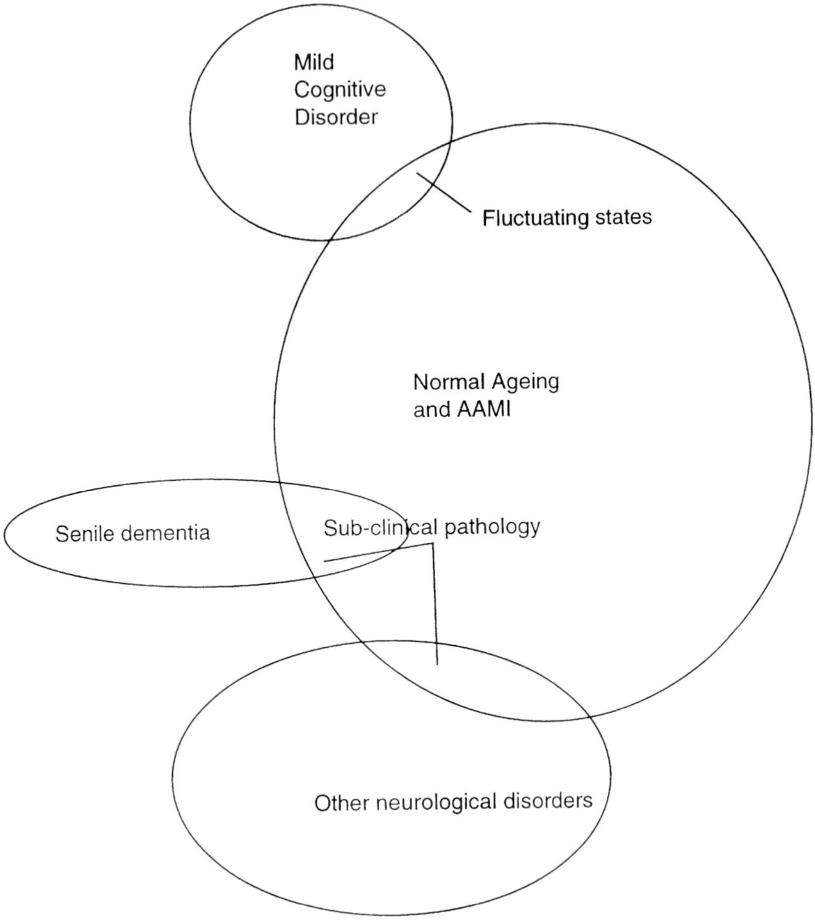

Figure 16.2 The medical model assumes that healthy and sick populations are qualitatively different with overlap occurring on measures of cognitive functioning due to marginal, fluctuating states and prodromal features of yet undiagnosed disorders. (AAMI = age-associated memory impairment.)

lary tangles, which are considered the principal criteria for the confirmed diagnosis of AD, are also found in normal aging, thus suggesting that the distinction is primarily qualitative. This position is further supported by internationally accepted neuropathologic criteria for AD, which provide age-adjusted threshold levels for plaques and tangles in specific parts of the brain based on density alone [28]. Other theorists have also proposed similar biological pathways to both normal aging and AD—for example, theories of programmed neuronal apoptosis [29], free radical neurotoxicity [30], and defective DNA repair [31].

A number of studies have, however, identified qualitative differences at a biological level but only as yet in small clinical samples. West and colleagues [32], for example, have demonstrated different patterns of neuronal loss in the hippocampus in AD and normal patients, consistent and significant loss being reported in the pyramidal cell layer of CA1 in AD only. The longitudinal cerebral imaging study of AD conducted by Jobst and colleagues [33] shows evidence of rapid, catastrophic atrophy occurring in specific areas of the medial temporal lobe inconsistent with the notion of a progressive aging process. Gómez-Isla and colleagues [34] also note distinctive profound loss of layer II entorhinal cortex neurons in very early AD that is not typical of normal aging.

Politoff and Monson [35] have demonstrated electrophysiologic differences between normal aging and AD. Normal aging is associated with posterior increases in the alpha band and decreases in the delta band in anterior regions in comparison with younger adults. According to the continuum hypothesis, AD subjects should demonstrate alpha and delta values that are extensions of these upward- and downward-turning curves. In fact, the AD subjects were found to show a trend in the opposite direction, suggesting that normal aging and AD affect different neuronal populations.

Brayne and Calloway [36] demonstrate a continuous distribution of scores on tests designed to evaluate cognitive disorders associated with AD. The lack of discontinuity is interpreted by the authors as proof that normal aging and dementia lie on a continuum. The study does not, however, take into account the existence of subclinical pathology occurring in early stages of AD that would erroneously classify AD subjects as normal and give an impression of continuity in a situation of discontinuity. The problem is well illustrated by the longitudinal study conducted by Storandt and colleagues [37] in which nine out of 20 control subjects used in a case-control study were found at autopsy to meet neuropathologic criteria for AD. Reallocation of false-negatives to the clinical group polarized cognitive test scores.

At a clinical level there is frequently very little to differentiate initially the complaints of elderly individuals with AD and those with benign impairment. Within a clinical context, diagnosis is often made by reference to deviation on cognitive tests from age-adjusted normative data. Longitudinal studies of cognitive performance in elderly cohorts have suggested many similar changes in normal and AD subjects, with AD being diagnosed beyond a critical threshold [38,39]. Laboratory studies of cognitive functioning in AD also suggest many similarities but also identify impairments that appear to be specific to AD—notably in the visuospatial and central executive components of short-term or primary memory [20,40,41] and semantic memory [42,43].

The very extensive literature on cognitive change in normal aging and AD have been summarized in Table 16.1. Cognitive functions are classified according to the degree of change that has been observed in laboratory studies of information processing. Change is classified as –2 (extensive deterioration), –1 (deterioration), 0 (no change), and 1 (improvement). Overall, the pattern of changes is suggestive of a pathologic process that both accelerates the process of normal cognitive aging and provokes significant decline in cortical areas normally relatively spared.

Caution should be applied in interpreting the results of cognitive tests. Cognitive test batteries used in population studies may be too crude to detect more subtle changes in cognitive subsystem functioning, and the small numbers used in clinical studies may have led to bias, particularly in the selection of normal control subjects. Again, such comparisons are often cross-sectional and may be confounded by cohort effects.

Table 16.1 Degree of cognitive change observed in normal and Alzheimer's disease subjects

Cognitive function	*Normal aging*	*Alzheimer's disease*
Motor speed	–2	–2
Decision-making speed	–1	–2
Focused attention	0	–1
Divided attention	–1	–2
Praxis	–1	–2
Visuospatial performance	–1	–2
Learning	–1	–2
Vocabulary	+1	–2
Verbal fluency	0	–2
Language comprehension	0	–2
Concept comprehension	0	–2
Primary memory	0	–1
Episodic memory	–1	–2
Semantic memory	0	–2
Long-term memory	0	–1
Implicit memory	0	0

–2 = extensive deterioration; –1 = deterioration; 0 = no change; 1 = improvement.

If AD is simply old age—a state we will all ultimately reach if we live long enough—then it is to be expected that at a population level, the prevalence and incidence of AD should increase with age, converging toward 100% at the extremes of life expectancy. Epidemiologic studies of AD have indeed consistently demonstrated that age is a highly significant risk factor for AD, with prevalence rates rising exponentially from age 60 onward [3,44], suggesting that increases in life expectancy may lead to "epidemics" of dementia [45]. The prevalence of senile dementia between ages 60 years and 90 years [3] appears to double every 6 years, and doubles for AD every 4 years according to the exponential relationship log: $P = -16.62 + 0.2(\text{age})$.

A meta-analysis of prevalence studies of senile dementia conducted on population studies that have examined rates at very high ages (85–100 years) has demonstrated a logistic relationship with age [46]—that is, the increase in dementia prevalence appears to slow down after age 80 years, flattening out to no increase at age 95 years, with a prevalence rate of 40%. This result is highly suggestive of an age-related rather than an aging-related disorder, in which a disease process with penetrance at higher ages is triggered by the aging process. Survivors older than age 95 years appear to have decreasing risk of being exposed to the relevant risk factor, be it genetic or environmental. This analysis is, however, based on prevalence data that do not take into account changes in survival rates. The finding requires verification from longitudinal studies of incidence.

Calculations of dementia-free life expectancy (Table 16.2), derived from the adjustment of population life tables by disease prevalence rates and thus taking survival into account in part, suggest a dimunition in dementia-free life expectancy with age [47]. The percentage of life expected to be lived by women falls by approximately 10% in the decade between the late 70s and late 80s in France and Australia, and up to 20% in the United Kingdom. Even at very high

Table 16.2 Dementia-free life expectancy as a proportion of life expectancy (%) for men and women at three different ages in France, Australia, and the United Kingdom

	France		*Australia*		*United Kingdom*	
Age	*Men*	*Women*	*Men*	*Women*	*Men*	*Women*
77	93	91	89	85	94	87
83	89	87	84	80	89	83
89	85	80	80	79	75	71

ages, however, the proportion of remaining life expected to be lived without dementia remains very high.

Using a regression model to project toward the upper limits of life expectancy [48], it was found for France, for example, that at age 97 years, life expectancy without dementia still occupies 67% of remaining life expectancy, and average human life expectancy would in fact have to go beyond 170 years of age under present survival conditions before dementia took up all life expectancy; suggesting that it is very unlikely that all persons will have dementia even if everyone lives to a very high age.

JC of Arles, France, who died in 1997 at the age of 122 years, was considered to be the oldest person in the history of the human race. She had no history of physical or mental illness and did not have AD or other neurologic disorder (she did not tremble). A computed tomography scan showed a degree of cortical atrophy consistent with her age. She had a normal young adult range in primary memory, and secondary memory abilities were reduced but a learning curve was apparent [49]. JC appeared to have escaped cardiovascular disease, cancer, and AD. Although she certainly did not represent average old age, she was nonetheless our best representative of normal (illness-free) cerebral aging.

Can we conclude that Alzheimer's disease is just old age? Present knowledge does not allow that conclusion, although there is perhaps more evidence in favor of a medical model of AD as a pathologic process that, although perhaps triggered by a critical loss of neuronal reserves related to normal aging, would appear to be related to independent etiologic factors. It is difficult to reach a conclusion given our present lack of understanding of the mechanisms involved in the development of AD. Perhaps the most difficult aspect of this question is the determination of normality. An age-related change may only come to be considered a pathology when treatment options become available. If a therapeutic intervention strategy is found tomorrow to halt the cascade of neurologic events leading toward AD, it will no doubt obtain the title of disease and screening methods will be put in place.

Jonathan Swift provides us with an eighteenth-century viewpoint on old age in *Gulliver's Travels*. His portrayal of the immortal Struldbruggs leads to an exploration of the mental health consequences of extending human life expectancy. A sure proponent of Kramer's [7] pandemic theory, Swift would appear to conclude in favor of a separation between dementia (dotage) and normal aging.

> When they come to fourscore years and ten, which is reckoned the extremity of living in this country . . . they have no remembrance of anything but what

they learned in their youth and middle age. . . . As soon as they have completed the term of eighty years, they are looked on as dead in law. . . . At ninety they lose their teeth and hair. . . . In talking they forget the common appellation of things, and the names of persons, even those who are their nearest friends and relations. . . . The least miserable among them appear to be those who turn to dotage, and entirely lose their memories; these meet with more pity and assistance, because they want many bad qualities which abound in others.

REFERENCES

1. Wyllie AH, Kerr JFR, Currie AR. Cell death: the significance of apoptosis. Int Rev Cyto 1980;68: 251–306.
2. Brody JA, Schneider EL. Disease and disorders of aging: an hypothesis. J Chronic Dis 1986;39: 871–876.
3. Ritchie K, Kildea D, Robine JM. The relationship between age and the prevalence of senile dementia: a meta-analysis of recent data. Int J Epidemiol 1992;21:763–769.
4. Forbes WF, Thompson ME. Age-related diseases and normal aging: the nature of the relationship. J Clin Epidemiol 1990;43:191–193.
5. Kohn RR. Causes of death in very old people. JAMA 1982;247:2793–2797.
6. Manton KG, Stallard E. Chronic Disease Modeling. London: Charles Griffin, 1988;97–115.
7. Kramer M. The rising pandemic of mental disorders and associated chronic diseases and disabilities. Acta Psychiatr Scand 1980;62:282–297.
8. Manton KG. Changing concepts of morbidity and mortality in the elderly population. Milbank Mem Fund Q Health Soc 1982;60:183–244.
9. Robine JM, Romieu I, Cambois E. Health expectancies and current research. Rev Clin Gerontol 1997;7:73–81.
10. Ritchie K, Ledésert B, Touchon J. The Eugéria study of cognitive aging: who are the "normal" elderly? Int J Geriatr Psychiatry 1993;8:969–977.
11. Williamson J, Stokoe IH, Gray S, et al. Old people at home: their unreported needs. Lancet 1964; 1:1117–1120.
12. Horvath TB, Davis EL. Central Nervous System Disorders in Aging. In EL Schneider, JW Rowe (eds), Handbook of the Biology of Aging. New York: Academic Press, 1990;270–281.
13. Hubbard BM, Anderson JM. A quantitative study of cerebral atrophy in old age and senile dementia. J Neurol Sci 1981;50:135–145.
14. Crookes TG. The Minnesota percepto-diagnostic test and presenile dementia. Clin Neuropsychol 1983;5:187–190.
15. Ska B, Nespoulous JL. Pantomimes and aging. J Clin Exp Neuropsychol 1987;9:754–766.
16. Inglis J, Caird WK. Age differences in successive responses to simultaneous stimulation. Can J Psychol 1963;17:98–105.
17. Craik FIM. Age Differences in Human Memory. In JE Birren, KW Schaie (eds), Handbook of the Psychology of Aging. New York: Van Nostrand, 1977;27–34.
18. Crook T, Ferris SH, McCarthy M. The misplaced-objects task: a brief test for memory dysfunction in the aged. J Am Geriatr Soc 1979;27:284–287.
19. Ferris SH, Crook T, Clark E, McCarthy M, Rae D. Facial recognition memory deficits in normal aging and senile dementia. J Gerontol 1980;35:707–714.
20. Baddeley AD, Logie R, Bressi S, Della Sala S, Spinnler H. Dementia and working memory. Q J Exp Psychol 1986;38:603–618.
21. Huff FJ, Corkin S, Growdon JH. Semantic impairment and anomia in Alzheimer's disease. Brain Lang 1986;28:235–249.
22. Schaie KW. The Seattle Longitudinal Study: A Twenty-One Year Exploration of Psychometric Intelligence in Adulthood. In Longitudinal Studies of Adult Psychological Development. New York: Guilford Press, 1983;64–135.
23. Schaie KW, Willis SL. Adult personality and psychomotor performance: cross-sectional and longitudinal analyses. J Gerontol 1991;46:275–284.

24. Ritchie K, Leibovici D, Ledésert B, Touchon J. A typology of sub-clinical cognitive disorder. Br J Psychiatry 1996;168:470–476.
25. Kral VA. Neuropsychiatric observations in an old people's home: studies of memory dysfunction in senescence. J Gerontol 1958;13:169–176.
26. Crook T, Bartus RT, Ferris SH. Age-associated memory impairment: proposed diagnostic criteria and measures of clinical change. Report of a National Institute of Mental Health Workgroup. Dev Neuropsychol 1986;2:261–276.
27. World Health Organization. The International Classification of Diseases (10th ed). Geneva: World Health Organization, 1992;318.
28. Khachaturian ZS. Diagnosis of Alzheimer's disease. Arch Neurol 1985;42:1097–1105.
29. Cotman CW, Anderson AJ. A potential role for apoptosis in neurodegeneration and Alzheimer's disease. Mol Neurobiol 1995;10:19–45.
30. Bondy SC. Reactive oxygen species: relation to aging and neurotoxic damage. Neurotoxicology 1992;13:87–100.
31. Itzhaki RF. Possible factors in the etiology of Alzheimer's disease. Mol Neurobiol 1994;9:1–13.
32. West MJ, Coleman PD, Flood DJ, Troncoso JC. Differences in the pattern of hippocampal neuronal loss in normal aging and Alzheimer's disease. Lancet 1994;344:769–772.
33. Jobst KA, Smith AD, Szatmari M, et al. Rapidly progressing atrophy of medial temporal lobe in Alzheimer's disease. Lancet 1994;343:829–830.
34. Gómez-Isla T, Price J, McKeel D, et al. Profound loss of layer II entorhinal cortex neurons occurs in very mild Alzheimer's disease. J Neurosci 1996;16:4491–4500.
35. Politoff AL, Monson N. Age vs. aging in the pathogenesis of senile dementia of the Alzheimer type: electrophysiological evidence. Dement Geriatr Cogn Disord 1997;8:18–25.
36. Brayne C, Calloway P. Normal aging, impaired cognitive function, and senile dementia of the Alzheimer's type: a continuum? Lancet 1988;4:1265–1269.
37. Storandt M, Morris JC, McKeel DW, Rubin EH, Grant EA. Psychometric test distinction of normal aging versus very mild Alzheimer's disease. International Psychogeriatric Association Workshop, Amsterdam, 1994.
38. Flicker C, Ferris SH, Reisberg B. A two-year longitudinal study of cognitive function in normal aging and Alzheimer's disease. J Geriatr Psychiatry Neurol 1993;6:84–96.
39. Albert MS. Age-Related Changes in Cognitive Function. In ML Albert, JE Knoefel (eds), Clinical Neurology of Aging. New York: Oxford University Press, 1994;314–328.
40. Morris RG. Short term forgetting in senile dementia of the Alzheimer's type. Cog Neuropsychol 1986;3:77–97.
41. Sahakian BJ, Morris RG, Evenden JL, et al. A comparative study of visuospatial memory and learning in Alzheimer-type dementia and Parkinson's disease. Brain 1988;111:695–718.
42. Appell J, Kertesz A, Fisman MA. A study of functioning in Alzheimer's disease. Brain Lang 1982; 17:73–91.
43. Martin A, Fedio P. Word production and comprehension in Alzheimer's disease: the breakdown in semantic knowledge. Brain Lang 1983;19:124–141.
44. Jorm AF, Korten AE, Henderson AS. The prevalence of dementia: a quantitative integration of the literature. Acta Psychiatr Scand 1987;76:465–479.
45. Ineichen B. Measuring the rising tide: how many dementia cases will there be by 2001? Br J Psychiatry 1987;150:193–200.
46. Ritchie K, Kildea D. Is senile dementia "age-related" or "aging-related"?—evidence from a meta-analysis of dementia prevalence in the oldest old. Lancet 1995;346:931–934.
47. Ritchie K. Dementia-Free Life Expectancy. In JM Robine, CD Mathers, MR Bone, I Romieu (eds), Calculation of Health Expectancies. Paris: John Libbey, 1993;271–279.
48. Ritchie K, Robine JM, Letenneur L, Dartigues JF. Dementia-free life expectancy in France. Am J Pub Health 1994;84:232–236.
49. Ritchie K. The mental status examination of an exceptional case of longevity: JC aged 118 years. Br J Psychiatry 1995;1:17–22.

17
Controversies in the Classification of Focal Lobar Atrophies

David Neary, David Mann, and Julie Snowden

Controversies in neurology and neuropathology, as with theological debates, often rest on terminologic confusions, traditionally held beliefs, and a degree of ancestor worship, not to say proprietorial politics. Current debate concerning the classification of the focal lobar atrophies exemplifies these common foundations.

The term *progressive focal cortical syndrome* refers to a relatively restricted psychological disorder that, although progressive, does not include other psychological deficits until relatively late in the evolution of disease. The particular neuropsychological syndrome is determined by the topographic distribution of the pathologic lesion and is reflected by highly localized or asymmetric atrophy and hypoperfusion demonstrated on structural and functional brain imaging. In one sense, all cortical atrophies leading to dementia syndromes are focal in that they have a preferential site of disease onset. For example, Alzheimer's disease has an affinity for the association areas of the parietotemporal cortex and limbic system leading to a characteristic syndrome of visuospatial disorientation, aphasia, and amnesia. Typically in Alzheimer's disease, however, highly selective deficits are short-lived and a constellation of characteristic neuropsychological deficits accrue within a relatively short time. In contrast, in non-Alzheimer forms of cerebral atrophy, psychological deficits can remain highly circumscribed and the march of pathology through the brain can remain relatively restricted and asymmetric for many years.

Recognition that degenerative cerebral disease may have a focal clinical presentation is not new. One hundred years ago Arnold Pick [1–4] described a series of patients with circumscribed disorders of language and behavior, occurring in association with focal atrophy of the frontal lobes, temporal lobes, or both. His was an anatomic observation, and the histology of ballooned cells and inclusion bodies, which now bears Pick's name, was only later described by Alzheimer [5]. The designation *Pick's disease*, suggesting a unique clinical and pathologic entity distinct from Alzheimer's disease gained coinage in the Continental literature, but in the English literature faded into near oblivion so that it became a clinical aphorism that Pick's disease could not be differentiated from Alzheimer's disease during life, and its existence as a separate entity even came into question.

FOCAL CORTICAL SYNDROMES

A resurgence of interest in focal cerebral atrophy has come from several sources. In 1982, Mesulam [6] described a group of patients with slowly progressive aphasia in association with left hemisphere atrophy. The assumption was that this focal neuropsychological syndrome may represent a novel entity, clinically and pathologically distinct from hitherto recognized forms of dementia. Subsequently, a host of case reports of patients with progressive disorders of language in association with circumscribed cerebral atrophy have surfaced [7–17]. These reports do not describe a uniform clinical syndrome. Mesulam's patients had a nonfluent aphasia, with predominant difficulty in verbal expression and phonologic errors in speech. Atrophy was most marked in left perisylvian regions. Other reports describe a fluent language disorder, in which the salient feature is a loss of word meaning, so that patients can no longer name, nor comprehend nominal terms [9,12,14]. Nonsemantic aspects of language in these patients, such as phonology and use of syntax, are well preserved. Prominent atrophy of the left temporal lobe is seen. Other patients share features of both syndromes or are distinct from both [14,17].

Focal neuropsychological disorders are not confined to the realm of language. In many patients with a fluent "semantic" form of aphasia, loss of meaning typically extends to nonverbal concepts, encompassing understanding of the meaning of visual percepts (objects and faces) as well as tastes, smells, and tactile stimuli. Nonsemantic aspects of visual perception and sensory discrimination are well preserved. The term *semantic dementia* [18] was used as a qualitative descriptor to encapsulate the multimodal nature of this circumscribed disorder of meaning and has been adopted by others [19]. Atrophy in such patients involves the temporal lobes bilaterally, affecting in particular inferior and middle temporal gyri [20]. In some patients, loss of meaning may initially be in the realms of visual perception, giving rise to the syndrome of progressive prosopagnosia [21,22]. Other focal syndromes include progressive apraxia, involving a selective apraxia affecting predominantly the upper limbs [23–25]; posterior cortical atrophy, comprising visual agnosia, agraphia, and spatial disorientation in the absence of memory loss [26,27]; and progressive visual agnosia, involving an apperceptive form of object agnosia [23]. Given the highly asymmetric distribution of pathology in the frontoparietal cortex as well as the basal ganglia, cortical–basal ganglionic degeneration [28], in which there is profound limb apraxia and other cortical signs, could reasonably be incorporated within the rubric of focal cortical atrophy. Authors of many of the reports of focal cortical syndromes, like Mesulam, have implied that the circumscribed disorder under discussion may represent a novel entity, clinically and pathologically distinct from established forms of dementia.

Although some focal syndromes, such as progressive apperceptive agnosia, selectively affect the posterior cerebral hemispheres, these are relatively rare in comparison with disorders affecting the frontal and anterior temporal lobes. Workers in Lund, Sweden [29,30], and Manchester, England [20,31], drew attention to a disorder of behavior characterized by profound personality change and breakdown in social conduct. The disorder, which has subsequently been described by others [32,33], has been termed variously as *frontal lobe dementia* and *dementia of frontal lobe type*, although a recent consensus statement [34] advocated the use of the term *frontotemporal dementia* (FTD) (see Chapter 2). In FTD, the form of the character change is not uniform. Patients may become disinhibited, overactive, and restless, with a fatuous, unconcerned affect. They may clown, pun, sing, and dance, usually conforming to a restricted, stereotyped repertoire. Alternatively, patients may become apathetic and inert, lacking in drive and initiative and showing little response to stimuli. The disinhibited and inert forms represent opposite poles of a spectrum of behavioral disorder. Patients who present with extreme overactivity and disinhibition may become increasingly apathetic and inert with disease progression. Altered preference for sweet foods, development of food fads, and oral exploration of inedible objects may occur. Stereotypic features, such as repeated wandering following an identical route, are common in FTD. In a minority of patients, however, the stereotypical ritualist nature of the patient's behavior is the dominant presenting feature. Such patients may develop elaborate rituals for dressing or toileting, adhere to a rigid daily routine, and may be unwilling, for example, to walk on cracks in the pavement. The presence or absence of a family history does not determine the behavioral pattern; familial cases occur in the disinhibited, inert, and stereotypical forms of the disorder. The differences in behavioral subtype reflect differences in the distribution of pathologic change within the frontal and anterior temporal lobes [20]. In overactive, disinhibited patients, degenerative change predominantly affects orbitofrontal and anterior temporal regions, whereas in apathetic, inert patients, atrophy is widespread throughout the frontal lobes and includes dorsolateral frontal cortex. In patients in whom behavioral stereotypies are prominent, atrophy is particularly accentuated in anterior temporal regions and striatum.

FTD may sometimes occur in association with the amyotrophic form of motor neuron disease [35], the physical signs of motor neuron disease typically emerging after the onset of behavioral change. The clinical picture most commonly conforms to the overactive, disinhibited type, and consistent with this finding, cerebral atrophy predominantly involves orbitomedial regions of the frontal lobes. Pathologic changes of motor neuron disease within brain stem cranial nerve nuclei and motor cortex at least are typically seen [36].

NOSOLOGIC ISSUES

A variety of nosologic issues have arisen in relation to these focal cortical syndromes. Does the focal symptomatology persist over many years or is it a precursor to a more global dementia [9,37]? Do the syndromes represent novel entities or focal presentations of established forms of dementia? What is the interrelationship between the diverse clinical syndromes? What is the relationship between clinical syndrome and underlying histology?

It is now well established that although focal cortical syndromes may be a presenting feature of Alzheimer's disease [38,39], a substantial proportion of patients have a non-Alzheimer pathology. Nevertheless, issues surrounding the nosologic status of these focal atrophies have not been readily resolved. Whether or not focal syndromes are manifestations of "established dementias" or represent "novel entities" has been hampered by uncertainties regarding the definition of those dementias, in particular what constitutes Pick's disease. Some authors assume that the key diagnostic feature of importance is the macroscopic finding of focal circumscribed frontotemporal atrophy [40,41], as highlighted by Pick himself, whereas others emphasize the diagnostic importance of the histologic characteristics of swollen neurons and intraneuronal inclusion bodies [42,43]. Some have proposed diagnostic criteria based on a combination of progressive dementia, lobar atrophy, and neuronal argentophilic inclusions [44,45]. The term *Pick's disease* is often used interchangeably to denote an ill-defined clinical syndrome or a pathology whose criteria are not agreed on. Implicit in these definitions are different assumptions about the key feature of etiologic significance.

Much of the confusion arises from the failure of terminology to honor different hierarchical levels of description. It is central to the debate about the classification of focal cerebral atrophies that conceptual distinctions need to be drawn between clinical syndrome, topography of brain pathology on which the clinical syndrome depends, and underlying histologic appearances, as each may ultimately contribute to the elucidation of etiology.

In the behavioral disorder of FTD, there are two characteristic underlying histologies [34,46–49]. The most common histologic change is loss of large cortical nerve cells (chiefly from layers III and V) and a spongiform degeneration or microvacuolation of the superficial neuropil (layer II); gliosis is minimal and restricted to subpial regions; layers III and V show no gliosis. No distinctive changes (swellings or inclusions) within remaining nerve cells are seen. The limbic system and the striatum are affected, but to a much lesser extent. The nonspecific large neuronal cell loss and spongiform appearances have been referred to by some authors as *dementia lacking histologic features* [50]. The second and less common histologic process is characterized by a loss of large cortical nerve cells with widespread and abundant gliosis but minimal or no spongiform change or microvacuolation. Swollen neurons or inclusions that are both *tau*- and ubiquitin-positive are present in some cases, and the limbic system and striatum are more seriously damaged. The two differing histologies nevertheless share a similar distribution within the frontal and temporal cortex and cannot be distinguished on the basis of the type of behavioral disorder or familial incidence. Patients with markedly stereotyped behavior and predominant striatal pathology share features of both histologic types. Similar patterns of histology have also been found in progressive aphasia and semantic dementia [8,14,20,51–53]. Pick-type histology has been found in patients with progressive apraxia [20]. If *Pick's disease* is taken to refer to a focal atrophic process affecting the frontal and temporal lobes, then all cases of FTD, as well as patients with progressive language disorders, would fulfill criteria for Pick's disease, whereas patients with progressive apraxia would not, because the distribution of pathologic lesions is outside the frontotemporal lobes. Conversely, if *Pick's disease* is defined in terms of the underlying pattern of histology, then only a small proportion of patients with focal cerebral atrophy, including some with parietal lobe pathology, would be so defined. Because it is currently unknown whether the apparently distinct histologies represent a spectrum of nonspecific changes or have distinct etiologic significance, an empirical approach has been adopted. In a consensus statement published by workers in Lund, Sweden, and Manchester, England, the changes associated with microvacuolation have been termed *frontal lobe degeneration–type* (FLD-type), whereas the gliotic appearances with or without inclusion bodies and swollen neurons have been denoted *Pick-type* histology [34]. Future molecular biological studies are likely to determine whether these histologies have a unique import or whether they represent different phenotypic pathologic variants of a common cause.

Conceptual confusion can be avoided by demarcating hierarchic levels of description. The term *frontotemporal lobar degeneration* has been used to indicate the anatomically circumscribed nature of a primary degenerative disease process affecting these brain regions, but without specifying the precise nature of the histologic changes [20]. It is the topographic distribution of pathology that determines the nature of the clinical syndrome(s) because distinct neuropsychological processes are dependent on regional cerebral functions. That more than one clinical syndrome can arise from frontotemporal lobar degeneration is due to variation and asymmetries in the distribution and march of pathology, both along a longitudinal (anterior-posterior) and horizontal (left-right) axis. There is a close, consistent relationship between clinical syndrome and anatomy. Bilateral frontal and anterior temporal lobe pathology gives rise to the clinical syndrome of FTD [20], characterized by profound behavioral disorder with change in personality and social conduct. The disinhibited, apathetic, and stereotypical subtypes reflect differential emphasis of degenerative change in orbitofrontal cortex, dorsolateral frontal cortex, and striatum. When the pathology is asymmetric, predominantly involving the perisylvian left hemisphere, a syndrome of progressive aphasia emerges. Semantic dementia, in which there is a multimodal loss of conceptual knowledge, resulting in failure to understand meanings of words and recognize objects, is associated with bilateral atrophy of temporal neocortex, particularly inferior and middle temporal gyri. Differential emphasis of pathology in the left or right temporal lobe reflects the relative severity of semantic loss for verbal or nonverbal information. Progressive prosopagnosia occurs when the right temporal lobe is principally affected. Inevitable overlaps between the prototypical syndromes occur. There is much less predictable relationship between clinical syndrome and histology. Both histologic types are associated with a variety of clinical syndromes. The non-Alzheimer pathology is associated with a high familial incidence so that there may be common genetic influences linking the different clinical syndromes. Indeed, links between the syndromes are exemplified by findings of different manifestations of focal cerebral atrophy occurring within a single family [54]. Two brothers were observed to present with a progressive nonfluent aphasia. One brother retained a selective disorder of language over many years, and at autopsy there was a markedly asymmetric distribution of atrophy affecting the left hemisphere. The other brother developed within a few months all the characteristic features of FTD, with gross personality change and breakdown in social conduct. Functional imaging and subsequent autopsy findings revealed spread of pathology into both frontal lobes. The link between distinct clinical syndromes is highlighted also by the finding that motor neuron disease may occur in association with progressive aphasia [55] as well as with FTD.

In general, the focal cerebral atrophies favor the anterior-superior cortex (frontotemporal and superior parietal lobes). The majority of instances of these anterior-superior atrophies will exhibit a non-Alzheimer form of cerebral atrophy. In Alzheimer's disease, in contrast, posterior-inferior cortex (inferior parietal-temporal lobes) is most often involved. It is perhaps not surprising that the posterior cortical atrophy syndrome and visual and perceptual disturbances have been associated with Alzheimer pathology [56–59].

The conceptual distinction between "focal cerebral atrophy" and Alzheimer's disease has rested in large part on the continuing focal nature of the psychological deficits in the former and the emergence of more diffuse abnormalities in the latter. Yet the distinction is relative rather than absolute. As implied above, Alzheimer's disease gives rise not to global impairments, but rather to constellations of deficits reflecting the predominant atrophy in limbic and temporoparietal cortex. In the non-Alzheimer focal cerebral atrophies, the focal nature of the underlying process is emphasized during life by structural and especially functional brain imaging that specifies the maximal area of cerebral dysfunction. Nevertheless, longitudinal clinical follow-up almost invariably demonstrates the acquisition of additional areas of deficit, in keeping with spread of pathology. Moreover, atrophy, although characteristically asymmetric, is found to involve both cerebral hemispheres at autopsy. The notion of focal cortical atrophy without dementia and the conceptual distinction between focal deficits and global dementia are spurious and misleading. When other psychological deficits arise in focal cerebral atrophy, they are often relatively circumscribed, and areas of functional preservation can be demonstrated. For example, even in end-stage examples of the different clinical forms of lobar atrophy, visuospatial functions, reflecting posterior hemispheric processes, are spared.

The selective site of onset and later spread of pathology is not the privilege of a particular histologic process, and to suggest that the Pick-type histology is associated with dementia, whereas non–Pick-type histology remains focal and therefore psychologically pure and localized, is invalid. Indeed, if dementia is conceived of as a generic term embracing the neuropsychological syndromes characteristic of particular brain diseases, rather than denoting end-stage and generalized brain failure, the apparent dichotomy of focal atrophy syndromes and dementia no longer holds.

CORTICOBASAL DEGENERATION AND FOCAL CEREBRAL ATROPHY

It has been suggested earlier that corticobasal degeneration may also be considered a focal cortical syndrome. The clinical syndrome of corticobasal degeneration [28] comprises progressive asymmetric limb akinesia and rigidity, dystonia and myoclonus with "cortical" sensory signs, apraxia and alien limb, gait disorder, and disequilibrium. The clinical entity is distinct and easily separable from the behavioral syndrome of FTD, the language disorder of progressive aphasia, and the disorder of word and object meaning of semantic dementia. It suggests a system degeneration of processes related to skilled movement involving the striatum and interrelated frontoparietal cortices. The question arises as to whether it is the manifestation of a unique neuropathology that can also be designated *corticobasal degeneration*.

The prototypical histopathology consists of swollen achromatic neurons in the parietal cortex and basophilic inclusion bodies in the substantia nigra and nucleus basalis. The clinical syndrome, however, has also been reported in association with a Pick-type histology, with inclusion bodies and swollen neurons [60,61]. Moreover, in a study of neuropathologically diagnosed corticobasal degeneration [62], neuropathologic overlap was demonstrated with Alzheimer's disease, progressive supranuclear palsy, and Parkinson's disease. Furthermore, the histology held to be prototypical of corticobasal degeneration has been demonstrated in patients who presented with a behavioral disorder suggestive of a frontal lobe syndrome and in whom striatal signs were a minor or late feature [28,63]. Thus, the distinct clinical syndrome of corticobasal degeneration can be associated with a range of histopathologies, whereas what is held to be the cardinal histology of corticobasal degeneration can, when differently distributed in the brain, lead to other clinical syndromes.

It has been suggested in a comparison of histology in corticobasal degeneration and Pick's disease [28] that whereas both share the presence of swollen achromatic neurons and basophilic inclusions in the substantia nigra, Pick bodies are not a feature of corticobasal degeneration. A further clinical pathologic study [64], however, described the coexistence of swollen achromatic cortical neurons, depigmentation of the substantia nigra containing basophilic inclusions, and also the presence of Pick inclusion bodies within the cerebral cortex. The clinical diagnosis in life was Steele-Richardson-Olszewski syndrome! The taxonomic confusion between clinical syndrome and pathologic type is well illustrated.

In corticobasal degeneration, as in other focal syndromes, conceptual distinctions need to be maintained between the clinical syndrome, the associated anatomic distribution of the lesions, and the underlying histologic changes. Because clinical syndromes are dependent on the topography rather than the histologic nature of the lesions, it is unsurprising that the clinical syndrome of corticobasal degeneration has been found to be associated with alternative histopathologies.

CONCLUSION

In defining the histopathologies associated with focal cerebral atrophies, advances in immunohistochemistry have engendered the exciting possibility of more refined pathologic diagnosis. When these techniques are divorced from precise accurate clinical neurologic and psychological definition of cases, however, more color than light can be shed on understanding. It may be that the brain has only a limited repertoire of response to a variety of degenerative processes of different etiologies and that the phenotypic pathologic changes simply require description rather than taxonomic designations that, in any case, are likely to be premature and will await advances in molecular biology for clarification. Already a wide range of clinical phenotypes of focal cerebral atrophy have been associated with a genetic defect on chromosome 17 [65–67] and many more will undoubtedly follow. Whether this will form the genetic basis for explaining lobar degenerations irrespective of histology or clinical phenotype remains to be seen. Future genetic advances, however, will never make redundant precise information concerning the clinical neuropsychological syndrome, the regional involvement within the brain, and the histologic phenotype in unraveling the etiology of these degenerative disorders. The temptation of both neurologists and neuropathologists has been to apply eponymous titles and the term *disease* to clinical syndromes or patterns of histology and then to use the designations interchangeably, generating such mysterious entities as the Pick form of Alzheimer's disease or the Alzheimer's-Pick complex. It is here argued that *splitting* rather than *lumping* remains the only way to unravel the taxonomy of the neurodegenerative disorders, and that classification of the focal cerebral atrophies that respects hierarchical levels of description provides the optimal foundation for future understanding of these degenerative disorders.

REFERENCES

1. Pick A. Uber die Beziehungen der senilen Hirnatrophie zur Aphasie. Prag Med Wochenschr 1892;17: 165–167.
2. Pick A. Senile Hirnatrophie als Grundlage von Herderscheinungen. Wien Klin Wochenschr 1901;14: 403–404.
3. Pick A. Zur Symptomatologie der linksseitigen Schlafenlappenatrophie. Monatsschr Psychiat Neurol 1904;16:378–388.
4. Pick A. Uber einen weiteren Symptomenkomplex in Rahmen der Dementia senilis, bedingt durch umschriebene starkere Hirnatrophie (gemischte Apraxie). Monatsschr Psychiat Neurol 1906;19:97–108.
5. Alzheimer A. Über eigenartige Krankheitsfälle des späteren Alters. Z Gesamte Neurol Psychiat 1911; 4:356–385.
6. Mesulam MM. Slowly progressive aphasia without generalized dementia. Ann Neurol 1982;11:592–598.
7. Chawluk JB, Mesulam MM, Hurtig H, et al. Slowly progressive aphasia without generalized dementia: studies with positron emission tomography. Ann Neurol 1986;19:68–74.
8. Kirshner HS, Tanridag O, Thurman L, Whetsell WO. Progressive aphasia without dementia: two cases with focal spongiform degeneration. Ann Neurol 1987;22:527–532.
9. Poeck K, Luzzatti C. Slowly progressive aphasia in three patients. The problem of accompanying neuropsychological deficit. Brain 1988;111:151–168.
10. Delecluse F, Andersen AR, Waldemar G, et al. Cerebral blood flow in progressive aphasia without dementia. Brain 1990;113:1395–1404.
11. Kempler D, Metter EJ, Riege WH, et al. Slowly progressive aphasia: three cases with language, memory, CT and PET data. J Neurol Neurosurg Psychiatry 1990;53:987–993.
12. Tyrrell PJ, Warrington EK, Frackowiak RSJ, Rossor MN. Heterogeneity in progressive aphasia due to focal cortical atrophy. A clinical and PET study. Brain 1990;113:1321–1336.
13. Yamamoto H, Tanabe H, Kashiwagi A, et al. A case of slowly progressive aphasia without generalized dementia in a Japanese patient. Acta Neurol Scand 1990;82:102–105.
14. Snowden JS, Neary D, Mann DMA, et al. Progressive language disorder due to lobar atrophy. Ann Neurol 1992;31:174–183.
15. Karbe H, Kertesz A, Polk M. Profiles of language impairment in primary progressive aphasia. Arch Neurol 1993;50:193–201.
16. Bianchetti A, Frisoni GB, Trabucchi M. Primary progressive aphasia and frontal lobe involvement. Neurology 1996;46:289–290.
17. Snowden JS, Griffiths HL, Neary D. Progressive language disorder associated with frontal lobe degeneration. Neurocase 1996;2:429–440.
18. Snowden JS, Goulding PJ, Neary D. Semantic dementia: a form of circumscribed cerebral atrophy. Behav Neurol 1989;2:167–182.
19. Hodges JR, Patterson K, Oxbury S, Funnell E. Semantic dementia. Progressive fluent aphasia with temporal lobe atrophy. Brain 1992;115:1783–1806.
20. Snowden JS, Neary D, Mann DMA. Fronto-Temporal Lobar Degeneration. London: Churchill Livingstone, 1996.
21. Tyrrell PJ, Warrington EK, Frackowiak RSJ, Rossor MN. Progressive degeneration of the right temporal lobe studied with positron emission tomography. J Neurol Neurosurg Psychiatry 1990;53:1046–1050.

22. Evans JJ, Heggs AJ, Antoun N, Hodges JR. Progressive prosopagnosia associated with selective right temporal lobe atrophy. A new syndrome? Brain 1995;118:1–13.
23. De Renzi E. Slowly progressive visual agnosia or apraxia without dementia. Cortex 1986;22:171–180.
24. Dick JPR, Snowden JS, Northen B, et al. Slowly progressive apraxia. Behav Neurol 1989;2:101–114.
25. Leger JM, Levasseur M, Benoit N, et al. Apraxie d'aggravation lentement progréssive: étude par IRM et tomographie à positions dans quatre cas. Rev Neurol (Paris) 1991;147:183–191.
26. Benson DF, Davis RJ, Snyder BD. Posterior cortical atrophy. Arch Neurol 1988;45:789–793.
27. Freedman L, Selchen DH, Black SE, et al. Posterior cortical dementia with alexia: neurobehavioural, MRI and PET findings. J Neurol Neurosurg Psychiatry 1991;54:443–448.
28. Rinne JO, Lee MS, Thompson PD, Marsden CD. Corticobasal degeneration. A clinical study of 36 cases. Brain 1994;117:1183–1196.
29. Gustafson L. Frontal lobe degeneration of non-Alzheimer type. II. Clinical picture and differential diagnosis. Arch Gerontol Geriatr 1987;6:209–223.
30. Gustafson L. Clinical picture of frontal lobe degeneration of non-Alzheimer type. Dementia, 1993;4: 143–148.
31. Neary D, Snowden JS, Northen B, Goulding PJ. Dementia of frontal lobe type. J Neurol Neurosurg Psychiatry 1988;51:353–361.
32. Jagust WJ, Reed BR, Seab JP, et al. Clinical-physiologic correlates of Alzheimer's disease and frontal lobe dementia. Am J Phys Imaging 1989;4:89–96.
33. Miller BL, Cummings JL, Villanueva-Meyer J, et al. Frontal lobe degeneration: clinical, neuropsychological and SPECT characteristics. Neurology 1991;41:1374–1382.
34. Brun A, Englund B, Gustafson L, et al. Consensus statement. Clinical and neuropathological criteria for fronto-temporal dementia. J Neurol Neurosurg Psychiatry 1994;4:416–418.
35. Neary D, Snowden JS, Mann DMA, et al. Frontal lobe dementia and motor neuron disease. J Neurol Neurosurg Psychiatry 1990;53:23–32.
36. Neary D, Mann DMA, Snowden JS. Frontotemporal Dementia with Motor Neurone Disease. In A Kertesz, D Munoz (eds), Pick's Disease and Pick Complex. New York: Wiley Liss, 1998.
37. Green J, Morris JC, Sandson J, et al. Progressive aphasia: a precursor of global dementia? Neurology 1990;40:423–429.
38. Crystal HA, Horoupian DS, Katzman R, Jotkowitz S. Biopsy-proven Alzheimer's disease presenting as a right parietal syndrome. Ann Neurol 1982;12:186–188.
39. Pogacar S, Williams RS. Alzheimer's disease presenting as a slowly progressive aphasia. R I Med 1984;67:181–185.
40. Constantinidis J, Richard J, Tissot R. Pick's disease: histological and clinical correlations. Eur Neurol 1974;11:208–217.
41. Tissot R, Constantinidis J, Richard J. Pick's Disease. In JAM Frederiks (ed), Handbook of Clinical Neurology: Neurobehavioural Disorders. Amsterdam: Elsevier, 1985;46:233–246.
42. Munoz-Garcia D, Ludwin SK. Classic and generalized variants of Pick's disease: a clinicopathological, ultrastructural, and immunocytochemical comparative study. Ann Neurol 1984;16:467–480.
43. Munoz-Garcia D, Ludwin SK. Clinicopathological studies of some non-Alzheimer dementing diseases. J Can Sci Neurol 1986;13:483–489.
44. Kim RC, Collins GH, Parisi JE, et al. Familial dementia of adult onset with pathological findings of a "non-specific" nature. Brain 1981;104:61–78.
45. Verity MA, Wechsler AF. Progressive subcortical gliosis of Neumann: a clinicopathological study of two cases with review. Arch Gerontol Geriatr 1987;6:245–261.
46. Brun A. Frontal lobe degeneration of non-Alzheimer type. I. Neuropathology. Arch Gerontol Geriatr 1987;6:193–208.
47. Brun A. Frontal lobe degeneration of non-Alzheimer type revisited. Dementia 1993;4:126–131.
48. Mann DMA, South PW. The topographic distribution of brain atrophy in frontal lobe dementia. Acta Neuropath 1993;85:334–340.
49. Mann DMA, South PW, Snowden JS, Neary D. Dementia of frontal lobe type: neuropathology and immunohistochemistry. J Neurol Neurosurg Psychiatry 1993;56:605–614.
50. Knopman DS, Mastri AR, Frey WH, et al. Dementia lacking distinctive histologic features: a common non-Alzheimer degenerative dementia. Neurology 1990;40:251–256.
51. Graff-Radford NR, Damasio AR, Hyman BT, et al. Progressive aphasia in a patient with Pick's disease: a neuropsychological, radiologic and anatomic study. Neurology 1990;40:620–626.
52. Kertesz A, Hudson L, Mackenzie IRA, Munoz DG. The pathology and nosology of primary progressive aphasia. Neurology 1994;44:2065–2072.
53. Turner RS, Kenyon LC, Trojanowski JQ, et al. Clinical, neuroimaging and pathologic features of progressive nonfluent aphasia. Ann Neurol 1996;39:166–173.

54. Neary D, Snowden JS, Mann DMA. Familial progressive aphasia: its relationship to other forms of lobar atrophy. J Neurol Neurosurg Psychiatry 1993:56:1122–1125.
55. Caselli RJ, Windebank AJ, Petersen RC, et al. Rapidly progressive aphasic dementia and motor neuron disease. Ann Neurol 1993;33:200–207.
56. Ross GW, Benson DF, Verity AM, Victoroff JI. Posterior cortical atrophy: neuropathological correlations. Neurology 1990;40(suppl 1):200.
57. Hof PR, Bouras C, Constantinidis J, Morrison JH. Selective disconnection of specific visual association pathways in cases of Alzheimer's disease presenting with Balint's syndrome. J Neuropath Exp Neurol 1990;49:168–184.
58. Hof PR, Archin N, Osmand AP, et al. Posterior cortical atrophy in Alzheimer's disease—analysis of a new case and re-evaluation of a historical report. Acta Neuropath 1993;86:215–223.
59. Levine DN, Lee JM, Fisher CM. The visual variant of Alzheimer's disease: a clinicopathologic study. Neurology 1993;43:305–313.
60. Cambier J, Masson M, Dairou R, Henin D. Etude anatomo-clinique d'une forme parietale de maladie de Pick. Rev Neurol 1981;137:33–38.
61. Lang AE, Bergeron C, Pollanen MS, Ashby P. Parietal Pick's disease mimicking cortical–basal ganglionic degeneration. Neurology 1994;44:1436–1440.
62. Schneider JA, Watts RL, Gearing M, et al. Corticobasal degeneration: neuropathologic and clinical heterogeneity. Neurology 1997;48:959–969.
63. Clark AW, Manz HJ, White CL, et al. Cortical degeneration with swollen chromatolytic neurons: its relationship to Pick's disease. J Neuropath Exp Neurol 1986;45:268–284.
64. Jendroska K, Rossor MN, Mathias CJ, Daniel SE. Morphological overlap between corticobasal degeneration and Pick's disease: a clinicopathological report. Mov Disord 1995;10:111–114.
65. Lynch T, Sano M, Marder KS, et al. Clinical characteristics of a family with chromosome 17–linked disinhibition-dementia-parkinsonism-amyotrophy complex. Neurology 1994;44:1878–1884.
66. Basun H, Almkvist O, Axelman K, et al. Clinical characteristics of a chromosome 17–linked rapidly progressive familial frontotemporal dementia. Arch Neurol 1997;54:539–544.
67. Foster NL, Wilhelmsen K, Sima AAF, et al. Frontotemporal dementia and parkinsonism linked to chromosome 17: a consensus conference. Ann Neurol 1997;41:706–715.

Index

Note: Page numbers followed by f indicate figures; page numbers followed by t indicate tables.